Lecture Notes in Artificial Intelligence 8637

Subseries of Lecture Notes in Computer Science

LNAI Series Editors

Randy Goebel
University of Alberta, Edmonton, Canada
Yuzuru Tanaka
Hokkaido University, Sapporo, Japan
Wolfgang Wahlster
DFKI and Saarland University, Saarbrücken, Germany

LNAI Founding Series Editor

Joerg Siekmann
DFKI and Saarland University, Saarbrücken, Germany

T0212215

Timothy Bickmore   Stacy Marsella
Candace Sidner (Eds.)

Intelligent Virtual Agents

14th International Conference, IVA 2014
Boston, MA, USA, August 27-29, 2014
Proceedings

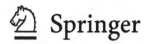 Springer

Volume Editors

Timothy Bickmore
Stacy Marsella
Northeastern University
College of Computer and Information Science
Boston, MA 02115, USA
E-mail: bickmore@ccs.neu.edu, s.marsella@neu.edu

Candace Sidner
Worcester Polytechnic Institute
Department of Computer Science
Worcester, MA 01609, USA
E-mail: sidner@wpi.edu

ISSN 0302-9743   e-ISSN 1611-3349
ISBN 978-3-319-09766-4   e-ISBN 978-3-319-09767-1
DOI 10.1007/978-3-319-09767-1
Springer Cham Heidelberg New York Dordrecht London

Library of Congress Control Number: 2014944748

LNCS Sublibrary: SL 7 – Artificial Intelligence

Typesetting: Camera-ready by author, data conversion by Scientific Publishing Services, Chennai, India

Printed on acid-free paper

Springer is part of Springer Science+Business Media (www.springer.com)

Preface

Intelligent virtual agents (IVAs) are autonomous, graphically embodied agents in an interactive 2D or 3D virtual environment. Although IVAs encompass a broader range of topics, there is a primary focus on simulating the verbal and nonverbal communicative behavior of animated humanoid agents, either among themselves or with one or more humans. The construction of such agents is an interdisciplinary endeavor, requiring the integration of theories and findings from linguistics, psychology, sociology, cognitive science, communication, and interactive media, in addition to the core disciplines of computer science and artificial intelligence. The end goal is to construct animated characters that exhibit realistic, life-like behavior when interacting with people in real or virtual environments.

The IVA conference was started in 1998 as a workshop at the European Conference on Artificial Intelligence on Intelligent Virtual Environments in Brighton, UK, which was followed by a similar one in 1999 in Salford, Manchester, UK. Then dedicated stand-alone IVA conferences took place in Madrid, Spain, in 2001, Irsee, Germany, in 2003, and Kos, Greece, in 2005. Since 2006 IVA has become a full-fledged annual international event, which was first held in Marina del Rey, California, then Paris, France, in 2007, Tokyo, Japan, in 2008, Amsterdam, The Netherlands, in 2009, Philadelphia, Pennsylvania, USA, in 2010, Reykjavik, Iceland, in 2011, Santa Cruz, USA, in 2012, and Edinburgh, UK, in 2013.

IVA 2014 was held in Boston, USA. The special topic of this conference was virtual agents in healthcare. With the world's aging population, increasing prevalence of chronic diseases and obesity in the developing world, and escalating health costs, health represents one of the most important research areas for societal impact. There is a growing body of research on technologies to promote healthy behavior, which has the promise to greatly improve the health of all populations. There has also been an increasing amount of work on IVAs designed to counsel and persuade users to exercise more, take their medication, perform physical rehabilitation exercises, and other health behaviors, as well as to provide companionship and social support, especially for the elderly. The conference was held at Northeastern University, which has a wide range of education and research programs in health informatics, and is situated near the Longwood Medical Area in Boston, home to Harvard Medical School and six world-renowned hospitals and medical research institutions, as well as Boston Medical Center, the site of multiple virtual agent health interventions. Two of the keynotes were given by physicians: Dr. Joseph Kvedar, director of the Partner's Center for Connected Health—the world's premier telemedicine organization, affiliated with Harvard Medical School—and Dr. Michael Paasche-Orlow, an internist at Boston Medical Center, and world expert on the problem of health literacy.

IVA 2014 received 78 submissions. Out of the 64 long paper submissions, only 14 were accepted for the long papers track. Furthermore, there were 24 short papers presented in the single-track paper session and 25 demo and poster papers were on display.

This year's IVA also included four workshops that focused on "Architectures and Standards for IVAs," "Affective Agents," "Models of Culture for Intelligent Virtual Agents," and "Playful Characters." There was also a Doctoral Consortium where PhD students received feedback from peers and established researchers.

IVA 2014 was locally organized by the College of Computer and Information Science (CCIS) at Northeastern University. We would like to thank the scientific committees that helped shape a quality conference program, the Senior Program Committee for taking on great responsibility and the Program Committee for their time and effort. We also want to thank our keynote speakers for crossing domains and sharing their insights with us. Furthermore, we would like to express thanks to Dina Utami who oversaw the poster session, Arno Hartholt, who oversaw the demo session, and Margot Lhommet, who organized the four workshops co-located with IVA. We are grateful for the logo design contributed by Zachary Berwaldt and the timely conference system support from Thomas Preuss. Finally, we would like to express our thanks to Lin Shi, who managed a significant portion of the conference organization and logistics.

June 2014   Timothy Bickmore
                                                        Stacy Marsella
                                                       Candace Sidner

Organization

Conference Co-chairs

Timothy Bickmore	Northeastern University, USA
Stacy Marsella	Northeastern University, USA
Candace Sidner	Worcester Polytechnic Institute, USA

Doctoral Consortium Chair

Magalie Ochs	CNRS LTCI Télécom ParisTech, France

Workshop Chair

Margot Lhommet	Northeastern University, USA

Poster Chairs

Dina Utami	Northeastern University, USA
Lin Shi	Northeastern University, USA

Demonstrations Chair

Arno Hartholt	Institute for Creative Technologies, University of Southern California, USA

Video Chair

Lazlo Ring	Northeastern University, USA

Senior Program Committee

Elisabeth Andre	University of Augsburg, Germany
Ruth Aylett	Heriot-Watt University, UK
Norman Badler	University of Pennsylvania, USA
Jonathan Gratch	University of Southern California, USA
Dirk Heylen	University of Twente, The Netherlands
Michael Kipp	Augsburg University of Applied Sciences, Germany
Stephan Kopp	University of Bielefeld, Germany
James Lester	North Carolina State University, USA
Jean-Claude Martin	Paris South University, France
Yukiko Nakano	Seikei University, Japan

Michael Neff	University of California, Davis, USA
Ana Paiva	Technical University of Lisbon, Portugal
Catherine Pelachaud	CNRS, TELECOM ParisTech, France
David Traum	Institute for Creative Technologies, USA
Hannes Vilhjálmsson	Reykjavík University, Iceland
Marilyn Walker	University of California, Santa Cruz, USA
R. Michael Young	North Carolina State University, USA

Program Committee

Jan Allbeck	George Mason University, USA
Christian Becker-Asano	Institut für Informatik, Germany
Kirsten Bergmann	Bielefeld University, Germany
Joost Broekens	TU Delft, The Netherlands
Donna Byron	IBM Watson Solutions Division, USA
Angelo Cafaro	CNRS-LTCI, TELECOM ParisTech, France
Ginevra Castellano	University of Birmingham, UK
Marc Cavazza	University of Teesside, UK
Yun-Gyung Cheong	IT University, Copenhagen, Denmark
Matthieu Courgeon	LabSTICC-University of South Brittany, France
Iwan de Kok	Sociable Agents, CITEC, Bielefeld University, Germany
Celso De Melo	USC Marshall School of Business, USA
David DeVault	Institute for Creative Technologies, USC, USA
Joao Dias	INESC-ID/IST, Portugal
Funda Durupinar	University of Pennsylvania, USA
Jens Edlund	KTH Speech, Music and Hearing, Sweden
Arjan Egges	Utrecht University, The Netherlands
Birgit Endrass	Augsburg University, Germany
Petros Faloutsos	York University, UK
Patrick Gebhard	DFKI, Germany
Sylvie Gibet	Université de Bretagne Sud, France
Marco Gillies	Goldsmiths, University of London, UK
Lynne Hall	The University of Sunderland, UK
Alexis Heloir	DFKI, Germany
Ian Horswill	Northwestern University, USA
Lewis Johnson	Alelo Inc., USA
Marcelo Kallmann	UC Merced, USA
Mubbasir Kapadia	Disney Research Zurich, Switzerland
Andrea Kleinsmith	University of Florida, USA
Tomoko Koda	Osaka Institute of Technology, Japan
Nicole Krämer	University of Duisburg-Essen, Germany
Brigitte Krenn	OFAI, Austria
H. Chad Lane	University of South California, USA
Margot Lhommet	Northeastern University, USA

Table of Contents

Using Virtual Doppelgängers to Increase Personal Relevance of Health Risk Communication

Sun Joo (Grace) Ahn[1], Jesse Fox[2], and Jung Min Hahm[1]

[1] University of Georgia, Athens, GA, USA
{sjahn,jungmin}@uga.edu
[2] The Ohio State University, Columbus, OH, USA
fox.775@osu.edu

Abstract. Virtual doppelgängers are human representations in virtual environments with photorealistic resemblance to individuals. Previous research has shown that doppelgängers can be effective in persuading users in the health domain. An experiment explored the potential of using virtual doppelgängers in addition to a traditional public health campaign message to heighten the perception of personal relevance and risk of sugar-sweetened beverages. Both virtual doppelgängers and an unfamiliar virtual human (i.e., virtual other) used in addition to a health pamphlet were effective in increasing risk perception compared to providing just the pamphlet. Virtual doppelgängers were more effective than virtual others in increasing perceived personal relevance to the health message. Self-referent thoughts and self presence were confirmed as mediators.

Keywords: Agents, Avatars, Health Technology, Virtual Environments, Presence.

Sugar-sweetened beverages (SSBs) have recently garnered much negative attention with the increasing concern for rising rates of obesity [1]. A flood of health promotion campaigns has been launched in an effort to counteract the prevalence of SSB consumption and some governments have even proposed a ban on large sized soft drinks in an attempt to assist the battle against obesity. Virtual health agents provide us with novel ways to address this health issue. Specifically, this study investigated how the use of virtual doppelgängers, or agents designed to look like the self [2], can be used to effectively change health behaviors.

1   Communicating Health Risk – Challenges for Personal Relevance

Perhaps one of the greatest challenges that health promotion campaigns face is communicating risks in a personally relevant way. Personal relevance is the extent to which an issue or topic has important personal consequences and/or intrinsic importance [3]. Some scholars have noted that there lies a social distance between the individual and the risk presented in the mediated message wherein the individual does not feel that the risk is relevant to the self, leading him or her to discredit the personal

T. Bickmore et al. (Eds.): IVA 2014, LNAI 8637, pp. 1–12, 2014.
© Springer International Publishing Switzerland 2014

relevance of the message [4]. This challenge is magnified by the tendency of individuals to underestimate the self's susceptibility to various health conditions relative to others [5].

In an effort to overcome this barrier, the focus of health message strategies has been placed on tailoring messages to individuals rather than expecting the same broad message to work for everyone [6,7]. By formulating messages that address individual differences, studies have demonstrated that the tailoring approach is more effective in promoting desired health behavioral outcomes compared to interventions targeted to an audience segment [6]. Tenets of the elaboration likelihood model [3] suggest that personal relevance is increased by way of tailoring, and that increased relevance, in turn, leads to greater attention and persuasion. Thus, increasing the perceived personal relevance of a health message seems to be critical in the promotion of desirable health behaviors and tailored messages seem to be significantly more successful at increasing the relevance compared to traditional means of audience targeting [6].

Computer-tailored messages vary in their modality, level of personalization, and richness [8]. Much of the existing research on tailoring has focused on emails, web portals, and text messaging. Virtual health agents provide novel ways to deliver tailored health information, however [9]. The current experiment aims to extend the state of research on computerized tailoring by using virtual human representations within immersive virtual environments as a tailoring strategy to maximize the perceived personal relevance of a health message, and ultimately, risk perception. By shedding light on the underlying mechanisms that render health messages personally relatable and drive effective risk perceptions, the current study aims to yield findings that are easily translatable to a wide range of health contexts.

2   Virtual Doppelgängers as a Tailoring Strategy

Virtual doppelgängers represent the user within immersive virtual environments (IVEs) and are created with digital photographs of the participant so that they bear photorealistic resemblance to the self [2]. Thus, by using virtual doppelgängers that share striking physical similarities with the self to depict realistic future negative consequences, participants may feel as if the negative consequence is actually happening to him or her. Watching the threat discussed in a health message actually occur to a virtual entity that looks like the self is likely to decrease the underestimation of the self's vulnerability to the risk.

Virtual agents are becoming popular across a variety of health contexts [9, 10, 11,12,13]. In some cases, health interventions using virtual human agents have been successfully tested for effectiveness in promoting health behaviors (e.g., [14,15]). Although interactive in nature, these virtual agents did not take advantage of tailoring and were presented as a single and generic identity for all users, often posing as guides or coaches. Given the success of tailoring in health messages as well as the success of virtual agents in health behavior change, combining both concepts to produce a tailored virtual agent for each user may combine the advantages of both intervention strategies to yield synergistic effects.

Only a few academic studies have explored the possibility of using virtual doppelgängers to persuade users in the health context, but these initial investigations suggest that the virtual doppelgängers may be a powerful vehicle of persuasion. Doppelgängers were more effective in promoting exercise behavior both immediately after and a day after seeing one's doppelgänger exercising [16]. These studies demonstrated that the visual stimulus of seeing a negative consequence occurring to the virtual doppelgänger is much more powerful in modifying attitudes and behaviors compared to seeing a negative consequence occurring to a virtual other (i.e., a virtual human representation of an unfamiliar other). Another study demonstrated that individuals become physiologically more aroused when they see virtual doppelgängers than when they see virtual others [17], which may explain their persuasiveness.

Another way of tailoring these health agents is by showing the consequences of a given health behavior, which can be key to behavior change [18]. IVEs provide a unique opportunity for users to experience the immediate and future rewards and punishments of healthy and unhealthy behaviors. For example, users in one study could watch their own body gain weight as they continuously consumed candy [19]. Another study found that showing one's doppelgänger gain weight from not exercising promoted more exercise behavior than showing a generic agent gaining weight [16].

These earlier findings evidence the potential to use virtual agents as change agents of health behavior by confirming health behavior changes in the real world following exposure to virtual treatments. The current study strives to extend the earlier work by applying virtual doppelgängers in a familiar, everyday healthcare context wherein the virtual doppelgängers may be used alongside more traditional health messages (i.e., pamphlets). Furthermore, the current study focuses on the investigation of underlying mechanisms that drive future health behavior changes. Insight into the perceptual and attitudinal influence factors that underlie behavior change will allow theorists and practitioners to apply the current findings to a wide range of health contexts, above and beyond the consumption of SSBs.

In this study, the first test will be to explore whether tailoring using virtual humans (i.e., both virtual doppelgängers and virtual others) in addition to a traditional healthcare pamphlet will be more effective in increasing risk perception of sugar added beverages compared to the influence of the traditional pamphlet alone. Earlier IVE studies have shown that the persuasive effects of IVE-based messages are stronger compared to traditional print messages [20], and thus we also anticipate that:

H1A: Participants will perceive higher risk when experiencing an IVE after reading a pamphlet compared to the pamphlet-only condition.

H2A: Participants will perceive higher personal relevance when experiencing an IVE after reading a pamphlet compared to the pamphlet-only condition.

In addition, as earlier IVE research demonstrates that virtual doppelgängers are more effective than virtual others in promoting a host of desirable attitudes and behaviors, seeing the negative future consequence of SSB consumption on a photorealistic virtual doppelgänger is anticipated to be more impactful than seeing it on a virtual other:

H1B: Participants will perceive higher risk when the future negative consequence of SSB consumption occurs to a virtual doppelgänger compared to a virtual other.

H2B: Participants will perceive higher personal relevance when the future negative consequence of SSB consumption occurs to their virtual doppelgänger compared to a virtual other.

3   The Mediating Roles of Self Thought and Self Presence

H1 and H2 explore the effectiveness of virtual doppelgängers, but perhaps a more interesting question is about the underlying mechanisms that drive the increase in perceived risk of negative consequences compared to virtual others. Often times, health treatments are found to be successful, but they can be difficult to extend or replicate if it is not clear *why* they are successful. Determining the mechanisms (i.e., mediators) driving increases in risk and relevance will clarify why virtual agents are or are not successful persuaders as well as provide the groundwork to progress theoretical developments on the effects of virtual doppelgängers.

A number of studies have demonstrated that increased perceived personal relevance and risk following messages lead to an increase in behavioral intent [4,5] but not many studies have investigated what drives this increase in perceived relevance. As perceived personal relevance is thought to be the main underlying mechanism driving tailoring effects and one of the main challenges of health message effectiveness [7], the current study will extend earlier research to explore the underlying processes of personal relevance. Thus, by identifying these mediators, we will glean a greater understanding of how and why virtual agents can make health messages seem more relevant to users.

Earlier findings, albeit in an advertising context, have confirmed that experiencing virtual simulations through a virtual human identified as the self triggered more self-referent thoughts (i.e., thinking about the self in relation to the virtual experiences) than experiencing those simulations through a virtual human unidentifiable as the self. These self-referent thoughts encouraged individuals to associate the experiences of the virtual self to the physical self [21] and resulted in stronger persuasive effects. Similarly, we posit that vicariously experiencing the negative consequence of SSB consumption via a virtual doppelgängers in addition to the traditional health message would lead individuals to more self-referent thoughts (i.e., thinking about the self in relation to the negative consequences) than vicariously experiencing the negative consequence via virtual others. Having self-referent thoughts is anticipated to lead to perceptions of personal relevance toward the message:

H3: Self-referent thoughts will mediate the relationship between experimental conditions (virtual doppelgänger vs. virtual other) and perceived personal relevance of the health message.

Furthermore, in order for participants to feel that a risk discussed in a health message is personally relevant, the negative consequence occurring to their virtual doppelgängers would have to feel genuine. Perceived realism of virtual experiences, or the sense of "being there" in the mediated environment [22], has been shown to favorably influence a wide range of outcomes. Specifically, presence has been shown to maximize the effects of doppelgängers [19]. Particularly relevant in the current context of increasing the personal relevance of health messages through virtual doppelgängers is the concept of self presence, or the close mental mapping of the user's physical body to a virtual body [23]. Thus, we expect that:

> **H4**: Self presence will serve as a mediator between experimental conditions (virtual doppelgänger vs. virtual other) and perceived personal relevance of the health message.

4   Methods

4.1   Sample and Procedure

The effect of three conditions on perceived personal relevance and risk of SSB consumption was assessed with a convenience sample of 47 participants (11 males, age $M = 17.70$, $SD = 7.54$) recruited from a large Southern university and offered course credit for participation. One week before the experiment, participants had their photograph taken for the creation of the virtual doppelgängers.

At the time of the experiment, all participants received the Pouring on the Pounds pamphlet and were instructed to read it carefully. After reading the pamphlet, participants were randomly assigned to one of three conditions: control ($n = 16$), virtual doppelgänger ($n = 16$), and virtual other ($n = 15$). Participants in the control condition completed survey measures after reading the pamphlet. Participants in the virtual doppelgänger and virtual other conditions were immersed in the IVE to vicariously experience the negative consequences of SSB consumption.

The IVE system used in the treatment conditions implemented a head-mounted display (HMD; VR2000 Ruggedized Pro) providing three-dimensional perception through stereoscopic views of the virtual world. The resolution was 1024 x 768 XGA with 45 degrees field of view. An orientation sensor with six degrees of freedom and an update rate of 125Hz was attached to the HMD to allow participants to control their field of view using naturalistic head movements. Finally, stereo audio information was delivered through the headphones of the HMD to present realistic sounds.

In the IVE, a virtual room was shown with either a virtual doppelgänger or a virtual other standing, consuming one soft drink a day for two years and consequently gaining weight. The virtual other was the representation of the participant preceding the current participant that matched in gender and ethnicity. As the virtual human consumed the soft drink, its body grew larger due to weight gain. The ten pounds a year in fat that the virtual human gained was also visually and aurally depicted as piles of fat splattering onto a digital scale. Figure 1 depicts the IVE treatment.

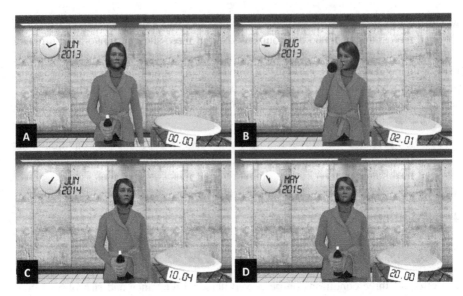

Fig. 1. Participants saw either a virtual doppelgänger or a virtual other standing in a room, holding a soft drink bottle (A). As the virtual human begins drinking from the bottle, the calendar and clock portray the rapid passing of time, and fat begins to fall on the digital scale (B). After one year of consuming soft drinks, the virtual human has gained ten pounds (C). At the end of two years, the virtual human has gained a total of 20 pounds as shown on the scale (D).

4.2   Dependent Measures

Risk Perception. Three 5-point interval scale items asked participants the extent to which they thought they and their friends were at risk of and concerned about gaining weight as a result of drinking SSBs. The three items were averaged to create a single index for risk perception (Cronbach's $\alpha = .72$).

Personal Relevance. A 5-point interval scale item asked participants how personally relevant the issue of gaining weight as a result of SSB consumption is to them.

Self-referent thoughts. Cognitive responses to the experimental stimuli were assessed using the thought-listing procedure [24]. Immediately following experimental treatments, participants were asked to freely write down as many thoughts as they had. The total number of self-referent thoughts (e.g., "I need to stop drinking Coke," "I should cut down on my soda consumption," "I hope I don't look like that") were counted and divided by the total number of thoughts ($Min = 1$, $Max = 12$, $M = 6.05$, $SD = 2.67$) in order to account for the individual differences in cognitive processes. This measure was only collected in the virtual doppelgänger and virtual other conditions.

Self Presence. Five 5-point interval scale items adapted from prior studies [19, 25] asked participants the extent to which they felt that if something happened to the virtual human it was happening to them; the virtual human was their own body; they were in the virtual human's body; the virtual human was an extension of them; and the virtual human was them. The five items had high reliability, with Cronbach's α = .90, and were averaged to create a single index of self presence. This measure was only collected in the virtual doppelgänger and virtual other conditions.

Game Play (Covariate). A single open-ended item asked participants the average number of hours a week they spend playing video, computer, mobile, and arcade games, and was controlled for in the ensuing analyses.

5   Results

H1A and H1B were tested with an ANCOVA with experimental condition as the independent variable, risk perception as the dependent variable, and game play as the covariate. Results revealed a significant main effect of condition, $F(1, 43) = 5.38$, $p = .008$, $\eta^2 = .20$. A post hoc analysis using Fisher's Least Significant Difference (LSD) revealed that both virtual doppelgängers ($M = 2.80$, $SD = .84$) and virtual others ($M = 3.02$, $SD = .90$) were equally influential in increasing perceived risk compared to the control group ($M = 2.18$, $SD = .49$). H1A was supported; H1B was not.

H2A and H2B were tested with an ANCOVA with experimental condition as the independent variable, personal relevance as the dependent variable, and game play as the covariate. Results revealed a significant main effect of experimental condition, $F(1, 43) = 3.56$, $p = .04$, $\eta^2 = .14$. A post hoc analysis using Fisher's LSD revealed that virtual doppelgängers ($M = 3.24$, $SD = 1.28$) promoted a significantly higher level of personal relevance to the health message compared to the control ($M = 2.20$, $SD = .83$) and the virtual other ($M = 2.47$, $SD = 1.24$) conditions, which did not significantly differ. Thus, H2A and H2B were both supported.

The PROCESS path-analysis macro for SPSS [26] was used to test the mediation models for H3 and H4. To test H3, experimental conditions were coded (*virtual others* = 0, *virtual doppelgängers* = 1) and entered as the independent variable; self-referent thought was entered as the mediator; personal relevance as the dependent variable; and game play as the control variable. Bootstrapping methods were used and results of the direct and indirect effects are reported in Table 1. Results indicated that self-referent thought has a strong relationship with relevance; thinking about the negative consequences in terms of the self encouraged participants to consider the health message to be personally relevant. Further, self-referent thought mediated the relationship between experimental condition and personal relevance. Seeing the virtual doppelgänger led to more self-referent thinking about negative consequences than seeing the virtual other, and thinking more about the self led to greater perceived relevance to the message. Thus, H3 was supported.

The PROCESS path-analysis macro was used again to test H4. Experimental condition was entered as the independent variable; self presence was entered as the mediator; personal relevance as the dependent variable; and game play as the control variable. Bootstrapping methods were used and results of the direct and indirect effects are reported in Table 2. Results indicated that self presence has a strong

Table 1. Regression Weights, Indirect Effects Showing Mediation, Bootstrap 95% Confidence Interval, Lower and Upper Bounds

Regression Weights	Coefficient	SE	Bootstrap 95% CI Lower	Upper
Direct Effects				
Condition → Self Thoughts[+]	.22	.12	-.022	.468
Condition → Relevance	.37	.46	-.586	1.320
Self Thoughts → Relevance*	1.75	.69	.330	3.171
Indirect Effects	Effect Size	*Bootstrap SE*		
Condition → Self Thoughts → Relevance*	.39	.23	.085	1.111

Note. SE = standard error; CI = confidence interval.
Bootstrap resampling = 1000. ** $p < .01$, * $p < .05$, [+] $p = .06$.

relationship with relevance; perceiving that the negative consequences occurring to the virtual human is real encouraged participants to consider the health message to be personally relevant. Self presence mediated the relationship between experimental condition and personal relevance. Therefore, experiencing presence while experiencing the negative consequence occurring to the virtual doppelgänger was more effective in heightening personal relevance compared to the virtual other. Thus, H4 was supported.

Table 2. Regression Weights, Indirect Effects Showing Mediation, Bootstrap 95% Confidence Interval, Lower and Upper Bounds

Regression Weights	Coefficient	SE	Bootstrap 95% CI Lower	Upper
Direct Effects				
Condition → Self Presence[+]	.55	.28	-.028	1.128
Condition → Relevance	.24	.43	-.646	1.130
Self Presence → Relevance**	.94	.27	.380	1.497
Indirect Effects	Effect Size	*Bootstrap SE*		
Condition → Self Presence → Relevance*	.52	.32	.060	1.470

Note. SE = standard error; CI = confidence interval.
Bootstrap resampling = 1000. ** $p < .01$, * $p < .05$, [+] $p = .06$.

6   Discussion

Using virtual humans within IVEs in addition to a traditional health pamphlet was more effective in heightening perceptions of personal relevance and risk than a non-tailored pamphlet developed for the general population. Furthermore, virtual doppelgängers were more influential than virtual others in increasing perceived personal relevance of the risk of SSB consumption as described in the pamphlet. Two underlying mechanisms seem to be driving the increase in perceived relevance—self-referent thoughts and self presence.

The findings suggested that using virtual humans, in general, to deliver vicarious experiences of future negative consequences augments the effects of traditional health messages by heightening perceived risk perceptions and is more effective than the baseline of using traditional media alone. As heightened risk perception has been considered as one of the main motivators of behavior change [27], these results imply that IVEs may be valuable contributors to public health campaigns.

Furthermore, the results yielded insight into the perception of personal relevance, which has been shown to encourage attention [6] and elaborated processing of information [3]. Although virtual humans in general were effective in increasing risk perception, virtual doppelgängers were significantly more effective in increasing the perception of personal relevance compared to virtual others. Because virtual doppelgängers display a photorealistic similarity with the individual, it may have been difficult to ignore or underestimate the self's vulnerability to the risk discussed in the message. Conversely, it may have been easier to discount the risk when the negative consequence occurred to an unfamiliar other, as is often the case with non-tailored health messages [5]. As perceived personal relevance is thought to be the main driver of tailoring effects [7], these results suggest that optimal tailoring effects may be reaped by photorealistically tailoring each virtual human to each individual.

The virtual doppelgängers' influence on perceived personal relevance was driven by both self-referent thoughts and self presence. Perceived realism of a mediated experience leading to heightened perceptions of personal relevance and risk in the context of health communication has also been demonstrated with traditional media [4]. Current results extend these earlier findings by indicating that it is not only the realism of the vicarious experience, but also the extent to which the experience brings forth self-referent thoughts that lead to increase in personal relevance. As Bandura [18] noted, it seems to be a combination of environmental stimuli and cognitive processing of the stimuli that leads to potential behavioral modification. This suggests that regardless of the realism of the material delivered by advanced digital media, the message may be ineffective if it fails to elicit self-referent thoughts in relation to the health issue discussed in the message.

The incorporation of virtual doppelgängers within traditional health promotion campaigns seems to be a timely endeavor. As only two digital photographs were used to create the virtual doppelgängers, and as social media users inundate the virtual space with photos of themselves, the implementation of virtual doppelgängers within the social media space is particularly feasible. The simplicity of the design of these virtual agents and simulations yields promising practical implications outside the virtual space as well. This is particularly true as participants in the current study were given only limited interactivity with the virtual simulation. The current findings suggest that virtual health agents may serve as effective change agents by having individuals merely view the negative health consequences of their virtual doppelgängers and may be easily applicable to a wide range of health contexts. For instance, these agents may be a simple, yet effective, health intervention technique to be used in doctor's offices along with traditional health pamphlets. By presenting patients with a brief simulation featuring a virtual agent that looks photorealistically like the patient in addition to the pamphlets typically offered during office visits, doctors might be able to effectively encourage the patients to think more seriously about the risk and how relevant it is to themselves. Furthermore, with the increasing popularity of gaming technology such as the Microsoft Kinect and the Oculus Rift, IVE systems are increasingly becoming accessible, affordable, and ubiquitous. Moreover, virtual doppelgängers offer high scalability and may be used across different media platforms ranging from mobile devices to desktop computers; applied in health messages dealing with a variety of topics; and sent to existing IVE systems at home en masse so that individuals may be exposed to valuable health messages in the comforts of their own homes.

One limitation is that the current study used a relative small sample comprised of college students. The relatively young sample of research participants is highly relevant for studying SSB consumption [28], and the partial eta-squared values suggest sufficient level of power despite the small sample size. However, future studies should investigate the effects of virtual doppelgängers across a wider range of populations and with a larger sample for greater accuracy and generalizability of results. This study also only included a single treatment. Longitudinal research should be pursued to examine the effects over time. Finally, in this study, we did not measure users' reactions to doppelgängers. In some cases, realistic virtual agents can fall into the uncanny valley, and users have aversive reactions [29], which would likely negate the effects of a health message.

In sum, virtual doppelgängers present a promising novel approach that fuses traditional tailoring strategies with advanced digital technology. Within the timely context of reducing SSB consumption, virtual doppelgängers offer a unique yet feasible and translatable solution in a world inundated with advertising and promotions. With the continuing advancement of digital media technologies, the capacity of virtual doppelgängers to serve as powerful amplifiers of message effects seems limitless.

References

1. Johnson, R.K., Appel, L.J., Brands, M., Howard, B.V., Lefevre, M., Lustig, R.H., Sacks, F., Steffen, L.M., Wylie-Rosett, J.: Dietary Sugars Intake and Cardiovascular Health: A Scientific Statement from the American Heart Association. Circulation 120, 1011–1020 (2009)
2. Fox, J., Bailenson, J.N.: The Use of Doppelgängers to Promote Health and Behavior Change. CyberTherapy & Rehabilitation 3, 16–17 (2010)
3. Petty, R.E., Cacioppo, J.T.: Communication and Persuasion: Central and Peripheral Routes to Attitude Change. Springer, New York (1986)
4. So, J., Nabi, R.: Reduction of Perceived Social Distance as an Explanation for Media's Influence on Personal Risk Perceptions: A Test of the Risk Convergence Model. Human Communication Research 39, 317–338 (2013)

5. Weinstein, N.D., Lyon, J.E.: Mindset, Optimistic Bias about Personal Risk and Health-Protective Behavior. British Journal of Health Psychology 4, 289–300 (1999)
6. Kreuter, M.W., Strecher, V.J., Glassman, B.: One Size Does Not Fit All: The Case for Tailoring Print Materials. Annals of Behavioral Medicine 21, 276–283 (1999)
7. Noar, S.M., Harrington, N.G., Aldrich, R.S.: The Role of Message Tailoring in the Development of Persuasive Health Communication Messages. In: Beck, C.S. (ed.) Communication Yearbook, pp. 73–133. Routledge (2009)
8. Noar, S.M., Harrington, N.G.: Computer-tailored interventions for improving health behaviors. In: Noar, S.M., Harrington, N.G. (eds.) eHealth Applications: Promising Strategies for Behavior Change, pp. 128–146. Routledge, New York (2012)
9. Fox, J.: Avatars in Health Communication Contexts. In: Noar, S.M., Harrington, N.G. (eds.) eHealth Applications: Promising Strategies for Behavior Change, pp. 96–109. Routledge, New York (2012)
10. Bickmore, T., Gruber, A.: Relational Agents in Clinical Psychiatry. Harvard Review of Psychiatry 18, 119–130 (2010)
11. Gaggioli, A., Mantovani, F., Castelnuovo, G., Wiederhold, B., Riva, G.: Avatars in Clinical Psychology: A Framework for the Clinical Use of Virtual Humans. Cyberpsychology & Behavior 6, 117–125 (2003)
12. Gratch, J., Morency, L.P., Scherer, S., Stratou, G., Boberg, J., Koenig, S., Rizzo, A.: User-State Sensing for Virtual Health Agents and TeleHealth Applications. Studies in Health Technology and Informatics 184, 151–157 (2012)
13. Ahn, S.J., Johnsen, K., Robertson, T., Moore, J., Brown, S., Marable, A., Basu, A.: Using Virtual Pets to Promote Physical Activity in Children: An Application of the Youth Physical Activity Promotion Model. Journal of Health Communication (in press)
14. Ijsselsteijn, W.A., Kort, Y.D., Westerink, J.H.D.M., Jager, M.D., Bonants, R.: Virtual Fitness: Stimulating Exercise Behavior Through Media Technology. Presence: Teleoperators and Virtual Environments 15, 688–698 (2006)
15. King, A.C., Bickmore, T.W., Campero, M.I., Pruitt, L., Yin, J.L.: Employing Virtual Advisors in Preventive Care for Underserved Communities: Results from the COMPASS Study. Journal of Health Communication 18, 1449–1464 (2013)
16. Fox, J., Bailenson, J.N.: Virtual Self-Modeling: The Effects of Vicarious Reinforcement and Identification on Exercise Behaviors. Media Psychology 12, 1–25 (2009)
17. Fox, J., Bailenson, J.N., Ricciardi, T.: Physiological Responses to Virtual Selves and Virtual Others. Journal of CyberTherapy & Rehabilitation 5, 69–72 (2010)
18. Bandura, A.: Social Foundations of Thought and Action. Prentice-Hall, Englewood Cliffs (1986)
19. Fox, J., Bailenson, J.N., Binney, J.: Virtual Experiences, Physical Behaviors: The Effect of Presence on Imitation of an Eating Avatar. PRESENCE: Teleoperators & Virtual Environments 18, 294–303 (2009)
20. Ahn, S.J., Bailenson, J., Park, D.: Short- and Long-Term Effects of Embodied Experiences in Immersive Virtual Environments on Environmental Locus of Control and Behavior. Computers in Human Behavior (in press)
21. Ahn, S.J., Bailenson, J.: Self-Endorsing Versus Other-Endorsing in Virtual Environments: The Effect on Brand Attitude and Purchase Intention. Journal of Advertising 42, 93–106 (2011)
22. Lombard, M., Ditton, T.: At the Heart of It All: The Concept of Presence. Journal of Computer-Mediated Communication 3 (1997)
23. Biocca, F.: The Cyborg's Dilemma: Progressive Embodiment in Virtual Environments. Journal of Computer-Mediated Communication 3 (1997)

24. Cacioppo, J.T., von Hippel, W., Ernst, J.M.: Mapping Cognitive Structures and Processes through Verbal Content: The Thought-Listing Technique. Journal of Consulting and Clinical Psychology 65, 928–940 (1997)
25. Ahn, S.J., Le, A.M.T., Bailenson, J.: The Effect of Embodied Experiences on Self-Other Merging, Attitude, and Helping Behavior. Media Psychology 16, 7–38 (2013)
26. Hayes, A.F.: PROCESS: A Versatile Computational Tool for Observed Variable Mediation, Moderation, and Conditional Process Modeling (2012)
27. Rimal, R.N., Real, K.: Perceived Risk and Efficacy Beliefs as Motivators of Change. Human Communication Research 29, 370–399 (2003)
28. West, D., Bursac, Z., Quimby, D., Prewitt, E., Spatz, T., Nash, C., Mays, G., Eddings, K.: Self-Reported Sugar-Sweetened Beverage Intake among College Students. Obesity 14, 1825–1831 (2006)
29. Mori, M., MacDorman, K.F., Kageki, N.: The Uncanny Valley (From the Field). IEEE Robotics & Automation Magazine 19, 98–100 (2012)

Luke, I am Your Father:
Dealing with Out-of-Domain
Requests by Using Movies Subtitles

David Ameixa[1], Luisa Coheur[1], Pedro Fialho[2], and Paulo Quaresma[2]

[1] Instituto Superior Técnico, Universidade de Lisboa/INESC-ID
[2] Universidade de Évora/INESC-ID
Rua Alves Redol n 9, 1000-029 Lisbon, Portugal
name.surname@inesc-id.pt

Abstract. Even when the role of a conversational agent is well known users persist in confronting them with Out-of-Domain input. This often results in inappropriate feedback, leaving the user unsatisfied. In this paper we explore the automatic creation/enrichment of conversational agents' knowledge bases by taking advantage of natural language interactions present in the Web, such as movies subtitles. Thus, we introduce Filipe, a chatbot that answers users' request by taking advantage of a corpus of turns obtained from movies subtitles (the Subtle corpus). Filipe is based on Say Something Smart, a tool responsible for indexing a corpus of turns and selecting the most appropriate answer, which we fully describe in this paper. Moreover, we show how this corpus of turns can help an existing conversational agent to answer Out-of-Domain interactions. A preliminary evaluation is also presented.

1 Introduction

The number of organisations providing virtual assistants is increasing. Examples of such assistants are Siri, from Apple, IKEA's Anna, or Monserrate's butler, Edgar Smith [5]. Yet, even when their roles are well known – for instance, answering questions about a specific domain or performing some pre determined task – users persist in confronting them with Out-of-Domain (OOD) input, that is, personal questions, requests about the weather, or about other topics unrelated with their tasks. Although it might be argued that such systems should only be focused in their own pre-defined functions, the fact is that people become more engaged with these applications if OOD requests are properly addressed [11]. Therefore, current approaches usually anticipate some OOD requests and handcraft answers for them. However, it should be clear that it is impossible to predict all the possible sentences that can be submitted to such agents.

An alternative solution to deal with OOD requests is to explore the (semi-)automatic creation/enrichment of the knowledge base of virtual assistants/chatbots by taking advantage of the vast amount of dialogues present in the web. Recently, Banchs and Li introduced *IRIS* [3], a chatbot that has in its knowledge base a corpus of interactions extracted from movie scripts (the *MovieDiC* corpus [2]). In this paper we take this idea one step further, and, instead of movie scripts, we propose the use of movie subtitles to

T. Bickmore et al. (Eds.): IVA 2014, LNAI 8637, pp. 13–21, 2014.
© Springer International Publishing Switzerland 2014

build a chatbot's knowledge base from scratch, and also to deal with the OOD requests of an existing conversational agent. Although less precise, Subtitles are easier to find and are available in almost every language; in addition, as large amounts of subtitles can be found, linguistic variability can be covered and redundancy can be taken into consideration (if a turn is repeatedly answered in the same way, that answer is probably a plausible answer to that turn). Therefore, in this paper we present Say Something Smart (SSS), a system that chooses an answer to a certain input, by taking into consideration a knowledge base of interactions – currently, the Subtle corpus [1], built from movies subtitles. We also show how this strategy can be applied to build a chatbot, Filipe (Figure 1)[1], and also to answer OOD requests posed by real users to Edgar Smith, the aforementioned Monserate's butler. Some preliminary results are also presented.

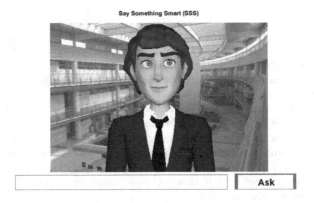

Fig. 1. Filipe, our chatbot based on SSS

This paper is organised as follows: in Section 2 we present some related work, in Section 3 we briefly describe the Subtle corpus, in Section 4 we detail SSS, and, in Section 5, we present a preliminary evaluation. Finally, in Section 6 we close the paper by providing some conclusions and pointing to some future work.

2 Related Work

Several conversational agents animate museums all over the world. Examples are: the 3D Hans Christian Andersen (HCA), which is capable of establishing multi-modal conversations about the namesake writer's life and tales [4]; Max, a virtual character employed as guide in the Heinz Nixdorf Museums Forum [12]; Sergeant Blackwell, installed in the Cooper-Hewitt National Design Museum in New York, and used by the U.S. Army Recruiting Command as a hi-tech attraction and information source [13]; the twins Ada and Grace, virtual guides in the Boston Museum of Science [15]. More recently, the virtual butler Edgar Smith [9,5] answers questions about Monserrate palace,

---
[1] Filipe can be tested in `http://www.l2f.inesc-id.pt/~pfialho/sss/`

in Sintra, Portugal, where he can be found. However, despite the sophisticated technologies behind all these systems, every single one reports the problem of having to
deal with OOD requests.

In order to cope with this, these conversational agents follow different strategies:
Edgar suggests questions when he is not able to understand an utterance, and starts
talking about the palace if he does not understand the user repeatedly. A feature in
his character also "excuses" some misunderstandings: as he is an old person, he does
not have a very acute hearing; HCA changes topic when he is lost in the conversation,
and also has an "excuse" for not answering some questions: the virtual HCA does not
remember (yet) everything that the real HCA once knew; Max consults a Web-weather
forecast for queries about this topic and uses Wikipedia to find answers to some factoid
questions [16]. However, despite all these stratagems, actualisations of these agents
knowledge bases, grounded in collected logs, still need to be performed on a regular
basis.

The idea of taking advantage of existing human requests to feed dialogue systems
emerges naturally from this context. Recently, the work presented in [3] describes a
chat-oriented dialogue system, which has in its knowledge sources MovieDiC [2], a
corpus extracted from movies scripts. In this paper we take this idea a little further and
take advantage of movies subtitles to answer users' requests. Contrary to movies scripts,
subtitles exist in much larger quantities and for almost every language.

Considering the process of choosing the answer, we use SSS, which is based in Information Extractions techniques and also in edit distance metrics. The process behind
SSS is somewhat similar to the one described in [6], where both a role-play (representing free-form human interactions) and a Wizard of Oz dialogue corpora (specific task
turns) are used to find answers: our approach also works at the lexical level, not using
any kind of dialogue act or semantic annotation. However, contrary to our approach,
context is already taken into consideration.

Finally, another related systems that should be mentioned, although developed with
other goal, is Say Anything [14] where the user and the computer take turns to write a
story. Say Anything is based on a corpus of millions of stories extracted from weblogs
and Lucene is also used by this system.

3   The Subtle Corpus

We follow [15] and envisage the use of knowledge bases constituted of turns. From
now on we will call *interactions* to each pair of sentences (T, A), where A (the *answer*)
corresponds to a response to T, from now on the *trigger*. The following are examples
of interactions.

Example 1. (T1: You know, I didn't catch your age. How old are you?, A1: 20)

Example 2. (T2: So how old are you?, A2: That's none of your business)

The Subtle corpus is a collection of interactions, extracted from four different movies
subtitles genres (Horror (H), Scifi (SF), Western (W) and Romance (R)), for Portuguese

Table 1. Number of available turns

#Interactions **Subtle – English**				
R	**SF**	**W**	**H**	**All**
1,392,569	625,233	333,776	1,000,902	3,352,480
#Interactions **Subtle – Portuguese**				
R	**SF**	**W**	**H**	**All**
627,368	477,521	129,081	696203	1,930,173

and English. Details on how this corpus was obtained from subtitles files can be found in [1]. Table 1 shows the number of available interactions for each genre.

It should be clear that as Subtle Interactions are obtained from subtitles' files based on the time elapsed between the dialogue lines, many turns in Subtle are not real dialogue pairs. In addition, some expected Interactions are not captured. This can be observed when Filipe is not able to answer *He told me YOU killed him.* with *No, I am your father*, a piece of dialogue from Star Wars[2]. This is due to the time elapsed between Darth Vader and Luke Skywalker lines that surpasses the time limit established to consider two turns as an interaction. Moreover, unexpected formats found in subtitles' files also led to false interactions. An example that illustrates this problem is: User: *Hasta la vista, babe*, SSS: *(CROWD CHEERING)*. Another example of unexpected information that can still be found in Subtle interactions is illustrated in the following, where the first turn shows a trigger with the name of the character that says it (PHILIP).

Example 3. (T3: PHILIP: How How are you?, A3: Fine.)

4   Say Something Smart

In the section we describe SSS. It takes as input the user request and returns an answer from the agent knowledge base. At the basis of this process there are several sentences comparisons. Thus, due to the large amount of interactions available, and because this selection needs to be done very fast (the user cannot wait long for an answer), a previous filtering step takes place in SSS before it selects an answer. In the following we detail these steps.

4.1   Indexing Subtle and Extracting Candidate Answers

We start by indexing the Subtle corpus through Lucene[3], a open-source, high-performance text search engine library, widely used by the Natural Language Processing/Information Extraction community. Then, given a user request, Lucene search engine is also used to retrieve a ranked set of interactions. Results returned by Lucene are based on an internal scoring algorithm[4] that takes into consideration the words present in the interactions and in the user request. Nevertheless, although the first interactions are usually

---

[2] Actually, *Luke, I'm your father* is a misquotation from Star Wars, parodied in other movies.
[3] http://lucene.apache.org
[4] http://www.lucenetutorial.com/advanced-topics/scoring.html

the most accurate, the fact is that several interactions in which the trigger is not semantically related with the user request, are also returned. For instance, given the user request *Do you have brothers?*, the following are examples of interactions returned by Lucene (in the first 20 positions).

Example 4. (T4: Brother! Do you've a cigarette?, A4: Take it.)

Example 5. (T5: Do you've any brothers?, A5: I'll manage the business)

Example 6. (T6: You don't have to go, brother., A6: I'm not your brother.)

Example 7. (T7: Brother, you don't have a clue., A7: What were you thinking about?)

Example 8. (T8: Didn't you have a brother in the war?, A8: Well, my brother Roy.)

In addition, SSS, as many Question/Answering systems (e.g. [7]), is based on the answers redundancy. That is, we assume that if an answer to a certain request is more frequent than others, it has a higher probability of being a plausible one. Thus, a "reasonable" number of interactions need to be returned by Lucene. Considering again time as a factor that needs to be taken into consideration, and after several preliminary experiments, we opt to ask Lucene for a maximum of 100 interactions, which guarantees redundancy but also allows SSS to obtain an answer to any question in less that one second (using an Intel Core i5-480M).

4.2   The Answer Selection Step

In order to choose an answer from the retrieved set of interactions, SSS performs two sequential tasks. As previously shown, many of the triggers from the interactions returned by Lucene might not be (semantically) related with the user request. Therefore, SSS starts by filtering the retrieved interactions, choosing only those where the triggers are similar to the user request, according to a given threshold. That is to say, all the retrieved interactions above the threshold are kept; all the others are discarded. Previous work [10] have shown us that a simple yet effective similarity measure is a combination between Jaccard similarity coefficient[5] and Overlap coefficient[6]. For Overlap we use bigrams with a minimum score of 0.4, and, for Jaccard, unigrams with minimum score of 0.7 (these values were empirically obtained). A weight-factor distributes the importance of both scores.

If no interactions is selected, a discarding answer such as *I'm sorry but I do not know how to answer your question* is given. Otherwise, SSS moves to a second step, where the answers of the remaining interactions are analysed. As previously said, as our approach is based on the answers redundancy, we check for the most frequent answer (see [8] for a review about answer selection in Question/Answering systems). Once again, we do not force exact matches, and answers are compared according with the previously mentioned similarity measure. If none of them is similar (above a threshold) to any of the remaining answers, a random answer is returned (which allows Filipe to sometimes provide different answers to the same input); otherwise, the most common answer, that is, the one that has the highest similar values concerning the other answers, is returned.

---

[5] http://en.wikipedia.org/wiki/Jaccard_index
[6] http://en.wikipedia.org/wiki/Overlap_coefficient

5   Preliminary Evaluation

5.1   Experimental Setup

We have at our disposal a corpus collected by the developers of Edgar Smith, representing requests posed by real people to Edgar. As expected, several OOD requests appear in these logs. From this corpus, the 58 questions unanswered by Edgar and marked as OOD were extracted and used in our first experiments, as described in the following.

5.2   Should We Take the Different Movies' Genres into Consideration?

Firstly, we wanted to understand how many OOD requests SSS was able to answer, and see if there was any significant difference in the capacity of the different movies genres to contribute with plausible answers. Therefore, we run SSS with the different partitions of the Subtle corpus, taking as input the previously mentioned 58 OOD requests. Results were labeled as:

- (Disc)arded, when SSS provides a discarding answer (e.g. User: *Why you talk so funny dude?* SSS: *I'm sorry, I'm not able to answer.*);
- OK when SSS returns a plausible answer (e.g. User: *Are you joking?* SSS: *Do I look like a joker?*);
- KO, when SSS supplies an inappropriate answer (e.g. User: *You have a big nose.* SSS: *I didn't say you kidnapped Megan*).

The attained results can be seen in Table 2.

Table 2. Evaluation of SSS answers

	Horror	Romance	Western	Sci-fi	All Genres
Disc	22	19	28	21	**16**
OK	20	21	17	23	**27**
KO	16	17	13	14	**15**

As expected, best results are obtained using the whole Subtle corpus (column **All Genres**). Answers from Westerns had the worst results and Sci-fi the best. Considering the all genres together, 72% of the requests are now answered (42 in 58), and, from these, about 65% are considered to be appropriate (27 in 58). The ones that were discarded pose no problem, as at the end the answer results in the same answer that Edgar would give: *I'm sorry, I'm not able to answer.*. Still, there are 26% of answers given that are not suitable to the users requests.

5.3 Answers Evaluation

From the 42 requests that did not return a discarded answer we selected 20 (from now on the test set), with the following criteria:

- Do not contain offensive language;
- From the 9 questions paraphrasing *How are you?* 3 where chosen randomly;
- Questions with only one word, like "here?" or "Where?", were rejected;
- From the remaining requests, we randomly chose them.

Then, we built a questionnaire, based on the answers provided by SSS to those 20 requests, and also on hand-crafted plausible answers. Then we divided this question-naire in two: each questionnaire had 10 questions of each type (generated by SSS and hand-crafted). To our 30 evaluators (adults with different ages and backgrounds, not necessarily working in computer science) we told that these requests were posed to Edgar and that the answers were its response. Evaluators should give them a 1-5 score according to how satisfied they were (being 5 the best score). A snippet of the question-naire can be found in Figure 2.

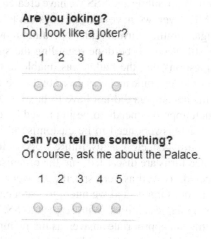

Fig. 2. Snippet from the questionnaire

To test the evaluators concordance we used the Cronbach α measure. The inter-rater agreement score was high, for both the SSS and the manual answers (0,80 and 0,84, respectively). People preferred the manual answers, as expected: SSS obtained a score of $2,9 \pm 1,37$ and manual answers of $4,3 \pm 0,84$.

The variation of results attained from SSS also show that some of the provided ques-tions are very good, and others are very bad. Five of our questions had an average rate of less than 1.9 points; in the other hand the remaining answers had an average rate of almost 4.0. Analysing the 5 answers with a very low rate, we can see that they are not related with the topic of the question or they not fit in the present context, like when is said *You have a big nose*, and the answer is *I didn't say you kidnapped Megan.* The same happens when is given the utterance *I said Hello!* and the answer is *I say shut up, you bilge rat, before I use you as an anchor.* and with the question *Are you a donkey?* that is answered with *Ok. Do one thing. Tell me the story of your journey to heaven once again. Only once.* Some answers, although "funny", are definitely not suitable to the environment where, for instance, Edgar is integrated (an elegant palace).

Thus, despite some problems related with the corpus itself, SSS strategy needs to be improved so that answers related with a very specific context are avoided.

Nevertheless, this strategy can easily provide answers to many (not so obvious) OOD requests. For instance, if Filipe is told *I like your hair* or *Are you a mutant?*, he will provide very reasonably answers.

6   Conclusions and Future Work

We have presented an approach to deal with OOD requests that takes advantage on movies subtitles. Thus, we have built SSS a tool that indexes the interactions from its knowledge base (the Subtle corpus, obtained from movies subtitles) and, given an user request, chooses an answer. With Subtle and SSS we have created Filipe, a virtual agent, implemented over SSS. Moreover, we have used this system to answer OOD requests asked by real users to Edgar Smith, a virtual butler operating in Monserrate palace.

Although much work still needs to be done regarding the subtle corpus and SSS, the fact is that several questions that the butler was unable to deal with can now be successfully answered; moreover, some answers given by Filipe are extremely interesting, if we consider that his developers did not have to hand-craft them. Nevertheless, it should be clear that such approach needs to be improved before being applied to a formal agent such as Edgar (answers need to be customise to be adequate to an old butler, slang needs to be eliminated, etc.). Thus, future work includes the refinement of Subtle, so that badly formed turns are discarded, and the organisation of the corpus, so that paraphrases are detected, as well as very specific answers. Moreover, normalisation of the corpus is one of our targets, and we intent to use a named entity recogniser to generalise turns involving names entities. With respect to SSS, a main concern is to extended its way of selecting an appropriate answer, as many important variables, such as context (as done in [6]) and the agent personality should be taken into account.

Acknowledgments. This work was supported by national funds through FCT – Fundação para a Ciência e a Tecnologia, under project PEst-OE/EEI/LA0021/2013.

References

1. Ameixa, D., Coheur, L.: From subtitles to human interactions: introducing the subtle corpus. Tech. rep., INESC-ID (November 2014)
2. Banchs, R.E.: Movie-dic: a movie dialogue corpus for research and development. In: Proceedings of the 50th Annual Meeting of the ACL, pp. 203–207. Association for Computational Linguistics, Jeju Island (2012)

3. Banchs, R.E., Li, H.: Iris: a chat-oriented dialogue system based on the vector space model. In: ACL (System Demonstrations), pp. 37–42 (2012)
4. Bernsen, N.O., Dybkjær, L.: Meet hans christian anderson. In: Proceedings of the Sixth SIG-dial Workshop on Discourse and Dialogue, pp. 237–241 (2005)
5. Fialho, P., Coheur, L., dos Santos Lopes Curto, S., Cládio, P.M.A.: Ângela Costa, Abad, A., Meinedo, H., Trancoso, I.: Meet edgar, a tutoring agent at monserrate. In: Proceedings of the 51st Annual Meeting of the Association for Computational Linguistics, ACL (August 2013)
6. Gandhe, S., Traum, D.: First steps towards dialogue modelling from an un-annotated human-human corpus. In: 5th Workshop on Knowledge and Reasoning in Practical Dialogue Systems, Hyderabad, India (January 2007)
7. Mendes, A.C., Coheur, L., Silva, J., Rodrigues, H.: Just.ask - a multi-pronged approach to question answering. International Journal on Artificial Intelligence Tools 22(1) (2013)
8. Mendes, A.C., Coheur, L.: When the answer comes into question in question-answering: survey and open issues. Natural Language Engineering 19(1), 1–32 (2013)
9. Moreira, C., Mendes, A.C., Coheur, L., Martins, B.: Towards the rapid development of a natural language understanding module. In: Vilhjálmsson, H.H., Kopp, S., Marsella, S., Thórisson, K.R. (eds.) IVA 2011. LNCS, vol. 6895, pp. 309–315. Springer, Heidelberg (2011)
10. Mota, P., Coheur, L., Curto, S., Fialho, P.: Natural language understanding: From laboratory predictions to real interactions. In: Sojka, P., Horák, A., Kopeček, I., Pala, K. (eds.) TSD 2012. LNCS, vol. 7499, pp. 640–647. Springer, Heidelberg (2012)
11. Patel, R., Leuski, A., Traum, D.R.: Dealing with out of domain questions in virtual characters. In: Gratch, J., Young, M., Aylett, R.S., Ballin, D., Olivier, P. (eds.) IVA 2006. LNCS (LNAI), vol. 4133, pp. 121–131. Springer, Heidelberg (2006)
12. Pfeiffer, T., Liguda, C., Wachsmuth, I., Stein, S.: Living with a virtual agent: Seven years with an embodied conversational agent at the heinz nixdorf museumsforum (2011)
13. Robinson, S., Traum, D.R., Ittycheriah, M., Henderer, J.: What would you ask a conversational agent? observations of human-agent dialogues in a museum setting. In: LREC. European Language Resources Association (2008)
14. Swanson, R., Gordon, A.S.: Say anything: A massively collaborative open domain story writing companion. In: First International Conference on Interactive Digital Storytelling, Erfurt, Germany (November 2008)
15. Traum, D., Aggarwal, P., Artstein, R., Foutz, S., Gerten, J., Katsamanis, A., Leuski, A., Noren, D., Swartout, W.: Ada and grace: Direct interaction with museum visitors. In: Nakano, Y., Neff, M., Paiva, A., Walker, M. (eds.) IVA 2012. LNCS, vol. 7502, pp. 245–251. Springer, Heidelberg (2012)
16. Waltinger, U., Breuing, A., Wachsmuth, I.: Interfacing virtual agents with collaborative knowledge: Open domain question answering using wikipedia-based topic models. In: Walsh, T. (ed.) Proceedings of the 22nd IJCAI, IJCAI 2011, Barcelona, Spain, July 16-22, pp. 1896–1902. IJCAI/AAAI (2011)

Animated Faces, Abstractions and Autism

Diana Arellano[1], Volker Helzle[1], Ulrich Max Schaller[2], and Reinhold Rauh[2]

[1] Filmakademie Baden-Wuerttemberg, Germany
{diana.arellano,volker.helzle}@filmakademie.de
[2] University Medical Center Freiburg, Germany
{ulrich.schaller,reinhold.rauh}@uniklinik-freiburg.de

Abstract. The Agent Framework is a real-time development platform designed for the rapid prototyping of graphical and agent-centric applications. Previous use cases show the potential of the Agent Framework, which is currently used in a project that combines facial animation, non-photorealistic rendering and their application in autism research.

Keywords: affective characters, facial animation, real-time, healthcare.

1 Introduction

Along the years, animated characters have found their way to numerous applications in entertainment, human-computer interaction and more recently in medical practices. One of the reasons is the flexibility in the manipulation and customization of these characters, so they could be re-used in different contexts.

This paper presents the Agent Framework, an open-source platform for the rapid creation and prototyping of animated virtual characters, where facial animations and head movements can be manipulated in real-time. In the following, we will introduce previous and current applications developed using the framework, with special emphasis in SARA, a project that brings together facial animation, abstractions and research on Autism.

2 Related Work

The widespread use of animated virtual characters has caused researchers to look for faster and more "comfortable" ways of creating and designing characters, such that it can also be done by non-experts. Nowadays several platforms, commercial and from academia, offer a wide range of functionality in order to create affective and believable characters. Some examples are the work of Magnenat-Thalmann and Thalmann [1], Greta [2], MARC [3], the Augsburg's Horde3D Game Engine [4], SmartBody [5], or EMBR [6], among many others. Harthold et al. [7] offers a very complete list of frameworks based on the Behavior Markup Language (BML). Jung et al. [8] also offers a very detailed state of the art of models and architectures that have been used for the creation of believable virtual characters.

T. Bickmore et al. (Eds.): IVA 2014, LNAI 8637, pp. 22–25, 2014.
© Springer International Publishing Switzerland 2014

3   Agent Framework

The Agent Framework is a set of functionalities within our open-source development platform, Frapper, for the creation of application prototypes that involve high-quality animated characters with believable facial animations. On its part, Frapper (Filmakademie Application Framework) [9] arose from the desire to be independent from the other platforms and have complete control over its development. The source code of Frapper is available under GNU LGPL v2.1.

One of the advantages of the Agent Framework is its modular structure, where each functionality is encapsulated in a C++ plugin that can be extended or created according to the developers requirements. In this way, 3rd-party libraries (commercial or not) can be integrated, bringing to the framework new functionalities like speech recognition, voice generation, alternative input devices and so on. For regular users, the framework as it is offers an intuitive node-based interface, where the existent functionalities can be visualized as nodes that can be connected among themselves to create the logic of the application. Fig. 1 depicts a set of nodes of the Agent Framework for emotional facial animation.

Two human-like characters, a young woman (Fig. 1) and an older man are provided with the Agent Framework, under a Creative Commons license. Both are animated using our Facial Animation Toolset (FAT) [10] and the Facial Action Coding System (FACS) [11]. In the case a new character needs to be added, it should be modeled and rigged in an external software (e.g. Maya® or 3Dd Max®) and imported into the framework using the Ogre Maya Exporter.

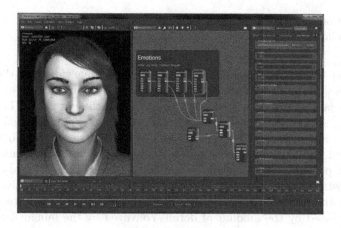

Fig. 1. The Agent Framework in Frapper

4   Applications

The Agent Framework has been successfully used in a number of applications. Together with FAT, an automatic speech recognizer (ASR) SemVox [12] and text-to-speech (TTS) SVOX [13] (both 3rd party software embedded in the framework), it allowed the creation of affective, interactive and believable characters.

One of the first use cases of the Agent Framework was the creation of Nikita, a "terminal agent conference guide" who not only replied to the questions formulated by the attendees in reference to the conference, but also showed sadness, anger and joy (Fig. 2(a)). The Muses of Poetry [14] is an interactive installation where animated characters transmit to an audience the intrinsic emotions conveyed in existent poems (Fig. 2(b)). Emote [15] is a web based messaging services, which converts plain text messages into animated ones (Fig. 2(c)). The Dynamic Emotion Categorization Test (DECT) [16] was a psychological computer-based experiment where four human actors and two virtual actors (animated characters) where used to examine the ability of emotion recognition with dynamic physical stimuli in children and teenagers with autism (Fig. 2(d)).

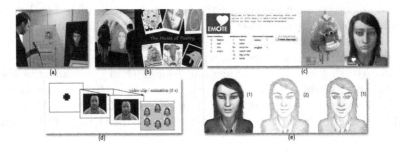

Fig. 2. (a) Conference Guide, (b) Muses of Poetry, (c) Emote, (d) DECT, (e) SARA: (1) Original image, (2) Water Color 'Joy', (3) Sketched 'Joy'

Based on the results achieved with the Agent Framework and the DECT test, SARA - Stylized Animations for Research on Autism intends to take the study of facial recognition in persons with autism to the next level. The goal of SARA is to study how abstraction in animated facial expressions affects their recognition, in comparison to their realistic versions. The abstractions will be implemented through non-photorealistic rendering (NPR) algorithms in order to simulate painting styles like watercolors or sketching. Fig. 2(e)) shows some levels of abstraction in a character expressing "joy". One of the motivations for SARA was the difficulty in emotions recognition in people with autism, which might be caused by the amount of details conveyed by the human face. Thus, with the Agent Framework the psychologists will have the possibility to abstract and simplify the level of detail of different regions of the face, and adapt them in real-time according to the feedback of the autistic person.

5   Conclusions and Future Work

The Agent Framework offers the users an intuitive interface, while giving the developers a powerful platform where they can add new functions and integrate new libraries or devices according to the needs of their deployments. The use cases showed the multidisciplinary character of the Agent Framework and its potential in medical fields like autism spectrum disorders (ASD). Moreover, the character animations can be of great aid in therapies and treatments for other conditions like eating or personality disorders, attention deficit, depression and social behavior problems. The current project SARA intends to bring the framework to the next level by offering the possibility to create abstracted facial animations in real-time, with multiple characters at the same time.

Acknowledgments. The SARA project (officially *Impact of non-photorealistic rendering for the understanding of emotional facial expressions by children and adolescents with high-functioning Autism Spectrum Disorders*) is funded by the German Research Foundation (DFG).

References

1. Kasap, Z., Ben Moussa, M., Chaudhuri, P., Magnenat-Thalmann, N.: Making Them Remember - Emotional Virtual Characters with Memory. IEEE Computer Graphics and Applications 29(2), 20–29 (2009)
2. Poggi, I., Pelachaud, C., de Rosis, F., Carofiglio, V., De Carolis, B.: GRETA. A Believable Embodied Conversational Agent. Multimodal Intelligent Information Presentation 27, 3–25 (2005)
3. Hoque, M., Courgeon, M., Martin, J.C., Mutlu, B., Picard, R.W.: MACH: My Automated Conversation coacH. In: UBICOMP 2013 (2013)
4. Bee, N., Falk, B., André, E.: Simplified Facial Animation Control Utilizing Novel Input Devices: A Comparative Study. In: IUI 2009, pp. 197–206 (2009)
5. Shapiro, A.: Building a Character Animation System. In: Allbeck, J.M., Faloutsos, P. (eds.) MIG 2011. LNCS, vol. 7060, pp. 98–109. Springer, Heidelberg (2011)
6. Heloir, A., Kipp, M.: EMBR – A Realtime Animation Engine for Interactive Embodied Agents. In: Ruttkay, Z., Kipp, M., Nijholt, A., Vilhjálmsson, H.H. (eds.) IVA 2009. LNCS (LNAI), vol. 5773, pp. 393–404. Springer, Heidelberg (2009)
7. Hartholt, A., Traum, D., Marsella, S.C., Shapiro, A., Stratou, G., Leuski, A., Morency, L.-P., Gratch, J.: All Together Now: Introducing the Virtual Human Toolkit. In: Aylett, R., Krenn, B., Pelachaud, C., Shimodaira, H. (eds.) IVA 2013. LNCS (LNAI), vol. 8108, pp. 368–381. Springer, Heidelberg (2013)
8. Jung, Y., Kuijper, A., Kipp, M., Miksatko, J., Gratch, J., Thalmann, D.: Believable Virtual Characters in Human-Computer Dialogs. In: EUROGRAPHICS, pp. 75–100 (2011)
9. Frapper, http://research.animationsinstitut.de/frapper/
10. Helzle, V., Biehn, C., Schlömer, T., Linner, F.: Adaptable Setup for Performance Driven Facial Animation. In: ACM SIGGRAPH 2004 Sketches, p. 54 (2004)
11. Ekman, P., Friesen, W.V., Hager, J.C.: The Facial Action Coding System. Weidenfeld & Nicolson, London (2002)
12. SEMVOX ASR, http://www.semvox.de/
13. SVOX TTS, http://www.nuance.de/products/SVOX/index.htm
14. Arellano, D., Helzle, V.: The muses of poetry. In: CHI EA 2014, pp. 383–386 (2014)
15. Helzle, V., Spielmann, S., Zweiling, N.: Emote, a new way of creating animated messages for web enabled devices. In: CVMP 2011 (2011)
16. Rauh, R., Schaller, U.M.: Categorical Perception of Emotional Facial Expressions in Video Clips with Natural and Artificial Actors: A Pilot Study. Technical Report ALU-KJPP-2009-001, University of Freiburg (2009)

Is That How Everyone Really Feels? Emotional Contagion with Masking for Virtual Crowds

Tim Balint and Jan M. Allbeck

Laboratory for Games and Intelligent Agents,
George Mason University, 4400 University Drive, MSN 4A5,
Fairfax, VA 22030, USA
{jbalint2,jallbeck}@gmu.edu

Abstract. Many simulations use emotional contagion to simulate how groups of humans behave in emotionally charged environments. These models either have each individual agent conform to a group emotion, or have emotional spirals. However, these models do not include well known phenomenon such as displaying and receiving emotions through different means of communication, or having emotions masked by an agent's desired display emotion. We create a model of emotional contagion that considers multiple channels to communicate on. We also provide a method for agents to mask their emotions, which is used to control the spread of contagion between agents, and can prevent emotional spirals. We demonstrate our model with a sample scenario, and show the effects of having multiple channels and emotional masking on the overall emotional contagion for several groups of agents.

Keywords: Group and Crowd Simulation, Personality and Emotion Models, Modeling and Animation Techniques, Applications in Games.

1 Introduction

Multi-agent simulations capture the interaction between groups of humans, and are used in applications such as games, movies, and civil design. These interactions attempt to model human behavior in varying situations, and include human characteristics such as emotion, which tend to be designed using either an appraisal system [1] or a valence system [2]. While these models attempt to explain how emotions arise individually, the propagation of emotions, known as emotional contagion, captures emotional interactions between groups of humans. Emotional contagion allows for group reactions to stimuli, even if not all members of that group receive the stimuli. For example, in a movie such as *Godzilla*, not all the people running away in fear have actually seen Godzilla. Some become afraid because they see others running away in fear. Having virtual agents with emotional contagion allows for scenes such as this to be more realistically rendered.

Hatfield et al. [3] has shown that contagion occurs through unconscious mimicking of other's emotional features, such as facial expressions. This is known

T. Bickmore et al. (Eds.): IVA 2014, LNAI 8637, pp. 26–35, 2014.
© Springer International Publishing Switzerland 2014

as momentary micro mimicry, which transfers a small amount of emotion. This can be amplified when continuously being exposed to the stimuli or occurring within a large group, and can lead to phenomenon such as emotional spirals, where the emotional amplitude grows out of control. While Hatfield et al. primarily focused on facial expressions, they mentioned several other channels with which emotion can be interpreted and mirrored. For example, if someone is in a large, aggressive stance, another person could momentarily shift their stance, becoming angrier in the process. Most current contagion implementations use proximity or group cohesion to determine the spread of emotion, however, using multiple channels would allow for more realistic human simulations, as physical humans have varying abilities to encode and decode their emotions on these different channels.

Emotional contagion is also an unconscious effect, and it would be fool-hardy to believe that it is not always present in crowds. However, there are many situations in which emotional spirals do not occur and contagion is at a minimum. People commuting home from work on the train do not experience emotional spirals, even though they are all essentially of the same group, and confined together for long periods of time. This is most likely due to the commuters outwardly displaying little to no emotion, which is known as emotional masking. Furthermore, the sender may not wish to convey their emotions, and so will send more obvious signals to convey a different, or false emotion. Someone who is sad may take on a neutral pose and expression, so that they do not betray their emotions to others, while still considering their inward emotion when interpreting the environment. While there has been much research on having virtual agents displaying emotions [4], most have their *display* emotion be their outward emotion.

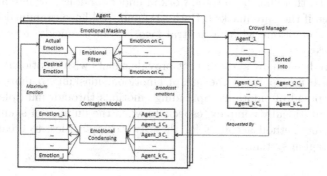

Fig. 1. A graphical representation of our system

To create more realistic multi-agent systems, we have developed a novel model of emotional contagion that incorporates emotional masking, and provides agents several methods of communicating and receiving emotions, depicted in Figure 1. Our agents use this novel masking to determine a display emotion, broad-casted on several channels. A crowd manager determines which agents can receive these broadcasts and appropriately directs the information into each agent's contagion model. This information is then condensed into bins, with the highest becoming the new emotion for each agent.

2   Related Work

There have been several models of emotional contagion for crowds of agents. [5] have contagion as an emergent effect inside part of a larger crowd simulation engine. A couple of other models [6, 7], use only one emotion, fear, and are used to predict human movement in fearful situations. These models were later validated from panic situations in [8]. Various other models use a small set of emotions [9–11], and model the inter-connectivity between emotions. Many of these models use either proximity or interpersonal connection between agents when determining the spread of emotions. This generates group emotions, and keeps contagion among those group members. However, there is a large swatch of psychology literature that also shows contagion happens between strangers [12, Chapter 3], [13]. Our method captures this emotional spread by passing emotions through several simulated virtual channels between groups of agents based on channel visibility.

Emotions have also been used for several other applications including negotiation [14]. Additionally, it has been shown that physical humans can understand emotions from virtual agent's facial expressions [15], body posture [16], vocal patterns, and gestures [17]. If physical humans use these different channels to understand each other's emotions, virtual humans should be able to as well. In the context of emotional contagion, these factors are what humans use to mimic each other and are the mechanism for conveying emotions between agents. Also in recent years, there has been some work in understanding how humans decode emotions even if they are masked. Both [18] and [19] have examined if humans can recognize emotions when a neutral face is shown quickly after seeing an emotional face.

There have been many systems that provide agents with emotional contagion but none have incorporated the use of emotional masking to more naturally control the spread of emotions. Spreading emotions through multiple channels can be computationally complex, especially when the number of agents is large and dense. Our method accounts for these two complexities, to create a more realistic contagion system.

3   Emotions and Agents

Emotional masking and contagion cannot take place in a group of agents if they lack an understanding of emotion. We adopt an approach, similar to [9, 11], using the emotional transition table developed by Adamatzky [13]; namely *happiness(H)*, *anger(A)*, *confusion(C)*, *sadness(S)*, which is referred to as *HACS* emotional states. We use Adamatzky's model because it simulates transistions between non-paired emotions, such as happiness and sadness. To represent low emotional states, we add a *neutral(N)* emotion for the agents to display. Emotions can be transitioned to from other states using the state transition diagram from Adamatzky and seen in Figure 2. Using the *HACS* model provides several advantages: that transitions occur in discrete event probabilities and that emotional coupling of a shared emotion does not change states, which can preserve emotional spirals.

Sending Receiving	H	A	C	S	N
H	H	C	C	C	N
A	C	A	A	A	N
C	A	C	C	C	N
S	A	S	S	S	N
N	H	A	C	S	N

Fig. 2. The transition diagram between agents using *HACS*. In this table, the transition is the most probable contagion response for an agent with their given emotion encountering another agent with a given emotion.

3.1 Emotional Contagion

Our system creates an emotional contagion model that operates on the *HACS* model of emotion. Using our model allows agents to spread and communicate their emotional state, using environmental variables that surpass mere proximity, and, with the correct necessary conditions, creating emergent effects like emotional spirals.

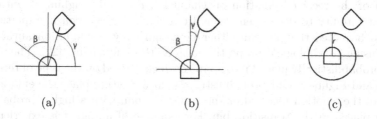

(a)   (b)   (c)

Fig. 3. Different methods of computing agent channels between two agents, with perception occurring from the center agent. (a)Computing non-reflexive channels using Equation 1, where β is half the field of view, and γ is the angle between agents. (b)Computing reflexive channels using Equation 1, where β is half the field of view, and γ is the angle between the agent's center of field of view. (c)Computing non-reflexive vocal channels using Equation 2.

The first step in our emotional contagion model determines the subset of agents and channels that an agent can perceive emotions from, and is performed by the crowd manager section of our model from Figure 1, and is similar to [20] in that we process which channels can be observed in a crowd management system. To determine a valid connection, a boolean function F_c, based on sensory perceptions like those found in [21]. Several of these perception channels are reflexive, in that if F_c is true for one agent, it is for both agents, and does not need to be repeated. We have three primary methods for determining channels. Specifically, we use non-reflexive equations for body posture and gestures seen in Figure 3a, reflexive functions for facial expressions and gaze seen in Figure 3b, and, vocal features based on Figure 3c. Using these equations, a crowd manager can construct a graph of all the channels each agent can perceive every other agent on, which, for large groups of agents, can become sparse. It can also be observed that, for large, dense areas, an agent should not be expected to momentarily mimic all other agents instantaneously. If a given agent is inside a crowd, the momentary micro mimicry should occur sequentially or between a small number of agents at a time. Using a sparse graph representation allows the agent to examine a small number of agents at a time, without having to section off agents or recompute calculations at every frame.

$$F_c = -\beta < \gamma < \beta \tag{1}$$

$$F_c = dist(agents) < r \tag{2}$$

The data from this sparse graph contains a list of emotions and channels, and each agent can request the list built for them from the crowd manager. By using a crowd manager to maintain the sparse graph, the number of computations are decreased by the number of reflexive channels. The received emotions from the list are processed by our emotional contagion engine, by determining the strength of the received emotion on channel i, e_{ci}, and weighing it with w_c, the agent's ability to decode emotions from channel c, as seen in Equation 3. It should be noted that w_c can either be assigned by a simulation author, or created using psychological properties such as those found in [22]. Then each e_{rc} are probabilistically placed into a bin $received_i$, based on the type of received emotion and Figure 2. Our probabilistic system will either place the emotion to the bin of the emotion received or the transition bin, with a higher probability of being placed in the transition bin. For example, if an agent is experiencing *happiness*, and attempts to decode an agent displaying *sadness*, then the happy agent has a likely chance to become confused, but may also become sad from it.

$$e_{rc} = e_{ci} * w_c \tag{3}$$

Once an agent probabilistically condenses all channels into $received_i$, it is added back into the agents emotion, as seen in Equation 4. A summation of all the perceived emotions is performed, which is then subtracted from each value of $received$. If most of the perceived emotions are neutral, this has the effect of lessening any perceived emotional contagion. We control the influence this summation has with a constant α, which controls the speed at which emotional spirals happen for single emotion simulations. Setting α greater then 1 keeps the system from always culminating in an emotional spiral.

$$e_i = received_i - \frac{\alpha * \sum_{i=0}^{n} e_i}{n} \qquad (4)$$

3.2 Emotional Masking

Most physical humans do not display their true emotional state all of the time. It can be inappropriate or unwise for a person to express their feelings in certain situations. Emotional masking attempts to hide the emotion being felt by a person through the display of another emotion, or by not displaying any emotion. An agent may decide to mask their emotion, or be told to by a simulation author, allowing an agent to have a *true* emotion used for other processes, such as decision making, and a *display* emotion that can be received by other agents. It has also been shown that the effectiveness of masking one emotion with another is emotion dependent [18].

To determine the type and intensity of the emotion displayed by an agent, we combine the actual and display emotion with an emotional filter, using Equation 5. This equation uses the true emotional intensity e_i, the desired display emotional intensity e_j, and a weight w_{ij} that represents how effective masking one emotion with another is, based on Rohr et al. [19], which determined that physical humans can easily mask anger, sadness, and confusion with one another, but cannot easily mask happiness. The agent then determines if the displayed emotion e_{dis} is positive, and if so, the agent can successfully mask their emotion using their desired display emotion. e_{dis} is then treated in the same manner as the true emotional intensity was in Section 3.1.

$$e_{dis} = e_i - w_{ij} * \frac{e_j}{1 + e_i} \qquad (5)$$

4 Experimentation

We examine the effects of emotional masking and using separate channels by implementing our model in a virtual agent system. Control of our agent's walking and gesture realization is provided by Smartbody [23]. All agent's channel weights are normally distributed. The intensity of each agent's displayed emotion is shown as the agent's primary color, with black representing no emotion and green, red, blue, and grey respectively representing an emotion from *HACS*.

We simulate a group of agents walking down the street on a normal day, much like commuters going home in the evening. Several agents are walking pass each other, all of which have been given various intensities of all five emotions between zero and half of the maximum intensity. Figure 4 shows the use of masking for agent contagion when simulating agents acting as commuters.

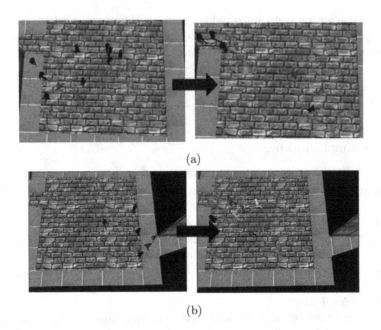

(a)

(b)

Fig. 4. A sample scenario of several agents walking through an environment. (a) Agents are masking their emotion with a neutral emotion. (b) Agents are not masking their emotions at all, resulting in an unnatural spread of emotions.

From Figure 4a, when agents mask their emotions with neutral emotions, the overall intensity of a displayed emotion is much less, as is the amount of contagion. This is to be expected, as agents that are hiding their emotion should not be passing their emotion onto others. When masking is taken away, the agents conform to a few emotions with much higher intensities. Specifically, many of the agents are either angry or confused. When examining Figure 2, this is to be expected. Most of the transitions in the table are either towards angry or confused, and these transitions are stable when angry agents perceive confused agents. Therefore, when these agents encounter each other, and decode each other's emotions we expect agents to display a high intensity when not masking. Combining contagion with masking gives a more realistic everyday scenario for physical humans, where most do not display emotion, and therefore, do not create these emotional spirals in crowds. This means our system allows a scenario author the flexibility to alter parameter settings and achieve the likelihood of emotional contagion they desire while maintaining plausible agent behaviors.

We also examine how emotional masking affects the total number of agents that outwardly display emotions, for both masked and open settings. Channel weights for each agent are determined from a uniform distribution, as are the type and strength of each agent's starting true emotion. Each agent is constrained to a fixed grid, and at the end of each iteration, may move one space over on that grid, or slightly change their orientation. This reduces the number of agents that form closed groups. When masking emotions, the agents use a neutral state, with an intensity between ten percent and half of the emotions maximum intensity. The results of fifty runs at 100 iterations is seen in Figure 5.

From Figure 5c it can be seen that with masking, the number of agents that display no emotion is much greater than any other set of emotions. This does not mean that emotional contagion is not occurring, as can be seem from Figure 5a. This shows contagion still occurs, as the number of happy agents rises as time goes on. This occurrence is much slower then without masking, seem in Figure 5b.

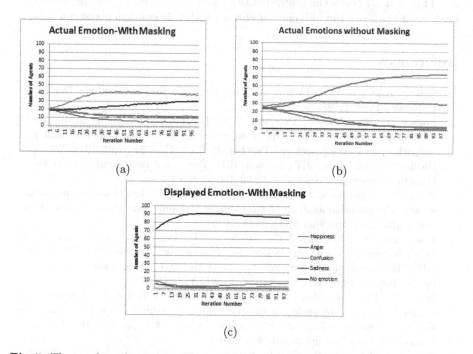

(a)   (b)

(c)

Fig. 5. The number of agents vs. the iteration number for multiple emotions. (a)The number of agents actually feeling each emotion when masking is enabled. (b)The number of agents displaying each emotion without masking. (c)The number of agents displaying each emotion when masking is enabled.

5   Conclusions

We present a model of emotional contagion that allows an agent to decode emotions on multiple channels. In order to do this, we created a system to encode and decode emotions on several channels, using a probabilistic transition between different types of emotions. To allow for downward emotional spiral and neutral scenes, we implemented a method for emotional masking that allows an agent to determine which emotion they wish to display, and mask their felt emotions, allowing for an over-abundance of neutral expression. A neutral expression causing a downward spiral is similar to the military coming to fight Godzilla, calming the populous with their stern emotional neutrality.

While our system adds several human characteristics to a contagion model, it also has several unrealistic limitations. Agents in our system display the same emotion on all channels, and these are always correctly interpreted by the surrounding agents. In realistic situations, this is not always the case and an interesting addition would be to examine mis-understandings of emotions. Also, our work is focused on having a contagion system where agents consciously control the display of their emotions, which we assume a group of agents would want to do. This is not always culturally realistic, and an interesting extension of this work would capture the influence of culture with this contagion system.

References

1. Ortony, A., Clore, G.L., Collins, A.: Cognitive Structure of Emotions. Cambridge University Press (1988)
2. Posner, J., Russell, J.A., Peterson, B.S.: The circumplex model of affect: An integrative approach to affective neuroscience, cognitive development, and psychopathology. Development and Psychopathology, 715–734 (September 2005)
3. Hatfield, E., Cacioppo, J.T., Rapson, R.L.: Emotional contagion. Current Directions in Psychological Science 2(3), 96–100 (1993)
4. Rumbell, T., Barnden, J., Denham, S., Wennekers, T.: Emotions in autonomous agents: Comparative analysis of mechanisms and functions. Autonomous Agents and Multi-Agent Systems 25(1), 1–45 (2012)
5. Pelechano, N., Allbeck, J.M., Badler, N.I.: Controlling individual agents in high-density crowd simulation. In: Proceedings of the 2007 ACM SIG-GRAPH/Eurographics Symposium on Computer Animation, SCA 2007, pp. 99–108. Eurographics Association, Aire-la-Ville (2007)
6. Bosse, T., Duell, R., Memon, Z.A., Treur, J., van der Wal, C.N.: A multi-agent model for mutual absorption of emotions. In: Proceedings of the 23rd European Conference on Modelling and Simulation, ECMS 2009, pp. 212–218. European Council on Modeling and Simulation (2009)
7. Tsai, J., Fridman, N., Bowring, E., Brown, M., Epstein, S., Kaminka, G., Marsella, S., Ogden, A., Rika, I., Sheel, A., Taylor, M.E., Wang, X., Zilka, A., Tambe, M.: Escapes: Evacuation simulation with children, authorities, parents, emotions, and social comparison. In: The 10th International Conference on Autonomous Agents and Multiagent Systems, AAMAS 2011, vol. 2, pp. 457–464. International Foundation for Autonomous Agents and Multiagent Systems, Richland (2011)
8. Tsai, J., Bowring, E., Marsella, S., Wood, W., Tambe, M.: A study of emotional contagion with virtual characters. In: Nakano, Y., Neff, M., Paiva, A., Walker, M. (eds.) IVA 2012. LNCS, vol. 7502, pp. 81–88. Springer, Heidelberg (2012)
9. Bispo, J., Paiva, A.: A model for emotional contagion based on the emotional contagion scale. In: 3rd International Conference on Affective Computing and Intelligent Interaction and Workshops, ACII 2009, pp. 1–6 (September 2009)
10. Dimas, J., Pereira, G., Santos, P.A., Prada, R., Paiva, A.: "i'm happy if you are happy": A model for emotional contagion in game characters. In: Proceedings of the 8th International Conference on Advances in Computer Entertainment Technology, ACE 2011, pp. 2:1–2:7. ACM, New York (2011)

11. Lhommet, M., Lourdeaux, D., Barthès, J.P.: Never alone in the crowd: A microscopic crowd model based on emotional contagion. In: Proceedings of the 2011 IEEE/WIC/ACM International Conferences on Web Intelligence and Intelligent Agent Technology, pp. 89–92. IEEE Computer Society Press, Washington, DC (2011)

12. Knapp, M.L., Hall, J.A.: Nonverbal Communication in Human Interaction. Hold, Rinehart, and Winston, Inc. (1997)

13. Adamatzky, A.: Dynamics of Crowd-Minds: Patterns of Irrationality in Emotions, Beliefs and Actions. World Scientific Series on Nonlinear Science. World Scientific (2005)

14. de Melo, C.M., Carnevale, P., Gratch, J.: The effect of virtual agents' emotion displays and appraisals on people's decision making in negotiation. In: Nakano, Y., Neff, M., Paiva, A., Walker, M. (eds.) IVA 2012. LNCS (LNAI), vol. 7502, pp. 53–66. Springer, Heidelberg (2012)

15. Sloan, R.J.S., Robinson, B., Scott-Brown, K., Moore, F., Cook, M.: A phenomenological study of facial expression animation. In: Proceedings of the 25th BCS Conference on Human-Computer Interaction, BCS-HCI 2011, pp. 177–186. British Computer Society, Swinton (2011)

16. Normoyle, A., Liu, F., Kapadia, M., Badler, N.I., Jörg, S.: The effect of posture and dynamics on the perception of emotion. In: Symposium on Applied Perception, pp. 91–98. ACM (2013)

17. Callejas, Z., López-Cózar, R., Àbalos, N., Griol, D.: Affective conversational agents: The role of personality and emotion in spoken interactions. In: Conversational Agents and Natural Language Interaction: Techniques and Effective Practices, pp. 203–217. Information Science Reference

18. Whalen, P.J., Raunch, S.L., Etcoff, N.L., McInerney, S.C., Lee, M.B., Jenike, M.A.: Masked presentations of emotional facial expressions modulate amygdala activity without explicit knowledge. The Journal of Neuroscience (1998)

19. Rohr, M., Degner, J., Wentura, D.: Masked emotional priming beyond global valence activations. Cognition and Emotion 26(2), 224–244 (2012)

20. Saunier, J., Jones, H.: Mixed agent/social dynamics for emotion computation. In: Autonomous Agents and Multiagent Systems, pp. 645–652. International Foundation for Autonomous Agents and Multiagent Systems (2014)

21. Balint, T., Allbeck, J.M.: What's going on? multi-sense attention for virtual agents. In: Aylett, R., Krenn, B., Pelachaud, C., Shimodaira, H. (eds.) IVA 2013. LNCS, vol. 8108, pp. 349–357. Springer, Heidelberg (2013)

22. Coenen, R., Broekens, J.: Modeling emotional contagion based on experimental evidence for moderating factors. In: Autonomous Agents and Multiagent Systems, pp. 26–33. International Foundation for Autonomous Agents and Multiagent Systems (2012)

23. Feng, A., Huang, Y., Xu, Y., Shapiro, A.: Automating the transfer of a generic set of behaviors onto a virtual character. In: Kallmann, M., Bekris, K. (eds.) MIG 2012. LNCS, vol. 7660, pp. 134–145. Springer, Heidelberg (2012)

Narrative Scenarios as a Testbed for Moral Agents

Cristina Battaglino[1] and Rossana Damiano[2]

[1] Dipartimento di Informatica, Università di Torino, Italy
battagli@di.unito.it
[2] Dipartimento di Informatica and CIRMA, Università di Torino, Italy
rossana@di.unito.it

Abstract. Moral emotions play an important role in the design and implementation of virtual agents, since they have implications not only for the agent's deliberation process but also for its interactional and social functions. In this paper, we propose an empirical methodology that leverages narrative situations to evaluate the emotional state felt by an intelligent agent.

1 Introduction

Moral emotions [9,13,8] deserve special attention in the design of virtual agents, since they play a crucial role in many agent's functions, ranging from self regulation [4] to the handling of social and interactional aspects [5]. Moral emotions have been integrated into a number of computational models of emotions, with approaches that range from the hard coding of moral standards in the emotional component [12,10], to the design of high level moral values to drive the generation of emotions [3]. In this paper, we propose a methodology for evaluating the generation of moral emotions that leverages the capability of narratives of exemplifying the connection between moral values and emotions.

2 Values and Emotions

In order to test the feasibility of the proposed methodology, in this paper we apply it to the emotional agent model described by [3], where a BDI agent is extended with emotions and moral values. In [3], agents have an explicit representation of their moral dimension based on a value system [6], and a motivational dimension given by the desires they want to pursue [2]. According to [1], the emotional state of the agent is the result of the appraisal and affect generation processes The appraisal process is based on goal and value processing and outputs a set of appraisal variables that are the input to the affect generation process. In particular, the appraisal process generates a *desirability or (undesirability)* variable when an agent's goal is achieved (or unachieved) in the state of the world as an effect of some action or event; it generates a *probability* variable depending on the probability that an agent's plan succeeds; finally, it generates a *praiseworthiness* (or *blameworthiness*) variable when an agent's value is balanced (or put at stake)by the execution of some action.

T. Bickmore et al. (Eds.): IVA 2014, LNAI 8637, pp. 36–39, 2014.

3   Experimental Protocol

The experiments we conducted to evaluate the moral emotional agent relied on narrative scenarios that we presented to participants in a text-based form though a web site[1]. Emotions were described trough text labels (e.g. "Hamlet feels *Reproach, Shame* and *Anger* towards Ophelia), without any colors. The scenarios were selected from famous works of fiction with the help of a drama expert, who identified them based on availability of well established critical interpretations of the emotions felt by the characters [11,7]. The selected scenes are taken from: *Hamlet*'s (Shakespeare), *The count of Monte Cristo* and *The Vicomte of Bragelonne:Ten years later* by Alexandre Dumas, *Thérèse Raquin* (Émile Zola). The methodology we followed to create the narrative scenarios is the following: first, we analyzed the structure of the narrative, then, with the help of the expert, we identified the cognitive states of the characters and we characterized their mental attitudes (i.e. beliefs, desires and values). By doing so, we also verified that the agent model under evaluation had the necessary expressiveness to model the selected narrative situations.

A convenience sample of twenty subjects, 9 female and 11 male, aged 24-35, participated in the study. In the web experiment, we assigned participants randomly to the test conditions (V+) and (V−). The (V+) group evaluated scenarios in which emotions are associated to characters following the model in [3], in which moral values and moral emotions are presented. The (V−) group evaluated scenarios with emotions related to goals, such as Joy and Distress. The primary hypotheses of the study are:

- H1: emotions in the V− condition are less believable than V+ condition (*believability*);
- H2: emotions in the V− condition are less complete than V+ condition (*completeness*);

For example, in the scenario of Hamlet, Hamlet feels Anger towards Ophelia because she lied, putting at stake Hamlet's value honesty (*blameworthy action*) and threatening Hamlet's goal of saving her from the corruption of the court (*undesirable event*). In the V+ group, we associated Anger, Reproach and Distress emotions to Hamlet because the V+ condition contemplates values. In the V− condition, we associate only Distress emotion because the V− condition doesn't provide values but only goals, so emotions related to values are not taken into account.

Given a scenario, participants first read the scenario and then he/she received the post questionnaire about the scenario. The believability and completeness measures of the affective states of characters involved in the scenario were assessed by direct questions in the post questionnaire, with a 5-item Likert scale response. We also asked to the participants to list the emotions they would felt if they were to identify with the story characters, using multiple-choice questions based on OCC categories of emotions [1].

---

[1] The web experiment is online at *www.ilnomedellarosa.it/Valutazione* - in Italian only.

4 Evaluation

In order to determine if there are differences in the variables under study (believability and completeness of the set of characters' emotions, H1 and H2 respectively) between the groups V+ and V−, we conducted the Mann-Whitney U test on the completeness and believability Likert scores. We run a series of tests considering all the scenarios, then we run the same tests on every scenario. In (Table 2, Table 1) we summarize the results of the Mann-Whitney U tests on the Likert scores.

Table 1. Mann Whitney U statistics for *complete* metric

Results	U	p (two tailed)	p (one tailed)
Hamlet	19	.01	.005
Count of Monte Cristo	13	.003	.001
Thérèse Raquin	33	.185	.09
Vicomte Bragelonne	6	.001	.0
All	277	.0	.0

Table 2. Mann Whitney U statistics for *believable* metric

Results	U	p (two tailed)	p (one tailed)
Hamlet	6	.0	.0
Count of Monte Cristo	19	.012	.006
Thérèse Raquin	32	.133	.133
Vicomte Bragelonne	45	.6	.3
All	453	.0	.0

Quantitative Results. Considering all scenarios, results show that the perceived level of believability and completeness of emotions in the V− condition were significantly lower than the V+ condition at $p < 0.01$. Regarding the specific scenarios, in the *Hamlet* and *Count of Monte Cristo* scenarios, the perceived level of believability of emotions in the V− condition was significantly lower than the scores in the V+ condition, while, in the *Hamlet, Count of Monte Cristo* and *Vicomte the Bragelonne*, the perceived level of completeness of emotions in the V− condition was significantly lower than the scores in the V+ condition (with significance at $p < 0.05$ in general). Results don't show statistical significance for the third scenario.

Discussion. The analysis of the results confirms the hypothesis H2 but not H1. However, the emotions associated with the V− condition were a subset of emotions in the V+ condition, so the lack of some of them may have been not perceived. We also observed that participants attributed to the characters the emotions predicted by the moral emotional agent model. The third scenario was not evaluated as complete, possibly because the characters' values were perceived by the participants.

5 Conclusion

In this paper, we proposed a methodology to evaluate the generation of moral emotions that relies on narrative scenarios, considered as paradigmatic cases of the interplay between emotions and moral values. By modeling the characters in each scenario as value-based emotional agents [3], we asked a set of testers to assess the adequacy of the characters' emotions to the given scenarios. The results suggest that the participants perceive as more believable the emotional states that encompass moral values and emotions, and that they agree with the generated emotions. This suggests that the users perceive the relevance of moral values – and of moral emotions – in narrative situations. As future work, we plan to design and run further tests to verify this hypothesis.

References

1. Collins, A., Ortony, A., Clore, G.L.: The cognitive structure of emotions. Cambridge University Press, Cambridge (1988)
2. Bratman, M.E.: Intention, plans, and practical reason. Harvard University Press, Cambridge (1987)
3. Lesmo, L., Battaglino, C., Damiano, R.: Emotional range in value-sensitive deliberation. In: AAMAS, pp. 769–776 (2013)
4. de Melo, C.M., Zheng, L., Gratch, J.: Expression of moral emotions in cooperating agents. In: Ruttkay, Z., Kipp, M., Nijholt, A., Vilhjálmsson, H.H. (eds.) IVA 2009. LNCS, vol. 5773, pp. 301–307. Springer, Heidelberg (2009)
5. de Melo, C.M., Carnevale, P., Gratch, J.: The influence of emotions in embodied agents on human decision-making. In: Safonova, A. (ed.) IVA 2010. LNCS (LNAI), vol. 6356, pp. 357–370. Springer, Heidelberg (2010)
6. Van Fraassen, B.C.: Values and the heart's command. Journal of Philosophy 70(1), 5–19 (1973)
7. Freytag, G.: Technique of the drama, an exposition of dramatic composition and art. S.C. Griggs and Company, Chicago (1985)
8. Garcia, A.E., Ostrosky-Solís, F.: From morality to moral emotions. International Journal of Psychology 41(5), 348–354 (2006)
9. Haidt, J.: The moral emotions. In: Handbook of Affective Sciences, pp. 852–870 (2003)
10. Marsella, S., Gratch, J.: Ema: A process model of appraisal dynamics. Cognitive Systems Research 10(1), 70–90 (2009)
11. Polti, G.: Les trente-six situations dramatiques. Mercure de France, Paris (1895)
12. Reilly, W.S., Bates, J.: Building emotional agents (1992)
13. Stark, S.: Emotions and the ontology of moral value. The Journal of Value Inquiry 38, 355–374 (2004), doi:10.1007/s10790-005-1341-y

On the Sociability of a Game-Playing Agent: A Software Framework and Empirical Study

Morteza Behrooz, Charles Rich, and Candace Sidner

Worcester Polytechnic Institute
Worcester, Massachusetts, USA
{mbehrooz,rich,sidner}@wpi.edu

Abstract. We report on the results of evaluating a virtual agent that plays games with automatically generated social comments and social gaze. The agent played either a card game (rummy) or a board game (checkers) with each of 31 participants. Based on objective and subjective measures, the agent using social comments and gaze was preferred to both a version of the agent using only social gaze and to playing the game interactively, but without a virtual agent. We have also developed a generic software framework for authoring social comments for any game based on the semantics of the game.

Keywords: social interaction, social game, social comment, social gaze, virtual agent, human-robot interaction.

1 Introduction

It is no secret: humans love playing games. Humans have figured out a way to create games with every emerging technology in history. In fact, games have often contributed to the expansion and deployment of many of those technologies. Today, there are millions of games with different rules and goals; they are played in many different circumstances by people of different cultures and various ages. However, there is a single element in most of these gaming experiences that goes beyond these differences, an element that makes people laugh while playing games and makes them play together to enjoy more than just what the game itself has to offer: This is the *social* element of playing games.

Nowadays, the role of social robots and virtual agents is rapidly expanding in daily activities and entertainment. One of these areas is games, where people traditionally play even simple card and board games as a means of socializing, especially if not gambling. Therefore, it seems desirable for an agent to be able to play games socially, as opposed to simply having the computer make the moves in a game application.

To achieve this goal and to create a human-like experience, verbal and non-verbal communication should be appropriate to the game events and human input, to create a human-like social experience. Moreover, a better social interaction can be created if the agent can adapt its game strategies in accordance with social criteria.

T. Bickmore et al. (Eds.): IVA 2014, LNAI 8637, pp. 40–53, 2014.

To facilitate social gameplay with as many different robots, virtual agents and games as possible, we have developed a generic software framework that supports the authoring and automatic generation of appropriate social comments based on the gameplay semantics, which includes the legal moves and states of the game and an evaluation of the relative strength of particular moves and states. We applied this generic framework to a card game (rummy) and a board game (checkers) and used the resulting systems in a user study that demonstrated that users enjoy the type of social interactions that the framework supports.

In the following, after laying out the related research, we will explain study setup and procedures, followed by the results and discussions. We will then introduce our framework and describe its architecture and functionality. Lastly, we will draw conclusions and discuss future directions.

2 Related Work

The most closely related work to this research is by Paiva et al. [1–3], using the iCat robot. They suggest that users' perception of the game increases when the iCat shows emotional behaviors that are influenced by the game state. They also indicate that by using affect recognition, the state and evolution of the game and display of facial expressions by the iCat significantly affects the user's emotional state and levels of engagement. Furthermore, in a study where an iCat observing the game behaves in an empathic manner toward one of two players in a chess game, and in neutral way toward the other, the authors report on higher companionship ratings by the player to whom the robot was empathic.

The same group introduced Fatima [4], an Agent Architecture with planning capabilities designed to use emotions and personality to influence the agent's behavior. Fatima has been used in different contexts including story-telling (e.g. FearNot! [5]) and education (e.g. ORIENT [6]). While this architecture would be extremely beneficial in bringing affect and emotion to games, it rightly has less direct focus on semantics inside the game, as it targets a general design that is suitable for many different contexts.

Paiva et al. have studied many social and emotional aspects of playing games with social robots and agents. Their work mostly focuses on empathy effects during games. While this was extremely valuable and inspiring to our research, we were more interested in focusing on the gaming side to create deeper connections between the gameplay semantics and social interactions, in a generic way.

McCoy et al. developed *Prom Week* [7], a social simulation game about the interpersonal lives of a group of high school students in the week leading up to their prom. Although in this work the virtual agents are not playing against the user, and therefore the associated social interactions are of a different nature, it clearly shows a successful application of modeling social interactions in games.

Many researchers report that social cues and emotions can make agents appear more believable. For instance, Bickmore et al. [8] report that displaying social cues by virtual agents resulted in agents being more believable in their experiments. Also, Canamero et al. [9] and Ogata et al. [10] conclude that emotions help facilitate more believable human-robot interactions.

Gonzlez-Pacheco et al. [11] introduced a robot (*Maggie*) for playing games socially. Although their system offers a great contribution on the robotic side, including the hardware and sensory capabilities and a software platform for controlling them, it has less focus on provide a generic software framework for facilitating social interactions during games.

In [12], Van Eck notes that simple games are more suitable than complex games for establishing empathic effects, since the cognitive load on the players in such games is much lower. This observation supports our choice of simple card and board games as the initial target of our work.

Beyond gaming, there are many contexts in which sociable agents and robots are popular [13], ranging from *Keepon* [14], a minimalistic musical robot particularly useful for treating children with autism, to much more complicated social agents. Whether it is therapeutic care [15], food delivery [16] or playing with toys [17], social interactions prove to be a crucial aspect of many experiences. In this work, we study such sociability in a game context.

3 User Study

In our user study, a virtual agent capable of speaking comments and performing social gaze behaviors (see Fig. 1), played checkers and rummy with participants. By incorporating two different games, we intended to assess the generality of our approach and framework.

Our general assumption was that a gaming experience that involves social behaviors inspired by the semantics of the game would be preferable to a gaming experience that does not. Two readily available social behaviors were making comments and introducing some social gaze. The gaze choices for the agent were limited to ones that involved the agent directing its gaze in three different ways, but did not include mutual gaze with the user because of the complexities of assessing mutual gaze. We suspected that users' non-verbal gestures might also be important. Because smiling is associated with pleasure in playing games, we hypothesized that smiles would more readily occur when the agent produced more types of social behavior.

In our hypotheses below, we are exploring the relationships between social behaviors (gaze and comments) and participants' preferences and smiling.

Hypothesis I: Participants will (a) *prefer* and (b) *smile more* playing checkers and rummy with a virtual agent that interacts using *both* social gaze and comments, compared to *either* a virtual agent using *only social gaze* or playing *without* a virtual agent.

Hypothesis II: Participants will (a) *prefer* and (b) *smile more* playing checkers and rummy with a virtual agent that interacts using *only social gaze*, compared to playing *without* a virtual agent.

3.1   Experimental Setup

Participants. There were 31 participants in the study, 12 males and 19 females. The average age of participants was 20.23 with a standard deviation of 3.67. All participants were offered course credits for their participation.

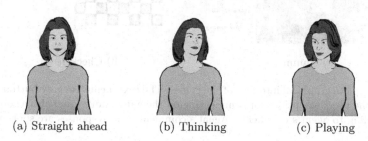

(a) Straight ahead   (b) Thinking   (c) Playing

Fig. 1. Different gaze directions of the agent

Interaction Elements. Our virtual agent is shown in Fig. 1. The agent was always located at the top-right part of the screen (see Fig. 2) and was able to speak and perform gazes in different directions. These gaze directions were straight ahead, thinking and playing. The thinking gaze was used before the agent played a move (for 2 to 3.5 seconds, depending on the game and move), and the playing gaze was used from 0.5 seconds before playing a move to 1 second after. The playing gaze was also used during user's turn and before user's move to reflect the anticipation of user's move in agent's expressions. A significant amount of effort was devoted to making the gaze animations and timing smooth and accurate. The rest of the time (e.g., when agent was speaking to user) the agent gazed straight ahead (during which time a face-tracking mode was activated to allow the agent's head to follow participant's face). During both gaze and face-tracking behaviors, the agent's eyes moved in synchrony with its head according to well-known rules for human gaze motions.

The agent was also capable of making social comments about its own or the human player's moves using the IVONA text-to-speech engine. After the agent's comment, the participant is given a chance to respond by choosing one of the text menus appearing on the right side of the screen. Participants also had a chance to make a social comment on either their own or the agent's moves, after which the agent would respond with another comment. After each played move, the commenting opportunity was given to one of the players randomly. A maximum of one comment and one optional response was possible each time. The participant had the ability to skip entering a comment, or a response, by either making a move in the game if it was his/her turn, or by selecting *"Your turn"* (Fig. 2a) which always appeared as menu choice when the agent's turn was coming up. See Sec. 4 for details on the generic framework and how social comments were chosen.

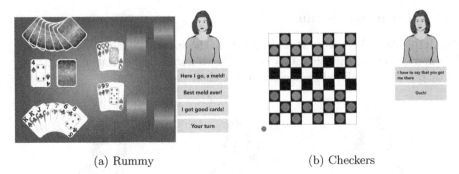

(a) Rummy   (b) Checkers

Fig. 2. Complete graphical interface of the games. The text menus (in gray buttons) are offered to the users as options for commenting on the game moves, and also as options for responding to agent's comments. Agent's comments and responses are spoken.

Conditions. The study contained three conditions as follows (in all conditions the gaming area of the interface was identical):

- **NoAgent:** *The screen space occupied by the agent in the other conditions was left blank and there were no social comments;*
- **GazeOnly:** *Agent with social gaze only;*
- **GazeComment:** *Agent with social gaze and comments.*

Procedure. As introduced earlier, we used rummy and checkers games in our study. The study was within-subject. Each participant was assigned one of the two games and played it in all three conditions, in a random order. At the start of the study, the participant was consented by the experimenter and told which game he/she was going to play. The participant was then asked if he/she needed a tutorial about how to play that game. The tutorials were short one-page documents in electronic format that explained the game rules, but did not contain any information about the agent or the conditions. The participant was given time to read the tutorial while the experimenter waited outside.

The computer used in the study was a touch-screen PC; participants used the touch input for gameplay.

In all conditions, the participant was told that he/she had an unlimited amount of time in order to play one round of the game. However, after 7 minutes, the participant was given the option to decide to continue the game or to move on to the next phase of the study. This was primarily done to avoid the overall study time from being too long. Participants were also told to notify the experimenter by knocking on the closed door, if they finished the game sooner than 7 minutes.

After playing in each condition (during which the experimenter waited outside) the participant was asked to fill out an electronic questionnaire. The questionnaire was identical for all conditions of both games. After completing three conditions and three questionnaires, the study was concluded.

During the study, we also used the Shore [18, 19] face detection engine to record the occurrences of participants' smiles.

Table 1. Questionnaire items and categories

Category 1: Working Alliance Inventory (6 questions)
· I can say that the opponent appreciated my gaming capabilities
· I believe that the opponent and I respect each other
· I believe the opponent was playing honestly
· I was frustrated by my interaction with the opponent in the game *
· I find our gaming experience with the opponent confusing *
· I think the opponent in the game and I trusted one another during the game

Category 2: Enjoyable (5 questions)
· The game was enjoyable
· I would have played the game longer
· I laughed during the game
· The game was fun
· The game was more fun than other similar computer games I have played

Category 3: Sociable (5 questions)
· The game was more social than other similar computer games I have played
· I felt that I had a social experience during the game
· I found the opponent in the game social
· I believe the game meant more than just winning to the opponent
· I believe the game became/was more than just winning for me

Category 4: Human-like and intelligent (3 questions)
· The game experience was natural and human-like
· I found the opponent in the game intelligent
· The game made me feel that I was playing with something more than just a CPU

Category 5: Game adoption (5 questions)
· I would show this game to my friends
· I can see myself getting used to playing this game on a daily basis
· I can see myself playing this game instead of some other more ordinary games
· I can see this game as a close replacement for playing with friends when that is not possible
· If I could, I would have asked for the same kinds of interaction in my other activities as the ones I had in the game

3.2   Results

Questionnaire. The questionnaire consisted of 24 items using a 7-point Likert scale from "strongly disagree" to "strongly agree", coded as 1 to 7, respectively. The items were 5 different categories which were not apparent in the questionnaire. These categories, and their items, can be found in Table 1. The questionnaire items were presented in an identical shuffled order to all participants.

One of the questionnaire categories consisted of items from the Working Alliance Inventory [20], a standard collection of statements used to measure the alliance between the two parties in an interaction. *Alliance* refers to the achievement of a collaborative relationship, meaning that there is a consensus and willingness in both parties to be engaged in the interaction.

Table 2 shows the results for each questionnaire category, along with the overall results, in an aggregated fashion. The answers to the 2 items marked with asterisk in Table 1 were subtracted from 7 because of their phrasings.

Smile Detection. As mentioned earlier, we used the Shore [18, 19] face detection engine to detect participants' smiles. We chose smiles because they could be reliably automated with no special apparatus for the user and also because

Table 2. Questionnaire results, showing the Mean and Standard Deviation (m(sd)) in an aggregated analysis over categories and overall for all conditions. p(x, y) shows the p-value from a paired two-tailed t-test between conditions x and y, where NA stands for NoAgent, GO for GazeOnly and GC for GazeComment.

Category	NoAgent	GazeOnly	GazeComment	p(NA, GO)	p(GO, GC)	p(NA, GC)
1	3.86(1.72)	4.13(1.67)	4.70(1.54)	$<$.05	$\ll$.001	$\ll$.001
2	4.02(1.74)	3.99(1.77)	5.14(1.49)	.8	$\ll$.001	$\ll$.001
3	2.25(1.59)	2.65(1.42)	4.39(1.81)	$\ll$.001	$\ll$.001	$\ll$.001
4	2.80(1.78)	3.68(1.67)	4.10(1.69)	$\ll$.001	.07	$\ll$.001
5	3.39(1.89)	3.65(1.59)	4.17(1.88)	.06	$<$.003	$\ll$.001
aggregate	3.33(1.86)	3.64(1.71)	4.54(1.72)	$\ll$.001	$\ll$.001	$\ll$.001

smiles are a facial expression associated with enjoyment in game playing. We did not have access to any other means of automatically collecting other facial expressions or body gestures that seemed relevant. In this process, Shore reported the "perceived happiness" of the participant's facial expression as a number in the range of [0, 100], which we recorded every 0.5 seconds. We later counted the number of times (h) that each participant's happiness value exceeded 50 in each condition. It should be mentioned that the creators of Shore have reported [18] a successful recognition rate of 95.3% for this feature of their engine.

We chose the threshold approach, which filters out low values in Shore's reported numbers, as opposed to other possible methods of analysis, such as summing or averaging, to be more certain that the h value better represents smiles that were most likely caused by the game interaction and not, for example, the constant smiles of cheerful people. We did not try to correlate the timing of the smiles with any particular events in the interaction.

The results for a paired two-tailed t-test between the recorded h values in three conditions along with the mean h values can be found in Table 3.

Table 3. Mean of h values for perceived happiness in three conditions. p(x, y) also shows the p-value from a paired two-tailed t-test between conditions x and y where NA stands for NoAgent, GO for GazeOnly and GC for GazeComment.

NoAgent	GazeOnly	GazeComment	p(NA, GO)	p(GO, GC)	p(NA, GC)
21.19	21.38	49.3	.9	$<$.002	$<$.001

To illustrate this distribution better, a three-dimensional area chart, showing the h values for every participant and in all conditions, can be found in Fig. 3.

Although we arbitrarily chose a threshold of 50 in our analysis, we observed that for any other threshold, ranging from 5 to 95, the average of h values in the GazeComment condition was consistently 2 to 3 times larger than that of other conditions, with similar p-values to the ones reported in Table 3.

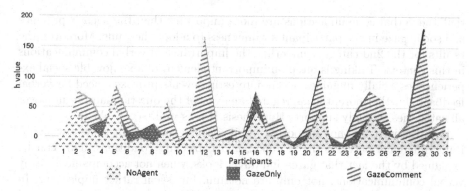

Fig. 3. In this chart, the Y-axis represent the h values (with a threshold of 50) for all three conditions, while the X-axis contains each study subject (31)

Other Results. As stated before, participants had the chance to continue playing the game after 7 minutes. Out of 93 plays in all conditions, 41 cases were finished before 7 minutes, 46 were stopped on 7 minutes and only 6 cases were extended (3 in the GazeOnly condition and 3 in the GazeComment condition).

When the same analyses were performed for the two individual games (checkers and rummy) separately, the results of questionnaire and smile detection were similar to the combined results.

3.3 Discussion

Hypothesis I-a (comparing preferences for the GazeComment condition to the other two conditions) is strongly supported by the questionnaire results in Table 2, except in the case of comparing the GazeOnly and GazeComment conditions in category 4 (human-like and intelligent), for which this hypothesis remains a trend. This shows that nothing stood out for the participants in terms of agent's intelligence and human-likeliness between these two conditions. However, comparing the NoAgent and GazeOnly conditions in category 4 shows statistical significance. Thus participants' perception of the agent's intelligence is greater in the GazeOnly and GazeComment conditions as compared to NoAgent, even though the agent was not *really* more intelligent, since we did not change its gaming strategies. This increase hints at the importance of sociability when an agent is intended to be perceived as intelligent.

Moreover, Hypothesis I-a is also fully supported in the aggregated analysis of the questionnaire results over all categories (see Table 2).

Hypothesis I-b is strongly supported by the results as well. Smile detection analysis suggests a significant increase in the number of smile occurrences during the gaming interactions in the GazeComment condition, compared to the others.

Hypothesis II-a (comparing the NoAgent and GazeOnly conditions) is supported in the 1st (alliance), 3rd (sociable) and 4th (human-like and intelligent) categories. It remains a trend for the 5th category (game adoption) and unsupported for the 2nd category (enjoyable). On the 5th category, the results suggest that the verbal communications are more important than the agent's presence and social gaze in the participant's willingness to adopt the game. Moreover, the results for the 2nd category underline the importance of verbal communications in this context. Talking is often an important element of an enjoyable social experience, especially in games, where interesting events provoke a need for verbal feedback. Furthermore, the aggregated analysis of the questionnaire results over all categories strongly supports Hypothesis II-a as well (see Table 2).

Hypothesis II-b is not supported. Smile occurrences do not show any significant difference between the NoAgent and GazeOnly conditions. This can be explained by the fact that gazes and direct looks, when not accompanied by any verbal communications, not only are not fun, but seem rather unpleasant. In fact, between humans, this kind of behavior usually bears a negative message of disengagement or dissatisfaction.

Notably, the smile detection results are consistent with the results from a related item of the questionnaire (the third item in 2nd category of Table 1) where p(NA, GC) and p(GO, GC) were both $\ll .001$ and p(NA, GO) was 0.8.

4   A Software Framework

All of the social comments in our user study were generated using a generic software framework (see Fig. 4) we developed. This framework brings to the gaming experience systematically authored social comments selected based on the semantics of the game. Since the architecture is game-independent, it enables a developer to create new social games for any robot or virtual agent. Please note that the gaze behaviors in the study were not generated by this framework. However, the study system supported BML-like markups for adding non-verbal behaviors which could be included in the commenting strings.

A High Level Tour of the Framework. The starting point is the *Legal Move Generator* which generates all the possible moves on every agent's turn. Then, the *Move Annotator* annotates the generated moves with a set of pre-defined annotations that have numeric and boolean values, such as *move strength* (how much a specific move will help the player win) and *novelty* or *bluffing*. If scenarios are used (see Sec. 4.2), the annotated moves will be first filtered by the *Scenario Filter* and then the move with the highest *move strength* will be chosen by the *Move Chooser* to be played by the agent. After each played move, one of the two players will randomly be selected to make a social comment, to which the other player can respond. User's commenting and responding options are presented as menus on the screen (see Fig. 2). In order to avoid overwhelming the user, on 25% of the moves, unless the move is significant (e.g., a double jump in checkers) or the game is in a significant state (e.g., win or lose), no comments are made. The *Comment Chooser* chooses a comment from the *Comment Library* based on the latest played move along with the *Game Logic State* (and the *Current Scenario*, if scenarios are used).

An author of a new game using this framework only has to implement the game-specific components in the architecture (gray boxes in Fig. 4) and optionally add extra generic or game-specific comments (and scenarios) to the libraries.

4.1 Commenting System

A main purpose of the framework is to generate social comments based on the semantics of the gameplay. This process involves the *Comment Library* and the *Comment Chooser*, which are explained below.

Comment Library. The *Comment Library* contains social comments authored in XML format (see Fig. 5). Each comment includes a set of attributes. Comment attributes are used to determine the best situation in which to use the comment. These attributes have boolean, numerical and string values. Examples include *competitiveness, regret, compliment, offensive* and *brag*. The *gameName* attribute restricts a comment to a specific game; the *gameType* attribute restricts a comment to a specific type of game such as *card* or *board*.

Comment Chooser. This component chooses an agent comment or choices for the user comment menu, in response to the most recent game move or comment. For commenting on a move, an algorithm finds the best matches for the current stage of the game out of all the comment library items using the annotations of the move and the game logic state (as well as the current scenario, in case scenarios are used). These comments must have the maximum similarity in their

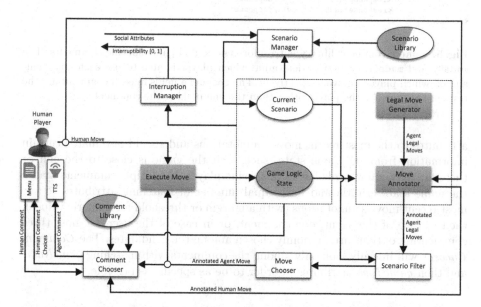

Fig. 4. Framework Architecture. Gray boxes indicate game-specific components while others are generic. Libraries have both generic and game-specific entries.

```
<comment competitiveness='0.2' tags="askHand" gameType="card" madeBy="agent"
    madeOn="agentMove">
                <content>How is your hand?</content>
                <response>Good!</response>
                <response>Not gonna tell you!</response>
                <response>Terrible</response>
</comment>
<comment competitiveness='0.3' tags="agentFewCardsLeft" gameType="card" madeBy="human"
    madeOn="agentMove">
                <content>Oh you got only a few cards left!</content>
                <response>Do not worry, too soon to tell</response>
                <response>Haha, I am gonna win</response>
</comment>
<comment competitiveness='0.8' tags="agentMeld/brag" gameName="rummy" madeBy="agent"
    madeOn="agentMove">
                <content>And that's how you make a meld!</content>
                <response>Well, wait for mine!</response>
                <response>Yes that was nice!</response>
</comment>
<comment competitiveness='0.7' tags="humanMultipleCapture" gameName="checkers" madeBy="human"
    madeOn="humanMove">
                <content>Wow! I seem to love jumping!</content>
                <response>Yea, you got me there!</response>
                <response>Oh Come on!</response>
                <response>Nice set of moves</response>
</comment>
<comment moveStrength='0.7' competitiveness='0.1' tags="humanMultipleCapture"
    gameType="generic" madeBy="agent" madeOn="humanMove">
                <content>I should say, you do play very well!</content>
                <response>Well, try to learn!</response>
                <response>Thank you, you do too</response>
</comment>
<comment competitiveness='0.6' tags="longTimeNoMeldByHuman" gameName="rummy"
    madeBy="agent" madeOn="humanMove">
                <content>You realize you have not made a meld in ages, haha!</content>
                <response>Wait for it!</response>
                <response>Yeah, I know!</response>
</comment>
```

Fig. 5. Sample comment library entries for generic and game specific comments. The madeBy and madeOn properties determine which player is able to use each comment, and on which player's move, respectively. The **response** fields in each comment are the response options for the player other than the one making the comment.

attributes to the most recent move's annotations and should also match certain information from the game state, such as if the game is close to the end or there are only a few cards left for a specific player. If multiple comments match the game state criteria and have equal number of matching attributes to the most recent move's annotations (with a margin or threshold for numeric values), then in case of the agent, one comment, or in case of the user, at most three commenting options are randomly chosen among the candidates. The *Comment Chooser* will initially look only among the comments with matching *gameName* and then *gameType* attributes in order to be as specific as possible.

4.2   Scenarios and Interruptibility

This section describes two mechanisms in the framework that were not utilized in our study, but we think may be useful in other applications that include longer-term use of our system.

Scenarios introduce the capability to not only control the verbal interaction in the game, but to also change the agent's gaming strategies in order to increase its sociability. A scenario includes a plan for choosing moves with specific kinds of annotations at different stages of its progress. Thus, the agent can, for example, start the game strongly or weakly to control the suspense. Scenarios can also generate attributes for the *Comment Chooser* to enforce a desired kind of comment that fits the scenario. For example, the agent can follow a *Self-Deprecating Humor* scenario in which it starts the game strongly and then loses on purpose after generating comments with the *bragging* attribute to create a humorous experience for the user or to boost the confidence in a novice player.

In Fig. 4 the *Current Scenario* is selected by the *Scenario Manager* from the *Scenario Library* at the the start of every session. This selection is made based on a set of *Social Attributes* that are imported from outside of the framework. Thus scenarios can be used to achieve social goals in gameplay.

Interruptibility is continuously reported as a numeric value in $[0, 1]$, where a higher value is an indication of the current moment being more appropriate for pausing the game, and, for example, initiating social chit-chat on topics other than game matters (generating such chit-chat is not part of this framework). For instance, when there is nothing significant about the current game state, this value is closer to 1, whereas if a player is about to win, it is closer to 0.

5   Conclusions and Future Work

Our results suggest that there is a great potential in bringing sociability to the gaming interactions of virtual agents and robots, and that we can do so in a systematic way, based on the semantics of the game. We observed that this sociability significantly improved the gaming experience for users and also caused the agent to be perceived as more intelligent.

This work offers two main contributions. First, we designed and developed a generic software framework which aims at enabling many virtual agents and robots to play games socially in the future through making deeply relevant social comments based on the game state and events. Second, in order to apply and evaluate our framework, we conducted a user study, during which we observed both subjective and objective measures of the effects of social gaze and comments. The gaming interactions proved to be significantly more social, human-like, intelligent, enjoyable and adoptable when social behaviors were employed. Moreover, the participants showed increased alliance [20] with a social gaming opponent. Furthermore, since facial expressions can be a strong indication of internal state, we measured the number of participants' smiles during the gameplay and observed that the participants smile significantly more when social behaviors were involved than when they were not.

A main limitation of our work may be the type of games used. Some more social but highly verbal games, such as charades, are perhaps beyond this approach. However, more complex games than rummy and checkers, such as Risk or Monopoly, would be worthwhile exploring in this framework.

It would also be valuable to explore if the scenarios and interruptibility in our framework (see Sec. 4.2) can influence gaming interactions and especially users' perception of the agent's sociability and intelligence.

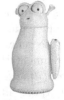

Fig. 6. Reeti

Another interesting future direction for this work is to use emotion modeling techniques (as in [2]) for generating our social comments, so that they are able to make use of the relation between different emotional states of the users and emotional expressions of the agent, in the presence of varying gaming events. This direction will be able to take good advantage of the scenario functionality of our framework (see Sec. 4.2).

Moreover, detecting and analyzing other facial expressions than smile could be worth investigating. Furthermore, this work could be expanded for games involving more players, including one or more agents. Lastly, using an expressive robot (e.g., Reeti in Fig. 6) could lead to new opportunities.

Acknowledgments. This work is supported in part by the National Science Foundation under award IIS-1012083. Any opinions, findings, and conclusions or recommendations expressed in this material are those of the authors and do not necessarily reflect the views of the National Science Foundation. Thanks to Prof. Tim Bickmore of Northeastern University for allowing us to use their virtual agent Karen in our user study. Also, thanks to Prof. Jeanine Skorinko of Worcester Polytechnic Institute for their help in recruiting participants.

References

1. Leite, I., Martinho, C., Pereira, A., Paiva, A.: iCat: an affective game buddy based on anticipatory mechanisms. In: Proc. of the 7th Int. Joint Conf. on Autonomous Agents and Multiagent Systems, pp. 1229–1232 (2008)
2. Leite, I., Pereira, A., Martinho, C., Paiva, A.: Are emotional robots more fun to play with? In: The 17th IEEE Int. Symposium on Robot and Human Interactive Communication, pp. 77–82. IEEE (2008)
3. Castellano, G., Leite, I., Pereira, A., Martinho, C., Paiva, A., McOwan, P.W.: It's all in the game: Towards an affect sensitive and context aware game companion. In: 3rd Int. Conf. on Affective Computing and Intelligent Interaction, pp. 1–8. IEEE (2009)
4. Dias, J., Mascarenhas, S., Paiva, A.: Fatima modular: Towards an agent architecture with a generic appraisal framework. In: Proc. of the Int. Workshop on Standards for Emotion Modeling (2011)
5. Paiva, A., Dias, J., Sobral, D., Aylett, R., Woods, S., Hall, L., Zoll, C.: Learning by feeling: Evoking empathy with synthetic characters. Applied Artificial Intelligence 19(3-4), 235–266 (2005)
6. Aylett, R., Vannini, N., Andre, E., Paiva, A., Enz, S., Hall, L.: But that was in another country: agents and intercultural empathy. In: Proc. of the 8th Int. Conf. on Autonomous Agents and Multiagent Systems, vol. 1, pp. 329–336 (2009)

7. McCoy, J., Treanor, M., Samuel, B., Mateas, M., Wardrip-Fruin, N.: Prom week: Social physics as gameplay. In: Proc. of the 6th Int. Conf. on Foundations of Digital Games, pp. 319–321. ACM (2011)

8. Bickmore, T.W., Picard, R.W.: Establishing and maintaining long-term human-computer relationships. ACM Transactions on Computer-Human Interaction 12(2), 293–327 (2005)

9. Cañamero, L., Fredslund, J.: I show you how I like you - Can you read it in my face? IEEE Transactions on Systems, Man and Cybernetics, Part A: Systems and Humans 31(5), 454–459 (2001)

10. Ogata, T., Sugano, S.: Emotional communication robot: Wamoeba-2r emotion model and evaluation experiments. In: Proc. of the Int. Conf. on Humanoid Robots (2000)

11. Gonzalez-Pacheco, V., Ramey, A., Alonso-Martin, F., Castro-Gonzalez, A., Salichs, M.A.: Maggie: A social robot as a gaming platform. Int. Journal of Social Robotics 3(4), 371–381 (2011)

12. Van Eck, R., Global, I.: Gaming and cognition: Theories and practice from the learning sciences. Information Science Reference (2010)

13. Fong, T., Nourbakhsh, I., Dautenhahn, K.: A survey of socially interactive robots. Robotics and Autonomous Systems 42(3), 143–166 (2003)

14. Kozima, H., Michalowski, M.P., Nakagawa, C.: Keepon. Int. Journal of Social Robotics 1(1), 3–18 (2009)

15. Shibata, T.: Importance of physical interaction between human and robot for therapy. In: Stephanidis, C. (ed.) Universal Access in HCI, Part IV, HCII 2011. LNCS, vol. 6768, pp. 437–447. Springer, Heidelberg (2011)

16. Lee, M.K., Forlizzi, J., Rybski, P.E., Crabbe, F., Chung, W., Finkle, J., Glaser, E., Kiesler, S.: The Snackbot: Documenting the design of a robot for long-term human-robot interaction. In: Int. Conf. on Human-Robot Interaction, pp. 7–14. IEEE (2009)

17. Steels, L., Kaplan, F.: Aibo's first words: The social learning of language and meaning. Evolution of Communication 4(1), 3–32 (2002)

18. Ruf, T., et al.: Face detection with the sophisticated high-speed object recognition engine (SHORE). In: Microelectronic Systems, pp. 243–252. Springer (2011)

19. Küblbeck, C., Ernst, A.: Face detection and tracking in video sequences using the modifiedcensus transformation. Image and Vision Computing 24(6), 564–572 (2006)

20. Horvath, A.O., Greenberg, L.S.: Development and validation of the working alliance inventory. Journal of Counseling Psychology 36(2), 223–233 (1989)

Effects of Coupling in Human-Virtual Agent Body Interaction

Elisabetta Bevacqua, Igor Stanković, Ayoub Maatallaoui,
Alexis Nédélec, and Pierre De Loor

UEB, Lab-STICC, ENIB, France
{bevacqua,stankovic,maatallaoui,nedelec,deloor}@enib.fr

Abstract. This paper presents a study of the dynamic coupling between a user and a virtual character during body interaction. Coupling is directly linked with other dimensions, such as co-presence, engagement, and believability, and was measured in an experiment that allowed users to describe their subjective feelings about those dimensions of interest. The experiment was based on a theatrical game involving the imitation of slow upper-body movements and the proposal of new movements by the user and virtual agent. The agent's behaviour varied in autonomy: the agent could limit itself to imitating the user's movements only, initiate new movements, or combine both behaviours. After the game, each participant completed a questionnaire regarding their engagement in the interaction, their subjective feeling about the co-presence of the agent, etc. Based on four main dimensions of interest, we tested several hypotheses against our experimental results, which are discussed here.

Keywords: Human-virtual agent interaction, coupling, co-presence and engagement measurement, experimental study.

1 Introduction

Coupling [1] is the continuous mutual influence between two individuals, and has a dynamic specific to the dyad. It possesses the capability to resist disturbance, and compensates by evolving the interaction. Disturbances come from both the environment and from within the individuals, depending on how they perceive the interaction. This definition is recursive since coupling exists because of the human effort to "recover" it as its quality decreases; this is why it is highly complex to reproduce when employing virtual agents. Coupling between two persons implies an *evolving equilibrium* between regularity and surprise, and it is a fundamental key to establish an interaction. Our assumption is that coupling and sense-making are tightly linked to a subjective feeling of several dimensions of interaction. In this paper we focus on co-presence, believability, and engagement as these are important dimensions frequently addressed by the virtual character community.

Many studies in the field of human-agent interaction have tried to develop believable, co-present, and/or engaging agents. If presence is addressed in virtual reality as the feeling of "being there" [2], co-presence is the feeling of "being

T. Bickmore et al. (Eds.): IVA 2014, LNAI 8637, pp. 54–63, 2014.

with" [3]. Believability is how an object or character fits a user's model, and engagement is a measure for being "into the game". The improvement of these subjective feelings must address two problems. The first is the multi-dimensionality of the interaction. Emotional feedback, expressed through facial expressions, is just one of the cues that helps agents build a better rapport with humans [4]. Also, back-channels are considered "the most accessible example of the real-time responsiveness that underpins many successful interpersonal interactions", and expressive feedback, such as a nod or an "a-ha" (which literally means "I am listening, tell me more"), given at the right moment, heightens the degree of convergence [5]. In addition, synchrony is also an important parameter in human-agent coupling [6]. The second problem is the difficulty of defining and evaluating the subjective feelings of users. There is much debate on the link between feeling, in the sense of "What is it like?", and physiological responses [7]. The debate about the notion of presence is well known [8]. Some researchers argue that co-presence is primarily subjective, so they try to define a "good" subjective questionnaire [9], while others stress that only physiological measures can provide progress on the understanding of presence [10]. It is also possible to find objective measures for believability [11], or to use subjective evaluation techniques [12], while engagement can be evaluated by feeling (e.g. of pleasure, or control), or through objective measures in terms of time before fatigue [13].

To study the links between coupling and the three dimensions (believability, co-presence, and engagement), we propose a body interaction experiment that allows us to vary the coupling between a human and a virtual character. We aim at improving the interaction experience by gathering insights into the principles necessary for implementing virtual characters. Additionally, the experiment could help us to better understand how "subjective feeling" should be evaluated.

Details on the experiment, its variations (the different condition scenarios), and tested hypotheses are given in Sect. 2, while Sect. 3 explains the methods utilized. Section 4 presents several result sets, which are discussed in Sect. 5. Conclusions are drawn in the final section (Sect. 6).

2   Experiment

An evaluation test was used to assess the dynamic coupling between a human user and virtual agent. In a theatrical exercise, two players facing each other imitated the other person's upper-body movements but introduced subtle changes by proposing, from time to time, new movements. This dyadic imitation game causes dynamic notions of coupling and interaction to emerge naturally from both players. Regularity (through the imitation of the other subject) and surprise (seen in the new movements) are intrinsic to the exercise, and are perfectly balanced. This game meets our needs perfectly, and the participants were asked to play it with a virtual agent.

Our system uses a motion capture device (Microsoft Kinect) to collect positional information about the user's body. Captured coordinates are passed through a simple averaging filter to reduce noise, and then sent onto a synthesis module built in Unity3D. It uses the body coordinates and inverse kinematics to make the virtual agent strictly imitate/follow the user's movements. A Wizard of Oz (WOZ) technique allows an agent to create new movements during the interaction. The WOZ, managed by one of the evaluators through keyboard controls, can change the agent's hands directions. No blending issues between old and new movements were perceivable since changes were quite slow. When the WOZ is disabled, the agent will again start strictly following the user's movements. To study only body movements and for artistic reasons, one of Joan Miró's colourful paintings involving a devil-like minimalist character made of black segments, was utilized as the agent (see Fig. 1). Participants interacted with the agent by utilizing one of three scenario conditions:

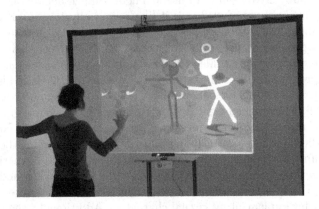

Fig. 1. Scene installation: When the user is detected, the devil-like character "jumps out" of the painting leaving a white empty shape, and the interaction starts

- 1st *condition (C1):* the agent's behaviour was a pure imitation of the user's.
- 2nd *condition (C2):* the agent's behaviour was partially driven by the WOZ.
- 3rd *condition (C3):* the agent's movements were controlled by a previously recorded motion capture file of another person playing the game.

The agent imitates the user's movement in cases C1 and C2 with a slight delay. Without such a delay, the agent almost instantly imitates the user's behaviour, which does not seem natural to the human participant, and makes the agent seem too obviously computer-driven. Pretests showed that employing a half second delay is a good solution to this problem.

Prior to our experiment, we formulated several hypotheses involving four dimensions of interest (coupling, co-presence, engagement, and believability) that will be measured through a questionnaire:

Hypothesis 1. The four dimensions would be most prominent in condition C2 rather than in C1 or C3. Also, since the agent does not react to human behaviour in C3, no connection would develop between the subject and the agent. This suggests that higher results would be expected in C1 than in C3.

Hypothesis 2. Level of engagement, sense of co-presence, and believability are due to a subtle equilibrium between surprise and regularity during an interaction. In other words, co-presence, engagement, and believability are connected to the level of coupling.

Hypothesis 3. Engagement and a feeling of co-presence are linked. Perceiving the co-presence of the agent makes the game more fun, and so more engaging.

3 Method

The experiment was conducted at a school during an exhibition about the links between art and science. We decided on an independent-measures design: each subject participated in just one condition scenario (C1, C2, or C3). Data from forty-one French-speaking subjects (20% women, 80% men) was collected: thirteen subjects, age from 18 to 30 (*Median* = 21), participated in C1; fifteen, age from 15 to 42 (*Median* = 21), participated in C2; thirteen participants, age from 19 to 46 (*Median* = 20), interacted with the agent under condition C3.

The exercise was explained to the subjects and they were invited to play the game with one of the evaluators. This introduction encouraged the participants to feel the type of connections that could occur in the game. The subjects did not know which condition they were playing, and to measure their level of engagement, no time limit was imposed. At the end of the interaction, each participant filled in a questionnaire (see Table 1) to judge their experience and the agent's behaviour.

Table 1. The sixteen statements in our questionnaire

Dimension	Question
Coupling	**q1.** I had the impression that the agent was proposing new movements.
	q2. I had the impression that the agent was following my movements.
	q3. I had the feeling that the agent's behaviour was connected to mine.
	q4. The agent did not take my movements into account.
	q5. I was able to make the agent follow me.
	q6. I was surprised by the agent's behaviour.
Co-presence	**q7.** I had the impression that I was in the presence of another being.
	q8. I had the feeling that the agent was aware of my presence.
	q9. I perceived the agent as a simple computer program.
	q10. The agent seemed aware of its own behaviour.
Engagement	**q11.** I enjoyed playing with the agent.
	q12. I had the feeling that I was really playing with the agent.
	q13. Playing the game with the agent was easy.
Believability	**q14.** The agent's behaviour made me think of human behaviour.
	q15. I don't think that the agent was behaving like a real person.
	q16. I had the impression that the agent was controlled by a human.

The questionnaire contained sixteen statements (each used a 6-point Likert scale: 1 = disagree strongly; 6 = agree strongly) grouped according to the four dimensions we have retained. Six of them are based on the definition of coupling presented in [1] and then they are related to the feeling of regularities and surprises during the interaction. Our evaluation of co-presence drew inspiration from a questionnaire proposed in [3]. Level of engagement was evaluated according to how enjoyable the agent interaction was for the participant, the ease of the interaction, and whether the user felt involved in the game. We also recorded the length of each interaction with the aim of collecting additional information on the users' engagement since more engaging interactions last longer. To assess the perceived believability of the agent's behaviour, the questionnaire addressed the closeness of the agent's behaviour to human actions.

4   Results

Each questionnaire was analysed by evaluating each statement within the context of the three condition scenarios (C1, C2, and C3). We compared the answers to each question pairwise, by considering each pair of different conditions. For this we utilized the Wilcoxon test, a non-parametric equivalent of the t-test. All our hypothesis analyses were one-tailed because the direction of each expected difference was specified. The results were significant for several of the statements, particularly for those that evaluated the feeling of coupling. Subjects easily recognized that the agent suggested fewer new movements ($q1$) in condition C1 than in C2 ($p < .01$) or C3 ($p < .01$), and less in C2 than in C3 ($p < .01$). They also noticed when the agent was following the user more closely ($q2$) in condition C1 rather than in C3 ($p < .01$), and more in C2 than in C3 ($p < .01$). Participants felt a stronger connection between their behaviour and the agent's ($q3$) in C1 than in C3 ($p < .01$), and in C2 rather than in C3 ($p < .01$). In $q4$ (question 4), the agent was judged as taking the subject's behaviour more into account in condition C1 than in C3 ($p < .01$), and more in C2 more than in C3 ($p < .01$). The subjects were more surprised by the agent's behaviour ($q6$) in C3 than in C1 ($p < .05$).

These results show that we did not find many significant differences between conditions C1 and C2. This is not surprising, particularly for those questions that asked the subjects if they felt that the agent was following them ($q2$ and $q5$), or if they felt a connection with the agent ($q3$), or if the agent was taking their movements into account ($q4$), since the agent imitates the subjects in both conditions. However, the agent imitates less in condition C2, and people do tend to feel it, as shown in the box plots diagrams in Fig. 2. The diagrams of $q2$ and $q5$ shows that the subjects were more aware of the agent imitation in condition C1 than in C2. The diagram for $q4$ shows that people tend to believe that the agent takes their movements into account less in condition C2 than in C1. The agent seems a little more surprising in C2 than in C1, as shown by the box plot diagram of $q6$. The diagram for $q3$ indicates that people feel slightly less connected to the agent in condition C2 than in C1. It is more surprising that the subjects also feel quite connected to the agent in condition C3 (even though there is a significant difference between the other two conditions). Perhaps this condition scenario forces people to try harder to play (since the agent doesn't interact at all), and the increased effort causes the players to imagine a connection that isn't there.

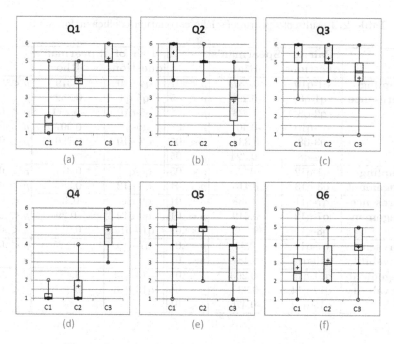

Fig. 2. Box plot diagrams of the coupling questions

None of the questions regarding agent believability produced significant results, and the questions regarding co-presence contained almost no significant results. Participants felt that the agent was aware of its own behaviour ($q10$) more in condition C3 than in C1 ($p < .01$) and C2 ($p < .05$), and more in C2 than in C1 ($p < .05$). No significant results were obtained for the feeling of engagement, except in question 12, where the subjects had the impression of playing with the agent more in condition C3 than in C1 ($p < .01$).

Co-presence and engagement are very hard to evaluate solely through a questionnaire, although we did hope to find that a feeling of co-presence and engagement are linked to the level of coupling between the human and the virtual agent. Consequently, we built a correlation matrix between all the questions (disregarding the condition) by utilizing Spearman's Rho correlation coefficient. The two-tailed significance level of the correlation was measured to determine if it was significantly different from a zero-correlation in the positive or negative directions. Indeed, some of the questions were correlated (see Table 2). We also checked for a correlation between the questions and interaction duration, but only a weak result (Rho=0.268, $p < .05$) was obtained for question 12. It seems that the subjects interacted longer when they had a stronger impression of "playing" with the agent. Even without significant results for the agent's believability, correlations were detected between the questions on co-presence and believability and the questions on engagement and believability.

Table 2. Results of Spearman's Rho correlation coefficient for N=41

	Pair of questions	Spearman's Rho		Pair of questions	Spearman's Rho	
coupling-	q1-q10	0.757	$p < .01$	q4-q10	0.319	$p < .05$
co-presence	q1-q8	-0.296	$p < .05$	q5-q8	0.352	$p < .05$
	q2-q8	0.428	$p < .01$	q5-q10	-0.299	$p < .05$
	q2-q10	-0.407	$p < .01$	q6-q7	0.507	$p < .01$
	q3-q8	0.334	$p < .05$	q6-q10	0.306	$p < .05$
	q4-q8	-0.324	$p < .05$			
coupling-	q1-q12	0.35	$p < .05$	q6-q11	0.311	$p < .05$
engagement	q3-q13	0.415	$p < .01$	q6-q12	0.383	$p < .01$
co-presence-	q7-q11	0.438	$p < .01$	q9-q11	-0.408	$p < .01$
engagement	q7-q12	0.619	$p < .01$	q9-q12	-0.29	$p < .05$
	q8-q11	0.283	$p < .05$	q10-q12	0.312	$p < .05$
co-presence-	q7-q14	0.33	$p < .05$	q7-q15	-0.375	$p < .01$
believability	q10-q14	0.481	$p < .01$			
engagement-	q11-q15	-0.263	$p < .05$	q13-q14	0.475	$p < .01$
believability	q12-q14	0.323	$p < .05$	q13-q16	0.367	$p < .05$
	q15-q12	-0.475	$p < .01$			

5 Discussion

As for the first hypothesis, the experimental setup clearly allows coupling to emerge, and C2 gives the users the best feeling of coupling. Another property of C2 is its balance between surprise and regularity. For instance, *q6* shows that C2 encourages more surprise than C1 and less than C3 (where the agent's behaviour is unconnected to the human's). Similarly, *q1* shows that C2's behaviour is felt to lie somewhere between that of a passive agent (C1) and a directed agent (C3). A consideration of the questions concerning believability, co-presence, and engagement shows that C2 represents a balance between low and high autonomous behaviours (*q10*). No other significant results concerning the discriminatory role of C2 were found, for which there are two possible explanations: 1.) feelings like co-presence and engagement are difficult to assess solely with a questionnaire, and 2.) some questions are victims of alternative interpretations, or were inadequate for discriminating our types of interaction. The second case was particularly true for the statements involving believability. All of our condition scenarios present agent behaviour intrinsically similar to that of a real human: the agent is solely driven by the user in C1, the agent partly reproduces the behaviour of the user in C2, and the agent plays back a behaviour generated by another human in condition C3. When considered this way, users can judge all the agent's behaviours to be human-like.

Condition C3 produced an interesting result. We did not expect any connection to be established between the subject and the agent, so initially thought that C1 and C2 would generate stronger engagements. However, $q12$'s results show that users believe they are playing with the agent more in C3 than in C1. It appears that when a subject is imitating the agent, they also believe that they are playing the game together, and so feel an increased connection. The subjects seem to actively *look for* this connection since it is the goal of the exercise. This indicates how a goal's role in this type of study can have a strong impact on the users' sense of engagement. There is a real difficulty in finding a balance between the fact that the subject must do something with the virtual character to induce coupling and how the user can become so focused on their role that the precise behaviour of the agent becomes less important. To test our last two hypotheses, we looked at the correlation between questions (independent of the experimental conditions). We examined the subjective links between human feelings, which are not necessarily related to the objective behaviour of the virtual character. Most of the questions about coupling correlate with one or more questions about co-presence (Table 2). From the user's point of view, the agent seems to be aware of the subjects' presence when it takes their movements into account and follows them, and this regularity is what people expect. Subjects feel the agent's presence strongly when its behaviour surprises them, so a balance between regularity and surprise increases a sense of co-presence. Even if people cannot objectively define what condition makes the feeling of co-presence stronger, they can subjectively feel that such a feeling has increased when coupling emerges. This confirms part of our second hypothesis. The other part, concerning the link between coupling and engagement, is harder to sustain since the only relevant correlations are between $q11$ and $q6$, and between $q12$ and $q6$. Clearly, surprise triggered by an agent's behaviour has an effect on a user's engagement because it increases the game's enjoyment, and heightens the impression of playing with the agent. This result may not be enough on its own to show a link between coupling and engagement, but it connects engagement with surprise as a component of coupling.

Table 2 shows several correlations between questions about co-presence and those on engagement. When a subject enjoys playing with the agent, they feel more involved in the game, feel the agent's presence, and form an impression that the agent is perceiving them. As a consequence, the agent is not seen as a simple computer program. Although there is a clear link between the feeling of co-presence and engagement, the subjects do not find it easy to judge which condition scenario provokes a stronger sense of co-presence and engagement, but they do subjectively connect these two dimensions. Our hypotheses did not consider how the feelings of co-presence and engagement can influence the believability of agent behaviour, but a strong correlation between questions on co-presence and engagement, and questions on co-presence and believability was found (see Table 2). When users feel the agent's presence, or enjoy playing with it, they also judge its behaviour to be more human-like.

These correlations stress the link between subjective feelings and objective conditions. For example, C2 and C3 are objectively different, but no statistical difference was found between them regarding the feeling of co-presence. However, there are correlations between the feeling of co-presence and the feeling of coupling. This can be explained by how a person will construct a feeling of coupling with an agent even when such a connection does not really exist (see Fig. 2.c). For instance, the agent in C3 is constantly proposing new movements, but because the participants knows that the goal of the game is to imitate and be imitated, they try to create a (fake) coupling. They feel coupling because they want to, and once they think they are coupled with the agent, they also begin to feel its presence. To confirm this notion, we checked the correlations between coupling and co-presence in C3 and several interesting results were revealed. For example, $q8$ ("I had the feeling that the agent was aware of my presence") correlates with almost all the questions on coupling: $q1$ (Rho=-0.541, $p < .05$), $q2$ (Rho=0.765, $p < .01$), $q4$ (Rho=-0.74, $p < .01$), and $q5$ (Rho=0.815, $p < .01$), for N=13; $q9$ and $q4$ also correlate (Rho=0.618, $p < .05$), indicating that the agent is perceived as less like a simple computer program when it takes the user's movements into account. The correlation between co-presence and coupling, which was found independent of the game condition, indicates that there is a "hidden" correlation phenomena at work. Perhaps there are two types of user: those who try to "play the game" by introducing a coupling, and so feel coupling and co-presence by the end of the experiment, and those users who do not "play the game" and so are denied those feelings.

6 Conclusions

We have presented a study on human-virtual agent body interaction with four dimensions investigated: coupling, co-presence, engagement, and believability. Our results show that coupling is easily recognized by the participants, but the other three dimensions are harder to assess solely through a questionnaire. However, result correlations were found between coupling and co-presence, and between coupling and engagement. It seems that people do feel a sense of co-presence and heightened involvement when they feel coupled with the agent. There is a link between co-presence and coupling for subjects who make an effort to create coupling. This desire for interaction provokes a fake feeling of coupling which improves the feeling of co-presence. There may be an objective measure of this "coupling willingness", developing such a measure presents our next challenge.

Our results suggest that cognitive architectures must include coupling capabilities, as in [6], in agents intended to engender a strong sense of co-presence and engagement with users. As our work shows, when these two dimensional values are increased, then so does the believability of the agent behaviour. We also introduced the importance of interaction willingness and we propose a link between action and co-presence.

Acknowledgement. This work was funded by the ANR INGREDIBLE project: ANR-12-CORD-001 (http://www.ingredible.fr).

References

1. De Loor, P., Bevacqua, E., Stanković, I., Maatallaoui, A., Nédélec, A., Buche, C.: Utilisation de la notion de couplage pour la modélisation d'agents virtuels interactifs socialement présents. In: Pevedic, B.L., Jost, C. (eds.) Actes de la deuxième conférence Intercompréhension de l'intraspécifique à l'interspécifique. Oxford University Press, Guidel (to appear, 2014)
2. Heeter, C.: Being There: The subjective experience of presence. Teleoperators and Virtual Environments (1992)
3. Bailenson, J.N., Guadagno, R.E., Aharoni, E., Dimov, A., Beall, A.C., Blascovich, J.: Comparing behavioral and self-report measures of embodied agents: Social presence in immersive virtual environments. In: Proceedings of the 7th Annual International Workshop on PRESENCE (2004)
4. Wong, J.W.E., McGee, K.: Frown More, Talk More: Effects of Facial Expressions in Establishing Conversational Rapport with Virtual Agents. In: Nakano, Y., Neff, M., Paiva, A., Walker, M. (eds.) IVA 2012. LNCS, vol. 7502, pp. 419–425. Springer, Heidelberg (2012)
5. Traum, D., DeVault, D., Lee, J., Wang, Z., Marsella, S.: Incremental Dialogue Understanding and Feedback for Multiparty, Multimodal Conversation. In: Nakano, Y., Neff, M., Paiva, A., Walker, M. (eds.) IVA 2012. LNCS, vol. 7502, pp. 275–288. Springer, Heidelberg (2012)
6. Prepin, K., Pelachaud, C.: Basics of Intersubjectivity Dynamics: Model of Synchrony Emergence When Dialogue Partners Understand Each Other. Agents and Artificial Intelligence 271, 302–318 (2013)
7. Insko, B.: Measuring presence: Subjective, behavioral and physiological methods. Emerging Communication (2003)
8. Schuemie, M., van der Straaten, P., Krijn, M., van der Mast, C.: Research on Presence in Virtual Reality: a Survey. CyberPsychology and Behavior 4(2), 183–201 (2001)
9. Witmer, B., Singer, M.: Measuring presence in virtual environments: A presence questionnaire. Presence 7(3), 225–240 (1998)
10. Slater, M.: How colorful was your day? Why questionnaires cannot assess presence in virtual environments. Presence: Teleoperators and Virtual Environments 13(4), 484–493 (2004)
11. Riedl, M.O., Young, R.M.: An objective character believability evaluation procedure for multi-agent story generation systems. In: Panayiotopoulos, T., Gratch, J., Aylett, R.S., Ballin, D., Olivier, P., Rist, T. (eds.) IVA 2005. LNCS (LNAI), vol. 3661, pp. 278–291. Springer, Heidelberg (2005)
12. Hingston, P. (ed.): Believable Bots: Can Computers Play Like People? Springer (2012)
13. O'Brien, H., Toms, E.: What is user engagement? A conceptual framework for defining user engagement with technology. American Society for Information Science & Technology 59, 938–955 (2008)

Improving Motion Classifier Robustness by Estimating Output Confidence

Durell Bouchard

Roanoke College, Salem VA 24153, USA

1 Introduction

Embodied conversational agents that can sense and respond to multiple modalities of user communication, like speech, gesture, and facial expressions, create a better impression and facilitate communication [1,2]. Responding to a user's gestures entails classifying the content and quality of each gesture, but classification performance is dependent on the selection of input sequence boundaries. Small changes in the boundaries of an input sequence can have a large effect on classifier output. Failing to correctly classify a user's gestures may cause an agent to respond incorrectly, which can negatively impact the agent's ability to communicate.

Motion classifiers must be robust to changes in input boundaries to create effective conversational agents. This poster outlines a method of modifying any learning based motion classifier to estimate the confidence of the classifier's output. The method calculates confidence by using multiple classifiers that are sensitive to different input sequence boundaries. Preliminary results show that the classification rate of a motion classifier improves by selecting input sequences with highest confidence estimation.

2 Model

The error rate of a motion classifier is dependent on the location of the input motion sequence's boundaries. A shift of a single frame in either the start or end boundary of an input motion sequence can have a negative impact on the classifier's error rate.

The effect of input sequence boundary shift on a motion classifier's error rate is a result of the selection of the boundaries of the training motion sequences. For example, if two identical classifiers are trained with the same motion sequences, except the start boundary of every training sequence is shifted by one frame forward or backward, then one classifier will have a lower classification error rate. If, however, the boundaries of input motion sequences are shifted the same way as the boundaries of the training motion sequences, then the output of the two classifiers is similar.

The similarity between two classifiers trained with the same motion sequences, but with different boundaries, can be used to estimate the confidence of a motion classifier. The less similar the outputs of the two classifiers are, the less likely it

T. Bickmore et al. (Eds.): IVA 2014, LNAI 8637, pp. 64–66, 2014.

Table 1. Classifier Error Rates

(a) Static Boundary		(b) Variable Boundary	
Training	Testing	Training	Testing
0.09	0.35	0.08	0.12

is that the outputs are correct. The similarity of the two outputs is a measure of the confidence of their combined output. Furthermore, if there are more than two classifiers, trained with different permutations of boundary shift, the probability that all of the classifiers will produce the same incorrect output is low.

A compound classifier, multiple motion classifiers trained with different permutations of boundary shift, is used to search for input sequence boundaries with the highest output confidence. The confidence of the compound classifier's output, c, is the reciprocal of the average deviation of all of the sub-classifiers and is calculated as

$$c = 121/(\sum_{i=1}^{11} \sum_{j=1}^{11} |a - o_{ij}|) \tag{1}$$

where o is the output of a sub-classifier and a is the average output of all of the sub-classifiers. The compound classifier uses 121 sub-classifiers because the effect of boundary shift plateaus at 5 frames of total boundary shift and there are 121 permutations of shifting an input sequence's start and end boundaries by 5 frames or less. The average output of the classifiers with the highest confidence is the final output of the variable boundary compound classifier.

3   Preliminary Results

The variable boundary compound classifier is tested with a feed-forward neural network that uses simple kinematic features, such as average velocity and initial acceleration, to classify Laban Movement Analysis (LMA) Effort factors of motion capture data. Zacharatos et al.[3] demonstrated the ability and utility of classifying the LMA Effort factors of movements.

Table 1 summarizes the 24-fold cross validation error rates of the variable-boundary compound classifier and the static-boundary simple classifier. The 288 non-emblematic training motions represent a diversity of movements as defined by LMA. Note that the error rates of the static-boundary classifier and variable-boundary classifier are similar for the training set but are different for the testing set.

The training set error rates of the two classifiers are similar because the classifiers are sensitive to the boundaries of the training motion sequences. The testing set error rates are different because the compound variable-boundary classifier is more robust to the segment boundary shifts in sequences on which it was not trained. Note that the difference between training and testing error rates is 0.26 for the static-boundary simple classifier, but is 0.04 for the variable-boundary compound classifier.

The variable-boundary compound classifier is more robust to variability in input sequence boundary selection for an LMA neural network classifier. Future work will evaluate the impact of interacting with a conversational agent that uses a variable-boundary compound classifier. The compound classifier's confidence may also be useful in creating more sophisticated conversation agents. For example, a conversational agent should respond differently to a user who is definitely nervous than to a user who is potentially nervous. Future work should also evaluate using classifier confidence to create more nuanced conversational agents.

References

1. Cafaro, A., Vilhjálmsson, H.H., Bickmore, T., Heylen, D., Jóhannsdóttir, K.R., Valgarðsson, G.S.: First impressions: Users' judgments of virtual agents' personality and interpersonal attitude in first encounters. In: Nakano, Y., Neff, M., Paiva, A., Walker, M. (eds.) IVA 2012. LNCS, vol. 7502, pp. 67–80. Springer, Heidelberg (2012)
2. Huang, L., Morency, L.-P., Gratch, J.: Virtual rapport 2.0. In: Vilhjálmsson, H.H., Kopp, S., Marsella, S., Thórisson, K.R. (eds.) IVA 2011. LNCS, vol. 6895, pp. 68–79. Springer, Heidelberg (2011)
3. Zacharatos, H., Gatzoulis, C., Chrysanthou, Y., Aristidou, A.: Emotion recognition for exergames using laban movement analysis. In: Proceedings of Motion on Games, pp. 39–44. ACM (2013)

A Method to Evaluate Response Models

Merijn Bruijnes, Sjoerd Wapperom, Rieks op den Akker, and Dirk Heylen

Human Media Interaction, University of Twente,
P.O. Box 217, 7500 AE, Enschede, The Netherlands
m.bruijnes@utwente.nl

Abstract. We are working towards computational models of mind of virtual characters that act as suspects in interview (interrogation) training of police officers. We implemented a model that calculates the responses of the virtual suspect based on theory and observation. We evaluated it by means of our test, the "Guess who you are talking to?" test. We show that this test can contribute to building response models for believable virtual agents.

Keywords: Response Model, Evaluation, Virtual Agent.

1 Introduction

We work towards a virtual agent that can play a suspect in a serious game that can be used by police students to hone their skills in police interviewing. A virtual agent needs three main components to be able to have a meaningful interaction. The actions of the user have to be sensed and interpreted (e.g. the user says "Confess, criminal!" which is dominant and aggressive behaviour). This interpretation provides the input to a response model that provides the reasoning of the agent (e.g. the user is dominant and aggressive which makes me sad and angry). A response model should take into account the specific role that the agent plays. In this case that is a suspect with all the tactics and psychological manoeuvring that is involved. A response model based on human behaviour can be used to make the behaviour of a virtual agent more believable to humans [5]. Based on the state of the response model the agent can select the most appropriate behaviour in its repertoire (e.g. make a sad face and say "You're not nice!"). The human responds to the agent and the cycle continues.

In this paper we discuss a method to evaluate response models. We focus on the consistency with which a response model (and thus an agent using this response model) can portray a personality. We present a way to evaluate only the response model, in an abstract interaction without actual linguistic content. We report the evaluation of a suspect response model based on the work in [3].

2 Method for Evaluation of Response Models

In this Section we present our method for evaluating response models and we show the viability of this method by evaluating a response model. The response

T. Bickmore et al. (Eds.): IVA 2014, LNAI 8637, pp. 67–70, 2014.

model is based on the work in [3] where we analysed the DPIT-corpus [1] to get insight into the social behaviour of police officers and suspects in the police interview setting. We collected terms that people use to describe the interactions in the corpus. A factor analysis revealed factors that could be interpreted as relating to the theories of *interpersonal stance* [4], *face* [2], and *rapport* [6] and the meta-concepts *information* and *strategy*. Our response model can portray a persona based on settings in the response model that are based on these theories.

We want to know whether a response model can portray a persona in a recognizable and consistent way using our "Guess who you are talking to?" test. Participants interact with the response model and have to guess which of a selection of personas is portrayed by the system. In our method, we evaluate the response model in an abstract manner, without the ambiguity of specific utterances that stem from the semantics of the utterances rather than the emotional and pragmatic variables that the model is intended to account for. Evaluating a response model using utterances that have a subjective quality introduces two sources of ambiguity related to the experiment: during the creation of the utterances (e.g. by the virtual agent) and during the interpretation of the utterance (e.g. by the user). The following examples show an interaction of two utterances (1u and 2u) that are ambiguous and the 'intended' interpretation of these utterances in terms of the response model (1i and 2i):

1u Police: "Why did you hide the body?"
1i Intention of the Police in terms of the response model: "Open Question, Dominant Stance, Politeness is Direct, Indication of Guilt, ..., Case Related Frame"
2u Suspect: "None of your business!"
2i Intention: "Aggressive Stance, Short Answer, Strategy Avoiding, ..., Unfriendly"

Some utterances leave room for interpretation and the reader might interpret these sentences different from how they should be interpreted according to the writer. In our method, participants interact with a response model in an abstract manner. This means the interaction takes place in the terms of the response model: the user is his own wizard of Oz. This way there is no confusion between what a writer meant and what he wrote down, and what the participant read and what he thought the writer meant. However, this comes at a cost. The participants need to be instructed on the abstract factors that the model uses and the personas that are portrayed by the model.

The participants have at least two sessions of interactions with the response model, once with one of the personas and once with a random response generator (not based on a persona or response model). During each session they are asked to indicate with which of the personas they think they are interacting. In addition, the participants are asked how confident they are about their choice, how realistic they found the interaction, and how familiar they are with the concepts and terms used in the response model. Finally, after each session they are asked about their experiences during the interaction.

Our Response Model Tester consists of two graphical frames that users see and use during interactions with the 'suspect agent'. These frames handle all input from and output generation to the user. The input the user gives in the police frame is the police contribution to the interaction. This input is given in the terms of the response model, see example 1i above. The input is passed to the response model that calculates the suspect behaviour. This suspect behaviour is depicted in the suspect frame again in terms of the response model, see example 2i above. All response model input and output, and the participant's choices, confidence, and realism ratings are logged.

2.1 Participants and Evaluation

For our evaluation, 48 participants (42 male, mean age 24.8 with SD 3.7) volunteered to take part in the study.

Three personas were created, based on personas from the DPIT-corpus [1,3]. Each persona was introduced in a short text. Participants received elaborate explanation of the factors in the response model (e.g. stance) and the aspects of the contributions of both the police and suspect (e.g. an aggressive stance). Each factor was explained and illustrated with several examples. Participants were encouraged to ask questions if something was unclear to them. Once everything was clear, they could start playing with the response model.

2.2 Results and Discussion

A total of 39 (81.25%) participants guessed correctly with which persona they were interacting after eight interactions. Participants who were correct were (significantly: $Z = -2.001, p < 0.1$) more confident (4.41) compared to the participants who were incorrect (3.67) (rated on a 5-point Likert scale (1=strongly disagree, 5=strongly agree)). The realism rating was similar: 3.90 for correct compared to 3.89 for incorrect. In the interactions where the responses of the system were random we might expect that each of the personas would be chosen an equal number of times (33%). However, the distribution of choices for the personas was 62.5%, 20.8%, and 16.7%. The average confidence level for interactions with personas was significantly higher 4.27 (SD = 0.76) compared to 3.46 (SD = 0.77) for the random interactions ($Z = -4.2, p < 0.00$). The average level of realism for personas was significantly higher 3.90 (SD = 0.52) compared to 3.35 for random rounds (SD = 0.89) ($Z = -3.7, p = 0.001$).

After the experiment, we informally asked participants about their experiences during the experiment. People who interviewed the *random generator first* reported that they started doubting their decision on the first persona after they had interacted with the second persona. They felt more confident about choice for the second persona. They also felt the first to be more random after they had interviewed the second. They reported the second persona met their expectations of one of the three personas. Some participants struggled with the feeling that when they had chosen a persona for the random output they felt they could not pick that persona again at their second run. They felt this way because the output was different from the first and they did feel some sort of confidence about their first choice. This led to some people mistakenly choosing a different persona from the one they chose earlier. People tended to base their decision on parts of the output generated by the persona, they did not always look at all the output. They tried to rationalize 'weird random output' and actively tried to find reasons to consider it as correct and realistic. Also, we asked on which aspects of the suspect response they based their decision. Most participants based their output only on parts of the suspect response. However, the part they focussed on differed and across all participants all of the suspect response output was used.

3   Conclusion

The results of this "Guess who you are talking to" test give an indication that our response model generates responses to user actions in such a way that the user is able to recognize a persona. This gives evidence of the validity of the response model and it promises that the model can be used in the implementation of believable virtual suspect characters with various personal characteristics as we encountered in our police interview corpus.

The method of evaluation of response models gives insight into the consistency with which a response model can portray a personality. It provides hints for improvements of the response model. Investigating which aspects of the model's response participants that 'guess wrong' focus on can provide hints for improvements of the model on these aspects. It is possible to investigate how each part of the response model's response contributes to a 'correct guess' of participants by showing only some parts to different participants and comparing their 'correct guess-scores'. In addition, when comparing several settings for a persona our evaluation method can show which setting is recognized most consistently as this persona, thus showing the 'optimal settings of the persona' in the response model.

Acknowledgements. This publication was supported by the Dutch national program COMMIT.

References

1. op den Akker, R., Bruijnes, M., Peters, R., Krikke, T.: Interpersonal stance in police interviews: content analysis. Computational Linguistics in the Netherlands Journal 3, 193–216 (2013)
2. Brown, P., Levinson, S.C.: Politeness: Some universals in language usage. Cambridge University Press, Cambridge (1987)
3. Bruijnes, M., Linssen, J., op den Akker, R., Theune, M., Wapperom, S., Broekema, C., Heylen, D.: Social behaviour in police interviews: Relating data to theories. In: Conflict and Negotiation: Social Research and Machine Intelligence (2014)
4. Leary, T.: Interpersonal Diagnosis of Personality: Functional Theory and Methodology for Personality Evaluation. Ronald Press, New York (1957)
5. Steunebrink, B.R., Dastani, M., Meyer, J.J.C.: A formal model of emotion triggers: an approach for BDI agents. Synthese 185(1), 83–129 (2012)
6. Tickle-Degnen, L., Rosenthal, R.: The nature of rapport and its nonverbal correlates. Psychological Inquiry 1(4), 285–293 (1990)

When to Elicit Feedback in Dialogue: Towards a Model Based on the Information Needs of Speakers

Hendrik Buschmeier and Stefan Kopp

Sociable Agents Group – CITEC and Faculty of Technology,
Bielefeld University, Bielefeld, Germany
{hbuschme,skopp}@uni-bielefeld.de

Abstract. Communicative feedback in dialogue is an important mechanism that helps interlocutors coordinate their interaction. Listeners pro-actively provide feedback when they think that it is important for the speaker to know their mental state, and speakers pro-actively seek listener feedback when they need information on whether a listener perceived, understood or accepted their message. This paper presents first steps towards a model for enabling attentive speaker agents to determine when to elicit feedback based on continuous assessment of their information needs about a user's listening state.

Keywords: Communicative feedback, feedback elicitation, dialogue.

1 Introduction

Much work has been directed towards producing 'active listening' behaviours in virtual conversational agents. Virtual agents, however, often also come to contribute and provide information in the role of the speaker in dialogue. In previous work, we described abilities that conversational agents need in order to be 'attentive speakers' [5]. Such agents should be able to attend to and to interpret multimodal communicative feedback (short verbal/vocal expressions such as 'uh-huh,' 'okay,' etc., head gestures, facial expressions and gaze) from their users. They should then be able to make inferences, based on these feedback signals, reason about the users' listening-related mental state and to adapt their ongoing utterances to the users' specific needs. If the evidence and information is insufficient, e.g., because a user is not a very active listener and gives only limited informative feedback, attentive speaker agents should also seek user-feedback pro-actively. That is, they should elicit communicative feedback from their users whenever knowledge of a user's state of dialogue processing might be helpful to their (the agent's and the user's) 'joint project' [7].

In this paper, we propose that one factor in determining *when* to elicit feedback from users is an agent's 'information needs.' Effective communicators tailor their utterances to their addressees, and want to make sure that their message is conveyed optimally at any point in time. The assumption is that an agent has a good understanding of how a message is likely to be received by the interaction partner. At given points in the dialogue, the agent may be sufficiently certain of a user's listening-related mental state. In these cases, additional feedback by the user might not actually be informative. In other situations, however, the agent's uncertainty about a user's listening state may

T. Bickmore et al. (Eds.): IVA 2014, LNAI 8637, pp. 71–80, 2014.

not warrant well-grounded choices in language generation, or may even be completely unknown. Furthermore, when choices for strategies and mechanisms for adaptive generation are limited, the agent needs to know in which – of a number of the states it knows how to deal with – a user can most likely be found. Given that such information needs occur, eliciting feedback from the user is one strategy to ensure and achieve an effective dialogue.

We present first steps towards a model that enables virtual conversational agents to determine *when* to elicit feedback by assessing their information needs about a user's mental state when processing an utterance. After reviewing research on feedback elicitation and explaining our current approach to modelling a user's listening-related mental state in Sect. 2, we present an extension of a model that captures the temporal dynamics of this process during ongoing utterances in Sect. 3. In Sect. 4 we then discuss approaches to utilising this dynamic model to quantify an attentive speaker agent's information needs and give an example of how these needs evolve over time in a simulated dialogue situation. Finally, in Sect. 5, we discuss the proposed model and conclude this paper.

2   Background

2.1   Feedback Elicitation

An assumption commonly made in research on backchannels and communicative feedback is that listeners in dialogue produce feedback, at least partly, in response to behavioural 'elicitation cues' by their interaction partners[1]. These cues have been analysed extensively. It has been found that acoustic features [9,12,22], syntactic information [9,12], gaze [3], as well as head gestures [10] play a role in eliciting feedback responses from listeners. The mechanism used to identify feedback elicitation cues used in these studies, however, is problematic for two reasons. Firstly, only cues that were actually followed by listener feedback were analysed (i.e., only those cues to which listeners responded). Secondly, speech that preceded listener feedback signals was assumed to contain a cue (i.e., the possibility that the listener produced the feedback signal without being cued by the speaker is not allowed). Consequently, these types of analyses miss some of the cues that speakers actually produced, while categorising behaviours as a cue that were not intended as such.

These problems have been addressed by having multiple listeners respond to the same speaker behaviour in either a 'parasocial interaction' setting [11] or by creating the illusion of being in a one-on-one interaction with the speaker for more than one listener simultaneously [13]. These methods seek to remedy the first problem by increasing the range of available cues (different listeners responding to different cues). Similarly, the second problem may be remedied by clustering feedback (places in the speaker's speech that are followed by feedback signals from multiple listeners are more likely to contain a cue). Nevertheless, the form-features in feedback elicitation cues

---

[1] It should be noted that communicative feedback serves functions for listeners as well, e.g., they can signal comprehension problems early on so that speakers can address them before they get worse.

have proven informative enough to enable automatic detection of feedback elicitation cues in audiovisual data-streams and have been successfully used to model the feedback behaviour of virtual agents [17,20].

A different line of research has shown that conversational agents producing synthetic feedback elicitation cues while speaking, received feedback responses from their human interaction partners. Elicitation cues were either generated using an HMM-based speech synthesis system trained on a corpus of acted speech containing elicitation cues at interpausal unit (IPU) boundaries [15,16], or by adding prosodic and non-verbal cues to the behaviour repertoire of a virtual agent [18].

What is not proposed by either of these two approaches – nor in the literature on feedback – is a theory of *when* and *why* speakers produce feedback elicitation cues. Empirically, this is due to the problems involved in identifying elicitation cues as described above. From a theoretical point of view, cues are produced at different levels of intentionality. They can be fully intentional, e.g., when the speaker wants to know whether the listener understood what was said. They can also be produced by convention, e.g., by inviting a backchannel at the end of an IPU. Additionally, they can also occur purely coincidentally, e.g., a breathing pause by the speaker might be taken as a backchannel opportunity. In the following, we will concentrate on intentional feedback elicitation cues strategically produced by speakers with the aim of obtaining more – possibly new – information about their listeners' state of understanding (i.e., cues produced out of 'information needs'), most likely to reduce the uncertainty about the state of the dialogue.

2.2 Attributed Listener State

Another common assumption is that communicative feedback and backchannels are one and the same, and that listeners, when giving feedback, merely communicate that speakers can continue speaking. Under this assumption, it would be sufficient for feedback elicitation cue placement to be governed by simple rules. Backchannels are, however, just one type of feedback (termed a *generic* listener response by Bavelas and colleagues [2]). Feedback signals can be much richer in their form [21] and often fulfil *specific* functions [2] that go beyond the backchannel. By strategically placing feedback elicitation cues in a turn, speakers can thus use them as a way of querying information from listeners.

According to Allwood and colleagues, listeners use feedback to communicate whether they are in contact with the speaker, whether they are willing and able to perceive what the speaker is saying, or whether they are willing and able to understand the speaker's message. They also convey attitudinal reactions such as acceptance or agreement with the speaker's message [1]. As such, listeners partially reveal their mental state – the 'listener state' [5,14] – which in turn allows speakers to reason about possible communication problems and common ground, and provides a basis for repair processes and adaptation of language to the listeners' needs. Based on this listening state, we proposed earlier [5,6] that an attentive speaker agent should maintain an 'attributed listener state' (ALS) about its dialogue partners that tracks their actual listener state based on an interpretation of their feedback behaviour and the dialogue context.

This ALS is modelled probabilistically as a Bayesian network consisting of five variables C, P, U, AC, AG. These variables represent whether the speaker agent believes the listener to be in contact, and whether it believes the listener to perceive, understand, or

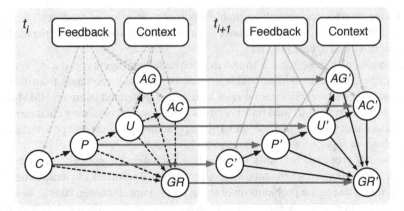

Fig. 1. Dynamic version of the Bayesian network model of the listener [6]. Posterior distributions of attributed listener state variables C, P, U, AC, AG, GR calculated at time t_i are taken as prior feedback [19] at time t_{i+1} and influence their corresponding variables $C', P', U', AC', AG', GR'$.

accept an utterance and to agree with its proposition, respectively. See Figure 1 – either the left or the right time slice – for a simplified graphical depiction of the model. The domain of each of the ALS-variables consists of three elements: *low*, *medium*, and *high*, and represent whether the listener's understanding (for example) is believed to be low, medium, or high, respectively (see [6] for details). A probability assigned to this element (e.g., $P(U = high) = 0.3$) is interpreted as a speaker's degree of belief that a listener's understanding is high. A probability distribution over this variable (e.g., $P(U = low) = 0.2$, $P(U = medium) = 0.5$, $P(U = high) = 0.3$) is thus considered to be a speaker's belief state about this variable.

The ALS-variables influence each other according to the hierarchy of feedback functions [1] and are influenced by variables that model the listener's behaviour, the speaker's utterances and expectations as well as the dialogue situation (for simplicity these factors are collapsed in the boxes 'feedback' and 'context' in Figure 1; see [6] for details). This allows for a context-sensitive interpretation of the listener's feedback behaviour. Furthermore, the five ALS-variables contribute to an inference about the grounding status of the utterance (GR) thus interpreting the listener's feedback as 'evidence of understanding' [8].

3 Temporal Dynamics of Attributed Listener State

A limitation in Buschmeier and Kopp's [6] Bayesian model of attributed listener state is that it analyses feedback signals and their dialogue context at independent intervals (increments of the speaker's utterance similar to intonation units). Listener state attribution is repeated for subsequent increments of the utterance [4], but information from previous increments is not carried over. Thus, the model assumes that a listener's mental state at a point t_i is independent from – i.e., has no influence on – the mental state at a subsequent point at time t_{i+1}.

This assumption is a considerable simplification. Consider a case where a listener does not provide feedback at a given interval. The model either needs to maintain the last belief state where feedback occurred (which becomes implausible when feedback is absent for several intervals) or immediately change to a default belief state (which is implausible if the previous belief state was decidedly positive or negative). A more plausible assumption would be a combination of these two behaviours, i.e., neither maintaining the last belief state indefinitely nor changing abruptly, but instead developing slowly and continuously from the last towards a default belief state. This behaviour would capture the intuition that listeners that understand well can be assumed to still have a good understanding even when not providing feedback for a certain period of time. If, however, feedback is absent for extended periods of time, the belief in their high understanding will vanish over time.

In order to track how a listener's mental state changes over time, we extend the static model of attributed listener state [6] to include a temporal dimension. This is achieved by transforming it into a *two time-slice dynamic Bayesian network* (see Figure 1). In this network, one slice represents the current point in time t_{i+1}, and the other slice represents the preceding point in time t_i. Temporal influences are modelled by linking some of the variables at time-slice t_{i+1} with variables at time-slice t_i: The five ALS-variables C, P, U, AC, and AG as well as the groundedness variable GR at time t_i serve as temporally persistent variables and are directly linked to their counterparts at time t_{i+1} (C', P', U', AC', AG', and GR'). Thus P', for example, is not just influenced by C', listener feedback and dialogue context, but also by P.

Development over time is modelled with a step-by-step *unrolling* of the network. At each step, Bayesian network inference is carried out on time-slice t_i, and the resulting

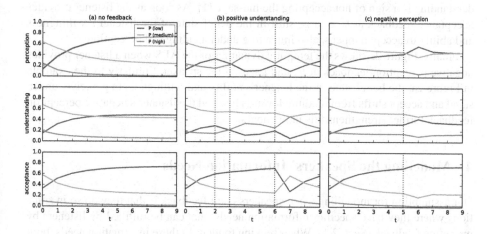

Fig. 2. Temporal dynamics of the speaker's degrees of belief in the ALS-variables P, U, and AC in three simulated feedback conditions. Dotted vertical lines visualise verbal-vocal listener feedback. (a) the listener does not provide feedback and looks away from the speaker; (b) the listener provides understanding feedback at t_2 and t_3, expressing a high certainty at t_3 and additionally gazing at the target object at t_3 and t_4, at t_6 the listener provides acceptance feedback; (c) the listener provides negative perception feedback at t_5 and gazes at the speaker at t_6.

marginal posterior probabilities of the temporally persistent variables are calculated. Since the network makes a first order Markov assumption, previous time slices are not considered further. Links to them, as well as to non-persistent variables are cut off. The calculated posterior distributions are then used as 'prior feedback' ([19]; i.e., simply interpreted as prior distributions of those variables that are used as evidence nodes) to the subsequent time slice t_{i+1}). The ALS-variables in time-slice t_i thus implicitly represent the history.

To demonstrate how this model simulates the temporal dynamics of the attributed listener state, Figure 2 shows three simulated examples of ten time steps each (only the variables P, U, and AC are plotted). Each graph shows how the probabilities for each of the different values of the respective variables change over time (magenta coloured lines show $P(X = \text{low})$, yellow coloured lines $P(X = \text{medium})$ and cyan coloured lines $P(X = \text{high})$ for $X \in P, U, AC$).

Figure 2a shows an interaction where the listener does not produce any feedback and even looks away from the speaker (these behaviours are fed into the input nodes). Over time, the degree of belief in the listener's ability and willingness to perceive quickly shifts from an initial guess of medium towards low perception. Similar shifts can be observed in the belief states of the listener's willingness and ability to understand and accept the speaker's message.

Figure 2b shows a more complex interaction in which the listener provides understanding feedback from t_2 to t_3, expressing high certainty at t_3, and additionally gazes at the target object in the visual domain at t_3 and t_4. Additionally, the listener provides acceptance feedback at t_6. As soon as feedback occurs, a medium to high level in perception and understanding becomes more likely. This level persists even when no feedback occurs at t_5. Acceptance, however remains low, as feedback of the type indicating understanding is a sign of not accepting the message [1]. As soon as the listener provides acceptance feedback at t_6, a large shift in the belief state of the listener's willingness and ability to accept happens, also impacting understanding and perception.

Finally, Figure 2c shows the temporal dynamics of the ALS when a listener provides negative perception feedback at t_5, and gazes at the speaker. Similarly to the example in Figure 2a, the belief state in the listener's ability and willingness to perceive, understand and accept shifts from medium towards low and the listener's negative perception feedback further strengthens this judgement.

4 Modelling the Speakers' Information Needs

Our assumption for modelling *when* speakers elicit feedback is that they do so in situations where they have specific 'information needs' that can be fulfilled by listeners by providing feedback (Sect. 2.1). When seeking to identify these information needs, both the attributed listener state at the current point in time, as well as how it developed into this state, are relevant. We propose the following three criteria for assessing whether an agent has an information need. It needs feedback from the user when

1. its belief about the user's mental state is not very informative (i.e., when the attributed listener state has high entropy);

2. its belief about the user's mental state is static over an extended period of time (i.e., when no feedback was received); or
3. its belief about the user's mental state is different from a desired mental state (e.g., sufficient understanding, high agreement) than is intended as the result of a specific communicative action by the agent or interactive adaptation in a previous utterance (i.e., when the attributed listener state diverges, by a given degree, from a given 'reference' state).

A maximal uncertainty about the mental state of a user would manifest in a uniform probability distribution across the elements of (one or more) variables, e.g., when $P(U = low) = 0.33, P(U = medium) = 0.33, P(U = high) = 0.33$. Conversely, uncertainty would be minimal in a maximally pointed distribution such as, e.g., $P(U = low) = 0.0, P(U = medium) = 0.0, P(U = high) = 1.0$. This way of measuring uncertainty, i.e., related to entropy, assumes that the underlying state of the user is of a discrete nature, rather than fuzzy and with considerable variance persisting over time. We therefore combine the first, entropy-based, criterion with an operationalisation of the third criterion by quantifying the distance between the probability distributions of the current state of a variable and a 'reference state' such as, for example, a state that represents very good or very bad understanding. This difference can be measured by the Kullback-Leibler divergence

$$D_{KL}(P||Q) = \sum_i P(i) \cdot \ln \frac{P(i)}{Q(i)}$$

which returns a scalar value greater or equal to zero, with $D_{KL}(P||Q) = 0$ for $P = Q$, i.e., the more similar the two distributions are, the smaller the KL-divergence.

Figure 3 shows an example of how the Kullback-Leibler divergence between the current ALS-variables and a reference state of these variables (one for positive: $P(P/U/AC = low) = 0.001, P(P/U/AC = medium) = 0.3, P(P/U/AC = high) = 0.69$; one for negative perception/understanding/acceptance: $P(P/U/AC = low) = 0.69, P(P/U/AC = medium) = 0.3, P(P/U/AC = high) = 0.01$) changes over time (b), alongside the temporal dynamics of the ALS-variables $P, U,$ and AC themselves (a). The listener gives positive understanding feedback at t_1 and gazes near the target object until t_2. No more feedback is received after this. The plots of the KL-divergence show that understanding is believed to be mediocre with a tilt towards low understanding and with some volatility at the beginning when feedback was received. The difference between the distributions of the variable U and the positive and negative reference distributions is not very large, however. In contrast, perception clearly changes toward low, and acceptance is believed to be low almost from the beginning. The KL-divergence with the negative reference distributions is almost 0.

Based on this, we can determine the speaker's information needs by looking for points where (1) the KL-divergence to a 'positive' reference distribution (representing an ALS with sufficient certainty and positive listener attributes) has a value higher by a given amount α than what is desired (criterion 3),

$$D_{KL}^t(\text{pdf}(P/U/AC), [0.01, 0.3, 0.69]) > \alpha, \quad \alpha = 1.0$$

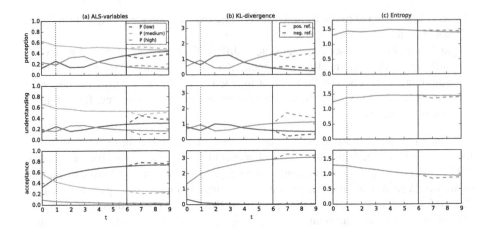

Fig. 3. (a) Temporal dynamics of the speaker's degrees of belief in the ALS-variables P, U, and AC in a simulated feedback condition where the listener provides understanding feedback of medium certainty at t_1 (visualised by the dotted vertical line), simultaneously gazing near the target object until t_2. (b) Kullback-Leibler divergence between the distribution of the ALS-variables and the positive/negative reference distributions. (c) Entropy of the ALS-variables. The solid vertical line at t_6 visualises a condition where the speaker can elicit feedback. Dashed lines show how the speaker's degrees of belief would develop when the listener immediately responds with non-understanding feedback of medium certainty while gazing towards the speaker.

and (2) where changes in the KL-divergence from one step to the next are smaller than a given value δ, i.e., when the values converge and the belief state becomes almost static (criterion 2):

$$D_{KL}^{t-1}(\text{pdf}(U), [0.01, 0.3, 0.69]) - D_{KL}^{t}(\text{pdf}(U), [0.01, 0.3, 0.69]) < \delta, \quad \delta = 0.1$$

These can be regarded as points where a speaker requires new information in order to know how to deal with the dialogue situation. This principle is applied to the example in Figure 3 to determine a point in time to elicit feedback. The criteria match at time t_6 with $\alpha = 1.03$ and $\delta = 0.077$ and result in a feedback elicitation cue being produced. Figure 3 also visualises the contrast in the development of the belief state in two situations: when the feedback elicitation cue is responded to by the listener with negative understanding feedback (solid lines), or when the elicitation cue does not result in feedback behaviour by the listener (dashed lines).

5   Conclusion

In this paper we have presented further steps towards creating attentive speaker agents that take into account their users' listening-related mental state, even while they are presenting information and making contributions to the dialogue. We have described an extension to our attributed listener state model [6] which enables it to deal with aspects of the temporal dynamics inherent to dialogue. The resulting dynamic Bayesian network keeps track of a listener's contact, perception, and understanding, as well as acceptance and agreement of the speaker agent's utterances. One goal here is to utilise this model to assess the information needs a speaker agent faces when it seeks to be cooperative in dialogue. When information about a user's mental state is insufficient or hints to upcoming problems that may lead to undesirable dialogue states (e.g., necessitating repair), the attentive speaker agent may use this information to decide when to elicit communicative feedback from the user in order to improve its own information basis and therefore take appropriate cooperative action.

We are currently implementing the model in a virtual conversational agent to enable user studies that can not only inform further development of the model, but also elucidate the coordination mechanisms required for attentive and pro-active dialogue agents.

Acknowledgements. This research is supported by the Deutsche Forschungsgemeinschaft (DFG) via the Center of Excellence EXC 277 'Cognitive Interaction Technology' (CITEC).

References

1. Allwood, J., Nivre, J., Ahlsén, E.: On the semantics and pragmatics of linguistic feedback. Journal of Semantics 9, 1–26 (1992)
2. Bavelas, J.B., Coates, L., Johnson, T.: Listeners as co-narrators. Journal of Personality and Social Psychology 79, 941–952 (2000)
3. Bavelas, J.B., Coates, L., Johnson, T.: Listener responses as a collaborative process: The role of gaze. Journal of Communication 52, 566–580 (2002)
4. Buschmeier, H., Baumann, T., Dosch, B., Kopp, S., Schlangen, D.: Combining incremental language generation and incremental speech synthesis for adaptive information presentation. In: Proceedings of the 13th Annual Meeting of the Special Interest Group on Discourse and Dialogue, Seoul, South Korea, pp. 295–303 (2012)
5. Buschmeier, H., Kopp, S.: Towards conversational agents that attend to and adapt to communicative user feedback. In: Vilhjálmsson, H.H., Kopp, S., Marsella, S., Thórisson, K.R. (eds.) IVA 2011. LNCS, vol. 6895, pp. 169–182. Springer, Heidelberg (2011)
6. Buschmeier, H., Kopp, S.: Using a Bayesian model of the listener to unveil the dialogue information state. In: SemDial 2012: Proceedings of the 16th Workshop on the Semantics and Pragmatics of Dialogue, Paris, France, pp. 12–20 (2012)
7. Clark, H.H.: Using Language. Cambridge University Press, Cambridge (1996)
8. Clark, H.H., Schaefer, E.F.: Contributing to discourse. Cognitive Science 13, 259–294 (1989)
9. Gravano, A., Hirschberg, J.: Turn-taking cues in task-oriented dialogue. Computer Speech and Language 25, 601–634 (2011)
10. Heylen, D.: Head gestures, gaze and the principle of conversational structure. International Journal of Humanoid Robotics 3, 241–267 (2006)
11. Huang, L., Morency, L.P., Gratch, J.: Parasocial consensus sampling: Combining multiple perspectives to learn virtual human behavior. In: Proceedings of the 9th International Conference on Autonomous Agents and Multiagent Systems, Toronto, Canada, pp. 1265–1272 (2010)
12. Koiso, H., Horiuchi, Y., Tutiya, S., Ichikawa, A., Den, Y.: An analysis of turn-taking and backchannels on prosodic and syntactic features in Japanese map task dialogs. Language and Speech 41(3-4), 295–321 (1998)

13. de Kok, I., Heylen, D.: Analyzing nonverbal listener responses using parallel recordings of multiple listeners. Cognitive Processing 13, 499–506 (2012)
14. Kopp, S., Allwood, J., Grammer, K., Ahlsen, E., Stocksmeier, T.: Modeling embodied feedback with virtual humans. In: Wachsmuth, I., Knoblich, G. (eds.) ZiF Research Group International Workshop. LNCS (LNAI), vol. 4930, pp. 18–37. Springer, Heidelberg (2008)
15. Misu, T., Mizukami, E., Shiga, Y., Kawamoto, S., Kawai, H., Nakamura, S.: Analysis on effects of text-to-speech and avatar agent in evoking users' spontaneous listener's reactions. In: Proceedings of the Workshop on Paralinguistic Information and its Integration in Spoken Dialogue Systems, Granada, Spain, pp. 77–89 (2011)
16. Misu, T., Mizukami, E., Shiga, Y., Kawamoto, S., Kawai, H., Nakamura, S.: Toward construction of spoken dialogue system that evokes users' spontaneous backchannels. In: Proceedings of the 12th Annual Meeting of the Special Interest Group on Discourse and Dialogue, Portland, OR, USA, pp. 259–265 (2011)
17. Morency, L.P., de Kok, I., Gratch, J.: A probabilistic multimodal approach for predicting listener backchannels. Autonomous Agents and Multiagent Systems 20, 70–84 (2010)
18. Reidsma, D., de Kok, I., Neiberg, D., Pammi, S., van Straalen, B., Truong, K., van Welbergen, H.: Continuous interaction with a virtual human. Journal on Multimodal User Interfaces 4, 97–118 (2011)
19. Robert, C.P.: Prior feedback: A Bayesian approach to maximum likelihood estimation. Computational Statistics 8, 279–294 (1993)
20. Schröder, M., Bevacqua, E., Cowie, R., et al.: Building autonomous sensitive artificial listeners. IEEE Transactions on Affective Computing 3, 165–183 (2012)
21. Ward, N.: Non-lexical conversational sounds in American English. Pragmatics & Cognition 14, 129–182 (2006)
22. Ward, N., Tsukahara, W.: Prosodic features which cue back-channel responses in English and Japanese. Journal of Pragmatics 38, 1177–1207 (2000)

Representing Communicative Functions in SAIBA with a Unified Function Markup Language

Angelo Cafaro[1], Hannes Högni Vilhjálmsson[2], Timothy Bickmore[3],
Dirk Heylen[4], and Catherine Pelachaud[1]

[1] CNRS-LTCI, Telecom ParisTech, France
{angelo.cafaro,catherine.pelachaud}@telecom-paristech.fr
[2] Center for Analysis and Design of Intelligent Agents, Reykjavik University, Iceland
hannes@ru.is
[3] College of Computer and Information Science, Northeastern University, USA
bickmore@ccs.neu.edu
[4] Human Media Interaction, University of Twente, The Netherlands
d.k.j.heylen@utwente.nl

Abstract. The SAIBA framework proposes two interface languages to represent separately an intelligent agent's communicative functions (or intents) and the multimodal behavior determining how the functions are accomplished with a particular multimodal realization. For the functional level, the Function Markup Language (FML) has been proposed. In this paper we summarize the current status of FML as discussed by the SAIBA community, we underline the major issues that need to be addressed to obtain a unified FML specification, we suggest further issues that we identified and we propose a new unified FML specification that addresses many of these issues.

Keywords: function markup language, communicative function, multimodal communication, embodied conversational agents.

1 Introduction

Over the past decade many Embodied Conversational Agent (ECA) systems [1,2,3,4,5,6] adopted an abstraction approach to multimodal behavior generation that separates communicative function or intent from its behavioral realization. This design and the need for sharing working components motivated the SAIBA framework [7]. SAIBA supports this separation through two interface languages named **Function Markup Language** (FML) [8] and **Behavior Markup Language** (BML) [7,9] respectively. A first version of BML has been adopted internationally [7,9], but a common unified FML specification has not yet emerged, although several specialized contributions exist [6,10,11]. There is an ongoing discussion about several issues that FML needs to address [8]. In this paper we summarize the status of FML based on discussions within the SAIBA community, we underline the major issues that need to be addressed to obtain a unified FML specification and suggest further issues that need to be tackled. Finally we propose a new unified FML specification that addresses many of these issues.

---

[1] Author conducted this research at CADIA, Reykjavik University.

T. Bickmore et al. (Eds.): IVA 2014, LNAI 8637, pp. 81–94, 2014.
© Springer International Publishing Switzerland 2014

2   Current Status of the FML Discussion

The first attempts to define the FML standard were based on various existing ECA systems. This included the REA system [1] and the systems that followed it: BEAT [3] and Spark [4]. Also the Multimodal Utterance Representation Markup Language (MURML) [12] used in the MAX system and the FML-APML mark-up language [11] developed for the Greta framework [2] provided inspiration. Other important systems that featured in the various discussions on FML were The Tactical Language and Culture Training System (TLCTS) [10] and the Virtual Human Toolkit [5] developed at the Institute of Creative Technologies (ICT) which uses FML-like concepts in the *Non-Verbal Behavior Generator* module. These systems attempted to adopt a clear separation between communicative function representation and corresponding behavior that would accomplish those functions. However, these systems focused on domain specific issues such as representation of emotions [11], cultural and other contextual information [6,10] and subsets of communicative functions [5]. In this paper we propose a new unified FML specification that builds on these earlier contributions and the current status of the FML discussion.

There has been an ongoing discussion about FML through a series of targeted workshops[1]. The work in [8] summarizes the discussions to date, and outlines the most important components of FML, including the following.

Contextual information and **person characteristics**. The former includes cultural and social setting, environmental information (e.g. time of the day), history of interactions and topics discussed. The latter, referring to a participant performing communicative functions, are organized in two main dimensions: person information (e.g. identifier, name, gender, role) and personality.

Communicative actions include dialogue acts, grounding actions and turn taking. Formal (logical) languages have been proposed to represent **propositional content** and a certain organization of propositions has emerged at both *sentence* level (emphasis, given/new information, theme/rheme) and *discourse* level (topics and rhetorical relations between different parts of the discourse). It is assumed that extra-linguistic or certain non-linguistic actions, such as picking up a glass of water, can also perform certain communicative functions.

Emotional and **mental states** are believed to contribute to the motivation of a communicative intent. Emotions are divided between *felt*, *faked* and *leaked*. Mental states are defined as cognitive processes such as *planning*, *thinking* or *remembering*.

Social psychological aspects and **relational goals** are also considered. The concepts of *interpersonal framing* (e.g. showing empathy in comforting interactions) and *relational stance* (e.g. warmth) functions are introduced to affect the behavior produced by an agent with those goals.

3   Outline of Important FML Issues

Defining and Separating Contextual Information. Some contextual information may be necessary, but how much and how should it be represented? Do we need a new

---
[1] At Reykjavik in 2005, AAMAS 2008, AAMAS 2009, ICT and Paris in 2010.

language to represent this information (e.g. CML as proposed in [10])? In addition to the two dimensions of person characteristics proposed earlier (*person information* and *personality*), what do we mean by enough context? The contextual parameters have been shown to be important for the generation of behavior, for example, with respect to the *environmental context* (greetings depending on the time of the day), *cultural background* or *socio-relational* goals. It is also important to consider how context could affect the planning of functions.

Defining and Classifying Functions. A communication function might arise from an action that does not have propositional content, these functions have been classified more generally as *communicative actions*. The main concern is what to consider as a communicative action. Choosing a classification scheme that embraces all prevailing perspectives on communicative function is not easy, but it will aid the designers of ECAs to use FML at different levels. At a higher level it will be possible to obtain a general outline of the human communicative capacity of a system by noting what general kinds of function specification are available. At a lower level, a designer can expect that functions belonging to the same category will share some specification characteristics and parametrization [13]. The main question that arises is how many groups and categories of functions are needed.

Characterizing and Separating Conscious vs. Unconscious Intents. Contextual information does not represent the only determinant for generating communicative functions. A broader distinction needs to be made between consciously planned intents and communicative functions resulting from unconscious determinants such as mental and emotional states. We may also want to support a direct path from perception to the realization of behavior as in FML-APML [11], but this raises the issue of possible conflict between unconscious/reactive intents and conscious planned intents.

Defining Temporal Constraints and a Prioritization Scheme. Assigning timing information to communicative functions and supporting the temporal coordination among them are important issues to consider as suggested by [11]. [13] suggested that temporal constraints at the functional level of description should be much more coarse-grained than those at lower levels since it becomes hard to specify exactly how long it will take to accomplish a specific function. In addition to supporting the specification of temporal constraints, an advantage of cutting FML in *"smaller chunks"* [14] or *"chunk plans"* [13] is that they could be processed separately allowing faster generation of corresponding BML compared to a larger FML input (i.e. containing several communicative functions). When dealing with real time reactions (e.g. back channel feedback) a large amount of communicative functions processed as a whole could create an unacceptable delay that would slow down the system's response and make the whole interaction feel unnatural from the user's point of view. However, assuming that FML chunks are adopted, several issues need to be resolved. First we have to come up with a precise definition of an FML chunk, keeping in mind what constitutes a useful semantic unit. Secondly, what timing primitives will suffice to temporally coordinate chunks? Finally, what kind of conflict resolution scheme is needed when chunks collide? For example, FML-APML proposed an *"importance"* attribute to help with this.

Defining an FML Representation Structure. Previous representation languages mainly adopted an XML-like syntax and assigned a nested structure to the specified set of tags (cf. [11,10]). While it is tempting to adopt a similar structure for a unified FML representation, one may wonder whether this is still a valid solution, and if so, what are the rules that govern the embedding of a set of tags into others. At the current stage of the work, the discussion has been kept on a theoretical level, but this is an important issue when it comes to practically defining a structure for an FML representation.

Single or Multiple Agents? An instance of FML could refer to a single or multiple ECAs. Dealing with individual ECAs might offer scalability and improved performance through distributed processing while mixing ECAs may require central processing, which does not scale well. But the latter makes it easier to solve complex highly co-ordinated interactions.

Multiple Interaction Floors and Roles of Participants. A person may be engaged in more than one conversation at the same time and assume different roles, including by-stander. This moves from dyadic settings towards more complex scenarios. Specifying the configuration of interactions at the functional level ensures that behaviors can take this into account. Some examples of configurations might be simple *1-to-1* interactions (for example dyadic), *1-to-many* (for example when describing a public speech) and *many-to-many* (two groups interacting as a whole with each other).

4   A Unified FML Specification

This section summarizes the complete proposed specification [2]. First some key terms:

Participant An entity (e.g. virtual agent or user) participating in an interaction and carrying out or being affected by communicative functions.

Floor A participant can be engaged in several interactions with other participants that we name *floors*. A metaphor for the social contract that binds participants together in the common purpose of interacting.

FML chunk The smallest unit of FML functions associated with a single participant that is ready to be turned into supporting BML-specified behavior.

4.1   Overview

Representation Structure and Target. A single FML representation instance includes functions that several participants want to accomplish. It is divided in two main sec-tions: a *declaration* (described in Section 4.2) and a *body* (Section 4.3), as illustrated in Figure 1. The declarations incorporate contextual information, whereas the body in-cludes all participants' generated functions grouped in FML chunks and belonging to

---

[2] See http://secom.ru.is/fml/ for full specification.

three different tracks (named interactional, performative and mental state) as a result of our functions categorization described below.

Contextual Information and Multiple Interaction Floors. We divided contextual information in two components: a *static* component describing participants information (e.g. gender, age, personality, etc...) and a *dynamic* component providing information about the active floors (e.g. participants in each floor and their attitudes). *Participant information* is labeled as *static* since it is meant to endure over time. It affects all active floors in which the participant is involved. This specification supports the co-existence of multiple active floors for each participant and each floor involving one or more participants. The *floors information* supports the specification of the active floors that the FML instance describes. It is labeled *dynamic* since the information included is meant to be temporarily associated with a particular floor.

Functions Categorization and Body Tracks. The body of an FML representation is divided into three sub-sections or *"tracks"*. This design reflects the choice of categorizing the communicative functions as suggested by [15]. The first category of functions (named **interactional**) deals with establishing, maintaining and closing the communication channel, instantiated with a floor, between participants. The second category (named **performative**) covers the actual content that gets exchanged across the communication channel. The third category deals with functions describing mental states and emotions (for simplicity it has been named **mental state**).

Temporal Constraints and FML Chunks. Splitting the body up into separate tracks requires an overall orchestration of the functions in relation to each other. The order of appearance of functions in the FML instance does not necessarily imply delivery time. Coarse-grained temporal constraints (described in Section 4.3) allow synchronization and relative timing among chunks across all the tracks.

Unconscious Intents. The mental state track assumes a particular meaning that addresses the issue of representing functions that are not deliberately planned by a participant. Every participant has a *ground state* that comprises his mental and emotional states (mood could be considered as well). Only functions in the mental state track can change the participant's ground state for a limited or unlimited time depending on the particular temporal constraint adopted. In essence, the ground state provides additional contextual information about the participant that can affect the generation and realization of multimodal behavior in the later stages of the SAIBA generation process.

4.2 FML Representation: Declaration

The declaration section stores contextual information in two separate sub-sections for participant's information and floors configurations as shown in Figure 2.

The **identikits tag** contains an `<identikit>` for each participant including person characteristics (e.g. a human readable *name* and *gender*). Each tag supports the inclusion of embedded information about the participant. We provide `<personality>` and `<relationship>` as examples. The former is based on the Big 5 [16] model dimensions (other models can be supported). The latter specifies a relationship level with other participants. The example scenario described in Section 4.4 shows the use of

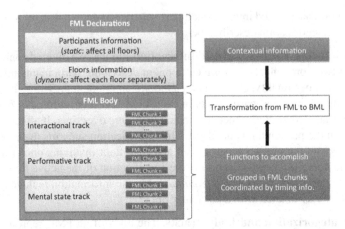

Fig. 1. An overview of our proposed FML specification. A representation instance is divided in declarations and body sections, respectively, for contextual information and communicative functions. Contextual information can affect all communication floors (participant information) or selected ones (floors information). The communicative functions are temporally coordinated in FML chunks.

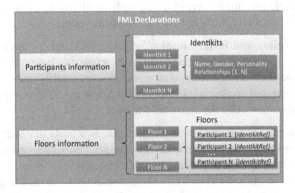

Fig. 2. The declarations section of an FML instance stores contextual information divided in participants information (identikits) and floors configurations (floors).

these tags. This part of the declaration section can be created once and then cached for later usage since it contains static information.

The floors tag describes each active floor in the FML instance. Each floor described has a *floor-cfg* attribute that specifies its configuration. We identified four possible configurations: *individual, unicast, broadcast* and *multicast* (naming inpsired by network protocols). An *individual* configuration describes a single entity (i.e. participant), *unicast* represents the classical dyadic interaction, *broadcast* describes an individual entity interacting with a group and *multicast* characterizes two groups, as a whole, interacting with each other.

A `<floor>` can include one or more `<participant>` tags depending on the number of participants involved. These tags have an *entity* attribute describing whether in the given floor configuration the participant is an *individual* or a *group*. A *role* attribute specifies the role assumed by the participant in the given floor, currently inpsired by Goffman's participation framework [17]. According to Goffman, participants can have a **speaker** or a **hearer** role. Two types of hearers are identified in this framework: *ratified* (official) and *unratified* (unofficial) participants. Ratified participants are subdivided into *addressed* and *unaddressed* recipients, and unratified participants or bystanders are subdivided into *eavesdroppers* and *overhearers*, based on their intent and degree of interest.

Furthermore, a `<participant>` tag can embed some contextual information. As an example, we defined `<attitude>` tags to specify the attitude that the participant has toward another participant in any given floor according to Argyle's status and affiliation model [18] (see the full example in Section 4.4).

4.3 FML Representation: Body

The body of an FML instance is divided in three tracks. Each track includes **FML Chunks** that are timed with relative **Temporal Constraints**. **FML Chunk tag:** Each `<fml-chunk>` refers to a single participant's identikit with the *participantRef* attribute. The first element within a chunk can be a single occurrence of a `<timing>` tag followed by any number of functions defined for the track in which the chunk appears. The `<timing>` tag temporally constrains the whole chunk relative to other chunks.

Temporal Constraints: Temporal constraints work on a chunk level with the following design principles: (1) the chunks' order of appearance in the body of an FML instance is not meaningful, (2) unless specified by the `<timing>` element an FML chunk should be scheduled for later processing (i.e. transformation to BML) "as soon as possible" and (3) the order of appearance of functions within a chunk is not meaningful and they will be considered in arbitrary order at later stages. The `<timing>` tag has a *primitive* attribute to specify the temporal relationship between the current chunk and the referenced one. Possible values are: *immediately, must_end_before, execute_anytime_during, start_immediately_after, start_sometime_after, start_together*.

FML Functions Specification: All FML functions tags have in common a unique identifier and a *floorID* attribute for referencing the floor in which the communicative function is meant to be accomplished.

Interactional track functions. This track supports the specification of a category of communicative functions that serve to coordinate a multimodal interaction. Table 1 shows the possible functions that can appear within an FML chunk in this track. The first column on the left side represents a broad category of interactional functions and it is also the name adopted for the corresponding tag. These tags have a common attribute named *type* that narrows down the specification of functions within the category. Some of the functions (marked with a "*") require the specification of the *addressee* attribute indicating the participant to which the function is addressed.

The initiation and closing categories describe the communicative functions, respectively, to manage the initial and termination phases of the interaction. In particular, the different available types of initiation and closing functions are based on the stages of a greeting encounter as suggested by Kendon's greeting model [19]. As starting point, the turn-taking, speech-act and grounding functions have type attribute values

Table 1. Interactional functions: suggested tag names on the left and possible type attribute values on the right. Functions marked with "*" have an *addressee* attribute.

Function Category	Type Attribute
initiation*	*react, recognize, salute-distant, salute-close, initiate*
closing*	*break-away, farewell*
turn-taking*	*take, give, keep, request, accept*
speech-act	*inform, ask, request*
grounding	*request-ack, ack, repair, cancel*

following the suggestions in [15]. All tags in this track can be linked to others in another track (e.g. speech acts linked with a performative tag) by using the temporal constraints.

Performative track functions. The various functions in this category can be divided across different organizational levels, from the largest organizational structure of a discourse down to the specification of each proposition. In our proposal, the performative track acts as place holder for further embedded extensions of FML specifically targeted to describe performative functions. Therefore, chunks in this track can host one or more `<performative-extension>` tags.

This tag is merely a stub and the description of an extension that will handle its contents is out of the scope of this paper, though we foresee an extension mechanism similar to BML's[3]. Following the recommendations in [15], Table 2 suggests a set of possible function categories and their specific types that could be included within this tag. Similarly to interactional functions, an *addressee* attribute specifies to which participant the included performative act is directed to.

Table 2. Performative functions: suggested tag names and type values

Function Category	Type Attribute
discourse-structure	*topic, segment, . . .*
rhetorical-structure	*elaborate, summarize, clarify, contrast, emphasize, . . .*
information-structure	*rheme, theme, given, new, . . .*
proposition	*any formal notation (e.g. "own(A,B)")*

Mental State Track Functions. Functions in this track are the only ones capable of changing the *ground state* of a participant. The concept of ground state is kept at abstract level in this proposal, but the idea is that it may affect the manner in which other functions get realized, thus modeling the unconscious side of a participant. We do not

---

[3] http://www.mindmakers.org/projects/bml-1-0/wiki#Extensions

specify how the ground state should be modeled and how it should affect the behavior generation and realization in later stages. However, we provide several design ideas as a starting point, we propose functions describing mental states and emotions (as shown in Table 3).

First, multiple functions can occur simultaneously in this track. We propose a *weight-Factor* attribute ranging from 0 to 1 to establish the impact that each single one has on the ground state. Secondly, we propose that every function appearing in this track gets sustained by default and unless specified with a temporal constraint (e.g. *must_end_before*), it changes the ground state permanently. However, reverting to a previous state or voiding the effect of a sustained emotion will be possible by specifying the same function again with the same *weightFactor* as it was before or zeroing it. Finally, by using the temporal constraints it is possible to sustain mental states or emotions only during the accomplishment of a function in another track.

Table 3. Mental and emotional state functions: suggested tag names and possible types

Function Category Type Attribute
cognitive-process *remember, infer, decide, idle ...*
emotion *anger, disgust, embarrassment, fear, happiness, sadness, surprise, shame ...*

We based the specification of the <**emotion**> tag on FML-APML [11]. So each <**emotion**> has two attributes that specify the *intensity* and *regulation* of the emotion. The regulation can be: *felt* (a felt emotion), *fake* (an emotion that the participant aims at simulating) and *inhibit* (the emotion is felt by the participant but is inhibited as much as possible).

4.4   Example Scenario

We now use the proposed specification to describe the communicative functions of an example scenario about ordering a cheeseburger in a diner, a scenario that has been subject of discussion in earlier FML workshops. The following declarations describe a two floors interaction among three individuals: Gilda, Pete and George. Gilda is a customer, Pete is the cashier taking orders and George makes the burgers.

We assume that Gilda, after having approached the cashier, has already placed her order. Thus, the FML describes a floor where Pete acknowledges the order just placed by Gilda and another floor where Pete requests George to make a cheeseburger. Gilda has a friendly attitude towards Pete and acts as by-stander in the second floor between Pete and George.

Declaration Section. First we show the declaration section in Listing 1.1. Contextual information appears in the participants' identikits. In particular, Pete's personality is defined as *LOW* for the extraversion trait and his relationships with other participants are specified. Both Pete and George work in the same place, therefore we assumed that they are friends. The relationship information of the other two participants is left out but can be specified similarly.

As for the floors, they describe a *unicast* configuration. In floor1 both Pete assumes the role of *speaker* and Gilda has *addressed-hearer* role. Furthermore, Gilda has a *FRIENDLY* attitude towards Pete. In floor2, Pete is the *speaker*, George is an *addressed-hearer* while Gilda is an *unaddressed-hearer*. They are all represented as *individual* entities in the two floors described.

```
<declarations>

<!-- Participants identikits -->
 <identikits>

   <identikit id="PET" name="Pete" gender="male">
   <personality extraversion="LOW"/>
   <relationships>
    <relationship level="STRANGER" with="GIL" />
    <relationship level="FRIEND" with="GEO" />
   </relationships>
   </identikit>

   <identikit id="GIL" name="Gilda" gender="female" />
   <identikit id="GEO" name="George" gender="male" />

 </identikits>

<!-- Floors configuration -->
 <floors>

   <!-- Floor1 is between Pete and Gilda -->
   <floor floorID="floor1" floor-cfg="unicast">
    <participant identikitRef="PET" role="speaker" entity="individual" />
    <participant identikitRef="GIL" role="addressed-hearer" entity="individual"
       >
     <attitude affiliation="FRIENDLY" status="NEUTRAL" towards="PET" />
    </participant>
   </floor>

   <!-- Floor2 is between Pete and George with Gilda as by-stander -->
   <floor floorID="floor2" floor-cfg="unicast">
   <participant identikitRef="PET" role="speaker" entity="individual"/>
   <participant identikitRef="GEO" role="addressed-hearer" entity="individual"/
       >
   <participant identikitRef="GIL" role="unaddressed-hearer" entity="individual
       "/>
   </floor>

 </floors>

</declarations>
```

Listing 1.1. The `<declarations>` section of the cheeseburger example

Body Section. Listing 1.2 shows the body section of our example. Pete *acknowledges* the order just placed by Gilda with a grounding function, as can be seen in the chunk at line 6. This *must_end_before* the beginning of the second chunk described at line 11. Within this second chunk, Pete switches to the floor with George, he *takes* the turn and performs a *speech act* in the form of a *request*.

Starting *immediately_after*, Pete tells George to make a cheeseburger as described in the performative track (see 26). The two chunks in the mental state track accomplish this function with a *fake* emotional state of *anger* (see at line 39). This Pete's emotional state is sustained only for the duration of the performative act, afterwards it gets voided as we can see at line 45. Finally, *immediately_after* that Pete requests George to make a cheeseburger, Pete *gives* the turn away as shown at line 17.

```
 1  <body>
 2
 3  <!— Interactional track —>
 4  <interactional>
 5
 6    <fml—chunk actID="ACT01" participantRef="PET" >
 7      <timing primitive="must_end_before" actRef="ACT02" />
 8        <grounding floorID="floor1" id="id1" type="ack" />
 9    </fml—chunk>
10
11    <fml—chunk actID="ACT02" participantRef="PET" >
12      <timing primitive="start_sometime_after" actRef="ACT01" />
13        <turn—taking floorID="floor2" id="id2" type="take" />
14        <speech—act floorID="floor2" id="id3" type="request"/>
15    </fml—chunk>
16
17    <fml—chunk actID="ACT03" participantRef="PET"  >
18      <timing primitive="start_immediately_after" actRef="ACT04" />
19        <turn—taking floorID="floor2" id="id4" type="give" />
20    </fml—chunk>
21
22  </interactional>
23
24  <!— Performative track —>
25  <performative>
26    <fml—chunk actID="ACT04" participantRef="PET" >
27      <timing primitive="start_immediately_after" actRef="ACT02"  />
28        <performative —extension id="id5" floorID="floor2" addressee="GEO">
29          <discourse—structure type="topic">
30          George make a <rhetorical—structure type="emphasis">cheesburger</
                          rhetorical—structure>
31          </discourse—structure>
32        </performative —extension>
33    </fml—chunk>
34  </performative>
35
36  <!— Mental state track —>
37  <mental—state>
38
39    <fml—chunk actID="ACT05" participantRef="PET" >
40      <timing primitive="start_together" actRef="ACT03"/>
41        <emotion floorID="floor2" id="id6" type="anger" regulation="fake"
42                     intensity="0.7" weightFactor="1.0" />
43    </fml—chunk>
44
45    <fml—chunk actID="ACT06" participantRef="PET">
46      <timing primitive="start_immediately_after" actRef="ACT03"/>
47        <emotion floorID="floor2" id="id7" type="anger" regulation="fake"
48                     weightFactor="0.0" />
49    </fml—chunk>
50
51  </mental—state>
52
53  </body>
```

Listing 1.2. The <body> section of the cheeseburger example

5 Conclusions and Future Work

In this paper we outlined the issues that an FML representation should address and we proposed a unified specification within the SAIBA framework. A preliminary interpreter for a subset of this specification has been implemented used to generate ECA behavior for a few sample scenarios [20].

The proposed FML specification is preliminary and has many limitations. The contextual information needs the inclusion of other important determinants discussed earlier, such as participant's culture and socio-relational goals. We think that the logical separation we have made in the declaration section will easily allow the inclusion of such information, for example culture and age could be part of the identikit, while socio-relational goals can be specified per floor basis.

We merely introduced the concept of *ground state* and we have suggested a simple mechanism (i.e. mental state track functions) to affect this state. However, where the ground state information is stored and the format needs to be defined. We introduced a simple prioritization schema for mental state functions with the *weightFactor* attribute, however an overall prioritization across the three tracks also needs to be defined.

The process of analyzing all the issues to address and the design of this specification led us to some final important considerations. First, modeling functions and categorizing them, separating and defining contextual information, and in general, dealing with all the aspects of human communicative functions when shaping this proposal required the adoption of a theoretical stance. For example, we adopted specific models of personality (Big 5) and interpersonal attitude (Argyle) to define contextual information. We also assumed that a communicative function can arise either from a consciously planned communicative intent that the participant aims to accomplish or unconsciously, for example, due to the participant's mental-emotional state. In either case (i.e. intentionally or unintentionally planned) our assumption is that a communicative function represents a goal to achieve in multimodal interaction and based on this assumption we designed our FML representation. These aspects certainly need agreement among the community, considering also the alternatives (for example other personality models) and the advantages of adopting specific models rather than others.

Secondly, we underlined that contextual information (or ground state of a participant) can have impact across different stages of the SAIBA framework. At functional level they can impact the production of functions (i.e. FML), at behavioral level they can impact the generation of multimodal behavior (i.e. BML) and how this behavior is realized (i.e. realization parameters). For this proposal we have chosen to deal with the last two when transforming from FML to BML. However, there seems to be a demand for inclusion in the SAIBA framework of an external standardized mechanism to handle this transformation and also a specification that goes beyond the mere representation of the two interface languages (FML and BML) is needed. In general, our recommendation is that SAIBA should not only provide standardized interface languages but also techniques and best practices that enable proper transfer between SAIBA components.

In conclusion, the FML specification proposed with this paper needs community feedback as part of an iterative process aimed at validating and improving it with further suggestions. We plan to keep working on top of this concrete specification and (1) add the missing tags to represent a wider set of communicative functions, (2) complete the specification of the *ground state* concept in the *mental state* track and possibly adopt a wider standard to express emotions (e.g. W3C EmotionML), and (3) provide a more detailed ontology to describe contextual information (e.g. incorporating participant's mood and environmental information to be used in case of iconic gestures).

Acknowledgements. This work was conducted at CADIA with support from the School of Computer Science at Reykjavik University and the Icelandic Research Fund (Learning Icelandic Language and Culture in Virtual Reykjavik). Further support provided by the EC FP7 (FP7/2007-2013) project VERVE and the Dutch national program COMMIT.

References

1. Cassell, J., Bickmore, T., Billinghurst, M., Campbell, L., Chang, K., Vilhjálmsson, H., Yan, H.: Embodiment in conversational interfaces: Rea. In: Proceedings of the SIGCHI Conference on Human Factors in Computing Systems, CHI 1999, pp. 520–527. ACM (1999)
2. Niewiadomski, R., Bevacqua, E., Mancini, M., Pelachaud, C.: Greta: an interactive expressive eca system. In: Proceedings of the 8th International Conference on Autonomous Agents and Multiagent Systems, vol. 2, pp. 1399–1400 (2009)
3. Cassell, J., Vilhjálmsson, H.H., Bickmore, T.: Beat: the behavior expression animation toolkit. In: Proceedings of the 28th Annual Conference on Computer Graphics and Interactive Techniques, SIGGRAPH 2001, pp. 477–486. ACM (2001)
4. Vilhjálmsson, H.H.: Augmenting online conversation through automated discourse tagging. In: Proceedings of the 38th Annual Hawaii International Conference on System Sciences (HICSS 2005) - Track 4, vol. 04, p. 109.1. IEEE Computer Society (2005)
5. Hartholt, A., Traum, D., Marsella, S.C., Shapiro, A., Stratou, G., Leuski, A., Morency, L.-P., Gratch, J.: All together now - introducing the virtual human toolkit. In: Aylett, R., Krenn, B., Pelachaud, C., Shimodaira, H. (eds.) IVA 2013. LNCS, vol. 8108, pp. 368–381. Springer, Heidelberg (2013)
6. van Oijen, J.: A framework to support the influence of culture on nonverbal behavior generation in embodied conversational agents. Master's thesis, University of Twente (2007)
7. Kopp, S., Krenn, B., Marsella, S.C., Marshall, A.N., Pelachaud, C., Pirker, H., Thórisson, K.R., Vilhjálmsson, H.H.: Towards a common framework for multimodal generation: The behavior markup language. In: Gratch, J., Young, M., Aylett, R.S., Ballin, D., Olivier, P. (eds.) IVA 2006. LNCS (LNAI), vol. 4133, pp. 205–217. Springer, Heidelberg (2006)
8. Heylen, D., Kopp, S., Marsella, S.C., Pelachaud, C., Vilhjálmsson, H.H.: The next step towards a function markup language. In: Prendinger, H., Lester, J.C., Ishizuka, M. (eds.) IVA 2008. LNCS (LNAI), vol. 5208, pp. 270–280. Springer, Heidelberg (2008)
9. Vilhjálmsson, H.H., et al.: The behavior markup language: Recent developments and challenges. In: Pelachaud, C., Martin, J.-C., André, E., Chollet, G., Karpouzis, K., Pelé, D. (eds.) IVA 2007. LNCS (LNAI), vol. 4722, pp. 99–111. Springer, Heidelberg (2007)
10. Samtani, P., Valente, A., Johnson, W.L.: Applying the saiba framework to the tactical language and culture training system. In: Workshop on Functional Representations for Generating Conversational Agent Behavior at AAMAS (2008)
11. Mancini, M., Pelachaud, C.: The fml-apml language. In: Workshop on Functional Representations for Generating Conversational Agents Behavior at AAMAS (2008)
12. Kranstedt, A., Kopp, S., Wachsmuth, I.: Murml: A multimodal utterance representation markup language for conversational agents. In: Proceedings of the AAMAS Workshop on Embodied Conversational Agents Let's Specify and Evaluate Them! (2002)

13. Thórisson, K.R., Vilhjálmsson, H.H.: Functional description of multimodal acts: A proposal. In: Proceedings of the 2nd Function Markup Language Workshop "Towards a Standard Markup Langauge for Embodied Dialogue Acts" at AAMAS (2009)
14. Bevacqua, E., Prepin, K., de Sevin, E., Niewiadomski, R., Pelachaud, C.: Reactive behaviors in saiba architecture. In: Proceedings of the 2nd Function Markup Language Workshop "Towards a Standard Markup Langauge for Embodied Dialogue Acts" at AAMAS (2009)
15. Vilhjálmsson, H.H.: Representing communicative function and behavior in multimodal communication. In: Esposito, A., Hussain, A., Marinaro, M., Martone, R. (eds.) COST Action 2102. LNCS, vol. 5398, pp. 47–59. Springer, Heidelberg (2009)
16. McCrae, R.R., Costa Jr., P.T.: Personality trait structure as a human universal. American Psychologist 52(5), 509–516 (1997)
17. Goffman, E.: Forms of Talk. University of Pennsylvania Press, Philadelphia (1981)
18. Argyle, M.: Bodily communication, 2nd edn. Methuen, New York (1988)
19. Kendon, A.: Conducting Interaction: Patterns of Behavior in Focused Encounters (Studies in Interactional Sociolinguistics). Cambridge University Press, New York (1990)
20. Cafaro, A.: First Impressions in Human-Agent Virtual Encounters. PhD thesis, Center for Analysis and Design of Intelligent Agents, Reykjavik University, Iceland (2014)

An Exploratory Analysis of ECA Characteristics

Adriana Camacho, Alex Rayon, Ivan Gris, and David Novick

Department of Computer Science, The University of Texas at El Paso
500 West University Avenue, El Paso, TX 79968-0518 USA
{accamacho2,amrayon2}@miners.utep.edu, {igris,novick}@utep.edu

Abstract. To help guide design and development of embodied conversational agents, this study reviews the evolving qualities of naturalistic agents by identifying and tracking their most relevant features. The study extends prior taxonomies of characteristics of ECAs, developing a rubric that distinguishes agents' visual and functional characteristics. The study applies the rubric to 15 agents representing different genres of games, distinguishing agents in terms of their naturalistic qualities. The study explores changes in qualities of agents as a function of time.

Keywords: Embodied conversational agent, taxonomy, rubric.

1 Introduction

Embodied conversational agents (ECAs) (Cassell, 2007) have changed the way humans interact with virtual environments and software products. In this paper, to help guide design and development of ECAs, we review the evolving qualities of naturalistic agents by identifying and tracking their most relevant features. In our study, we examined what qualities make a more naturalistic agent by assessing ECAs from video games based on their visual appearance and their functionality. We then assigned weights to the most important capabilities and compared 15 representative ECAs.

The qualities of embodied conversational agents have been analyzed independently (e.g., Pelachaud, 2005; Isbister & Doyle, 2002), but our review did not disclose a comparison of these qualities that developed a comprehensive set of guidelines for evaluation across agents. Existing rubrics include perception domain (context-related), interaction domain (turn-taking), and generation domain (display of expressive synchronized visual and acoustic behaviors) (Pelachaud, 2005). A proposed taxonomy of "Design and Evaluation of Embodied Conversational Agents" suggested measures for describing and evaluating ECAs (Isbister & Doyle, 2002). However, some of the measures were subjective or non-quantifiable, and no agents were evaluated. We propose an improved taxonomy that adds quantitative categories, and we use the taxonomy to evaluate a set of representative agents. Our taxonomy groups the features into two categories, visual and functional. In applying the taxonomy, we weight feature scores to reflect the features' importance and to account for composite features that can only exist in conjunction with others.

T. Bickmore et al. (Eds.): IVA 2014, LNAI 8637, pp. 95–98, 2014.
© Springer International Publishing Switzerland 2014

2   Methodology

We look first at the visual features of ECAs. We identified five key visual features: human likeness, realism, facial expressions, first vs. third person, and motion. Second, we look at the functional features of ECAs. We identified eight key functional features: non-scripted dialogue, verbal communication, level of interaction, group social skills, artificial intelligence level, environment interaction, persona, and nonverbal reaction.

Some agents had been updated across different versions of the games and others remained the same. For example, the agent Navi from the game "The Legend of Zelda" remained constant from its first incarnation at the game's release in 1998 through its last release in 2012. As different versions of the game were released, the agent's characteristics (and our assessment of the agent's realism) did not change. The first version of Navi apparently served its purpose and did not require updates of its appearance or functionality. Other agents were updated. For instance, the agent Cortana from the videogame "Halo" has had several appearance updates that increased her quality as an agent, becoming more realistic in her looks. In considering Cortana, we evaluated both the original and updated versions.

We applied our taxonomy of characteristics to 15 ECAs; the agents selected are presented in Figures 1 and 2. We chose agents based on how representative they were in their specific genre and whether they represented milestones in the game industry when they were introduced. Our evaluation of an ECA was based on our personal experiences of interacting with it and, when an ECA was not available for personal gameplay, on recorded gameplay. The games we were able to play were played in their entirety to provide a full basis for judging agents' quality. We also considered reviews by game critics and the consensus from players generally. From our 8 key visual and 15 key functional features, we developed a qualities rubric. Agents with scores of 5 for the visual features and 8 for the functional features, for a total of 13 points, would represent the highest-quality, most naturalistic agent.

3   Results

Figure 1 presents a scatter plot for the 15 agents in terms of their visual and functional scores, with the points in plot coded by color for the year the agent was originally released. Darker colors represent more recently released agents. Figure 2 presents a similar scatter plot for the agents in their latest release.

We calculated the mean visual, functional and total scores for the agents' original and latest versions. Bearing in mind that the evaluated agents do not represent a random sample of the population of commercial ECAs, we note that the agents, on average, improved modestly in visual, functional, and total quality. This improvement, though, came entirely from 3 of the 15 agents: Cortana, Glados, and Milo had a mean increase in score of 0.92 points, while the other agents had no increase in score.

To determine whether the quality of an agent was a function of its year of release, we calculated the correlations between the visual, functional and total scores and the years of original release and latest release. For the agents as originally released, the data suggest that agent quality—visually, functionally, and overall—has increased over time as new agents were developed. That is, newer agents tend to be better agents. But for the agents in their latest versions, there appears to be no significant relationship between quality and time, probably because most recent releases of all but three of the agents were basically the same as their original versions.

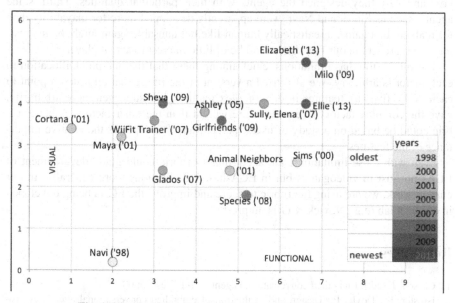

Fig. 1. Visual and functional scores of agents' original version

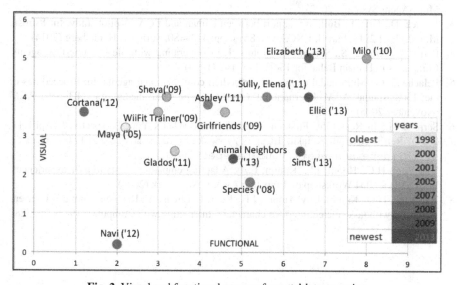

Fig. 2. Visual and functional scores of agents' latest version

Our analysis is subject to several limitations. First, the choice of agents was personal, reflecting the our impressions of game genres and of development milestones for ECAs. The agents we analyzed likely do not represent a true cross-section of ECAs. Indeed, defining such a cross-section would be difficult. A wider range of agents could have presented a fuller picture of characteristics of agents in video games. Second, we did not contact the agents' developers to obtain explanations of how and why they designed the agents with their particular qualities. Third, some agents, such as Sheva and Navi, were apparently developed more for playability than for realism. In a game, a realistically human-like but unusable agent might be interesting to researchers in our field but would be of little interest to actual players.

The rubric, too, has limitations, chief among these that the one-point allocation to each factor is arbitrary. We also tried a version of the rubric that allocated a point to each of the five sub-features in the complex features, but this, even more arbitrarily, gave the complex factors five times more weight than the other factors. A better rubric could be based on a study of users' perceptions that explores the relative importance of the features.

Even with these limitations, the agent-quality rubric could guide development of ECAs not just in videogames but in ECA-based applications more generally. In our current work, we are using the rubric to score and improve the ECAs being developed in our own lab (e.g., Novick & Gris, in press).

References

1. Cassell, J. (ed.): Embodied conversational agents. MIT Press (2000)
2. Isbister, K., Doyle, P.: Design and evaluation of embodied conversational agents: A proposed taxonomy. In: The First International Joint Conference on Autonomous Agents & Multi-Agent Systems (2002)
3. Novick, D., Gris, I.: Building rapport between human and ECA: A pilot study. In: Kurosu, M. (ed.) HCI 2014, Part II. LNCS, vol. 8511, pp. 472–480. Springer, Heidelberg (2014)
4. Parise, S., Kiesler, S., Sproull, L., Waters, K.: Cooperating with life-like interface agents. Computers in Human Behavior 15(2), 123–142 (1999)
5. Pelachaud, C.: Multimodal expressive embodied conversational agents. In: Proceedings of the 13th Annual ACM International Conference on Multimedia, pp. 683–689. ACM (November 2005)
6. Serrels, M.: In Real Life: First Or Third Person - What's Your Perspective? (April 18, 2011), Retrieved from Kotaku: http://www.kotaku.com.au/2011/04/first-or-third-person-whats-your-perspective/
7. Van Vugt, H.C., Hoorn, J.F., Konijn, E.A.: Adapting empathic agents to user experiences. In: AAMAS 2004 Workshop on Empathic Agents, New York (2004)
8. Van Vugt, H.C., Konijn, E.A., Hoorn, J.F., Keur, I., Eliéns, A.: Realism is not all! User engagement with task-related interface characters. Interacting with Computers 19(2), 267–280 (2007)

Motion Parameterization and Adaptation Strategies for Virtual Therapists

Carlo Camporesi[1], Anthony Popelar[1], Marcelo Kallmann[1], and Jay Han[2]

[1] School of Engineering, University of California Merced, USA
[2] Department of Physical Medicine and Rehabilitation,
University of California Davis, USA

Abstract. We propose in this paper new techniques for correction and parameterization of motion capture sequences containing upper-body exercises for physical therapy. By relying on motion capture sequences we allow therapists to easily record new patient-customized exercises intuitively by direct demonstration. The proposed correction and parameterization techniques allow the modification of recorded sequences in order to 1) correct and modify properties such as alignments and constraints, 2) customize prescribed exercises by modifying parameterized properties such as speed, wait times and exercise amplitudes, and 3) to achieve real-time adaptation by monitoring user performances and updating the parameters of each exercise for improving the therapy delivery. The proposed techniques allow autonomous virtual therapists to improve the whole therapy process, from exercise definition to delivery.

Keywords: virtual therapists, motion capture, virtual humans.

1 Introduction

The motivation of this work is to improve the usability of virtual humans serving as virtual therapists autonomously delivering physical therapy exercises to patients. We focus on the problem of automatic correction and parameterization of motion capture sequences defining upper-body exercises. Customized exercises per patient can be intuitively recorded from therapists by direct demonstration using the Kinect sensor or any other suitable motion capture device. Given a captured exercise, we propose correction and parameterization techniques that allow 1) fine-tuning of key characteristics of the exercise such as alignments and constraints, 2) customization of the exercises by modifying parameterized properties such as speed, wait times and amplitudes, and 3) real-time adaptation by monitoring user performances and updating exercise parameters in order to improve therapy delivery.

The presented techniques greatly facilitate the process of defining exercises by demonstration, allowing the customization of exercises to specific patients. We focus on providing parameterization while at the same time reproducing, to the desired degree, any small imperfections that are captured in the motion in order to maintain the humanlike behavior of the virtual therapist during therapy delivery. As a result the proposed methods produce realistic continuous motions

T. Bickmore et al. (Eds.): IVA 2014, LNAI 8637, pp. 99–108, 2014.

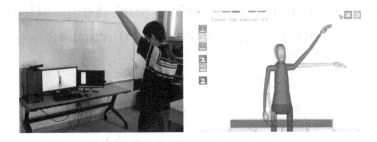

Fig. 1. Illustration of the system being used in practice

that can adapt to user responses in order to improve the overall experience of performing the exercises.

2   Related Work

The use of new technologies to overcome the limitations of standard approaches to physiotherapy is becoming increasingly popular. A typical approach in some applications is to track user movements while a virtual character displays the exercises to be executed. The representations of the user and virtual trainer are usually displayed side by side or superimposed to display motion differences, improving the learning process and the understanding of the movements [5,16].

Automated systems often allow parameterization capabilities. For instance, Lange et al. [7] describe core elements that a VR-based intervention should address, indicating that clinicians and therapists have critical roles to play and VR systems are tools that must reflect their decisions in terms of a person's ability to interact with a system, types of tasks, rates of progression, etc [8,4].

The key benefit of adopting a programming by demonstration approach is to allow the intuitive definition of new exercises as needed. The overall approach has been adopted in many areas [2,14,10], and it involves the need to automatically process captured motions according to the goals of the system.

Velloso et al. [15] propose a system that extracts a movement model from a demonstrated motion to then provide high-level feedback during delivery, however without motion adaptation to the user performances. The YouMove system [1] trains the user through a series of stages while providing guidance, however also not incorporating motion adaptation to the user performances.

We propose new motion processing approaches to achieve adaptive motions that are both controllable and realistic. While motion blending techniques with motion capture data [12,6,11,2] provide powerful interpolation-based approaches for parameterizing motions, they require the definition of several motion examples in order to achieve parameterization. In contrast our proposed techniques are simple and are designed to provide parameterization of a given single exercise motion. We rely both on structural knowledge of exercises and on generic constraint detection techniques, such as detection of fixed points [9,13] and motion processing with Principal Component Analysis (PCA) [3].

3   Detection of Constraints and Parameterizations

Given a new exercise motion demonstrated to the system, the system will analyze the motion and detect the parameterizations that can be employed. An input motion is represented as a collection of frames $M_i, i \in \{1, \ldots, n\}$, where each frame M_i is a vector containing the position and the joint angles that define one posture of the character in time.

3.1   Detection of Geometrical Constraints

Our constraint detection mechanism is designed for three specific purposes: to inform motion parameterization, to help correcting artifacts and noise in the motions, and to provide metrics for quantifying motion compliance. The metrics are used to provide visual feedback to the user, to inform the correctness of per-formed motions, to make decisions during the real-time adaptation mechanism, and to achieve an overall user performance score for each session.

Appropriate constraints are not constraints which are to be absolutely fol-lowed. Recorded motions may have unintended movements and imperfections introduced by the capture system. Constraints must be detected despite these fluctuations, and should be softly enforced so the motion can be made to look correct and also natural.

We analyze the position in space of a specific joint with respect to a frame of reference F which can be placed at any ancestor joint in the skeleton structure. The detection framework can accommodate any desired type of constraint but in this paper we focus on two types of constraints: Point and Planar.

- A Point Constraint (Fig-ure 2) describes a child joint that is static relative to its parent. Let's $P_i, i \in \{l, \ldots, k\}$ be the cloud of points formed by a joint tra-jectory with respect to a lo-cal frame F generated by re-sampling linearly the motion frames with constant frame rate. The standard deviation of the cloud of points σ is calculated and subsequently checked against a specific threshold α. When the condi-tion is met the current joint

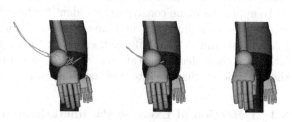

Fig. 2. Point Constraint. The yellow sphere repre-sents the detection of a point constraint at the elbow joint. From left to right: the wrist motion trajectory (depicted in green) is corrected to the mean point with 0%, 50%, and 100% correction.

is marked as a point constraint and it is represented by the specific point located at the mean μ. When a point constraint is detected the ancestor(s) can be then adjusted to enforce the constraint.

• A Plane Constraint (Figure 3) detects if a joint moves approximately within a plane. Similarly to the point constraint detection a point cloud is first generated. Then, PCA is applied to the set of points to determine a proper orthogonal decomposition considering the resulting Eigenspace from the covariance. A planar surface is then re-

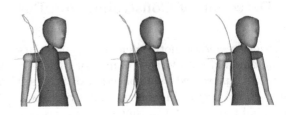

Fig. 3. Plane Constraint. The blue axis is the normal direction of the detected plane constraint affecting the shoulder joint. From left to right: correction level (from 0% to 100%) where the elbow trajectory (green trajectories) is gradually collapsed into a plane.

trieved considering the two Eigenvectors with higher Eigenvalue λ (the magnitude of λ is used to validate the plane). The average distance of the points from this plane is then checked against a threshold β to determine if a plane constraint is appropriate for the given joint.

3.2   Geometrical Constraint Alignment

Let i be the index of the frame currently evaluated. Let p_i be the position in space of the current joint and q_i be a quaternion representing the current local orientation. A point constraint is defined considering the orientation q_m in the local orientation frame that represents the vector defined by the local point constraint. A point constraint is enforced through spherical linear interpolation between q_i and q_m. Figure 2 shows the trajectories generated by the wrist joint collapsing into a point constraint.

To apply the plane constraint, we identify the orientation defined by the projection of each point p_i to the plane discovered during the detection phase. The plane constraint is then enforced, similarly to the point constraint, by interpolating the equivalent orientations. Figure 3 shows the trajectories generated by the elbow joint aligning into a plane constraint.

3.3   Detection of Exercise Parameterization

Consider a typical shoulder flexion exercise where the arm is raised until it reaches the vertical position or more (initial phase); subsequently the arm is hold for a few seconds (hold phase) and then it relaxes back to a rest position (return phase). This is the type of exercise that we seek to parameterize.

The analysis procedure makes the following assumptions: a) each motion M represents one cycle of a cyclic arm exercise; b) the first frame of a motion contains a posture representing the starting point of the exercise; c) the exercise will have distinct phases: the initial phase (M_{init}) is when the arm moves from the initial posture towards a posture of maximum exercise amplitude, then the exercise may or not have a hold phase (M_{hold}) but at some point the exercise

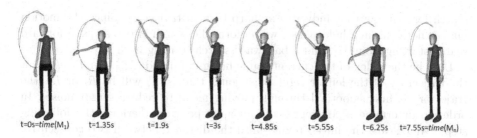

t=0s=*time(M₁)*   t=1.35s   t=1.9s   t=3s   t=4.85s   t=5.55s   t=6.25s   t=7.55s=*time(Mₙ)*

Fig. 4. Example of a typical exercise captured from a therapist in one of our tests with the system. The shown trajectory is the trajectory of the right wrist joint along the entire motion. The initial phase happens between t=0s and t=3s. Then, between t=3s and t=4.85s there is a hold phase at maximum amplitude where the therapist is static (but small posture variations are always noticeable). Then, between t=4.85s and t=7.55s we can observe the return phase.

must enter the return phase (M_{end}), where the exercise returns to a posture similar to the starting posture. In addition, if the motion contains a hold phase at the point of maximum amplitude, it will mean that an approximately static pose of some duration (the hold phase duration) exists at the maximum amplitude point. We also consider an optional 4th phase that can be added to any exercise, the wait phase (M_{wait}), which is an optional period of time where the character just waits in its rest pose before performing a new repetition of the exercise. Figure 4 illustrates a typical exercise that fits our assumptions.

The analysis if the exercise can be parameterized has two main steps: first the arm to be parameterized is detected; and then the two *motion apices* are detected. The apices, or the points of maximum amplitude, are the intersection points between the initial and return phases with the hold phase (frames $t = 3s$ and $t = 4.85$ in Figure 4). These points will be a single apex point if the motion has no hold phase in it. If the phases above are executed successfully the input motion is segmented in initial, return and an optional hold phase, and the motion can be parameterized.

In order to detect which arm to parameterize we extract the global positions of the left and right wrists along their trajectories. Let L_i and R_i respectively denote these positions. Since our focus is on arm exercises the wrist represents an obvious distal joint of the arm kinematic chain to use in our parameterization analysis algorithm. For each wrist trajectory L and R we compute the 3D bounding box of the 3D trajectory. The bounding box dimension is used to determine which arm is moving and if the motion can be parameterized. As a result of this process, the analysis will return one of the following four options: a) the motion cannot be parameterized; b) the motion will be parameterized by the left/right arm; or d) the motion will be parameterized by both arms (targeting symmetrical exercises).

4   Exercise Parameterization

If the motion can be parameterized and its type is determined, we then search the motion for the points of maximum amplitude. To detect one apex point we search for a frame that indicates a sharp turn in trajectory. Since the motion may or not contain a hold phase, we perform the search in two steps: a forward search starting from M_1, and a backward search starting from M_n.

Let i be the index of the current frame being evaluated (M_i). Let T represent the trajectory of the left or right wrist joint, that is, T_i will be R_i or L_i (the trajectory is first smoothed through moving mean to reduce sensor noise). In order to determine if M_i represents an apex point we perform the following steps. We discard the initial points until the distance between two consecutive points becomes greater than a specific threshold d_t (a threshold of 5cm worked well in practice). We first compute the incoming and outgoing direction vectors with respect to T_i, respectively: $a = T_i - T_{i-1}$, and $b = T_{i+1} - T_i$. If a or b is a null vector, that means we are in a stationary pose and we therefore skip frame M_i and no apex is detected at position i. Otherwise, the angle α between vectors a and b is computed and used to determine if there is a sharp change in direction at position i. If α is greater than a threshold angle, frame i is considered a probable apex point, otherwise we skip and proceed with the search. We are using a threshold of 75 degrees and this value has worked well in all our examples with clear detections achieved. To mark an apex to be definitive we consider the distance between the following k frames to be less than d_t.

The test described above is first employed for finding the first apex point by searching forward all frames (starting from the first frame). The first apex found is called Apex 1 and its frame index is denoted as a_1. If no apex is found the

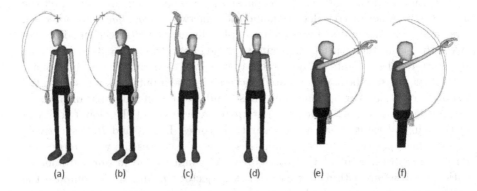

(a)   (b)   (c)   (d)   (e)   (f)

Fig. 5. The red trajectory shows the initial phase M_{init}. The blue trajectory shows the return phase M_{ret}. The input motion is the same as Figure 4. (a) The full (100%) amplitude of the input motion is shown by the trajectories. Two black crosses at the end of the trajectories (in almost identical positions) mark the positions of Apex 1 and Apex 2. (b) The two black crosses now mark the maximum amplitude points in the initial and return trajectories at 75% amplitude. (c,d) In this frontal view it is possible to notice that the postures at 75% amplitude in the initial and return phases are different. The hold phase will start by holding the posture shown in (c), and when the hold phase is over, we blend into the return motion at the posture shown in (d) in order to produce a smooth transition into the return phase. (e,f) Lateral view.

motion cannot be parameterized. If Apex 1 is successfully found, then the search is employed backwards starting from the last frame, however not allowing passing beyond Apex 1. The second apex found is called Apex 2 (a_2). Note that Apex 2 may be the same as Apex 1, in which case no holding phase is present in the input motion. After the described analysis, the main three portions of the motion have been detected: a) the initial phase is defined by frames $\{1, 2, \ldots, a_1\}$ (motion segment M_{init}); b) the hold phase is defined by frames $\{a_1, a_1 + 1, \ldots, a_2\}$, if $a_2 > a_1$, and nonexistent otherwise; and c) the return phase is defined by frames $\{a_2, a_2 + 1, \ldots, n\}$ (motion segment M_{ret}). Once an input motion M is successfully segmented, it can then be parameterized.

Amplitude and Hold Phase Parameterization. We parameterize amplitude in terms of a percentage of the wrist trajectory: 100% means that the full amplitude observed in the input motion M is to be preserved, if 80% is given then the produced parameterized motion should go into hold or return phase when 80% of the original amplitude is reached, and so on. Let h be the time duration in seconds of the desired hold duration. When the target amplitude is reached, the posture at the target amplitude is maintained for the given duration h of the desired hold phase. When the hold phase ends, the posture is blended into the return motion M_{ret} at the current amplitude point towards the final frame of M_{ret}. See Figure 5. The described operations are enough to achieve a continuous parameterized motion, however two undesired effects may happen: a noticeable abrupt stop of M_{init} or an unnatural start of M_{ret}, because the parameterization may suddenly blend motions to transition at points with some significant velocity. To correct this we re-time the segments so that motion phases always exhibit ease-in or ease-out profiles.

Behavior During Hold and Wait Phases. In order to improve the realism, we add a small oscillatory spine movement mimicking a breathing motion, which is applied to spine joints during the hold and wait phases. One particular problem that is addressed here is to produce an oscillatory motion that ends with no contribution to the original pose at the end of the oscillation period. This is needed so that, after the oscillation period, the motion can naturally continue towards its next phase and without additional blending operations. We thus have to produce oscillations of controlled amplitude and period. This is accomplished with the following function: $f(t) = d \sin(t\pi/d)$, if $d < 1$, and $\sin(t\pi/(d/floor(d)))$ otherwise; where $d > 0$ is the duration of the oscillation period, which in our case will be the duration of the hold or wait periods.

At the beginning of a hold or wait phase we save the joint angles of the spine in a vector s, and then apply to the spine joints the values of $s + cf(t)$, where $t \in [0, d]$, and c is an amplitude constant. We obtained good behavior with $c = 0.007$, and only operating on one degree of freedom of two spine joints: one near the root of the character hierarchy, and one about the center of the torso. The used degree of freedom is the one that produces rotations on the sagittal plane of the character. The achieved breathing behavior can be observed in the video accompanying this paper.

Overall Parameterization. The described procedures allow us to parameterize an input motion M with respect to up to four parameters: amplitude a (in percentage), hold time h (in seconds), wait time w (in seconds), and speed s (as a multiplier to the original time parameterization). Given a set of parameters (a, h, w, s), the input motion can be prepared for parameterization very efficiently and then, during execution of the parameterized motion, only trivial blending operations are performed in real-time.

5   Real-Time Adaptation

When the adaptation mechanism is enabled the system collects information from the patient's performance in real-time and adapts the current exercise in its next repetition. In addition, visual feedback is also provided: arrows showing direction of correction for improving motion compliance, constraint violation feedback and also an overall performance score with explanatory text (see Figure 6).

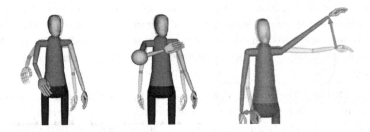

Fig. 6. The red character displays the user's motion and the blue one the target exercise. Left: no violated constraints. Center: user is reminded to correct the elbow. Right: arrows show direction of correction to improve compliance.

Four types of adaptation mechanisms are provided:

• **Amplitude Adaptation** The range can vary from 75% to 100% of the target amplitude. The system tracks the distance between the patient's active end-effector and the apex at the target amplitude position. If the minimum distance is larger than the amplitude compliance parameter specified by the therapist, the next exercise execution will have the target amplitude lowered to become within the compliance range. If in a subsequent repetition the user reaches the current (reduced) target amplitude, then the next target amplitude will be increased towards the original target amplitude.

• **Hold Time** The hold phase adaptation is designed to adapt the time at hold stance to improve resistance, usually in a posture that becomes difficult to maintain over time. The maximum distance between the target hold point and the performed end-effector position is computed. If above a threshold, the patient is having difficulty in maintaining the posture and the next exercise repetition will have a shorter hold phase duration. If in a subsequent repetition the patient is able to well maintain the hold posture, then the hold duration is gradually increased back to its previous value.

• **Speed Execution** During patient monitoring, the active position of the patient's end-effector is tracked and its distance to the demonstrated exercise end-effector is computed for every frame. If the average distance computed across the entire exercise is above a given trajecory compliance threshold (see Figure 7), the next exercise execution speed is decreased. If in a subsequent repetition the difference is under the threshold the speed will be gradually adjusted back.

• **Wait-Time Between Exercises** The initial wait time specified by the therapist is decreased or increased in order to allow the patient to have an appropriate time to rest between exercises. A performance metric based on averaging the trajectory compliance and the hold phase completion metrics is used to determine how well the patient is being able to follow an exercise. If the user is well performing the exercises a shorter wait time is selected, otherwise a longer wait time is preferred. In this way wait times are related to the experienced difficulty in each exercise, and they adapt to specific individuals and progress rates.

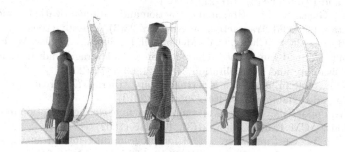

Fig. 7. From left to right: high, medium and low trajectory compliance

6 Results and Conclusions

The described algorithms have been tested for constraint detection and motion parameterization with a variety of arm exercises and different users. The obtained results were always as expected, within reasonable compliance with the defined exercise structure. All presented methods are very efficient for real-time computation. While this paper focuses on motion processing techniques, the described adaptation strategies have been specified from many discussions with therapists according to their needs while experimenting with our prototype system. Many variations and adjustments are possible, a final version will only be determined after the system and its several features are evaluated in practice. A supplemental video is available to demonstrate the obtained results. In summary, we present contributions on new motion processing approaches for single motion parameterization, and as well on novel strategies for motion adaptation to users during real-time exercise delivery.

Acknowledgments. This work was partially supported by NSF Award CNS-1305196 and by a HSRI San Joaquin Valley eHealth Network seed grant funded by AT&T.

References

1. Anderson, F., Grossman, T., Matejka, J., Fitzmaurice, G.W.: YouMove: enhancing movement training with an augmented reality mirror. In: Proceedings of User Interface Software and Technology (UIST), pp. 311–320. ACM (2013)
2. Camporesi, C., Huang, Y., Kallmann, M.: Interactive motion modeling and parameterization by direct demonstration. In: Allbeck, J., Badler, N., Bickmore, T., Pelachaud, C., Safonova, A. (eds.) IVA 2010. LNCS (LNAI), vol. 6356, pp. 77–90. Springer, Heidelberg (2010)
3. Glardon, P., Boulic, R., Thalmann, D.: A coherent locomotion engine extrapolating beyond experimental data. In: Proceedings of Computer Animation and Social Agent, pp. 73–84 (2004)
4. Grealy, M., Nasser, B.: The use of virtual reality in assisting rehabilitation. Advances in Clinical Neuroscience and Rehabilitation 13(9), 19–20 (2013)
5. Holden, M.K.: Virtual environments for motor rehabilitation: review. Cyberpsichology and Behavior 8(3), 187–211 (2005)
6. Kovar, L., Gleicher, M.: Automated extraction and parameterization of motions in large data sets. ACM Transaction on Graphics 23(3), 559–568 (2004)
7. Lange, B., Koenig, S., Chang, C.Y., McConnell, E., Suma, E., Bolas, M., Rizzo, A.: Designing informed game-based rehabilitation tasks leveraging advances in virtual reality. Disability and Rehabilitation 34(22), 1863–1870 (2012)
8. Levac, D.E., Galvin, J.: When is virtual reality "therapy?". Archives of Physical Medicine and Rehabilitation 94(4), 795–798 (2013)
9. Liu, C.K., Popović, Z.: Synthesis of complex dynamic character motion from simple animations. ACM Trans. Graph. 21(3), 408–416 (2002)
10. Lü, H., Li, Y.: Gesture coder: a tool for programming multi-touch gestures by demonstration. In: Proceedings of the 2012 ACM Annual Conference on Human Factors in Computing Systems, pp. 2875–2884. ACM (2012)
11. Ma, W., Xia, S., Hodgins, J.K., Yang, X., Li, C., Wang, Z.: Modeling style and variation in human motion. In: Proceedings of the ACM SIGGRAPH/Eurographics Symposium on Computer Animation, SCA (2010)
12. RoseIII, C.F., Sloan, P.P.J., Cohen, M.F.: Artist-directed inverse-kinematics using radial basis function interpolation. Computer Graphics Forum (Proceedings of Eurographics) 20(3), 239–250 (2001)
13. Salvati, M., Le Callennec, B., Boulic, R.: A Generic Method for Geometric Contraints Detection. In: Eurographics (2004)
14. Skoglund, A., Iliev, B., Palm, R.: Programming-by-demonstration of reaching motions - a next-state-planner approach. Robotics and Aut. Systems 58(5) (2010)
15. Velloso, E., Bulling, A., Gellersen, H.: Motionma: Motion modelling and analysis by demonstration. In: Proceedings of the SIGCHI Conference on Human Factors in Computing Systems, CHI 2013, pp. 1309–1318. ACM, New York (2013)
16. Wollersheim, D., Merkes, M., Shields, N., Liamputtong, P., Wallis, L., Reynolds, F., Koh, L.: Physical and psychosocial effects of Wii video game use among older women. Intl Journal of Emerging Technologies and Society 8(2), 85–98 (2010)

Corpus Creation and Perceptual Evaluation of Expressive Theatrical Gestures

Pamela Carreno-Medrano, Sylvie Gibet,
Caroline Larboulette, and Pierre-François Marteau

Université de Bretagne Sud, IRISA, Bâtiment ENSIBS,
F-56017 Vannes, France
{Pamela.Carreno-Medrano,Sylvie.Gibet,Caroline.Larboulette,
Pierre-Francois.Marteau}@irisa.fr

Abstract. While human communication involves rich, complex and expressive gestures, available corpora of captured motions used for the animation of virtual characters contain actions ranging from locomotion to everyday life motions. We aim at creating a novel corpus of expressive and meaningful gestures, and we focus on body movements and gestures involved in theatrical scenarios. In this paper we propose a methodology for building a corpus of full-body theatrical gestures based on a magician show enriched with affective content.

We then validate the constructed corpus of theatrical gestures and sequences through several perceptual studies focusing on the complexity of the produced movements as well as the recognizability of the additional affective content.

1 Introduction

Gestures and movements are increasingly exploited in advanced interactive systems populated with virtual agents. Application domains include entertainment, pedagogy and artistic performance. However, while human-to-human communication involves rich, complex and expressive gestures, often linked to verbal languages [11], available corpora of captured motion used for virtual characters usually comprise actions such as locomotion or everyday life motions, but not a large range of examples of expressive gestures.

Our aim is to study these so-called expressive gestures, i.e., gestures conveying some meaningful information and *expressive content*. Expressive content refers to aspects of motion related to feelings, moods, affect, or intensity of emotional experience. Analysis of expressive content has been conducted for artistic performances [4], everyday actions such as knocking or drinking [19], and interactive embodied conversational agents [17]. More specifically, we focus on theatrical gestures because they have to constantly and deliberately attract attention and use body language to express some meaningful scenarios with an emotional intent [12]. We are also interested in the spatio-temporal properties of those gestures, as we make the assumption that they have a richer and enhanced kinematics compared to everyday life actions.

T. Bickmore et al. (Eds.): IVA 2014, LNAI 8637, pp. 109–119, 2014.

In this paper we propose a methodology for designing a corpus of theatrical gestures in the context of three magic tricks. Experiments have been defined to carry out perceptual evaluations in order to select and characterize relevant gestures and their expressiveness for further analysis and synthesis studies.

The outline of the paper is as follows: section 2 briefly summarizes the existing expressive and non-expressive motion capture databases. Sec. 3 describes the composition and the capture protocol of the theatrical mocap corpus we propose. Sec. 4 describes the perceptual evaluations used to validate our corpus and protocol. Finally Sec. 5 summarizes our contributions.

2   Related Work

Different motion capture databases have been designed to study human behavior. Among them, we can identify those publicly available and largely used by the academic research community for motion analysis, recognition, or synthesis: the HDM05 database [16] provided by the Max Planck Institute, the CMU database provided by the Carnegie-Mellon University [5], and the UTA database provided by the University of Texas at Arlington [24]. These databases comprise a wide range of mocap data from diverse categories including locomotion, sport activities, and everyday life motions.

Even though these databases are useful for analyzing the social and relational behaviors of virtual agents, they lack of expressive data carrying information about the meaning conveyed by body movements [6] and the expressive content. Recently, an increased interest for expressive variations of body movements has led to the design and construction of affective motion capture databases. Among them, two categories may be considered: *i.) Portrayed emotional gestures*, where expressions are produced by actors upon instructions. This category consists of explicit affective archetype gestures where the subjects are instructed to perform short actions or adopt postures that explicitly represent a given emotion [10], [23]. *ii.) Induced emotional expressions occurring in a controlled setting*. In this category we find databases recorded for emotional dance studies, used either for emotion detection [18] or style synthesis [22], and databases used for emotion recognition [3], [13]. Our research objectives belong to the latter. More specifically, we focus on full-body gestures and their varying forms in theatrical scenarios. The gestures are regarded as actions that manifest deliberate expressiveness induced by the emotional state of the actors.

3   Building the Corpus of Expressive Theatrical Gestures

When designing our expressive gesture corpus, we started by defining a theatrical context. A motion lexicon was defined as well as sequences of actions following a meaningful body language associated to a narrative scenario. In this section, we present the reasons that form the basis of our work and describe the selected theatrical scenario.

3.1   Motivation

Identifying and producing *expressive gestures*, i.e., body movements carrying expression, meaning and intent, can be a highly subjective and context-dependent process. Gestures that are meaningful for one observer in a given situation can also be considered movements with no expression by a different observer.

When looking for possible sources of widely known *expressive gestures*, the performing arts (theater, dance, magic, mime, etc.) are a good starting point [12] since they aim at expressing emotions and thoughts through different means (e.g. body, voice, objects). As our primary interest is full-body motion as a medium for expressing affect and meaning, we propose a mime theatrical scenario where stories, ideas, and feelings can be solely conveyed by bodily movements [8].

In addition to providing a new source of expressive gestures in a mime theater context, we also aim to provide a new motion capture dataset that will be useful for research in human motion analysis, recognition and synthesis. This goal has strongly influenced many of the decisions that will be presented in this section.

3.2   Selected Scenario and Gestures

We propose a mime theatrical scenario based on a magician performance. The reasons behind this choice of context are threefold. Firstly, by constraining the actors to portray ideas, emotions and meanings through their body only, we expect they will perform gestures for which the main purpose is to be seen and understood by the whole audience. We assume that those gestures will carry more information and thus involve a higher kinematic and dynamic complexity [12].

Secondly, classical mime performances use bodily movements and facial expressions to portray a character and his emotions [2]. As we are solely interested in body, we need a scenario in which everything has to be shown through hand and body motions. Lastly, a magician is an artist of misdirection. He must thus master and use his entire body to mislead the senses of the spectator while performing [9], [14]. Therefore, we consider it an interesting trial case for the kind of scenario we are looking for.

We developed a scenario in which a magician will perform 3 magic tricks: *the disappearing box, pulling a rabbit from a hat*, and *appearing scarves in an empty jacket*. Each magic trick involves 3 stages: *i) Introduction:* the magician makes his appearance and introduces him-self to the audience. *ii) Preparation:* the magician shows each object he is going to use in his magic trick to the public. This stage ends when the magician invokes his magical powers. *iii) Conclusion:* the magician shows the result of his trick and makes a bow to the audience. In total the proposed scenario has 3 sequences consisting of 17 isolated gestures.

3.3   Expressive Variations

As stated before, we think that the gestures in our scenario are spatially and temporally more significant, because they must convey meaning, emotion and intent through bodily movements. In order to enhance this kinematic diversity, it is possible to introduce new sources of variation into the corpus by taking into account the style, personality and emotional state of the actor. Although we cannot directly influence the style and personality of the actor, we think that it is possible to elicit certain emotional responses that will produce additional spatio-temporal characteristics. Those characteristics may affect the spatiality, the timing, or the fluidity of the performed gestures. Thus, through eliciting different emotions in the performance of the actor we can increase the diversity and expressive richness of the proposed scenario and corpus. A set of 4 emotional states was chosen using the circumplex model of affect proposed by Russell [21]: *happy, sad, stress, and relaxed*. A *neutral* state was added to categorize the motions in which no emotion was intended.

3.4   Experimental Motion Capture Protocol

To produce a new motion capture database that can be used for the analysis, recognition and synthesis of expressive gestures, special care must be given to the number and variety of recorded gestures and sequences.

Technical Setup: the understandability and expressiveness of gestures require accuracy and high definition in the recording of captured motion. A Qualisys motion capture system composed of 8 Oqus400 cameras [20] was used. All full-body actions and hand movements inside a 2.5mx2mx2m volume were recorded. A total of 64 passive markers were placed on the body of the actor including 5 markers on each hand and 2 facial markers. The markers on the hands enabled capturing all the grasping movements involved in a magic performance, and the facial markers gave a more accurate idea of the direction of the head of the actor. We used a 200Hz capture frequency to correctly capture hand motion, since this kind of motion requires a higher accuracy.

Number of Actors and Repetitions: for the analysis and recognition of human motion, numerous repetitions of a set of actions performed by several subjects are needed. Each magic trick was recorded twice per emotional state. In addition, the most representative gestures (8 in total) were selected among the initial 17. For each selected gesture, 2 sequences of 5 repetitions per emotional state were recorded. Currently, our database contains the motions of 2 skilled amateur actors (1 man and 1 woman). For each actor, 110 motion capture files were produced. We intend to further record 8 additional actors.

Emotion Elicitation: another challenge concerns how the instructions for performing the scenario are given to the actor and how the emotional state is induced. First, a video of each magic trick was presented to the actors the day before the capture. This made possible for the actors to learn the gestures and perform more fluently. Second, on the day of the capture, the actors were asked to perform each magic trick several times before we started to record. By doing so, we could correct all possible doubts about how each gesture should be performed. Last, an emotional state was randomly chosen and the emotion elicitation was done using an imagination mood induction procedure. During the elicitation process, each actor was instructed to remember an emotional event in their lives that corresponded to the selected emotion. After performing the whole scenario, i.e., the 3 sequences plus the 8 isolated gestures in a given emotional state, a debriefing was done to re-establish the initial emotional state of the actor

4   Experiments and Results

Three perceptual experiments were performed to validate the suitability of the chosen scenario, and the effectiveness and efficiency of our experimental motion capture protocol. The experimental setup also enabled evaluating the usability of the produced mocap data for tasks such as motion analysis, motion recognition and motion synthesis. We were aiming to answer the following questions:

1. Do people perceive theatrical gestures as being more kinematically and dynamically significant than daily actions? Do people perceive theatrical gestures as motions conveying more information?

2. Can observers associate the spatio-temporal variations introduced through the elicitation of emotional states to one of the five selected emotions? If they can do so, how expressive do they find the theatrical gestures?

4.1   Stimuli Creation

For the theatrical gestures, 1 realization for 8 theatrical gestures and for 2 magic tricks were chosen per emotion and per actor. Additionally, the actors were asked to perform 8 daily actions that we consider are the most frequently found in available mocap databases (cf. Table 1 for a list of the chosen stimuli).

Table 1. Stimuli used for the perceptual evaluations

Daily gestures	Theatrical gestures	Sequences
Lifting	Show empty jacket	The disappearing box
Waving	Take scarves out of jacket	Scarves appear in a jacket
Kicking	Invoke magic with wand	
Hand shake	Show box disappeared	
Walking	Cover box	
Knocking	Invoke magic with hand	
Throwing	Introduction bow	
Punching	Final bow	

All stimuli were played on a of point-light like character (cf. Figure 1). We chose this kind of representation as we did not want to convey any additional information about the avatar's gender and appearance that might influence the categorization of the selected emotions. Additionally, previous studies have shown that this type of representation does not stop observers from perceiving any emotional state at any intensity [1], [15].

For the theatrical gestures and the daily actions, individual video clips of the same duration (10s) were created at 25Hz. For the magic trick sequences videos

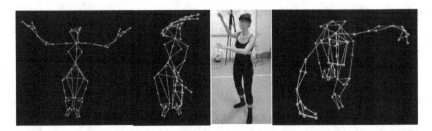

Fig. 1. Marker set and posture examples

of 42s were also produced. The character was displayed in the center of the screen, facing forward at the beginning of each clip. Video clips were presented at 1280x1024 resolution and 116 videos were generated in total.

4.2 Participants and Duration of Each Study

Twenty participants took part in the studies we will detail in the following section, a total of 100 different individuals contributed to our experiments. Participants came from various educational backgrounds and were all naive to the purpose of the experiment. They only knew they would watch some avatar videos and answer a few questions about what they perceived from those videos. Detailed informations about the gender and age distribution of each group of participants and the duration of each study are presented in Table 2.

Table 2. Information about each study's participants and duration in minutes

Study	Gender	Mean age	Duration
Daily actions vs theatrical gestures	11M, 9F	24.0+10.0	15
Isolated gestures (emotions male actor)	10M, 10F	23.5+6.0	40
Isolated gestures (emotions female actor)	15M, 5F	23+7.0	40
Gestures sequences (emotions male actor)	13M, 7F	21.6+7.5	15
Gestures sequences (emotions female actor)	13M, 7F	25.0+13.0	15

4.3 First Experiment: Everyday Life Movements vs. Skilled Theatrical Movements

In our first experiment we wished to determine whether observers perceived theatrical movements as more kinematically and dynamically significant than everyday life movements. Additionally, we wished to investigate whether participants regarded theatrical gestures as motions conveying more information compared to everyday life actions.

For this study, we presented participants with 32 video clips of 10s duration, depicting 8 daily actions and 8 theatrical movements for each actor. Participants viewed each video clip in a random order, played it as many times as they wished, and after each clip were asked to rate on a scale of 1-7 whether the performed action was considered as current, spontaneous and habitual (1 on the scale) or as skilled, meaningful and elaborated (7 on the scale).

Since the answers of the participants were nominal variables, we did not think the data fits the assumptions of an ANOVA. Results for this study were analyzed using Kruskal-Wallis one-way of variance and paired T-Tests for all post-hoc analyses. We found that the gender of the participants and actors had no effect on the ratings of daily actions and theatrical gestures. A significant difference ($H = 158.5377, 1d.f, p < 0.001$) between the mean rank scores of the two types of gestures was found. As we confirmed a significant divergence between the two categories of gestures, we were then interested in identifying which particular motions were considered more kinematically significant and conveying more information. The results of the Kruskal-Wallis test ($H = 270.15, 15d.f, p < 0.001$) were significant; the mean ranks scores of 7 of our 8 theatrical gestures were significantly different among the 16 different movements presented to the participants. For daily gestures, we found that *kicking* and *punching* gestures were perceived as the most kinematically significant actions among the everyday motions. A possible reason for this could be that both actions are considered more sportive actions than everyday motions, thus a higher kinematic variance can be attributed to them. Mean rank scores for both categories and for the 16 gestures are shown in Figure 2.

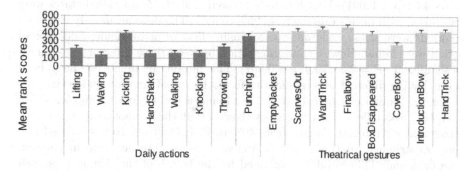

Fig. 2. Mean ranks scores for each category and each one of the sixteen presented actions

4.4 Second and Third Experiment: Perception of Emotion in Isolated Gestures and Sequences

In this study, we take into account the fact that emotional states are expressed differently depending on the subjects and that such states might be more easily recognized over longer stimuli. For this reason, we used 4 separated groups. Two groups rated the emotions of our male character and female character over isolated gestures, and the 2 other groups did the same over the sequences.

We wished to determine whether the 5 emotions portrayed in our theatrical gestures could be recognized among a 6 non-forced-choice list of emotions (the 5 emotions already listed plus the *other* option). Additionally, we wished to investigate the intensity with which each emotion was perceived.

For the isolated gestures, we presented participants with 8 video clips of 10s, representing our 8 theatrical gestures (cf. Table 1 for a detailed list) in each one of the 5 emotional states, where each gesture was presented twice. Participants viewed each video clip in a random order as many times as they wished and were asked to choose an emotion among the 6 possible options (also randomly presented). They were also asked to rate the intensity of the selected emotion on a scale from 1 (not intense) to 7 (very intense)

For the magic trick sequences, we followed the same methodology applied in the evaluation of isolated gestures. However, instead of using short videos of a unique gesture, we presented participants with a whole realization of a magic trick. For this study only the recordings of *the disappearing box* and *appearing scarves in an empty jacket* were considered.

Results for these studies were analyzed using standard analysis of variance (ANOVA) and paired T-Tests for all post-hoc analysis. As done in [7], we calculated and analyzed the accuracy rate for emotion, i.e., how many emotions were correctly recognized for each participant. We found no effect of participants and actors gender on the accuracy of emotion identification.

For the isolated gestures experiment we found a main effect of emotion ($F = 18.68, 4d.f, p < 0.001$). Post-hoc tests showed that the 5 emotional states were recognized with means ranging from 29% to 64%. The most accurately identified emotions were *stress* and *sadness*. No main effect of actor gender and type of action were found. However, an interaction between these 2 factors was shown as significant ($F = 2.81, 7d.f, p < 0.007$). This interaction might be due to both actors having different acting qualities for each type of emotion and action.

For the sequences experiment we also found a main effect of emotion ($F = 6.04, 4d.f, p < 0.001$). Post-hoc tests showed that the 5 emotional states were recognized with means ranging from 40% to 70%. Contrary to the isolated gestures experiment, in this study participants were more accurate in emotion categorization. This could be explained by the length of the stimuli presented to participants. We found that the most accurately identified emotional states were *stress* and *sadness*, followed by *relaxed* and *neutral*. As for the isolated gestures, no main effect for actor gender and action type were found. However, an interaction between the emotion and actor factors was again observed ($F = 4.75, 4d.f, p < 0.001$). We believe this interaction might be due to the acting qualities of our two actors.

To have a better insight of where the miscategorizations happened, the confusion matrices of both studies is shown in Table 3. For both studies, the accuracy rate of the participants is above chance (16.6%) and the results obtained for *neutral* and *sad* emotional states are consistent with previous works [7], [25]. Additionally, *stress*, an emotional state that is not frequently used, has the highest recognition rate. However, the *happy* and *relaxed* emotional states were

Table 3. Confusion matrices

Isolated gestures						
Correct answer	Relaxed	Happy	Neutral	Sad	Stress	Other
Relaxed	**29.22%**	13.44%	28.13%	14.06%	5%	10.16%
Happy	16.41%	**35.31%**	16.72%	2.03%	16.09%	13.44%
Neutral	17.03%	18.44%	**38.91%**	5%	10.16%	10.47%
Sad	8.44%	1.56%	15.63%	**49.84%**	8.91%	15.63%
Stress	2.81%	6.72%	5.47%	2.34%	**64.69%**	17.97%
Sequences						
Correct answer	Relaxed	Happy	Neutral	Sad	Stress	Other
Relaxed	**50.63%**	10%	13.13%	11.88%	4.38%	10%
Happy	11.88%	**52.50%**	13.75%	1.25%	13.75%	6.88%
Neutral	20%	19.38%	**40%**	3.13%	7.5%	10%
Sad	11.88%	1.88%	13.75%	**53.13%**	1.88%	17.50%
Stress	8.13%	7.50%	6.88%	2.50%	**70.63%**	4.38%

frequently misclassified between them or with the *neutral* state. We think possible reasons for this could be the proximity of these 3 emotional states in the circumplex model [21], the utilization of gestures whose sole purpose is not to convey emotional cues, and the recording of non-professional actors. Furthermore, as we are using gestures that are already spatially and temporally rich, we think it is also possible that the variations added by those 3 emotional states were perceived by the participants as indistinct.

To identify possible significant differences in the intensity of the emotional states, Kruskal-Willis tests were applied. We found no difference between the emotional intensities portrayed for both actors and for each action or sequence. For both studies, the emotions rated as the most intense are those the most accurately categorized ($H = 30.82, 4d.f, p < 0.001$ for the isolated gestures and $H = 14.09, 4d.f, p < 0.001$ for the sequences).

5   Conclusions

To date the existing motion capture databases consist of everyday actions with few expressive variations. In this paper, we have proposed a new motion capture corpus composed of 17 theatrical gestures, in the context of a magic performance, into which emotional variations were added.

Three perceptual studies were conducted in order to validate the suitability and usability of our mocap data as well as the relevance of the capture protocol. We found that theatrical gestures can be globally considered more skilled, meaningful and elaborated gestures compared to everyday life actions. We also established that for the selected theatrical scenario, emotional states can be successfully elicited in the laboratory setting, and most importantly that our recognition results are very close to those of previous studies in which archetypal affective actions and more complete visual clues were used [15].

We will improve our set of emotional states and our emotional elicitation procedure. We plan on recording more actors in order to provide a better insight about the influence of acting skills, gender and personal style in the perception of the expressiveness of theatrical gestures.

References

1. Atkinson, A.P., Dittrich, W.H., Gemmell, A.J., Young, A.W.: Emotion perception from dynamic and static body expressions in point-light and full-light displays. Perception 33, 717–746 (2004)
2. Aubert, C.: The art of pantomime. Dover Publications, Inc. (2003)
3. Bernhardt, D., Robinson, P.: Detecting emotions from connected action sequences. In: Badioze Zaman, H., Robinson, P., Petrou, M., Olivier, P., Schröder, H., Shih, T.K. (eds.) IVIC 2009. LNCS, vol. 5857, pp. 1–11. Springer, Heidelberg (2009)
4. Camurri, A., Mazzarino, B., Ricchetti, M., Timmers, R., Volpe, G.: Multimodal Analysis of Expressive Gesture in Music and Dance Performances. In: Camurri, A., Volpe, G. (eds.) GW 2003. LNCS (LNAI), vol. 2915, pp. 20–39. Springer, Heidelberg (2004)
5. Carnegie Mellon University: Motion capture database (2003), http://mocap.cs.cmu.edu/
6. Cowie, R., Douglas-Cowie, E., Cox, C.: Beyond emotion archetypes: Databases for emotion modelling using neural networks. Neural Networks 18(4), 371–388 (2005)
7. Ennis, C., Hoyet, L., Egges, A., McDonnell, R.: Emotion capture: Emotionally expressive characters for games. In: Proceedings of Motion on Games, MIG 2013, pp. 31:53–31:60 (2013)
8. Examinations, L.: Mime matters. Tech. rep., London Academy of Music & Dramatic Art (2012)
9. Jones, G.M.: Trade of the Tricks: Inside the Magician's Craft. University of California Press (2011)
10. Kapur, A., Kapur, A., Virji-Babul, N., Tzanetakis, G., Driessen, P.F.: Gesture-based affective computing on motion capture data. In: Tao, J., Tan, T., Picard, R.W. (eds.) ACII 2005. LNCS, vol. 3784, pp. 1–7. Springer, Heidelberg (2005)
11. Kendon, A.: Gesture: visible action as utterance. Cambridge University Press (2004)
12. Lecoq, J.: Theater of movement and gesture. Taylor & Francis (2006)
13. Ma, Y., Paterson, H.M., Pollick, F.E.: A motion capture library for the study of identity, gender, and emotion perception from biological motion. Behavior Research Methods 38(1), 134–141 (2006)
14. Macknik, S.L., King, M., Randi, J., Robbins, A., Thompson, J., Martinez-Conde, S., et al.: Attention and awareness in stage magic: turning tricks into research. Nature Reviews Neuroscience 9(11), 871–879 (2008)
15. McDonnell, R., Jörg, S., McHugh, J., Newell, F.N., O'Sullivan, C.: Investigating the role of body shape on the perception of emotion. ACM TAP 6(3), 14 (2009)
16. Müller, M., Röder, T., Clausen, M., Eberhardt, B., Krüger, B., Weber, A.: Documentation mocap database hdm05. Tech. rep., Universität Bonn (2007)
17. Niewiadomski, R., Bevacqua, E., Mancini, M., Pelachaud, C.: Greta: An interactive expressive eca system. In: AAMAS 2009, vol. 2, pp. 1399–1400 (2009)
18. Piana, S., Stagliano, A., Odone, F., Verri, A., Camurri, A.: Real-time automatic emotion recognition from body gestures. CoRR (2014)

19. Pollick, F., Paterson, H., Bruderlin, A., Sanford, A.: Perceiving affect from arm movement. Cognition 82(2), B51–B61 (2001)
20. Qualisys AB: Qualisys motion capture systems, http://www.qualisys.com/
21. Russell, J.A.: A circumplex model of affect. Journal of Personality and Social Psychology 39(6), 1161 (1980)
22. Torresani, L., Hackney, P., Bregler, C.: Learning motion style synthesis from perceptual observations. In: NIPS, pp. 1393–1400 (2006)
23. University College London: UCLIC Affective body posture and motion database, http://web4.cs.ucl.ac.uk/uclic/people/n.berthouze/AffectME.html
24. University of Texas at Arlington: Human motion database (2011), http://smile.uta.edu/hmd/
25. Zibrek, K., Hoyet, L., Ruhland, K., McDonnell, R.: Evaluating the effect of emotion on gender recognition in virtual humans. In: SAP 2013, pp. 45–49 (2013)

From Non-verbal Signals Sequence Mining to Bayesian Networks for Interpersonal Attitudes Expression

Mathieu Chollet[1], Magalie Ochs[2], and Catherine Pelachaud[2]

[1] Institut Mines-Telecom, Telecom Paristech, CNRS-LTCI,
46 rue Barrault, 75013 Paris, France
[2] CNRS-LTCI, Telecom Paristech, 46 rue Barrault, 75013 Paris, France
{mathieu.chollet,magalie.ochs,catherine.pelachaud}@telecom-paristech.fr

Abstract. In this paper, we present a model and its evaluation for expressing attitudes through sequences of non-verbal signals for Embodied Conversational Agents. To build our model, a corpus of job interviews has been annotated at two levels: the non-verbal behavior of the recruiters as well as their expressed attitudes was annotated. Using a sequence mining method, sequences of non-verbal signals characterizing different interpersonal attitudes were automatically extracted from the corpus. From this data, a probabilistic graphical model was built. The probabilistic model is used to select the most appropriate sequences of non-verbal signals that an ECA should display to convey a particular attitude. The results of a perceptive evaluation of sequences generated by the model show that such a model can be used to express interpersonal attitudes.

1 Introduction

Embodied Conversational Agents (ECAs) are increasingly used in training and social coaching, in applications such as science teaching [17] or education against bullying [5]. Empathic ECAs have been proposed [28] and it was shown that they can be successful in regulating the emotional state of users in a learning context, effectively affecting the learning outcome of the users [29].

In the TARDIS project[1], we aim at building a virtual recruiter to train job seekers to improve their social skills. Such a virtual recruiter should be able to convey different *interpersonal attitudes* (or *interpersonal stances*). Interpersonal attitudes can be defined as "*spontaneous or strategically employed affective styles that colour interpersonal exchanges*" [34]. A common representation for interpersonal stances is Argyle's bi-dimensional model of attitudes [3], with an affiliation dimension ranging from hostile to friendly, and a status dimension ranging from submissive to dominant.

Most modalities of the body are involved when conveying interpersonal attitudes [9]. Smiles can be signs of friendliness [9], performing large gestures may be a sign of dominance, and a head directed upwards can be interpreted with

---

[1] www.tardis-project.eu

T. Bickmore et al. (Eds.): IVA 2014, LNAI 8637, pp. 120–133, 2014.
© Springer International Publishing Switzerland 2014

a dominant stance [11]. However, when interpreting non-verbal behavior, the sequencing of non-verbal signals can be significant: for instance, while a smile is a sign of friendliness, a smile followed by a gaze and head aversion conveys embarassment [21]. While it has been observed that the sequencing of non-verbal signals influences how they are perceived [37], the literature on the topic is still limited. In this paper, our goal is to build a model for non-verbal behavior generation, which computes a sequence of non-verbal signals that an ECA should display given an input attitude to express and an input text that the ECA should say.

To build a model that takes the sequencing of signals into account, we use a data mining technique to extract sequences of non-verbal signals from a corpus of job interviews we annotated at two levels: the non-verbal behavior and the expressed attitude of the recruiter. The generation model uses a probabilistic framework to compute a set of candidate sequences and then selects the best sequence for expressing the given attitude using a classification method based on the frequent sequences previously extracted from the corpus. The model was evaluated with an perceptual experiment.

The paper is organized as follows. In Section 2, we present related models of interpersonal attitude expression for ECAs and their limitations. We then describe in Section 3 the multimodal corpus we collected and how it was annotated. Section 4 details the data mining process we used to gather knowledge about how sequences of non-verbal behavior are perceived. Section 5 discusses a method for generating and selecting behavior sequences using the extracted data. In Section 6, we describe the study we conducted to evaluate whether the generated sequences convey the desired attitude. Finally, the results of the evaluation study are discussed in Section 7.

2   Related Work

Models of interpersonal attitude expression for virtual agents have already been proposed. For instance, in the Demeanour project [6], postures corresponding to a given attitude were automatically generated for a dyad of agents. Lee and Marsella used Argyle's attitude dimensions, along with other factors such as conversational roles and communicative acts, to analyze and model behaviors of side participants and bystanders [23]. Cafaro et al. [10] conducted a study on how smile, gaze and proximity cues displayed by an agent influence the first impressions that the users form on the agent's interpersonal attitude and personality. Ravenet et al. [33] proposed a user-created corpus-based methodology for choosing the behaviors of an agent conveying an attitude along with a communicative intention. The Laura agent [7] was used to develop long term relationships with users, and would adapt the frequency of its gestures and facial signals as the relationship with the user grew. However, dominance was not investigated, and the users' behaviors were not taken into account as they used a menu-based interface when interacting with the agent. Prepin et al. [32] have investigated how smile alignment and synchronisation can contribute to stance building in a dyad of agents. These models, however, only consider the expression of a few signals at a given time, and do not consider how signals are sequenced.

The importance of the dynamic features of expressions has been highlighted in previous works. Keltner *et al.* [21] found that the sequencing of head aversion, gaze aversion and smile differentiate between embarassment, amusement and shame. With [37] found unique characteristic behavioral sequences for the expression of enjoyment, hostility, embarassment, surprise and sadness. Recently, models for displaying emotions for ECAs as sequences of signals have been proposed. Niewiadomski *et al.* [30] propose a representation for multimodal sequences of signals based on temporal constraints between signals, for instance $signal_1$ *precedes* $signal_2$. Their representation schema, applied to annotated videos, allows a virtual agent to express several emotions. Pan *et al.* [31] proposed another approach that makes use of motion graphs. In such graphs, arcs are motion clips (possibly containing facial expressions and/or head movements) and nodes are transitions between them. They trained a motion graph using video clips labelled with mental states (*e.g.* interest), and appropriate paths in the graph for each mental state are selected using dynamic programming. Finally, Lee and Marsella [24] proposed a model of head nods prediction based on Hidden Markov Models (HMM). The input of these HMMs is a sequence of words with associated linguistic features (*e.g.* part of speech, emotion label, noun phrase start...). Using an annotated corpus, they trained the prediction of head nods on trigrams, *i.e.* sequences of three words. Though they effectively adopted a sequential representation for their model, the sequential relationship between different head behaviors was not modelled (only linguistic features), and their work was limited to head movements.

Even though models of interpersonal attitude expression for ECA have already been proposed, they typically do not consider how the sequencing of signals influence attitudes, and only consider a limited number of modalities. In the next section, we present the corpus of job interviews we collected and annotated, and which was used subsequently to extract frequent sequences of non-verbal signals expressing interpersonal attitudes.

3   Multimodal Corpus

As part of the TARDIS[1] project, a corpus of simulation of job interviews between human resources practitioners and youngsters was collected. We decided to use these videos to investigate the sequences of non-verbal signals the recruiters use when conveying interpersonal attitudes. The non-verbal behavior of the recruiters, their perceived attitudes and the turn taking were then annotated manually on 3 videos, for a total of slightly more than 50 minutes. Our sequence mining method (see Section 4) being relatively simple, we found this amount of data to be sufficient for our purpose. Of course, more data would allow for achieving more precision and for using more complex models.

For the non-verbal behavior annotation, we adapted the MUMIN multimodal coding scheme [2] to our task and our corpus. The following modalities were considered : gestures (*e.g.* adaptors, deictics), hands rest positions (*e.g.* over or under table, arms crossed), postures (*e.g.* leaning backwards), head movements (*e.g.* nods, head tilted downwards), gaze (*e.g.* looking at interlocutor, downwards), facial expressions (since the videos were recorded from the side, we only considered simple facial expressions, *e.g.* smiles, eyebrow movements). Full details on the coding scheme can be found in [12]. We used Praat [8] for the annotation of the audio stream and the Elan annotation tool [38] for the visual annotations. A single annotator fully annotated the non-verbal behavior for the three videos. A second annotation on 10% of the total annotated video length was performed one month after the initial annotation to measure the reliability of the coding. Cohen's Kappa measures were computed across the two annotations and were found to be mostly satisfactory: *e.g.* $\kappa = 0.80$ for gestures, $\kappa = 0.93$ for postures. The lowest score was found for eyebrow movements ($\kappa = 0.62$), which we had anticipated considering the video setup (the video camera captured the full scene, thus the faces of the people are small in the video).

As the interpersonal attitudes of the recruiters vary through the videos, we chose to use GTrace, successor to FeelTrace [14]. GTrace is a tool that allows for the annotation of continuous dimensions over time. We adapted the software for the interpersonal attitude dimensions we considered. The speech was rendered unintelligible, as we focus on non-verbal behavior and did not want the content of the recruiters' utterances to affect the annotators' perception of attitudes. We asked 12 persons to annotate the videos with this tool. Each annotator had the task of annotating one dimension for one video, though some volunteered to annotate more videos. With this process, we collected two to three annotation files per attitude dimension per video. More details about the attitude annotation can be found in [13]

In a nutshell, the corpus has been annotated at two levels: the non-verbal behavior of the recruiters and their perceived attitudes. Our next step was to identify which sequences of non-verbal signals characterize interpersonal attitudes. As a first step, we have focused on the non-verbal signals sequences expressed by the recruiters when they are speaking. In the next section, we describe a method for extracting frequent non-verbal signals sequences from the multimodal corpus.

4 Mining Frequent Sequences Characterizing Attitudes

In order to extract significant sequences of non-verbal signals conveying interpersonal attitudes from our corpus, we chose to use a *sequence mining* technique. Such techniques have been widely used in tasks such as protein classification [15], and they have been recently used in computer-human interaction to find sequences of video game players' key presses correlated with affects such as frustration [27]. To the best of our knowledge, this technique has not yet been applied to analyse sequences of non-verbal signals.

Frequent sequence mining techniques require a dataset of sequences. Since we investigate which sequences of signals convey attitudes, we decided to segment the non-verbal behavior data using the timestamps in the annotations files where an attitude dimension begins to vary. We call these instants *attitude variation events*. Once the data was segmented with these events, we kept only the

Table 1. Cluster centers, segment counts per cluster and frequent sequences per cluster

	Large Decrease	Small Decrease	Small Increase	Large Increase
Friendliness	0.34 / 68 / 86	0.12 / 66 / 72	-0.11 / 77 / 104	-0.32 / 36 / 67
Dominance	0.23 / 49 / 141	0.09 / 66 / 244	-0.13 / 80 / 134	-0.34 / 24 / 361

segments where the recruiter is speaking. Since we found that the attitude variation events came with a wide range of values, we chose to differentiate between small and strong attitude displays. Therefore we used a K-means clustering algorithm with $k = 4$ to identify clusters corresponding to small increases, strong increases, small decreases and strong decreases. The amount of segments per attitude variation type and the associated clusters are described in table 1.

The next step consisted of applying a frequent sequence mining algorithm to each set of segments. We used the Generalized Sequence Pattern (GSP) frequent sequence mining algorithm described in [35]. This algorithm extracts sequences without temporal information, *i.e.* it only represents that behaviors happened after another. It is not be able to differentiate between short and long gestures. It also cannot represent simultaneous events (*e.g.* a smile and a nod happening simultaneously). More recent sequence mining techniques exist that take temporal information into account [16], [18]. However, as a first step, we decided to choose a simpler model and focus on the sequential representation, as a higher model complexity would require more data to learn and would be harder to apply to our generation problem. Our model could potentially be complemented by related works considering simultaneous signals, such as [33]. The GSP algorithm requires as an input a minimum support, *i.e.* the minimal number of times that a sequence has to be present in the corpus to be considered frequent, and its output is a set of sequences along with their support. For instance, using a minimum support of 3, every sequence that is present at least 3 times in the data will be extracted. The GSP algorithm based on the *Apriori* algorithm [1] follows two steps: first, it identifies the frequent individual items in the data and then extends them into larger sequences by iteratively adding other items, pruning out the sequences that are not frequent enough. Having acquired a set of frequent sequences for each type of attitude variation, we can characterize each of these sequences with several *quality measures*: *Support*, that is how many times the sequence appears in the data ($[0; \infty] \in \mathbb{N}$) ; *Confidence*, which represents the proportion of a sequence's occurrences that happen before a particular type of attitude variation ($[0; 1] \in \mathbb{R}$, 1 meaning this sequence only occurs before this attitude variation) ; *Lift*, which can be seen as how strong the confidence of a sequence is, compared to the random co-occurrence of sequence and the attitude variation, given their individual support ($[0; \infty] \in \mathbb{R}$, a higher value representing a stronger association).

In Table 2 we show examples of extracted sequences. The *Sup* column corresponds to the support of the sequence and the *Conf* column to the confidence of the sequence. Using a minimum support of 10, we extracted a set of 879 sequences for dominance variations and 329 for friendliness variations. In the next section, we describe an algorithm for generating non-verbal signals sequences

Table 2. Example sequences obtained with the sequence mining process

Sequence	Attitude Variation	*Sup*	*Conf*	*Lift*
BodyStraight -> ObjectManip	Friendliness Large Decrease	13	0.31	2.09
HeadNod -> Smile	Friendliness Large Increase	32	0.59	2.09
HeadNod -> RestHandsTogether -> Smile	Dominance Large Decrease	13	0.31	2.90
EyebrowsUp -> RestOverTable	Dominance Large Increase	21	0.33	1.54

conveying attitudes, that makes use of the frequent sequences we presented in this section.

5   Model of Non-verbal Signals Sequences Generation for Expressing Attitudes

Given an input attitude that an ECA should express and an input utterance tagged with communicative intentions that the ECA should say, the objective of our model is to generate a sequence of non-verbal signals that conveys the desired attitude. We place ourselves within the SAIBA framework [36], where our model fulfils the role of the *Behavior Planner* module, whose role is to translate communicative intentions into multimodal behaviors and to schedule them. Input utterances and intentions are defined in the Functional Markup Language (FML) [25], and output sequences of scheduled non-verbal signals are defined in the Behavior Markup Language (BML) format [36].

In a nutshell, our algorithm follows three steps, which are detailed in the following subsections. First, for each communicative intention contained in the input FML message, we retrieve all the signals that can express this intention, and build all the possible combinations of signals that can express the input's communicative intentions (Section 5.1). Secondly, for each of these combinations, the algorithm then finds all the time intervals where additional signals can be inserted, and builds a set of larger sequences by inserting additional signals in the available time intervals using a probabilistic framework (Section 5.2). These signals will enable the agent to display its interpersonal attitude. The third step (Section 5.3) consists of selecting the best sequence out of all these candidate sequences, by using a classification method trained on the frequent sequences that were extracted using the method described in Section 4.

5.1   Building Minimal Sequences Expressing the Input FML

In a conversation, communicative intentions can be expressed through non-verbal behavior as well as through speech. For instance, in Western culture, it is possible to convey uncertainty by squinting the eyelids, tilting the head, or performing a particular hesitation gesture. When emphasizing a word, it is common to make a quick head movement downwards, and to raise one's eyebrows.

The FML language [25] represents such communicative intentions. The first step in our algorithm consists of retrieving all the possible non-verbal signals that can be used to express the intentions contained in the input FML message. For this purpose, we used Mancini's framework [26], in which each communicative intention is characterized by a *behavior set*. A behavior set is the specification of the different non-verbal signals that can be displayed by an ECA to express a communicative intention. We can build a non-verbal signals sequence expressing an input message by selecting one signal in the behavior set of each communicative intention of the input message. Such a resulting sequence is called a *minimal sequence*. In our model, we only consider communicative intentions for altering the speech prosody (*i.e.* pitch accents and boundaries) and communicative intentions related to the speech semantics (*i.e.* spatio-temporal information which will trigger deictic gestures, particular meaning which will trigger iconic gestures, and performatives such as asking a question). Once all the minimal sequences have been computed (*i.e.* all the different combinations of signals from the behavior sets have been collected), the next step consists of enriching these sequences with additional signals to convey the interpersonal attitude.

5.2   Generating New Sequences

For every minimal sequence obtained in the previous step, we start by looking at all the time intervals where it is possible to insert other signals. For instance, if there is enough time between two head signals, we might insert a head nod, or a head shake. Since the signals chosen for the minimal sequences are only related to speech prosody or to certain speech semantics, we make the hypothesis that the inserted signals will not conflict with the original communicative intentions, and that only the inserted additional signals will contribute to expressing attitudes.

For this purpose, we represent the extracted frequent sequences (Section 4) with a probabilistic model: a Bayesian Network (BN). The nodes of the network represents the non-verbal signals and the interpersonal attitudes (Figure 1). The edges define a conditional dependence between two variables. The Bayesian Networks enable us to represent the causal and non deterministic relation of the attitudes on the signals (*e.g.* there might be more smiles for friendliness increases, or more arms crossed for friendliness decreases) and the sequences of signals (*e.g.* hands rest pose changes typically appear after a gesture). In our case, we note that $P(S_{i+1}|S_i, S_{i-1}, ..., S_1, A) = P(S_{i+1}|S_i, A)$, where S represents signals, i is the index of a signal in the sequence, and A is the chosen attitude variation. Note that some paths are impossible (*e.g. HeadAt → HeadAt* or *BodyStraight → BodyStraight*), and we made sure that such paths do not exist in the network.

An interesting feature of this model is that non-verbal signals sequences that did not occur in our data can still be generated, and their likelihood can be evaluated. Indeed, the representation of the sequences might lead to new sequences in the network. These new sequences are valuable as they can help improving the variability of the recruiter's behavior beyond the sequences that were observed in the corpus. To evaluate a new sequence, we can use the method described in [20] which classifies a new sequence with a majority-voting technique using its k sub-sequences contained in the new sequence that have the highest confidence score in the corpus. We trained a BN for dominance variations and another BN

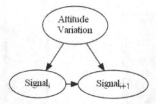

Fig. 1. A "rolled" representation of the Bayesian Networks we use for generating new sequences of behavior.

for friendliness variations. As a first step, we consider the attitudes of friendliness and dominance independently. A next step will consist in analysing how to combine attitude variations in the two dimensions simultaneously. We used the Weka open-source machine learning software [19] to train the networks, using our multimodal corpus as input data. The constructed models are then used to compute the sequences of non-verbal signals conveying a particular attitude.

The generation of the sequences starts with the minimal sequences obtained after the previous step (Section 5.1), and uses the Bayesian Networks to add new signals in the available intervals. Thus, it is ensured that every generated sequence contains signals that express every input communicative intentions. Also, the maximum sequence length (*i.e.* how far we "unroll") is the amount of time intervals contained in the original FML message. In order to reduce computing time and to sort out sequences that are too unlikely, we compute the overall probability of every generated sequence, and only keep those whose probability is above a certain threshold λ. For our evaluation, we chose λ to be equal to $P(minimal\,sequence) * \alpha$ where $P(minimal\,sequence)$ is the probability of the original minimal sequence and α is a coefficient, which we set to 0.005 after trial-and-error showed it to be an adequate compromise between the amount of generated sequences and computing time. The generated sequences that are left after this pruning process are called *candidate sequences*. Having computed all the candidate sequences, the final step consists of selecting the one that is most likely to convey the input attitude.

5.3   Selecting the Final Sequence

For selecting the final sequence, we compromise between having a sequence with a high likelihood to appear in the data, and a high confidence for conveying the appropriate attitude. We defined a score variable of a candidate sequence s as $Sc(s) = P(s) * Conf(s)$, where $P(s)$ is the probability of s computed by the appropriate Bayesian Network (BN for dominance or friendliness depending on the input attitude). If the sequence s has been extracted in the frequent sequence mining process, then $Conf(s)$ is equal to the sequence's confidence (see Section 4). If not, we compute $Conf(s')$ for every subsequence s' contained in s, and we define $Conf(s) = \Sigma Conf(s')/n$ where n is the number of subsequences of s. Finally, we select the sequence with the highest score Sc. Note that for a particular input utterance, the chosen sequence will always be the same with

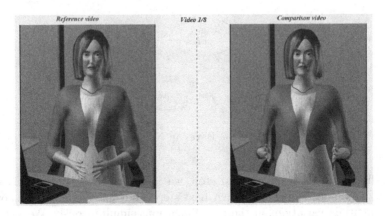

Fig. 2. The main screen of the online study.

this method. In the future, we plan to add a factor to weigh down sequences very similar to previously played sequences.

In the next section, we present an evaluation study we realized to assess whether the generated sequences convey the expected attitudes.

6   Evaluation

In order to evaluate our model, we conducted a study to verify that non-verbal signals sequences generated by the model with a certain input attitude are perceived as conveying the same attitude , and are perceived with the same intensity. In the following sections, we describe the study design and we then report the results of the study.

6.1   Study Design

The study was conducted online. The platform of the study was developed using Adobe Flash technology. Participants were asked to compare 8 pairs of videos of a virtual character acting as a job recruiter expressing non-verbal signals when speaking (see Figure 2). For every pair of videos, the virtual recruiter said a different job interview question (*e.g.* "In your previous professional experiences, did you ever have to deal with difficult situations?"). The 8 different questions were always presented to the users in the same order. The character's speech was identical in both videos, and was produced in English with the Cereproc Text-To-Speech engine [4]. The non-verbal behavior of the recruiter was however different in the two videos of every pair. Since the speech content was identical in both videos, and since we asked user the difference in attitude between both videos, we considered the utterances' content did not have an impact on the results.

Each of these 8 pairs of videos corresponded to a testing condition, namely one of the 8 following attitudes: *high dominance, low dominance, low submissiveness, high submissiveness, high friendliness, low friendliness, low hostility, high hostility*. On the right video (Figure 2), the ECA displayed sequences of non-verbal signals generated with our model. To generate a sequence for a given condition, we used as an input the corresponding attitude variation, for instance for *low hostility* our input was *small friendliness decrease*. On the left video, the virtual character's behavior was generated with a neutral attitude. For this purpose, our model only went through the first step of our algorithm (Section 5.1), and selected randomly one of the minimal sequences for the input question. While such a sequence could effectively express an attitude, we hypothesised that the attitude expressed in these videos would be considered more neutral than the attitude expressed in the videos generated with the attitude model. All in all, 64 distinct sequences were evaluated with our study (8 questions said by the ECA ∗ 8 attitudes), and 72 videos were generated for this purpose: (64 + 8 neutral). For every pair of videos, the participants answered the following questions: *Q1: "Compared to the Reference Video (left), the character on the Comparison video (right) is:"*, with the possible answers being : "Much less dominant", "Less dominant", "Equivalent", "More dominant", "Much more dominant", "Undecided" (resp. friendly). If they had not chosen "Undecided", they would then be asked to give their opinion on the next question: *Q2: "The intensity of the expressed attitude on the Comparison video (right) is:"*, with the possible answers being : "Very low", "Low", "Medium", "High", "Very high". In the following section, we present the results of this study.

6.2 Results

Eighty-one participants took part in our study (43 Female, 38 Male). The participants were mostly French (88%), and the mean age of the population was 32.4 years old (*StdDev*: 12.8).

In Table 3, we report the frequency table for participants' answers for *Q1*. The *Mean* values are computed by considering the answers are on an ordinal scale (Much less friendly = 1, Much more friendly = 5, *etc.*). To assess the statistical significance of our results, we performed χ^2 tests for every condition, and all were found to be significant (for all conditions $\chi^2 > 23.5$, $p < 0.0001$).

For *Q2*, we performed Student's T-tests between pairs of conditions of the same type (*i.e.* increase or decrease of dominance or friendliness) but different intensity (*i.e.* small or large). There was only a significant difference between perceived intensity of large (*Mean* = 2.97) and small (*Mean* = 3.31) decreases in friendliness ($p = 0.016 < 0.05$). Differences between increases in friendliness ($p = 0.62$), decreases in dominance ($p = 0.48$) and increases in dominance ($p = 0.73$) were not found to be significant.

7 Discussion

Our evaluation study aimed at assessing whether our model can generate sequences of non-verbal signals that convey the appropriate attitude, and if the generated sequences are perceived with the appropriate intensity.

Table 3. Percentages table for attitude rankings for the 8 conditions

	Friendliness Decrease	Friendliness Increase	Dominance Decrease	Dominance Increase
Much less (1)	3.73%	3.68%	2.26%	0.78%
Less (2)	**45.5%**	24.3%	24.1%	14.7%
Equivalent (3)	24.6%	**38.2%**	**39.1%**	20.9%
More (4)	20.9%	25.7%	27.1%	**52.7%**
Much more (5)	3.73%	8.09%	5.26%	9.30%
Undecided	1.04%	0%	2.26%	1.55%
Mean	2.71	3.10	3.02	3.50
$\chi^2(4)$	120.7	91.8	98.9	146.0

The results of *Q1* indicate that expressions of dominance were indeed perceived as such. However, sequences for submissive attitudes were perceived as equivalent to the neutral expression. Expressions of hostile attitudes were perceived as less friendly than the neutral one. Moreover, the expressions of friendliness were perceived as conveying a more friendly attitude than the neutral non-verbal behavior. In other words, the results of the study validate partially our model. Indeed, our model seems to generate appropriate non-verbal signals sequences for the expression of dominance, friendliness and hostility. However, the model cannot be used to convey submissiveness.

For *Q2*, the only significant difference was found between intensity of large and small decreases in friendliness, however the videos generated for smaller variations were found to be more intense than the videos generated for larger variations. Therefore, it seems that our model cannot simulate attitudes of different intensities.

The analysis of the results brings some interesting considerations. One factor that might have influenced the results of *Q1*, is that speaking in a job interview context can be viewed as a form of asserting control over the interaction. Therefore it might be argued that a virtual recruiter cannot express submissiveness while speaking. Similarly, interactions are not a one-way exchange, and the behaviors of the recruiter when the interviewee is speaking are certainly critical to express friendliness. For instance, it is known that mimicking the behaviors of an interlocutor is a sign of friendliness [22]. However, our evaluation protocol did not allow us to study this effect. Moreover, while the non-verbal signals and their sequencing were different between compared and reference videos, there was no difference in behavior expressivity (*e.g.* gesture amplitude, smile intensity). Also, the notion of *intensity* mentioned in *Q2* could have been interpreted in other ways that we had anticipated (*e.g.* intensity of behaviors, whereas we studied intensity of attitudes). These two factors might have been influenced the participants in rating the videos with similar intensities. Finally, one caveat in our evaluation protocol is that our model considers attitude variations, whereas our study could only compare differences in attitude expression with neutral behavior. To really assess whether the model can express attitude variations, we need to measure participants' appraisals of our virtual recruiter's attitude in full length, uninterrupted job interviews.

8   Conclusion

In this paper, we presented a corpus-based model for expression of attitudes by Embodied Conversational Agents and an evaluation study. From an annotated corpus of job interview, frequent sequences for different types of attitude expressions were extracted using a sequence mining technique. These were then used as data for building our sequence generation model based on Bayesian Networks.

The evaluation study validated that our model can generate non-verbal signals sequences for appearing friendly, hostile and dominant. However, the model was not able to express different attitude intensities. In future work, we plan on taking our model one step further by considering the listening behavior of the recruiter, and how the recruiter should react to behaviors of the interviewee. We also want to investigate how behavior expressivity, such as gesture amplitude or smile duration, is related to expressions of attitude and implement this in our model. Extensions of the sequence mining method considering temporal information will be considered. We will also extend our sequence generation and selection model to allow for simultaneously expressing variations of attitude along both dimensions, dominance and friendliness. Finally, we plan on evaluating our model in full-length, uninterrupted simulated job interviews, to assess whether our model can express attitude variations through the course of an interpersonal interaction. To this end, we will define a measure of similarity between sequences, which will be used when selecting a new sequence to ensure that the behavior remains varied.

Acknowledgements. This research has been partially supported by the European Community Seventh Framework Program (FP7/2007-2013), under grant agreement no. 288578 (TARDIS).

References

1. Agrawal, R., Srikant, R.: Fast algorithms for mining association rules in large databases. In: Very Large Data Bases, pp. 487–499. Morgan Kaufmann Publishers Inc., San Francisco (1994)
2. Allwood, J., Kopp, S., Grammer, K., Ahlsen, E., Oberzaucher, E., Koppensteiner, M.: The analysis of embodied communicative feedback in multimodal corpora: a prerequisite for behavior simulation. Language Resources and Evaluation 41, 255–272 (2007)
3. Argyle, M.: Bodily Communication. University paperbacks. Methuen (1988)
4. Aylett, M.P., Pidcock, C.J.: The CereVoice Characterful Speech Synthesiser SDK. In: Pelachaud, C., Martin, J.-C., André, E., Chollet, G., Karpouzis, K., Pelé, D. (eds.) IVA 2007. LNCS (LNAI), vol. 4722, pp. 413–414. Springer, Heidelberg (2007)
5. Aylett, R., Paiva, A., Dias, J., Hall, L., Woods, S.: Affective agents for education against bullying. In: Affective Information Processing, pp. 75–90. Springer (2009)

6. Ballin, D., Gillies, M., Crabtree, B.: A framework for interpersonal attitude and non-verbal communication in improvisational visual media production. In: First European Conference on Visual Media Production, pp. 203–210 (2004)

7. Bickmore, T.W., Picard, R.W.: Establishing and maintaining long-term human-computer relationships. ACM Transactions in Computer-Human Interaction 12(2), 293–327 (2005)

8. Boersma, P., Weenink, D.: Praat, a system for doing phonetics by computer. Glot International 5(9/10), 341–345 (2001)

9. Burgoon, J.K., Buller, D.B., Hale, J.L., de Turck, M.A.: Relational Messages Associated with Nonverbal Behaviors. Human Communication Research 10(3), 351–378 (1984)

10. Cafaro, A., Vilhjálmsson, H.H., Bickmore, T., Heylen, D., Jóhannsdóttir, K.R., Valgarðsson, G.S.: First impressions: Users' judgments of virtual agents' personality and interpersonal attitude in first encounters. In: Nakano, Y., Neff, M., Paiva, A., Walker, M. (eds.) IVA 2012. LNCS, vol. 7502, pp. 67–80. Springer, Heidelberg (2012)

11. Carney, D.R., Hall, J.A., LeBeau, L.S.: Beliefs about the nonverbal expression of social power. Journal of Nonverbal Behavior 29(2), 105–123 (2005)

12. Chollet, M., Ochs, M., Clavel, C., Pelachaud, C.: A multimodal corpus approach to the design of virtual recruiters. In: 2013 Humaine Association Conference on Affective Computing and Intelligent Interaction, ACII 2013, pp. 19–24 (2013)

13. Chollet, M., Ochs, M., Pelachaud, C.: A multimodal corpus approach to the design of virtual recruiters. In: Workshop Multimodal Corpora, Intelligent Virtual Agents, IVA 2013, pp. 36–41 (2013)

14. Cowie, R., Cox, C., Martin, J.C., Batliner, A., Heylen, D., Karpouzis, K.: Issues in data labelling. In: Cowie, R., Pelachaud, C., Petta, P. (eds.) Emotion-Oriented Systems. Cognitive Technologies, pp. 213–241. Springer, Heidelberg (2011)

15. Ferreira, P.G., Azevedo, P.J.: Protein sequence classification through relevant sequence mining and bayes classifiers. In: Bento, C., Cardoso, A., Dias, G. (eds.) EPIA 2005. LNCS (LNAI), vol. 3808, pp. 236–247. Springer, Heidelberg (2005)

16. Fricker, D., Zhang, H., Yu, C.: Sequential pattern mining of multimodal data streams in dyadic interactions. In: 2011 IEEE International Conference on Development and Learning (ICDL), vol. 2, pp. 1–6 (2011)

17. Graesser, A., Chipman, P., King, B., McDaniel, B., D'Mello, S.: Emotions and learning with autotutor. In: Proceedings of the 2007 conference on Artificial Intelligence in Education: Building Technology Rich Learning Contexts That Work, pp. 569–571. IOS Press, Amsterdam (2007)

18. Guillame-Bert, M., Crowley, J.L.: Learning temporal association rules on symbolic time sequences. In: Proceedings of the 4th Asian Conference on Machine Learning, pp. 159–174 (2012)

19. Hall, M., Frank, E., Holmes, G., Pfahringer, B., Reutemann, P., Witten, I.H.: The WEKA data mining software: An update. Association for Computing Machinery's Special Interest Group on Knowledge Discovery and Data Mining Explorations Newsletter 11(1), 10–18 (2009)

20. Jaillet, S., Laurent, A., Teisseire, M.: Sequential patterns for text categorization. Intelligent Data Analysis 10(3), 199–214 (2006)

21. Keltner, D.: Signs of appeasement: Evidence for the distinct displays of embarrassment, amusement, and shame. Journal of Personality and Social Psychology 68, 441–454 (1995)

22. LaFrance, M.: Posture mirroring and rapport. In: Davis, M. (ed.) Interaction Rhythms: Periodicity in Communicative Behavior, pp. 279–299. Human Sciences Press, New York (1982)
23. Lee, J., Marsella, S.: Modeling side participants and bystanders: The importance of being a laugh track. In: Vilhjálmsson, H.H., Kopp, S., Marsella, S., Thórisson, K.R. (eds.) IVA 2011. LNCS, vol. 6895, pp. 240–247. Springer, Heidelberg (2011)
24. Lee, J., Marsella, S.C.: Predicting speaker head nods and the effects of affective information. IEEE Transactions on Multimedia, 552–562 (2010)
25. Mancini, M., Pelachaud, C.: Dynamic behavior qualifiers for conversational agents. In: Pelachaud, C., Martin, J.-C., André, E., Chollet, G., Karpouzis, K., Pelé, D. (eds.) IVA 2007. LNCS (LNAI), vol. 4722, pp. 112–124. Springer, Heidelberg (2007)
26. Mancini, M., Pelachaud, C.: The FML - APML language. In: The First FML Workshop, AAMAS 2008, Estoril, Portugal (May 2008)
27. Martínez, H.P., Yannakakis, G.N.: Mining multimodal sequential patterns: a case study on affect detection. In: Proceedings of the 13th International Conference on Multimodal Interfaces, pp. 3–10. ACM, New York (2011)
28. McQuiggan, S.W., Robison, J.L., Phillips, R., Lester, J.C.: Modeling parallel and reactive empathy in virtual agents: An inductive approach. In: Proceedings of 7th International Conference on Autonomous Agents and Multiagent Systems, pp. 167–174 (2008)
29. Moridis, C.N., Economides, A.A.: Affective learning: Empathetic agents with emotional facial and tone of voice expressions. IEEE Transactions on Affective Computing 3(3), 260–272 (2012)
30. Niewiadomski, R., Hyniewska, S.J., Pelachaud, C.: Constraint-based model for synthesis of multimodal sequential expressions of emotions. IEEE Transaction on Affective Computing 2(3), 134–146 (2011)
31. Pan, X., Gillies, M., Sezgin, T.M., Loscos, C.: Expressing complex mental states through facial expressions. In: Paiva, A.C.R., Prada, R., Picard, R.W. (eds.) ACII 2007. LNCS, vol. 4738, pp. 745–746. Springer, Heidelberg (2007)
32. Prepin, K., Ochs, M., Pelachaud, C.: Beyond backchannels: co-construction of dyadic stancce by reciprocal reinforcement of smiles between virtual agents. In: Proceedings of the 35th Annual Meeting of the Cognitive Science Society (2013)
33. Ravenet, B., Ochs, M., Pelachaud, C.: From a user-created corpus of virtual agent's non-verbal behavior to a computational model of interpersonal attitudes. In: Aylett, R., Krenn, B., Pelachaud, C., Shimodaira, H. (eds.) IVA 2013. LNCS (LNAI), vol. 8108, pp. 263–274. Springer, Heidelberg (2013)
34. Scherer, K.R.: What are emotions? and how can they be measured? Social Science Information 44, 695–729 (2005)
35. Srikant, R., Agrawal, R.: Mining sequential patterns: Generalizations and performance improvements. In: Apers, P.M.G., Bouzeghoub, M., Gardarin, G. (eds.) EDBT 1996. LNCS, vol. 1057, pp. 1–17. Springer, Heidelberg (1996)
36. Vilhjálmsson, H.H., et al.: The behavior markup language: Recent developments and challenges. In: Pelachaud, C., Martin, J.-C., André, E., Chollet, G., Karpouzis, K., Pelé, D. (eds.) IVA 2007. LNCS (LNAI), vol. 4722, pp. 99–111. Springer, Heidelberg (2007)
37. With, S.: Structural analysis of temporal patterns of facial actions: Measurement and implications for the study of emotion perception through facial expressions. Ph.D. thesis, University of Geneva (2010)
38. Wittenburg, P., Brugman, H., Russel, A., Klassmann, A., Sloetjes, H.: Elan: a professional framework for multimodality research. In: Language Resources and Evaluation (2006)

ERiSA: Building Emotionally Realistic Social Game-Agents Companions

Andry Chowanda[1,2], Peter Blanchfield[1], Martin Flintham[1],
and Michel Valstar[1]

[1] School of Computer Science, The University of Nottingham, Nottingham, UK-GB
{psxac6,peter.blanchfield,martin.flintham,michel.valstar}@nottingham.ac.uk
[2] School of Computer Science, Bina Nusantara University, Jakarta, ID

Abstract. We propose an integrated framework for social and emotional
game-agents to enhance their believability and quality of interaction, in
particular by allowing an agent to forge social relations and make appropriate use of social signals. The framework is modular including sensing,
interpretation, behaviour generation, and game components. We propose
a generic formulation of action selection rules based on observed social
and emotional signals, the agent's personality, and the social relation between agent and player. The rules are formulated such that its variables
can easily be obtained from real data. We illustrate and evaluate our
framework using a simple social game called *The Smile Game*.

Keywords: Social Relationship, Framework, Game-Agents, Interactions.

1 Introduction

Taking Alan Turing's famous question "Can machines think?" [16] to it's logical
next step, researchers in computer science have started to challenge themselves
to build not only computers that can think but also ones that have a virtual
embodiment, can communicate and interact with humans, and "live" in a virtual world. Such embodied conversational agents are applied in a wide range of
applications areas covering training and education [4], government and military
[5], medical and health [3], films, and gaming [11].

In the area of gaming, Intelligent Virtual Agents (IVAs) research has led to
major improvements in their believability. This is generally achieved by improving their visual appearance and more recently by making their behaviour more
realistic. Yet there remain a number of improvements and contributions to be
made including more natural expression of emotions [2], enhanced role of personality and social relations in the selection of the agent's behaviour [11], and
better use of social signal processing [18] to drive the interaction.

In gaming applications, IVAs can be particularly interesting potential vehicles
of affect, because players naturally engage with agents as part of a game. Over
time, a pattern of interactions between player and agents may translate into a
relationship if the game and its IVAs are designed to allow for this. It is this

T. Bickmore et al. (Eds.): IVA 2014, LNAI 8637, pp. 134–143, 2014.
© Springer International Publishing Switzerland 2014

evolving relationship, expressed in terms of social signal that we propose to include in our IVA architecture.

In the real world, social interaction between people involve the encoding and decoding of social signals [18]. These signals are displayed through facial expressions, body gestures, and voice. We propose to model our game agents exactly like this: they will perceive and generate behaviour as we do, both when interacting with a user as well as when interacting with other IVAs.

While a number of works have moved towards building realistic IVAs in games (e.g. [11,15]), so far there exists no fully integrated framework for a social and emotional game-agent, complete with the ability to develop simple social relations over time. Hence, in this paper we propose such a framework. In addition, we propose a formulation of action selection rules based on the IVA's personality, the social relation between player and agent, and the perceived (non-)verbal actions to enhance the agents' believability and the user's interaction in a game context. The rules are formulated so that they can be easily learned from data.

To illustrate the efficiency of our framework, we implemented a simple game called the Smile Game. In this game, the player can play, interact, and build a relationship with the agents (see Section 5).

2   Related Work

A number of IVA frameworks have been proposed to improve the social capabilities of agents. For example: The SSI (Social Signal Interpretation) framework [19] aims to integrate multi-modal affect recognition and interpretation. The framework consists of several components that enabled affect recognition and interpretation using tools that can recognise and interpret a user's social signals conveyed by their voice and face. The results of the recognition and interpretation can be processed as sensing information by the agents.

Another example of a fully integrated IVA framework is the SEMAINE framework [14] [10]. SEMAINE is an open-standards-based framework for building emotion oriented systems. It consists of a number of components that communicate with each other using XML based messages. This framework emphasises nonverbal behaviour, turn-taking, and back-channelling rather than understanding the topics of conversation verbally.

A similar framework is the ICT Virtual Human [7] framework. It contains a number of components that cover automatic speech recognition, emotion sensors, natural language processing, and behaviour generation. This framework is more complex than the SEMAINE Framework, incorporating a large number of modules developed both by ICT USC as well as by third parties. Similar to SEMAINE, it uses XML messages in an ActiveMQ framework as the means of communication between components.

A framework developed specifically for the gaming context is Koko [15]. Koko describes a conceptual framework to integrate affect recognition into games. The framework has seven components which communicate using arrays of vectors. With these components, the framework allows the game system to manage the

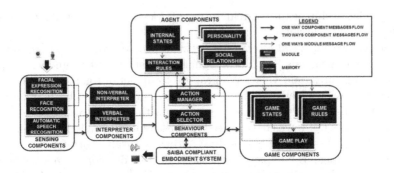

Fig. 1. Overview of the ERiSA Framework

agent's moods, user's emotional state, and game environment information. Unfortunately, this framework can only serve as an architectural connector between a game framework and other affective modules/frameworks, hence by itself it is not sufficient for building complex games.

In addition to building a framework to improve the capability of the agents, a formal model of the agents' behaviour is essential to allow agents to reason about their own behaviour. Ochs et al. proposed such a dynamic model for Non-Player Characters (NPCs) in computer games [11], which studied the dynamics of emotions, personality, and social relationship between the NPCs. In this model, the agent's behaviour is influenced by their emotions which in turn are affected by their personality. For example: a negative emotion in i induced by j decreases the value of liking i has for j and vice versa. However, this model does not define how the player's relationship to the agents comes about in the first place.

In summary, while the existing frameworks focus on generic models of IVAs, none are capable of modelling evolving social relations between users and agents, and use these to generate behaviour rules.

3   The ERiSA Framework

We propose a framework for game-agents that extends existing frameworks such as SEMAINE or the ICT Virtual Human framework by including social relationship as a variable as well as the ability to learn social interaction rules from data. We adapt the framework for a game environment by adding components that manage the game play dynamically. The framework consists of modular components including sensing, interpretation, and behaviour planning (see Fig. 1).

The functions of the main components are as follows:

- The **Sensing Component** provides modules for Facial Expression Recognition (FACS and six basic emotions [1]), Automatic Speech Recognition, and Face Recognition. The Face Recognition module is used to recognise a player's face based on which an agent can build and interpret a social relationship with a player.

- The **Interpreter Component** receives data about the player's utterances, facial expressions, and identity. The player's utterances are interpreted in the Verbal Interpreter module, while the user's emotions are interpreted by the Non-Verbal Interpreter module.
- The **Behaviour Component** proposes an agent behaviour based on the information of both verbal and non-verbal interpretation and the Interaction Rules. The proposed behaviour is then sent to a SAIBA compliant embodied system [9] by the Action Selector Module. Afterwards, the Action Manager module updates all the states and rules including Internal States, Game States, Interaction Rules, Game Rules, and Social Relationship.
- The **Agent Components** consist of Memories and a Social Relationship module. Memories include Internal States, Internal Rules, and Personality. The Interaction Rules are influenced by the agent's internal states such as personality, relationship , and emotion. The Social Relationship module manages the relationship status between two entities such as agent A-player I, player I - player II, or agent A-agent B.
- The **Game Components** consists of a Game Play module and related Memories including Game Rules, and Game States. The Game Play module regulates the game play from the Memories. The game play changes dynamically based on the agent's internal states.

An example in which the social relation is used in a game scenario is as follows: In an RPG game a player's mission is to convince guard Maximus to let the player pass the gate. The player has to do this by building a positive relationship, avoiding conflict. Suppose the player has met Maximus three times before, has a positive relationship with him, and Maximus has a high value of extraversion. The player greets the guard with a smile while saying "hello". The player's utterance and facial expression are captured and processed in the Sensing Components, and interpreted in the Interpreter Components. The Action Manager updates the values of the social relationship and the guard's internal states. In this case emotion is set to be more positive and the value of the social relationship is increased as well. Finally, Maximus reacts based on the information from the Interpreter Components and Interaction Rules.

4   Automatic Behaviour Modelling

Personality. We based our model on the OCEAN personality model [13]. This model has been used in several works in the area of IVAs [11]. The values of the traits are represented by a set of real numbers between -1 to 1, where 1 represents the strongest possible value in that particular trait. For example: if the agent has personality with an extraversion value of 0.65 and conscientiousness of -0.65 then the agent tends to be talkative and shows a lack of self-discipline.

$$\mathcal{P} = \{O, C, E, A, N\} \in [-1, 1] \tag{1}$$

Social Relationship. In the social relationship model, we highlight 2 variables of social relationship: *Likes* and *Knows*. The change in the degree of *Likes* ($Likes_t \in [-1, 1]$) at time t depends on the emotion E_t of the agent towards the player at that time (explained below), so a negative emotion at time t will lead to the decrease of *Likes*. The degree of *Knows* depends on how many times the agent and the player met, which in our game scenario is measured in terms of how often they played the game. The value of *Knows* is normalised to a real number between 0 to 1 ($Knows_{curr} \in [0, 1]$). The value of the Social Relationship at time t ($\mathcal{R}_t$) is calculated as:

$$\mathcal{R}_t = (Likes_t \times Knows) \tag{2}$$

where

$$Like_t = Likes_{t-1} + E_t \times a \tag{3}$$

Emotion. Both personality and emotion play a role in the individual's behaviour [8,12]. For example: an individual with high extraversion tends to express and perceive positive emotions, while an individual with high neuroticism trait tends to express and perceive negative emotions. In addition to personality, the social relationship also plays a role in the individual's emotional behaviour.

Subsequently, the agent's emotion at time t (E_t) is computed based on the average of events Evt_i at that time in addition to personality ($\mathcal{P}_E$ for extraversion and $\mathcal{P}_E$ for neuroticism) and social relationship at time t ($\mathcal{R}_t$). To model the dynamic properties of emotion perception in a simple yet convincing way, we implemented a decay function to our model. In the absence of any emotion evoking stimuli, the value of an affective dimension is assumed to decay over time [12]. The value of the decay rate r is set based on the agent's personality.

$$E_t = E_{t-1} \times e^{-rt} + V_t \tag{4}$$

where

$$V_t = \frac{\sum_{i=1}^{n} Evt_{(i,t)}}{n} \times (\mathcal{P}_E - \mathcal{P}_N + \mathcal{R}_t) \tag{5}$$

5   Experimental Methodology: The Smile Game

We implemented the proposed framework to create a simple game called *The Smile Game*. The main aim of this project is neither to detect nor synthesise laughter but to implement and evaluate the proposed framework and model that considers the relation between personality, social relationship, and emotion to enhance the agent's believability and quality of user interaction. Recent work in detecting and synthesising laughter can be found in the Ilhaire project [1] [17].

---

[1] http://www.ilhaire.eu/

The Smile Game is inspired by the "Don't Smile" game that has two people facing each other. The goal of the game is simple: make your opponent laugh with jokes, and funny facial expression. The first person to smile uncontrollably loses. In *The Smile Game*, we replace one of the players with an ECA. We use two SEMAINE characters, Poppy and Spike [10] as the game agents. Poppy has a high extraversion and low neuroticism personality ($\mathcal{P}_E = 0.5, \mathcal{P}_N = -0.1$, while Spike has a high neuroticism and low extraversion personality ($\mathcal{P}_E = 0.2, \mathcal{P}_N = 0.5$). This game is considered to be a good case study since the game play is simple yet elicits rich non-verbal interactions between the agents and the player.

5.1   The Smile Game Recordings

In order to study what type of behaviour people playing the Smile Game would exhibit, we performed an experiment in which two people at a time play the game whilst being video recorded. This will allow us to model typical behaviour and replicate it in the agents. We recruited 10 participants, all of whom are students in our institute (5 male; 6 Asian, 4 Caucasian). We conducted five recording sessions, with a different number of games played per session.

During the game, there were three cameras recording both visual and audio information. The first and second camera each record a player from the front while the third camera records a profile perspective of both players. The images are used for facial expressions analysis and the audio recording for discourse analysis (i.e. presence of conversation, and who spoke first).

We annotated the recordings using the Facial Action Coding System (FACS) [6] for the players' facial expressions and created a transcript of the players' utterances[2]. Next we selected utterances and facial expression that were used for attacks to make the opponent laugh. These attack behaviours were then implemented in the agent.

There were a total of 14 distinct FACS combinations that succeeded in making the opponent smile/laugh. Unfortunately, not all FACS combinations can be generated by the agents. There were ten utterances that succeeded in making the opponent smile/laugh. Hence, we push all these utterances to the agents' attack vocabulary. In addition we added twenty additional funny sentences from various sources on the internet, such as "I feel like such a homo sapiens right now" or "Don't you have something better to do?".

5.2   The Smile Game Flow

An overview of the game flow is shown in Fig. (2). When the system starts, it searches for a face. When a face is detected, the agent tries if it can recognise it from the current library of faces. Based on this, the agent greets the player using the Welcome Dialogue Set. If the face is not recognised, the agent will ask for the player's name and will initialise a new entry in the face library as well as a relationship value $\mathcal{R}$. If the system recognises the face, it searches for the

---

[2] The utterances in session 4 were in Indonesian, hence, we did a translation to English.

corresponding relationship value $\mathcal{R}$ and updates it. Afterwards, the agent starts a conversation using common topics such as the weather or news using the Chit-Chat Dialogue Set. After a fixed period of time, the agent will ask whether the player would like to play a game with the agent. If so, the game will commence and continues until someone smiles. The player can also asks the agent to play a game with them. When the game ends, the result of the game is saved by the agent, in addition to updating the value of $\mathcal{R}$. Both agent and player can ask to repeat the game, if the player does not want to repeat the game, the agent closes the interaction using its Goodbye Dialogue Set.

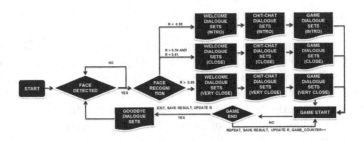

Fig. 2. Game flow. Action streams are selected based on the social relation value $\mathcal{R}$ which is either 'very close', 'close'. 'Intro' is used when the user is unknown.

In addition to the personality, relationship, and emotion model from subsection 4, we define a model to determine when the agent will smile. The agent's urge to smile S is derived from the model of emotion E from subsection 4. The difference is that while the model of emotion E considers all the possible player's verbal and non-verbal actions, the model of smile S only considers the possible player's verbal and non-verbal actions that could trigger the agent to smile. Currently, the same rules used by the agent to attack an opponent will incur an increase in S when observed by the agent.

To model the dynamic properties of the agent's smile in a simple yet convincing way, we again included a decay function to our model. This way the agent's urge to smile will diminish over time unless reactivated. Similar to the emotion model, the value of the decay rate r on this model is also set based on the agent's personality.

$$S_t = S_{t-1} \times e^{-rt} + V_t \qquad (6)$$

5.3   Evaluation

Before evaluating the system with real players, we created a simulation of the game. We experimented with two SEMAINE characters: Poppy and Spike [10]. The relationship value R between the simulated player and the agent is set to 0.65 and decay rate r to 0.02 for both agents. We performed random attacks to both characters for a certain time. Both characters were receiving the same sequence of attacks.

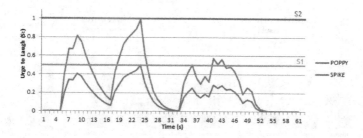

Fig. 3. Smile Simulation. The blue and purple lines show the character's urge to smile for Poppy and Spike, respectively. The orange line indicates the threshold to display a small smile and the purple line the threshold for smiling uncontrollably.

Figure 3 shows the result of the simulation of the both characters urge to laugh (S_t) as a result of three strikes. The first strike was a series of medium intensity attacks from the user from $t = 13$ to 17 s, the second one was a series of high intensity attacks from the user from $t = 25$ to 31 s, and the last strike was a series of low intensity attacks from the user from $t = 41$ to 57 s.

The S1 line indicates the threshold of generating a small smile by the agent, while the S2 line indicates the threshold for an uncontrollable smile, which means the agent loses the game. In this simulation, we used the same value of both thresholds for both agents. As we can see in the figure 3, from $t = 6$ to 11 s, Poppy who has a high extraversion value showed a small smile, and in the $t = 23$ s, Poppy was unable to hold her smile, and she lost, while Spike who has a high neuroticism only just showed a small smile at the second attack.

User Evaluation. In addition to the simulation, we performed a user evaluation of the game. We recruited 16 participants (9 male; all Asian; mean age = 24.440; age standard deviation = 3.759). All participants are students in our institute. Each participant played two sessions of the game, and in each session they played against both characters (Poppy and Spike). After the game, they were asked to fill in a questionnaire to rate their perceived relationship with the agent, the naturalness of the interaction during the conversation and the game, and the agent's response time. In addition, we also asked the participant to rate the agent's personality.

Figure 4 (a) and (b) shows the average scores for the social relationship and the naturalness of the interaction during the conversation and the game, while Fig. 4 (c) shows the score of the agents personality. A score of 1 is the lowest score, 3 indicates average score, and 5 is the highest score. Except for the rating of 'Social Relation', all scores were identical for session 1 and 2.

From the limited questionnaire results, we can tentatively draw two conclusions. Firstly, the users perceived the two characters to largely display the personality that we intended them to. Poppy was perceived to be twice as extrovert as neurotic, and Spike the other way around (see Fig. 4 (c)) Secondly, and more importantly, the participants were able to tell the changes in their social relationship with both characters over time. The average user score for the social

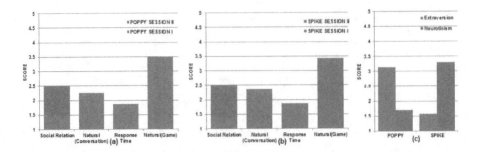

Fig. 4. User Evaluation results of the smile game. Sub-figures (a) and (b) show the perceived social relation, naturalness of behaviour, response time, and naturalness of the game for the game characters Poppy and Spike, respectively. Sub-figure (c) shows the results for perceived personality.

relationship between the agent and the player went from an average of about 1.5 at the first encounter, to 2.5 for the second encounter, when the agent was able to recognise the player and used the relevant dialogues for people it knows. However, the changes in the relationship are not very high because the participants only play with each character twice.

The rating of the naturalness in the interaction during the conversation is quite low for both of the characters due to the response time of the agents. Upon further analysis of the problem it turned out that this was caused by the low performance of the Speech Recognition module. In contrast, participants gave quite high scores for the naturalness of the interaction rating during the game.

6   Conclusion and Future Work

In this paper, we have presented an integrated framework for a social and emotional embodied game-agent. It has been evaluated in *The Smile Game*, a social game where the first person to smile loses. The results show that we successfully built an agent that is capable of creating and using the beginnings of a social relation with a player. However, we achieved quite low ratings for the naturalness in interaction during the conversation due to the low performance of the Speech Recognition module. We aim to explore better context-specific sensing components to enhance the interaction in our future work. Currently the agent's reactions are determined by simple hand-crafted interaction rules. In future work we aim for automatic interaction rule generation and adaptation by learning from (real-time) data obtained from actual interactions between the player and the game-agents.

References

1. Almaev, T.R., Valstar, M.F.: Local gabor binary patterns from three orthogonal planes for automatic facial expression recognition. In: Affective Computing and Intelligent Interaction (ACII 2013), pp. 356–361 (September 2013)

2. Bates, J.: The role of emotion in believable agents. Commun. ACM 37(7), 122–125 (1994)
3. Bickmore, T., Vardoulakis, L., Jack, B., Paasche-Orlow, M.: Automated promotion of technology acceptance by clinicians using relational agents. In: Aylett, R., Krenn, B., Pelachaud, C., Shimodaira, H. (eds.) IVA 2013. LNCS, vol. 8108, pp. 68–78. Springer, Heidelberg (2013)
4. Bogdanovych, A., Ijaz, K., Simoff, S.: The city of uruk: Teaching ancient history in a virtual world. In: Nakano, Y., Neff, M., Paiva, A., Walker, M. (eds.) IVA 2012. LNCS, vol. 7502, pp. 28–35. Springer, Heidelberg (2012)
5. Campbell, J., Core, M., Artstein, R., et al.: Developing inots to support interpersonal skills practice. In: Aerospace Conference, pp. 1–14 (March 2011)
6. Ekman, P., Friesen, W.V., Hager, J.C.: Facial Action Coding System (FACS): Manual. A Human Face, Salt Lake City, USA (2002)
7. Hartholt, A., Traum, D., Marsella, S.C., Shapiro, A., Stratou, G., Leuski, A., Morency, L.-P., Gratch, J.: All together now: Introducing the virtual human toolkit. In: Aylett, R., Krenn, B., Pelachaud, C., Shimodaira, H. (eds.) IVA 2013. LNCS, vol. 8108, pp. 368–381. Springer, Heidelberg (2013)
8. Hilgard, E.R.: Introduction to psychology. Harcourt, Brace (1953)
9. Kopp, S., Krenn, B., Marsella, S.C., Marshall, A.N., Pelachaud, C., Pirker, H., Thórisson, K.R., Vilhjálmsson, H.H.: Towards a common framework for multimodal generation: The behavior markup language. In: Gratch, J., Young, M., Aylett, R.S., Ballin, D., Olivier, P. (eds.) IVA 2006. LNCS (LNAI), vol. 4133, pp. 205–217. Springer, Heidelberg (2006)
10. McKeown, G., Valstar, M.F., Cowie, R., Pantic, M., Schröder, M.: The semaine database: Annotated multimodal records of emotionally coloured conversations between a person and a limited agent. T. Affective Computing 3(1), 5–17 (2012)
11. Ochs, M., Sabouret, N., Corruble, V.: Simulation of the dynamics of nonplayer characters' emotions and social relations in games. IEEE Transactions on Computational Intelligence and AI in Games 1(4), 281–297 (2009)
12. Picard, R.W.: Affective Computing. MIT Press, Cambridge (1997)
13. Saucier, G., Goldberg, L.R.: The language of personality: Lexical perspectives on the five-factor model. In: Wiggins, J.S. (ed.) The Five-Factor Model of Personality: Theoretical Perspectives, pp. 21–50. Guilford, New York (1996)
14. Schröder, M.: The SEMAINE API: Towards a standards-based framework for building emotion-oriented systems. In: Advances in Human-Computer Interaction, Article ID 319406 (2010)
15. Sollenberger, D.J., Singh, M.P.: Koko: An architecture for affect-aware games. Autonomous Agents and Multi-Agent Systems 24(2), 255–286 (2012)
16. Turing, A.M.: Computing machinery and intelligence. Mind 59(236), 433–460 (1950)
17. Urbain, J., Niewiadomski, R., Mancini, M., Griffin, H., Çakmak, H., Ach, L., Volpe, G.: Multimodal analysis of laughter for an interactive system. In: Mancas, M., d' Alessandro, N., Siebert, X., Gosselin, B., Valderrama, C., Dutoit, T. (eds.) INTETAIN 2013. LNICST, vol. 124, pp. 183–192. Springer, Heidelberg (2013)
18. Vinciarelli, A., Pantic, M., Bourlard, H.: Social signal processing: Survey of an emerging domain. Image Vision Comput. 27(12), 1743–1759 (2009)
19. Wagner, J., Lingenfelser, F., Baur, T., Damian, I., Kistler, F., André, E.: The social signal interpretation (ssi) framework: multimodal signal processing and recognition in real-time. In: ACM Multimedia, pp. 831–834. ACM (2013)

Building Virtual Humans with Back Stories: Training Interpersonal Communication Skills in Medical Students

Andrew Cordar[1], Michael Borish[1], Adriana Foster[2], and Benjamin Lok[1]

[1] Computer Information Science and Engineering, University of Florida, USA
[2] Psychiatry and Health Behavior, Georgia Regents University, USA
{acordar,mborish,lok}@cise.ufl.edu, afoster@gru.edu

Abstract. We conducted a study which investigated if we could overcome challenges associated with interpersonal communication skills training by building a virtual human with back story. Eighteen students interacted with a virtual human who provided back story, and seventeen students interacted with the same virtual human who did not provide back story. Back story was achieved through the use of cutscenes which played throughout the virtual human interaction. Cutscenes were created with The Sims 3 and depicted short moments that occurred in the virtual human's life. We found medical students who interacted with a virtual human with a back story, when interacting with a standardized patient, were perceived by the standardized patient as more empathetic compared to the students who interacted with the virtual human without a back story. The results have practical implications for building virtual human experiences to train interpersonal skills. Providing back story appears to be an effective method to overcome challenges associated with training interpersonal skills with virtual humans.

Keywords: virtual humans, back story, cutscenes, empathy.

1 Introduction

Virtual human experiences can be a useful tool for training interpersonal communication skills. An important component of interpersonal skills is empathy, which is the ability to understand the feelings of another and be able to communicate that understanding. Empathy plays an important role in medical education and is considered a core learning objective in a student's medical education [1]. Encouraging empathy with virtual humans is challenging. Prior research has shown that medical students empathize with virtual humans with less sincerity and frequency than with a real human [2].

In the medical field, one approach to foster empathy in medical students' is through Patient Shadowing: a technique in which medical students follow patients through their clinical visits [3]. Patient Shadowing provides context to a patient's daily life typically not seen by medical students. Shadowing is a powerful tool; however, it requires patient consent and willingness to share private experiences.

T. Bickmore et al. (Eds.): IVA 2014, LNAI 8637, pp. 144–153, 2014.
© Springer International Publishing Switzerland 2014

Informed by Patient Shadowing in the medical field, we wanted to apply this concept to virtual humans. If virtual humans were given context to their personal life, would this improve interpersonal communication skills? To investigate this, we added back story to our virtual human. Back story was added to our virtual human through cutscenes. Cutscenes, created with *The Sims 3*, are user-triggered and depict short moments that occurred in the virtual human's life.

We conducted a study in which 35 1st year medical students interviewed a virtual human depression followed by interviewing a standardized patient actor with depression. Eighteen students interacted with a virtual human with a back story (VH-Backstory), and seventeen students interacted with the same virtual human without a back story (VH-Control). The results show students in VH-Backstory group, when interacting with the standardized patient, were perceived by the standardized patient as more empathetic compared to the students in the VH-Control group.

While the research presented in this paper considers only virtual patients with back stories, the results presented have practical implications for building any type of virtual human experience to train interpersonal skills. Providing back story appears to be an effective way to overcome challenges associated with training interpersonal skills with virtual humans.

2   Related Work

2.1   Patient Shadowing

Patient shadowing is an initiative by Patient and Family Centered Care Innovation Center to produce a low-cost and effective way to follow (or shadow) patients as they receive medical care [3].

The advantage of shadowing is that the shadowers see a side of patient care they do not often see: the perspective of the patient in real-time. Patient shadowing is very powerful because medical students have the opportunity to see patients as more than just a diagnosis. Shadowing is the closest real-world counterpart to our approach of providing back story through the use of cutscenes.

2.2   Virtual Humans with Back Story

Bickmore et al developed virtual humans with back story to increase user engagement [4]. Participants were found to be more engaged with the virtual human when the virtual human told a story in the first-person as opposed the story being told in third-person. Back story was generated through text-based dialog and the study investigated more into user reaction to virtual humans with back story.

2.3   Cutscenes

Cutscenes are heavily used in video games as a way to drive the narrative forward. Cutscenes are almost always non-interactive, and just as in our system, are always triggered by the user in some way. Cutscenes in our virtual human interactions are triggered when the user elicits a response from the virtual human that is also associated with a cutscene. In video games, cutscenes can be triggered in many ways: starting/finishing a level, reaching a checkpoint, or initiating a conversation with a non-playable character.

2.4   Virtual to Real Behavioral Change

Another area of research looks at improving pro-social behavior through virtual experiences. Rosenberg et al looked at how giving participants virtual "super powers" would affect real world behavior [5]. Participants traversed a virtual city either flying in a helicopter or having the power of flight. Participants were assigned to either help a virtual diabetic child or just tour the city. Rosenberg found that participants who were given the power of flight were more likely to help the experimenter in the real world pick up spilled pens than participants who did not receive the power of flight.

3   Background

This research enhances pre-existing virtual human technology with cutscenes made from the video game *The Sims 3*. There are many forms of virtual humans; however, we use what are known as virtual patients.

The goal of this enhancement was to improve interpersonal communication skills in medical students. In particular, empathy was the most important targeted skill.

Cutscenes were made to depict various moments from the virtual patient's daily life in order to properly convey how the patient's medical condition was affecting them. The following sections will discuss virtual patients, empathy, and *The Sims*.

3.1   Empathy

Empathy, in the context of patient care, is defined as "a predominantly cognitive (rather than emotional) attribute that involves an understanding (rather than feeling) of experience, concerns and perspectives of the patient combined with a capacity to communicate this understanding" [6].

Empathy is a very important interpersonal skill for everyone to have; however, it is especially important for medical students to have strong empathy skills by the time they begin their medical profession. A key motivator for doctors to have strong empathy skills is that empathy is considered one of the best ways to improve patient compliance as well as reduce medical malpractice lawsuits [7].

3.2   The Sims

The Sims is a life-simulation game in which the player creates and maintains a family of Sims [8]. *The Sims* has various needs that reflect what humans need in the real world. They need to eat, go to the bathroom, get a job, etc. *The Sims* features robust character creation allowing users to create virtual humans of different age, weight, height, etc. In addition to the game component of *The Sims*, the game features a movie making component in which players can record Sims living their virtual life. The movie making tool was used to create the cutscenes for the virtual human.

4   Study

We conducted the use of cutscenes in virtual human interactions as part of a study involving 35 first year medical students. As seen in Figure 1, eighteen of the students interacted with a virtual human suffering depression with a back story provided by cutscenes and seventeen interacted with the same virtual human without a backstory. All 35 medical students, immediately after interacting with a virtual human, interacted with a human standardized patient actor who also suffered from depression. Because the study involves both a virtual and real component, the following sections will discuss each component.

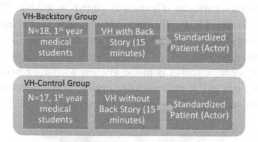

Fig. 1. Study Flow

4.1   Scenarios

Virtual. All students interacted with the same virtual patient suffering from depression. The virtual patient's name is Cynthia Young. Cynthia is a 21 year old college student whose depression has been affecting her life. Her cousin had recently passed 8 months ago. Cynthia Young has been used as a virtual patient in prior research [9].

All students were instructed to spend 15 minutes interacting with Cynthia and use their best communication skills to obtain a patient history. Students interacted with Cynthia using an online text-based interface. They conduct interviews as they normally would; however, they type want they want to say rather than speak it. The virtual patient built for this study had approximately 500 unique character speeches and approximately 4500 speech triggers for the speech matching algorithm to process user input.

Students were randomly assigned to one of two groups: a virtual patient interaction enhanced with backstory (VH-Backstory) or a virtual patient interaction without backstory (VH-Control).

Real. After interacting with Cynthia Young, all 35 students interacted with Ryan Higgins, a standardized patient actor. Ryan Higgins is a 25 year old soldier who has been experiencing symptoms of major depression. His sister had recently died 3 months ago.

4.2   Cutscenes

Four cutscenes were incorporated with the virtual human and are listed below:

- Introduction: This cutscenes serves as an introduction to Cynthia Young. It opens with Cynthia struggling to get out of bed in the morning. She is clearly sad and does not really want to get ready for class. The introduction cutscene is 46 seconds long and is played at the beginning of every cutscene enhanced virtual patient interaction.
- Weight Gain: Cynthia is shown getting ice cream from the refrigerator to eat, and after, she decides to take a nap. This cutscene is 14 seconds long and is played when students ask about her eating habits or whether she has been gaining weight.
- Watching TV: In this cutscene, Cynthia is shown watching TV and eventually falling asleep while the TV is still on. This cutscene is 12 seconds long and is shown when students ask Cynthia about what she does when she wakes up or what she does during the day.
- Crying: In this cutscene, Cynthia is in the kitchen washing her hands. After washing her hands, she sits at the kitchen table crying. This video is 15 seconds long and is shown when students ask about her general mood.

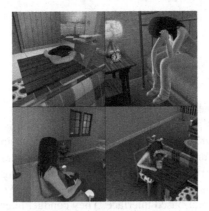

Fig. 2. Scenes from four cutscenes created

With the exception of the introduction, all cutscenes were triggered when the student asked a question that had an associated cutscene to accompany the response. 32 of Cynthia's responses had one of the three other cutscenes associated with it. 22 of those 32 responses would play the "Crying" cutscene, 8 responses would play the "Weight Gain" cutscene, and 2 responses would play the "Watching TV" cutscene.

For example, a user could ask "Have you been gaining weight recently?" in which Cynthia responds: "It feels like all I do is eat and sleep." The weight gain cutscene plays along with her response. This example is shown in Figure 3.

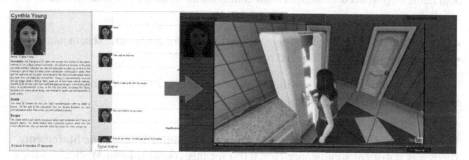

Fig. 3. Chat Interface (Left) and Cutscene triggering during interaction (Right)

4.3   Evaluation

Empathy Rating. All students' empathic responses to opportunities from patient interactions (virtual and real) were rated with the Empathic Communication Coding System (ECCS) [10]. Raters achieved an inter-rater reliability greater than 0.8 and all interaction transcripts were blinded before rating began. The ECCS scale is a 0-6 scale in which 0 is a denial of patient perspective and 6 is a statement of shared feeling or experience.

It is important to note that these empathy ratings were obtained from text-based transcripts only. No non-verbal component was considered when rating students' empathy.

Standardized Patient Communication Checklist. The standardized patients completed a communication checklist for all students which contained fourteen items rating the medical students' professional appearance, behavior, empathy, and rapport. Checklists are a common way of evaluating medical students' performance in an interview setting, and some have become a part of the US Medical Licensing Examination [11]. Elements of this checklist were based on the Medical Student Interviewing Performance Questionnaire which is a valid questionnaire for assessing medical student performance in psychiatric patient interviews [12].

5   Results

All results are based on ECCS scores and the communication checklist. For ECCS data, we ran a t-test between the 2 groups to compare means. For the checklist, Fisher's exact and the Mann-Whitney U tests were performed.

5.1   Standardized Patient Communication Checklist

There was statistical significance on two items of the communication checklist, and both items were related to interpersonal communication skills. The checklist items are as follows:

- The examinee offered encouraging, supportive, and/or empathetic statements.
- The students appeared warm and caring.

Although not statistically significant, there was also a difference for the item: "The examinee developed a good rapport with me."

The Examinee Offered Encouraging, Supportive, and/or Empathetic Statements. There was statistical significance ($p < 0.05$) for this checklist item. Medical students in the VH-Backstory group were more likely to offer encouraging, supportive, and/or empathetic statements.

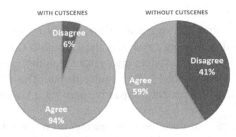

Fig. 4. Results for "The examinee offered encouraging, supportive, and/or empathetic statements"

As seen in Figure 4, approximately 94% of students in the VH-Backstory group offered empathetic statements as opposed to only approximately 59% of students in VH-Control. Additionally, only one participant did not offer empathetic statements in the VH-Backstory group. Seven participants in the other group did not offer empathetic statements.

The Student Appeared Warm and Caring. There was statistical significance ($p < 0.01$) for "The student appeared warm and caring" checklist item. Medical students in the VH-Backstory group were more likely to appear warm and caring to the standardized patient.

As seen in Figure 5, approximately 67% (twelve students) in VH-Backstory appeared warm and caring whereas approximately 35% (six students) in VH-Control appeared warm and caring.

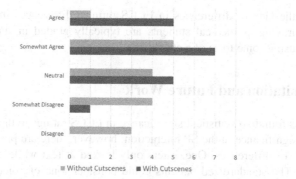

Fig. 5. Results for "The student appeared warm and caring."

The Examinee Developed a Good Rapport with Me. While not statistically significant (p=0.18), there were some differences between groups for this checklist item.

About 94% of students in VH-Backstory developed a good rapport with the standardized patient as opposed the VH-Control group where only 76% of students developed a good rapport. Again, only one student in VH-Backstory did not develop a good rapport with the standardized patient whereas 4 students in VH-Control did not develop good rapport.

5.2   ECCS

ECCS results showed no statistical significance (p=0.89) in student empathy during the standardized patient interaction. Students in VH-Backstory had a mean ECCS rating of 2.26 while students in VH-Control had a mean ECCS rating of 2.29.

6   Discussion

The standardized patients perceived the students who interacted with a virtual human with back story as more empathetic, and marginally better at developing rapport. These results suggest that using cutscenes to tell back story in a virtual setting can affect a person's perceived interpersonal skills in a real-world setting.

The standardized patient was unaware as to what condition the student belonged to. Given that the standardized patient considered the VH-Backstory group as more empathetic and was blind to the conditions, this further supports the cutscenes' efficacy in telling back story and improving interpersonal communication skills.

Since the cutscenes' total length was approximately 90 seconds, there is also evidence to suggest that this form of telling back story requires very little alteration to the original virtual experience to have a desired effect.

Students also did not know beforehand that they were going to interact with a VH who provided back story. Furthermore, students were never made directly aware that these cutscenes were depicting personal moments from the VH's life. Based on the results, this seems to indicate that students were able to use their gained insights from the back story and apply that directly in the standardized patient interaction.

Despite the lack of differences in ECCS ratings, differences in the checklist are more encouraging as medical students are typically graded in standardized patient encounters using some form of a checklist.

7   Limitation and Future Work

Our analysis found no statistical significance in ECCS ratings in the VP interaction as well as no significance in the SP interaction; however, there are possible explanations for the lack of differences. One, raters only looked at text while coding the student transcripts. The standardized patients could consider tone of voice as well as other non-verbal components such as eye contact and body language that play an important role in interpersonal communication.

We do not have any self-reported empathy of the students; however, all students were first year medical students who have received the same training. All students had taken an 8 hours "Communication skills lab" which emphasized the importance of empathy in the medical interview.

The results presented only look at the effect on interpersonal skills over a short period of time. We would also like to see how much of an impact back stories have on their interpersonal skills over time. For example, a future study could look at if whether students came back at a later for another standardized patient interaction would they still be more empathetic because of the back story provided by the virtual human.

8   Conclusion

Providing back story to virtual humans is a simple and effective way to affect students' perceived real world interpersonal communication skills. Using back story, we found that students were more likely to be empathetic with a standardized patient (a real human actor) than students who did not have back story.

Our approach of building virtual humans with back story enhances the interaction. Additionally, our method of providing back story, cutscenes, was only 90 seconds of video which does not prolong the interaction. Just as in patient shadowing, we were able to provide a way to show medical students that patients can be greatly impacted by their ailments. The virtual human is given more character with back story, and for medical students, helps convey to them that the virtual human is more than just a diagnosis or puzzle for them to solve.

Our results suggest that building virtual humans with back stories is an effective training tool for interpersonal communication skills. Skills such as empathy are essential in various domains. Virtual human training simulations that span military, education, or medicine application areas would likely benefit from virtual humans with back stories. For each domain, the context gained by back stories can help people become better communicators by applying what they learned in the virtual experience to real experiences.

Acknowledgements. The authors would like to acknowledge Dr. James Murphy, Dr. Thomas Kim, Neelam Chaudary, and Dr. Andrea Kleinsmith for providing ECCS coding. This research was funded by Arnold P Gold Foundation Grant F1-12-010 and UF Graduate Student Fellowships.

References

1. Anderson, B.: Learning objectives for medical student education – guidelines for medical schools: report I of the Medical School Objectives Project. Academic medicine: Journal of the Association of American Medical Colleges 74(1), 13–18 (1999)
2. Deladisma, A., et al.: Do medical students respond empathetically to a virtual patient? American Journal of Surgery 193(6), 756–760
3. Patient and Family Centered Care. Patient Shadowing (2013), http://www.pfcc.org
4. Bickmore, T., Schulman, D., Yin, L.: Engagement vs. Deceit: Virtual Humans with Human Autobiographies. In: Ruttkay, Z., Kipp, M., Nijholt, A., Vilhjálmsson, H.H. (eds.) IVA 2009. LNCS, vol. 5773, pp. 6–19. Springer, Heidelberg (2009)
5. Rosenberg, R.S., Baughman, S.L., Bailenson, J.: Virtual Superheroes: Using Superpowers in Virtual Reality to Encourage Prosocial Behavior. PLoS ONE 8(1), e55003 (2013)
6. Hojat, M.: A Definition and Key Features of Empathy in Patient Care. In: Eampthy in Patient Care, pp. 77–85. Springer, Heidelberg (2007)
7. Kim, S.S., et al.: The Effects of Physician Empathy on Patient Satisfaction and Compliance. Evaluation & the Health Professions, 237–251 (2004)
8. Maxis. The Sims 3 [Video Game] (2009), http://www.thesims.com
9. Shah, H., et al.: Interactive Virtual-Patient Scenarios: An Evolving Tool in Psychiatric Education. Journal. Academic Psychiatry, 146–150 (2012)
10. Bylund, C., Makoul, G.: Empathic communication and gender in the physician-patient encounter. Patient Education and Counseling, 207–216 (2002)
11. Turner, J.L., Dankoski, M.E.: Objective structured clinical exams: a critical review. Family Medicine, 574–578 (2008)
12. Black, A.E., Church, M.: Assessing medical student effectiveness from the psychiatric patient's perspective: the Medical Student Interviewing Performance Questionnaire. Medical Education, 472–478 (1998)

Agents Behavior Semi-automatic Analysis through Their Comparison to Human Behavior Clustering

Kévin Darty[1], Julien Saunier[2], and Nicolas Sabouret[3]

[1] Laboratory for Road Operations, Perception, Simulators and Simulations, French Institute of Science and Technology for Transport, Development and Networks, France
[2] Computer Science, Information Processing and Systems Laboratory, INSA of Rouen, France
[3] Computer Sciences Laboratory for Mechanics and Engineering Sciences, CNRS, France

Abstract. This paper presents a generic method to evaluate virtual agents that aim at reproducing humans behaviors in an immersive virtual environment. We first use automated clustering of simulation logs to extract humans behaviors. We then propose an aggregation of the agents logs into those clusters to analyze the credibility of agents behaviors in terms of capacities, lacks, and errors by comparing them to humans ones. We complete this analysis with a subjective evaluation based on a questionnaire filled by human annotators to draw categories of users, making their behaviors explicit. We illustrate this method in the context of immersive driving simulation.

Keywords: Virtual autonomous agent, virtual environment, behavior analysis, clustering and aggregation, logs explicitation.

1 Introduction

Intelligent virtual agents (*IVAs*) are used in several fields such as crowd simulation [1] and virtual human listener [12]. In these simulations, agents have to produce realistic behaviors. The notion of behavior can cover different views, from low level actions (*e.g.* action units on human face [6]) to complex emerging movements in crowds [1]. One specific aspect of *IVAs* is that they interact directly with human users in virtual environments (*VEs*). In this context, providing realistic behavior is a key issue to avoid breaking immersion in the *VE* [10].

In the domain of *IVAs*, several studies have already addressed the questions of believability or credibility of *IVAs* behaviors. For instance, Campano et al. [4] proposed evaluation methods for affective models. Pelachaud et al. [14] proposed a credibility evaluation of the agent affective behavior model. These methods rely on evaluation studies using participants judgment of the agent behavior credibility. Only few research rely on "objective" analysis of simulation data, and are mostly coming from the multi-agent systems (*MAS*) domain (*e.g.* [2]) in which the interaction context is very different.

T. Bickmore et al. (Eds.): IVA 2014, LNAI 8637, pp. 154–163, 2014.

We propose a method for the analysis of the agents credibility that combines human expertise and simulation logs analysis. We consider the specific case of agents aiming at reproducing human behaviors in an immersive VE. We propose to analyze the agents behaviors in terms of capacities, lacks, and errors with respect to humans. First, human participants act in the VE. Their behavior is logged and analyzed using objective methods from AI. IVAs are then evaluated by comparing their behaviors with the human participants ones in the same situation. We complete this analysis with a Human Sciences evaluation.

The next section presents related works in the domain of objective and subjective evaluation that was used in our research. Section 3 presents our method based on data clustering and aggregation algorithms. Section 4 illustrates the potential of this method in the context of a driving simulation.

2   Related Works

In our work, we want to evaluate the agents behavior at a strategic level: we consider that the behavior is based on a choice of tactics and that it evolves according to the dynamics of the environment, and to the mental state of the person [9]. For this reason, we will distinguish action logs, which are only traces of the behavior, from the behavior itself as it can be analyzed by a human. The work presented in this section relate to this level of behavior.

2.1   Objective Approach

Analysis of simulation data for the evaluation of the behavior credibility is widely used in the field of MAS. It consists in verifying through quantitative data that agents behave as in a "real" situation. This validation method is generally used at the macroscopic level [1]. However, having a valid collective behavior does not imply that the individuals behaviors are realistic. This is the reason why other researchers proposed to focus on the validation at the microscopic level. Caillou [2] showed that data analysis is more complex at this scale and cannot be done directly on the simulation logs due to the semantic gap between the noisy raw data and the sought behaviors. Field experts are generally consulted to determine high-level variables that describe the behavior to be analyzed through the data. An automated clustering algorithm can then be used to classify the agents behaviors [2]. For generic methods, as one does not have any information on the domain-specific behaviors, they are unpredefined. Therefore, the clustering method has to be unsupervised with a free number of clusters.

It is also worth noting that, in the domain of interaction, Delaherche and Chetouani proposed behavior traces clustering methods for the study of synchrony [8]. However, their goal is not to evaluate the realism of an IVA.

The main limitation of this approach is that while it allows to see the difference between categories of behaviors, extracted from the logs (i.e. behavior log clusters), it does not provide information beyond the used variables: it cannot give a meaning to the obtained clusters. On the contrary, the subjective approach, which relies on a higher-level analysis, offers this possibility.

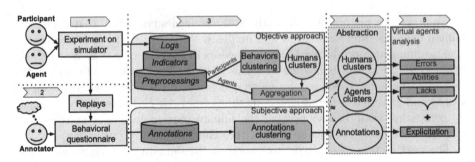

Fig. 1. Behavior analysis and evaluation method

2.2 Subjective Approach

The subjective approach for the evaluation of behavior similarity with human beings has been widely used in the domain of *IVAs* [11,14]. It consists in evaluating immersion quality through questionnaires. When it comes to *IVAs* and behavior analysis, the studies focus on the behavioral credibility [13], *i.e.* the evaluation of how human and *IVA* behaviors appear similar.

In this approach, the *IVAs* are observed by the immersed participant. The strength of this subjective approach is to characterize the adopted behaviors via questionnaires and to catch high-level behaviors through human participants annotations. One can regroup these behaviors based on these high-level descriptions. We shall then speak of *annotated behavior clusters*.

However, it is difficult to process hundreds of agents with such a method, since it requires a strong involvement of human participants.

Both logs clusters and annotations clusters aim at evaluating the adopted behaviors. For this reason, objective and subjective approaches through simulation data analysis and human expertise, complement each other. In our method, we propose to combine them: we use automated data analysis and aggregation method to build behavior log clusters, and human observers fill out a questionnaire about the adopted behaviors to build annotated behavior clusters.

3   Behavior Analysis and Evaluation Method

The method we propose is based on the combination of simulation logs analysis (objective part) and answers to a behavior questionnaire (subjective part). The simulation data are classified into behavior logs clusters. The behavior questionnaire allows us to define situation-specific users categories for both participants and agents. We then evaluate the agents by analyzing the behaviors logs clustering composition and make the behaviors explicit via the annotation clusters.

The general method is described in the Figure 1. It consists of 5 main steps: 1) collection of data in simulation and 2) annotation of these data, 3) data preprocessing and automatic clustering, then 4) clusters comparison, and finally 5) composition analysis and explicitation.

In the following subsections, we present these different steps.

Steps 1 and 2: Experiments

We use the human behaviors as the reference behaviors to analyze agents ones. This is why the first step of our method is the collection of quantitative data about human participants from an immersive simulation in a *VE*. We also produce new simulations in which the participant is replaced by an agent (*i.e.* placed in an identical situation to that presented to participants) and then collect the very same logs as for the participants. Different types of agents are generated by exploring the parameter space such as normativity, experience, decision parameters... We call *main actors* both humans and *IVAs* gathered together. The raw data from main actors experiments in the simulator are called *simulation logs.*

The second step is the subjective evaluation of the main actors behaviors. A different set of participants annotates the video replays of all main actors simulations via the behavior questionnaire. This step produces a set of annotations.

Step 3a: Logs Clustering

The first objective of the third step is to compare participants behaviors and agents behaviors so as to report on the capability of the agents to reproduce human behaviors. Our goal is to compute behavior categories that serve as abstractions to the logs: each cluster shall regroup different logs representative of the same type of high level behavior (see Figure 1).

To begin with, field experts are consulted to identify important domain-specific indicators. The values for these indicators are computed from the simulation logs and then turned into scalars within a series of preprocessing as described on the left part of figure 2.

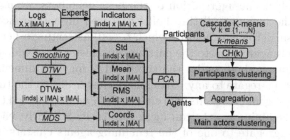

Fig. 2. Logs preprocessing, clustering, and aggregation with the time (T), the number of variables (X), of indicators ($|inds|$), and of main actors ($|MA|$)

The reason for this pre-processing it that most of the indicators are temporal and an identical behavior adopted by several main actors can occur with a temporal offset. In order to take this into account, we use the Dynamic Time Warping [16] algorithm (DTW) which computes mutual distances. The K-means algorithm need the data to be in a dimensional space for which axes are perpendicular. So as to include DTW similarities as new variables describing the main actors, we use a Multi-Dimensional Scaling algorithm (*MDS*) to place each main actor in a dimensional space. We then process a *Principal Component Analysis* to project the data on a hyperplane with non-correlated axes. The outcome of this process is a set of indicators. In order to draw the behavior categories, we use an automatic unsupervised clustering algorithm on these indicators. The number of clusters is not defined a priori: we apply the *K-means* clustering algorithm on the participants indicators, and use the *Variance Ratio Criterion* [3] to determine the appropriate number of clusters K.

This first part of step 3 has already been published and more information can be found in [7]. In this paper, we add a further building block to this method: the aggregation of agents to the participants clusters.

Step 3b: Cluster Aggregation

During the clustering process, the addition of a main actor modifies the clusters shape and may change the affectations. However, agents and humans should not be considered with the same view, since the humans behaviors represent the target to which we want to compare our agents behaviors. For this reason, we do not want agents to modify the humans clustering. In order to keep the human clusters intact, the k-means algorithm is applied on participants only. The agents are then aggregated to the fixed human clusters if close enough or classified into new agents clusters.

Our method works as follows. We define for each participants cluster $C_i \in C$ a threshold t_i above which the agent a is considered as being too far from the centroid m_i to be aggregated. This threshold t_i is defined on each dimension (*i.e.* on each indicator ind) as the distance between the centroid m_i and the farthest participant p: $t_i^{ind} = \forall\ p,\ max(|m_i^{ind} - p^{ind}|)$.

In order to allow the aggregation of the near neighbors, we enlarge t_i by a percentage of the mean of all thresholds t_i, based on a tolerance rate ϵ: this allows to have singleton clusters (for which $t_i = 0$) attracting other main actors.

Each agent a is aggregated to the participants cluster C_i of which the centroid is the closest among those under the threshold t_i for each dimension. If some agent(s) did not aggregate to any participants cluster due to the thresholds, the first "remaining" agent creates its own cluster C_{k+1} which is added to the clusters set C so that remaining agents can aggregate to it. Similarly, each remaining agent tries to aggregate to one of the remaining agents clusters, following the same threshold rule as for human clusters, or creates its own cluster if this is not possible. Thus, as shown in Figure 2, we obtain a clustering composed of all the main actors.

Step 3c: Annotation Clustering

The second objective is to analyze the behaviors through annotations, following the subjective approach. We use the same methodology as for logs clustering: identification of key indicators, unsupervised clustering on those indicators for the human participants and aggregation of *IVAs* to the human clusters.

The subjective approach requires manual annotation of replays: when the number of *IVAs* increases, it becomes impracticable to annotate them all. Yet, under the hypothesis that agents aggregated to a logs cluster of participants should have been annotated in the same way as the participants of this cluster, it is still possible to make these agents behaviors explicit via the participants annotation. In this case, the combination of the objective approach and the subjective one allows us to compare any number of agents and any number of agent models with human participants. However, clusters composed only of agents can no longer be explicited. For this reason, in the experiment presented hereafter, and considering that we had only a limited number of agents, we used manual annotation of all main actors.

The second difficulty for annotation clustering is to choose the right set of indicators. We want these indicators to be both field-specific and situation-specific. In general, behavior questionnaires allow to characterize the participant general behavior, while the participant can adopt a specific (and different) behavior in a local situation. For this reason, as will be shown in the next section, we adapt domain-specific behaviors questionnaires to define the indicators for the situation annotation. Scale scores of questionnaires are calculated by adding the scale-related questions, and normalized between 0 and 1.

We then classify the participants scores using the *K-means* algorithm with the agents aggregation, which builds our annotation clusters.

Steps 4 and 5: Clusters Analysis

The fourth step of our method is the comparison of the two clusterings (logs clusters with annotations clusters). As both evaluate behaviors, having a strong similarity between them in terms of composition is a partial verification that the logs clustering is meaningful in terms of situation-specific user categories, and thus corresponds to task-related high-level behaviors. We evaluate the similarity between them (dashed arrow) with the *Rand Index* (*RI*).

The fifth and final step consists in analyzing the *IVAs*. It is possible to distinguish three cluster types in terms of participant and agent composition: 1) The clusters containing both humans and agents : They correspond to high-level behaviors that are correctly reproduced by the agents. 2) Those consisting of simulated agents only: They correspond to behaviors that were produced only by the agents. In most cases it reflects simulation errors, but it can also be due to a too small participants sample. 3) Those consisting of participants only: They correspond to behaviors that have not been replicated by the agents. Thus, they are either lacks in the agent model or due to a too small agents sample in the parameter space. We then combine this human-agent comparison with the annotation analysis to give explicit information (*i.e.* high-level characteristics) about those agents behaviors and about the missing behaviors if any.

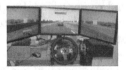 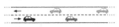

(a) The driving sim-   (b) Scenario of the
ulator device   driving experiment

Fig. 3. Application to the study of driving simulation

4   Evaluation

This section illustrates our method with an application to the study of driving simulation, and then presents the data analysis and discusses the results.

4.1   Case Study

We used the *ARCHISIM* road traffic simulator [5]. We want to evaluate the realism and credibility of the agents driving behaviors. To do this, the participants drive a car on a road containing simulated vehicles. The circuit (shown in Figure 3b) provides a driving situation on a single carriage way with two opposing lanes. It corresponds to about 1 minute of driving. The main actor encounters a vehicle at low speed on the right lane and oncoming vehicles on the left lane with increasing distances between them.

The *Driving Behavior Questionnaire (DBQ)* [15] collects data about drivers habits. In order to have a situation-specific questionnaire, we chose to base the annotation on the *DBQ* scales. The annotation questionnaire provides 5 *Likert*-type scales: *slips, lapses, mistakes, unintended* and *deliberate violations*. In addition, it supplies a scale related to the accident risk.

During the simulation we collect the main actors logs. We collect each 300 *ms* several variables such as the cap to the lane axis, the speed, and the topology. The road traffic experts chose both high-level indicators (*e.g.* the inter-vehicles distance, the time to collision, and the number of lane changings) and low-level variables (like speed, acceleration, and lateral distance).

The 22 participants of our driving simulation experiment are regular drivers aged from 24 to 59. Our experiment is carried out on a device comprising a steering wheel, a set of pedals, a gearbox and 3 screens (see Figure 3a).

Firstly, a test without simulated traffic is performed for the participant to get accustomed to the *VE*. Then, the participant performs the scenario, this time in interaction with simulated vehicles. It should be noted that as the behavior of simulated vehicles is not scripted, situations differ more or less depending on the main actors behavior. The data are then recorded for the processing phase and a video is made for the replay. Finally, 6 other participants fills the annotations questionnaire after viewing the video replays (22 participants and 14 agents).

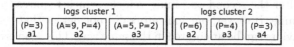

Fig. 4. Comparison of main actors between logs clustering (with participants P and agents A), and annotations clustering grouped together with the cluster numbers $(a\#)$ being written just bellow the composition.

4.2 Results

We have compared the logs clustering and the annotations clustering (see Figure 4). The Rand Index between the two clusterings is 0.51. There are 2 behavior log clusters and 4 behavior annotation clusters.

Logs cluster 1 contains 9 participants and all the 14 agents. The *number of lane changings* indicator value is 0 meaning that these main actors did not try to overtake the vehicle at low speed and preferred to follow it. As this cluster is composed of both agents and participants, it is therefore a capacity of the agent model to reproduce a human behavior which is to choose not to overtake.

Logs cluster 2 is only composed of participants. These 13 participants overtake the vehicle at low speed after the 2nd or the 3rd oncoming vehicle. As there are only participants, this human behavior can be considered as a lack in the agent model: the agents cannot choose to overtake as some human do.

Annotation cluster 1 contains 3 participants and no agent. The annotators consider that they are the more dangerous drivers with very high scores on each scale and especially on the *judgment* scale. Since no agent was considered that dangerous, and as the aim of the agents is to reproduce the most complete panel of human behaviors, there is a lack of unsafe behaviors in the model.

Annotation cluster 2 is composed of both participants and agents. They are annotated as very cautious drivers with the smallest scores on each scale. The space parameter of these agents ensure more respect for the highway code and smoother driving. The normative human behavior can therefore be considered as partly reproduced.

Annotation cluster 3 is a smaller cluster composed of participants and agents. The annotators considered them as ordinary drivers with medium scores. As for the previous cluster, the average behavior is reproduced in this situation.

Annotation cluster 4 is only composed of participants. It has some high scores on the specific *memory* and *judgment* scales. This behavior considered as slightly dangerous is also not reproduced by agents.

4.3 Discussion

In the *logs cluster 1*, the indicators were not able to distinguish the *annotations cluster 1* from the rest of the main actors. The judgment scale is very high and a video replay shows that these participants tried to overtake several times unsuccessfully. Likewise, the participants of the *annotations cluster 4* were not separated from *logs cluster 2*. This might be due to the fact that they dared to overtake just after the second oncoming vehicle, which requires to pull back in a short time frame. However, our indicators did not detect that difference.

Several behaviors can be annotated in the same way. This is an issue to analyze the similarity between the annotations clustering and the logs clustering with the *RI* measure. A solution could be compute the *RI* on logs clustering for which logs clusters annotated in the same way will be merged into one cluster.

We have a significant similarity between annotations and logs clusterings, meaning that we are able to classify our logs data into high-level behavior clusters which are meaningful in terms of driving annotations. Nevertheless the two clusterings are not identical with regard to the clusters composition. This could be due to the few number of annotators. This problem may also come from the clustering algorithm which is a classic but basic one. However, we already tried other algorithms such as *EM* and *HAC* without better results. We have to test with time-series based algorithms. Also, the experts of the domain have to be consulted to understand what missing indicator could catch these differences.

The third type of cluster (which does not appear in this experiment) is composed of agents only. In that case, we can consider - as no participant adopted this behavior - that the agents behavior is inaccurate (*i.e.* is an error) and should be investigated further. The method has to be applied in other situations in order to verify this particular case.

5   Conclusion and Perspectives

This paper presents a method to study *IVAs* behaviors through an experiment in a *VE*. This validation is original in coupling an objective analysis of the agents behaviors through simulation logs, with a subjective analysis, coming from Human Sciences, of the situation-specific user categories through an annotation done by participants. The objective analysis uses an unsupervised clustering algorithm applied on simulation logs in order to classify participants behaviors, and an aggregation method to compare agents behaviors to humans ones. This comparison allows us to evaluate the agents behaviors credibility in terms of capacities, lacks, and errors. It also provides an analysis of which *IVA* parameter space produces which perceived behavior. The method is generic for *VEs* where agents aim at reproducing human behaviors. When applied to a new domain, some of the tools have to be adapted, such as the choice of the behavior questionnaire which is domain-specific.

Our validation method was applied to the road traffic simulation. This experiment showed that the methodology is usable for mixed and complex *VEs* and that it is possible to obtain high-level behaviors from the logs via our abstraction.

Several tracks for further work remain to explore. On the clustering part, the evaluation of multiple time series based algorithms should help classifying the temporal data. On the aggregation part, the automation of the parameter calibration will be beneficial to the agents aggregation accuracy.

Another research open issue is how the behaviors clustering evolve through multiple situations of a longer scenario, whether the participants clusters remain stable or change in number or composition.

References

1. Bosse, T., Hoogendoorn, M., Klein, M.C.A., Treur, J., van der Wal, C.N.: Agent-based analysis of patterns in crowd behaviour involving contagion of mental states. In: Mehrotra, K.G., Mohan, C.K., Oh, J.C., Varshney, P.K., Ali, M. (eds.) IEA/AIE 2011, Part II. LNCS, vol. 6704, pp. 566–577. Springer, Heidelberg (2011)
2. Caillou, P., Gil-Quijano, J.: Simanalyzer: Automated description of groups dynamics in agent-based simulations. In: Proceedings of the 11th International Conference on Autonomous Agents and Multiagent Systems, vol. 3, pp. 1353–1354. International Foundation for Autonomous Agents and Multiagent Systems (2012)
3. Caliński, T., Harabasz, J.: A dendrite method for cluster analysis. Communications in Statistics-theory and Methods 3(1), 1–27 (1974)
4. Campano, S., Sabouret, N., Sevin, E.d., Corruble, V.: An evaluation of the core computational model for affective behaviors. In: Proceedings of the 2013 International Conference on Autonomous Agents and Multi-Agent Systems, pp. 745–752. International Foundation for Autonomous Agents and Multiagent Systems (2013)
5. Champion, A., Éspié, S., Auberlet, J.M.: Behavioral road traffic simulation with archisim. In: Summer Computer Simulation Conference, pp. 359–364. Society for Computer Simulation International (1998, 2001)
6. Courgeon, M., Martin, J.-C., Jacquemin, C.: Multimodal affective and reactive character. In: 1st Workshop on Affective Interaction in Natural Environments (2008)
7. Darty, K., Saunier, J., Sabouret, N.: A method for semi-automatic explicitation of agent's behavior: application to the study of an immersive driving simulator. In: The 6th International Conference on Agents and Artificial Intelligence (ICAART 2014), pp. 81–91. SciTePress (2014)
8. Delaherche, E., Chetouani, M., Mahdhaoui, A., Saint-Georges, C., Viaux, S., Cohen, D.: Interpersonal synchrony: A survey of evaluation methods across disciplines. IEEE Transactions on Affective Computing 3(3), 349–365 (2012)
9. Fisher, D.L., Rizzo, M., Caird, J.K.: Handbook of driving simulation for engineering, medicine, and psychology. CRC Press (2011)
10. Fontaine, G.: The experience of a sense of presence in intercultural and international encounters. Presence: Teleoperators and VEs 1(4), 482–490 (1992)
11. Gratch, J., Marsella, S.: Evaluating a computational model of emotion. Autonomous Agents and Multi-Agent Systems 11(1), 23–43 (2005)
12. Gratch, J., Wang, N., Gerten, J., Fast, E., Duffy, R.: Creating rapport with virtual agents. In: Pelachaud, C., Martin, J.-C., André, E., Chollet, G., Karpouzis, K., Pelé, D. (eds.) IVA 2007. LNCS (LNAI), vol. 4722, pp. 125–138. Springer, Heidelberg (2007)
13. Lester, J.C., A., S., Converse, o.: The persona effect: affective impact of animated pedagogical agents. In: Proceedings of the SIGCHI Conference on Human Factors in Computing Systems, pp. 359–366. ACM (1997)
14. Pelachaud, C.: Modelling multimodal expression of emotion in a virtual agent. Phil. Trans. R. Soc. B: Biological Sciences 364(1535), 3539–3548 (2009)
15. Reason, J., Manstead, A., Stradling, S., Baxter, J., Campbell, K.: Errors and violations on the roads: a real distinction? Ergonomics 33(10-11), 1315–1332 (1990)
16. Salvador, S., Chan, P.: Toward accurate dynamic time warping in linear time and space. Intelligent Data Analysis 11(5), 561–580 (2007)

Upper Body Animation Synthesis
for a Laughing Character

Yu Ding[1], Jing Huang[1], Nesrine Fourati[1],
Thierry Artières[2], and Catherine Pelachaud[1,3]

[1] Institut Mines-TELECOM, TELECOM ParisTech, Paris, France
[2] Université Pierre et Marie Curie (LIP6), Paris, France
[3] CNRS - LTCI UMR 5141, Paris, France

Abstract. Laughter is an important social signal in human communication. This paper proposes a statistical framework for generating laughter upper body animations. These animations are driven by two types of input signals, namely the acoustic segmentation of laughter as pseudo-phoneme sequence and acoustic features. During the training step, our statistical framework learns the relationship between the laughter human motion and the input signals. During the synthesis step, our trained framework synthesizes automatically natural head and torso animations from the input signals. Objective and subjective evaluations were conducted to validate this framework. The results show that our proposed framework is capable of generating laughing upper body movements.

Keywords: virtual character, head motion synthesis, torso motion synthesis, Hidden Markov model, laughter, character animation.

1 Introduction

Embodied conversational agents, ECAs, are autonomous software characters with a human-like appearance and communicative capabilities. Several models of ECAs have been proposed [1],[2] but very few works focus on animation synthesis for laughing.

Laughter is frequently used in human communication. Laughter is strongly linked to positive emotions and even more to cheerful mood [3]. Humans laugh at humorous stimuli or to mark their pleasure when receiving praised statements[4]; they also laugh to mask embarrassment[5] or to be cynical. Laughter can act also as social indicator of in-group belonging; it can work as speech regulator during conversation; it can also be used to elicit laughter in interlocutors as it is very contagious [4].

Laughter morphology involves facial expressions, body movements and vocalizations [6]. For hilarious laughter [5], muscular activities include mainly the zygomatic major, mouth opening and jaw movement. Eyebrows may be raised or even frown in very intense laughter [6]. Saccadic movements affect the whole body. Torso may bend back and forth and shoulder may shake. Changes in respiration patterns are also prominent. Inhalation and exhalation phases are very

T. Bickmore et al. (Eds.): IVA 2014, LNAI 8637, pp. 164–173, 2014.

noticeable. All these movements are done very rhythmically and they are also highly correlated. Indeed they arise from the same physiological processes [6].

Darwin reported "During excessive laughter the whole body is often thrown backward and shakes, or is almost convulsed" [7]. Ruch and Ekman [6] described laughter movements as "rhythmic patterns", "rock violently sideways, or more often back and forth", "nervous tremor ... over the body", "twitch or tremble convulsively". Melo et al. [8] built a virtual character which "convulses the chest with each chuckle". It means that periodic motions of head and body are important and well-known features during laughter. The periodicity of body motion was used to distinguish between laughters in[9]. Ruch and Ekman [6] reported that rhythmical patterns during laughter were usually characterized by frequency around 5 Hz. Mancini et al. [9] observed 8 videos, which show people laughing while watching funny images. Laughing persons produce rhythmic body movements with frequencies in the range of [$1.27Hz$ $3.66Hz$]. Using such findings of laughing behaviours, our main objective is to build an animation synthesis model of upper body movement during laughter.

The aim of this paper is to report head and torso animation synthesis for a hilarious laughing character. To achieve our aim, a data-driven animation model is proposed to first learn, from a collected laughter corpus, the relationship linking the input signals and human motions; then, this trained statistical model can be used as generator of laughter head and torso animations.

2   Dataset

We created a multimodal dataset of laughter. Three human subjects participated in the collection of laughter data. During recording session, the subjects watched funny movies for about 25-40 minutes. Since laughter motion occurs mainly during social interactions [10], [11], we propose an interactive setup where two subjects watch funny videos together. Only the movement of one person was gathered. Three-dimensional torso and head movements and audio signal are recorded by a motion capture system at 125 frames per second (fps) and a microphone at 44100 Hz, which were synchronized using the approach described in [12]. During data processing, all laughter episodes were manually extracted. In total, we obtain 259 laughter episodes; each one lasts from 1 to 37 seconds. Then phonetic transcription is extracted by Urbain et al [13], in which 12 laughter pseudo-phonemes are defined in reference to speech phoneme. Laughter involves very specific sounds that cannot be translated as speech phonemes. For simplicity, laughter pseudo-phoneme is called phoneme in this paper. Phonetic transcription contains phoneme (text signal) and its duration. An intensity value is also provided for each phoneme. Notice that, if one phoneme occurs successively several times, the sum of phoneme lasting time is viewed as one phoneme duration. Finally, PRAAT [13] is used to extract acoustic signals at 125 fps including pitch and energy.

3   Head and Torso Motion Synthesis

We propose a system to produce head and torso motions featured by 3D rotation angles (hence a 6 dimensional signal) from a number of input signals which are: the pseudo-phoneme sequence together with their duration and their intensity (low or high), and audio features (we use pitch and energy).

Animation Generator. To do so we consider building one model of generating animation for every (*phoneme, intensity*) pair, we name a model for each pair an Animation Generator (AG). Since *silence* phoneme is not labelled by intensity and the other 11 phonemes are labelled by low or high intensities, we build 23 AGs. Each of these 23 AGs is learned independently from the training corpus of corresponding (input, output) pairs where the input stands for all the above input features and the ouput stands for a sequence of animation motion for the 6 data streams we want to learn to synthesize (the 6 dimensions of the animation signal). Our modeling framework is based on three ideas that we detail now.

- Modeling one dimensional shaking-like movement with what we call *Loop HMM*.
- Introducing speech influence on motion through transition probability parameterization, yielding what we call Transition Parameterized Loop HMM (TPLHMM).
- Taking into account the dependencies between the 6 dimensions of the animation movements with coupled HMMs, yielding Coupled TPLHMM (CT-PLHMM).

Modelling Shaking Motion with a Loop HMM. We propose a specific HMM that we call a Loop HMM (LHMM) to model (and synthesize) a one-dimensional shaking-like (and/or trembling) signal (Figure 1). It has an approximate left-to-right chain structure where transitions are allowed from one state to itself, to the previous and to the next state. Yet it is intended that the transition probability from one state to the previous state be very small so that a likely state sequence will depict the entire chain form the first state to the last state with some *hesitation* corresponding to few back transitions.

The HMM is designed so that an observation sequence produced along such a state sequence will correspond to one shake pattern (with some trembling effect coming from back transitions). There is one Gaussian distribution associated to each state of the chain, which are set by hand rather than learned, as follows. We first divide the range of the signal value in N intervals and define N Gaussian Probability Density Function (PDF), one for each interval. The mean of the Gaussian distribution for a given interval is the mean of this interval and its variance is defined according to the width of this interval. Then we assign one of the PDF to every state of the left-right HMM so that going from the first state to the last state corresponds to a trajectory of a shaking movement. For instance in Figure 1, the first state has PDF p_2 which outputs intermediate values in the observation space, the second state has PDF p_3 which outputs higher values, it is followed by a state with PDF p_2, then by a state with PDF p_1 which outputs lower values. If a signal is produced by this HMM along a state sequence that goes from the first (left) to the last (right) state it will correspond to a shaking-like motion.

Finally, there is a loop from the last state to the first state to enable the repetition of such a shaking and trembling pattern. Figure 1 (top) shows one example of a synthesized motion stream by a LHMM. As can be seen, the animation inferred by a LHMM shows the repetition of a pattern.

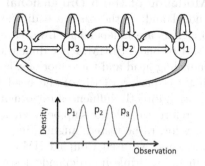

Fig. 1. A Loop HMM whose manual design allows us to model shaking and trembling one dimensional movements

Taking into Account the Dependency with Speech. Some evidence about the motion pattern may be gained from taking into account the dependencies between audio signal and motion during laughter [14]. Audio signal (we use pitch and energy) may then be used to shape the synthesized animation stream. In addition to introducing some variability in the inferred animation such a strategy makes animation look more realistic because of an increased consistency with the audio signal.

To exploit such a correlation between speech and movements we developed an extension of our LHMM, whose state transition probabilities depend on acoustic features. We call these models Transition Parameterized Loop HMM (TPLHMM). They may be used to model and synthesize one dimensional shaking movements that are linked in some way with speech. We implemented this idea in a similar way as proposed previously by [15] to take into account the dependency of observations sequences in the HMM framework to what was called contextual or external variables. The difference lies in that, while in [15] contextual variables were used to alter Gaussian PDF means, we use the speech features to alter the transition probabilities in our TPLHMMM. We consider that transition probablities from state i to state j at time t are defined according to:

$$a_{i,j}(t) = \frac{e^{W_{i,j}\theta_t}}{\sum_{j'} e^{W_{i,j'}\theta_t}} \tag{1}$$

where θ_t and W' are c-dimensional vectors. θ_t stands for contextual features at time t (e.g. pitch and energy) and W's are parameter matrices (to be learned from data) associated to each possible transition. The parameters of a TPLHMM (the W's) are learned via likelihood maximization with a Generalized EM algorithm. To ease learning it is initialized with a trained LHMM (HMM).

Isolated and Joint Modeling of the 6 Dimensional Animation Signal. A first possibility to model and synthesize the 6 dimensional animation signal is to assume the 6 signals are independent from each others and to learn independently one LHMM or one TPLHMM per dimension. Alternatively one could consider jointly modeling head and torso motions. For example, Ruch and Ekman [6] reported that the backward tilt of the head facilitates the forced exhalations, while exhalation directly influences torso motion as being done in DiLorenzo et al. [14]. Therefore, the relationship between head and torso motions should be modeled jointly for, to be tested, augmenting naturalness of synthesized animations. In our work, we used Coupled HMMs (CHMM) [16] which have been designed to model multiple interdependent streams of observations. In a CHMM with K streams of observations, there is one HMM per stream and transition probabilities account for transiting from K-tuple of states (one state in each stream's HMM) to another K-tuple of states. In our experiments we use 6 trained TPLHMMs to initialize one CHMM, we then get a Coupled TPLHMM, whose transitions are parameterized with speech features. After initialization it is retrained through maximum likelihood estimation.

Animation Synthesis. Given a phoneme sequence of length T, together with their intensity and duration, we independently synthesize T segments of appropriate duration. Each of the segment is synthesized with the corresponding model of the (phoneme, intensity) pair, which is either a set of 6 LHMMs, or a set of 6 TPLHMMs, or a CTPLHMM with 6 streams. In case TPLHMMs or CTPLHMM are used the acoustic features are exploited to alter the transition probabilities.

Whatever the models used, the synthesis is performed simply by randomly generating a state sequence according to transition probability distribution, then by synthesizing the most likely observation sequence given the state sequence, which consists in the sequence of the means of the Gaussian distribution of the states in the sequence.

4   Experiments

Animation synthesis model is built from human data of 2 subjects. The data contains 205 laugh sequences and 25625 frames in total. Human data from another subject is used for validation through subjective and objective evaluation studies. It contains 54 laugh sequences and 6750 frames. Objective and subjective evaluations are conducted to validate the proposed animation synthesis model.

4.1 Objective Evaluation

As described in Section 3, LHMM and TPLHMM treat separately each dimension motion of head and torso, while the coupled model can simulate the relationship between them. We first investigate whether such a coupling is relevant; then we compare the animations synthesized by LHMM, TPLHMM and CTPLHMM with respect to few quantitative criterion.

Investigating Relation between Head and Torso. To investigate the relevance of joint modeling of the 6 dimensions animation we tested the probabilistic independency between the 6 random variables corresponding to the states that are occupied at the same time in the 6 streams' LHMMs. For each pair of streams we built a contingency table for the two random variables of being in a state in the HMM for stream 1 while being in a state in the HMM for stream 2, then we computed a χ^2 test to evaluate the independency between the two random variables. We found that whatever the two streams are and whatever the model is, i.e whatever the pair (phoneme, intensity) is, the two random variables were found statistically dependent at a p-value lower than 0.001. This means jointly modeling the multiple streams is actually relevant and should lead to improved animation.

Furthermore to quantify the degree of dependency between the multiple streams we computed relative mutual information. The mutual information between two random variables X and Y, $I(X,Y)$, equals the difference between the entropy of X, $H(X)$ and the conditional entropy of X given Y, $H(X|Y)$. If X and Y are independent, Y does not bring any information about X and $I(X,Y) = 0$. Alternatively, if Y includes some information about X, the uncertainty on X is reduced when knowing Y so that the conditional entropy $H(X|Y)$ is lower than $H(X)$ and $I(X,Y) > 0$. Furthermore one can measure the amount of information Y brings on X by computing a normalized mutual information $\hat{I}(X,Y) = I(X,Y)/H(X)$ where $H(X)$ is the entropy of X. The normalized mutual information belongs to the range $[0,1]$. It equals 0 if X and Y are fully independent, while it equals 1 if X may be deterministically predicted from Y.

In all the tests we performed we obtained normalized mutual information between 17% and 22% which shows that some uncertainty exists between the 6 dimensions of the animation but that it is not fully random either.

As a conclusion, the 6 dimensions of the animation are not independent. Hence, independent modeling of the 6 streams would be suboptimal, and these are not deterministically linked, meaning that a pure synchronous modeling of the 6 streams in a single LHMM or a single TPLHMM would not be a good option either. Finally these resuts justify our choice of modeling the 6 dimensional animation signal within a coupled HMM that enables modeling a weak dependency between the streams.

Similarity between Synthesized and Real Animations. We compared our models by computing 3 criteria which allow evaluating the similarity between a synthesized signal and a real signal. Basically we consider the quality of the synthesized signal with respect to three features: the main frequency of the signal, as extracted by the Periodicity Algorithm [17], the amplitude of this main frequency, and the energy of this frequency. These criteria allow investigating if the main features of a shaking-like movement are well modeled by the synthesis system.

For each of the three features we computed a normalized error (e.g. $\left|\frac{f^s - f^h}{f^h}\right|$ for the frequency feature, where f^s and f^h stand for the frequency of the synthesized and of the human animation signals averaged over all phonemes realizations. The lower such a measure is the closer the synthesized signal is from the original one. The frequency, amplitude and energy errors obtained for our various models are reported in Figure 1. According to these measures, TPLHMM and CTPLHMM do perform much better than LHMM while the difference of performance between TPLHMM and CTPLHMM is less clear.

Table 1. Performance of the models with respect to the synthesis quality (frequency, amplitude and energy errors). Performances are averaged results gained on 54 test sequences (standard deviations are given in brackets).

Model	frequency	amplitude	energy
LHMM	0.21 (0.074)	0.24 (0.100)	0.41 (0.071)
TPLHMM	0.17 (0.063)	0.19 (0.066)	0.34 (0.057)
CTPLHMM	0.17 (0.061)	0.20 (0.059)	0.31 (0.052)

4.2 Subjective Evaluation

Two subjective evaluations were conducted through an online web application. First, we compare the animations synthesized by TPLHMM and CTPLHMM; then the best one is compared to human data. The participants were invited to watch 5 videos of laughing virtual character and to answer few questions for each video. They could control when to start the videos and could watch them as many times as they wish. Our aim is to evaluate the behaviors animation and not the appearance of the virtual agent. We used the same virtual agent to display motion data for both subjective evaluations. Motion data displayed with the virtual character consists of head and torso movements (motion capture or generated data) and facial expression. Facial expression of laughter was computed using our previous approach [18]. The 5 videos used in both subjective studies last respectively 9s, 10s, 18s, 26s and 27s.

TPLHMM and CTPLHMM Comparison. To compare TPLHMM and CT-PLHMM, both trained models were applied to the 5 test samples. For each test sample, a pair of videos was recorded in which the virtual agent's head and torso motions were driven respectively by these models. Each pair of video clips was displayed on the same web page and randomly arranged on the right or on the left. After watching each pair of video clips, participants were invited to select the best animation along four dimensions: naturalness of the animation, synchronization of head and torso movements with laugh sound, correlation of laughter intensity and torso movements, inter-correlation of head and torso movement.

This evaluation study involved 120 participants, 67 males and 53 females with age ranging from 18 to 65 years old (Mean=33.5 years, SD=9.6 years). We computed 95% confidence intervals that show that CTPLHMM is significantly better than TPLHMMs with respect to the 4 questions: we obtained a confidence interval equal to [66% 77%] for CTPLHMM being better than TPLHMMS with respect to Naturalness, [60% 72%] for Synchronisation, [58% 70%] for Intensity correlation and [63% 74%] for Head and Torso inter-correlation.

Synthesized and Human Data Comparison. With respect to the results above, CTPLHMM is perceived as the best animation synthesis framework; so we use the animations obtained with CTPLHMM in the comparison test with human data. This subjective evaluation was conducted to investigate how similar is the perception of the virtual agent displaying head and torso motions synthesized by CTPLHMM to the perception of the virtual agent displaying head and torso motions synthesized by CTPLHMM is similar to the perception of the virtual agent animated directly by human data. As the previous study, a comparison test was conducted.

In total, there were 80 participants consisting of 46 males and 34 females with age ranging from 12 to 78 (M=40.65 years, SD=17.91 years). To verify the hypothesis, 2 versions (conditions) of the virtual agent animations were created for each selected test sample. They are human and synthesized motions. There are a total of 10 video clips (5 input samples × 2 conditions). Each participant watched 5 video clips, each of which is randomly selected from the 2 conditions. Each video clip has been evaluated 40 times (i.e., by 40 participants). After watching each video clip, each participant was invited to answer the same four questions as in the first evaluation study, but this time the participant answered using a 5 point Likert scale.

The results are shown in Figure 2. As can be seen, synthesized motion obtains score less than human motions along the four dimensions: naturalness, synchronization, correlation of laughter intensity and torso movements, inter-correlation of head and torso movement. T-test shows that there are significant differences in all terms between human and synthesized data.

4.3   Discussion

The objective evaluation for comparing LHMM, TPLHMM and CTPLHMM shows that TPLHMM and CTPLHMM perform better than LHMM. It highlights that acoustic features and motions are linked. Thus acoustic features can

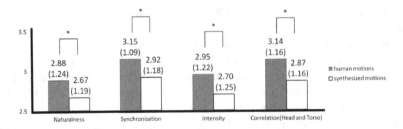

Fig. 2. Averaged values of virtual agent animated by animations from human and synthesized. Significant differences are identified by ⋆ ($P < .05$). The averaged values are shown with an histogram and the standard deviation is specified in parenthesis.

be used to capture motion trajectories. In LHMM, inputs of text signals, such as phoneme, intensity and duration, are global-level features. They do not contain enough information to characterize dynamic motion variance at each time frame. While, in TPLHMM and CTPLHMM, for each time frame, additional acoustic features are used to characterize dynamic variance of human motion. In LHMM and TPLHMM models, head and torso motions are modelled separately. In other words, they are considered as being independent. However, through the objective evaluation investigating the relation between head and torso, we found that head and torso motions are dependent with each other; relationship which is ignored in the other two models. In our work, coupled model is used to learn this dependent relation between head and torso movements.

The subjective evaluation compared TPLHMM and CTPLHMM. CTPLHMM obtains higher score than TPLHMM. In the subjective evaluation on comparing synthesized and human motions, human data is perceived significantly better than synthesized data in terms of naturalness, synchronisation, intensity and correlation of head and torso movements. However the difference in perception is not so severe (less than 1 on a 5 likert scale). This suggests that the proposed CTPLHMM is somehow capable of synthesizing human-like head and body motions.

5   Conclusion

In this paper we have presented an approach to model laughter head and torso movements, which are very rhythmic and show saccadic patterns. To capture laughter motion characteristics, we have developed a statistical approach to reproduce frequency movements, such as shaking and trembling. Our statistical model takes as input such phoneme sequences and acoustic features of laughter sound. Then it outputs the head and torso animations of the virtual agent. In the training model, not only the relation between input and output features is modelled, but also the relation between head and torso movements is captured. Experiments show that our model is able to capture the dynamism of laughter movement, but do not overcome animation from human data.

References

1. Marsella, S., Xu, Y., Lhommet, M., Feng, A., Scherer, S., Shapiro, A.: Virtual character performance from speech. In: Proceedings of the 12th ACM SIGGRAPH/Eurographics Symposium on Computer Animation, pp. 25–35 (2013)
2. Cassell, J., Vilhjálmsson, H., Bickmore, T.: Beat: The behavior expression animation toolkit. In: Proceedings of SIGGRAPH, pp. 477–486 (2001)
3. Ruch, W., Kohler, G., Van Thriel, C.: Assessing the 'humorous temperament': Construction of the facet and standard trait forms of the state-trait-cheerfulness-inventory - stci. Humor: International Journal of Humor Research 9, 303–339 (1996)
4. Provine, R.R.: Laughter: A scientific investigation. Penguin Books Edn. (2001)
5. Huber, T., Ruch, W.: Laughter as a uniform category? A historic analysis of different types of laughter. In: Congress of the Swiss Society of Psychology (2007)
6. Ruch, W., Ekman, P.: The Expressive Pattern of Laughter. Emotion Qualia, and Consciousness, 426–443 (2001)
7. Darwin, C.: The expression of the emotions in man and animals. John Murray, London (1872)
8. de Melo, C.M., Kenny, P.G., Gratch, J.: Real-time expression of affect through respiration. Computer Animation and Virtual Worlds 21(3-4), 225–234 (2010)
9. Mancini, M., Varni, G., Glowinski, D., Volpe, G.: Computing and evaluating the body laughter index. In: Salah, A.A., Ruiz-del-Solar, J., Meriçli, Ç., Oudeyer, P.-Y. (eds.) HBU 2012. LNCS, vol. 7559, pp. 90–98. Springer, Heidelberg (2012)
10. McKeown, G., Curran, W., McLoughlin, C., Griffin, H.J., Bianchi-Berthouze, N.: Laughter induction techniques suitable for generating motion capture data of laughter associated body movements. In: FG, pp. 1–5 (2013)
11. Niewiadomski, R., Mancini, M., Baur, T., Varni, G., Griffin, H., Aung, M.S.H.: MMLI: Multimodal multiperson corpus of laughter in interaction. In: Salah, A.A., Hung, H., Aran, O., Gunes, H. (eds.) HBU 2013. LNCS, vol. 8212, pp. 184–195. Springer, Heidelberg (2013)
12. Fourati, N., Pelachaud, C.: Emilya: Emotional body expression in daily actions database. In: LREC 2014, The 9th International Conference on Language Resources and Evaluation, Reykjavik, Iceland, pp. 3486–3493 (2014)
13. Urbain, J., Çakmak, H., Dutoit, T.: Automatic phonetic transcription of laughter and its application to laughter synthesis. In: Proceedings of Affective Computing and Intelligent Interaction, pp. 153–158 (2013)
14. DiLorenzo, P.C., Zordan, V.B., Sanders, B.L.: Laughing out loud: control for modeling anatomically inspired laughter using audio. ACM Trans. Graph. 27(5), 125 (2008)
15. Wilson, A., Bobick, A.: Parametric hidden markov models for gesture recognition. IEEE Transactions on Pattern Analysis and Machine Intelligence 21(9), 884–900 (1999)
16. Brand, M.: Coupled hidden markov models for modeling interacting processes. Technical report (1997)
17. Sethares, W., Staley, T.: Periodicity transforms. IEEE Transactions on Signal Processing 47(11), 2953–2964 (1999)
18. Ding, Y., Prepin, K., Huang, J., Pelachaud, C., Artières, T.: Laughter animation synthesis. In: Proceedings of the 2014 International Conference on Autonomous Agents and Multi-Agent Systems, pp. 773–780 (2014)

Simulating Deceptive Cues of Joy
in Humanoid Robots

Birgit Endrass[1], Markus Haering[1], Gasser Akila[2], and Elisabeth André[1]

[1] Human Centered Multimedia, Augsburg University, Germany
{endrass,haering,andre}@hcm-lab.de
[2] Media Engineering and Technology Dept., The German University in Cairo, Egypt

Abstract. Although generally not appreciated, lying constitutes a great part of human conversation. Thereby the nonverbal behavior plays a crucial role, as so-called deception cues can reveal the real intention or emotion by facial expressions or body movements. In this paper, we examine facial cues of deception and present a preliminary perception study with a humanoid robot that exhibits these cues. Initial results indicate that the shown expressions affect the observer's impression.

Keywords: Social Robots, Affective Computing, Facial Expressions.

1 Introduction

Most people would spontaneously not admit that they lie on a daily basis or that they would appreciate being lied to. DePaulo and colleagues [1] investigated this phenomena in more detail by testing daily deceptive situations. *"As predicted, lying was an everyday event."* Their results reveal, amongst others, that *"students reported lying in approximately one out of every three of their social interactions"*[1].

When humans lie, deception cues often show unintentionally in their nonverbal behavior. In principle, a humanoid robot could conduct a perfect lie, meaning that no cues would show on its face or in its body movements. In this contribution we address the question whether it is possible to convey subtle cues as shown during lies with the limited channels of expression of humanoid robots. It should be noted that a robot should not touch the domain of *serious lies* which could be harmful to a human user. However, so-called *social lies*, as commonly used for politeness reasons, might be a desirable feature of a humanoid robot.

Most related work on deceiving robots takes a game-theoretic approach to model the robot's strategic behavior by enhancing their decision by a deceptive layer. Work has been carried out by Wagner and Arkin, e.g. [2], who developed an algorithm to determine for an artificial system whether deception is warranted in a social situation. Other work investigates the question whether a robot can successfully deceive humans and presents studies where a robot showed behavior against the user's prediction [3]. In contrast, we do not target strategic lies but focus on simulating socially desired behaviors. To the best of our knowledge,

T. Bickmore et al. (Eds.): IVA 2014, LNAI 8637, pp. 174–177, 2014.
© Springer International Publishing Switzerland 2014

no research has been carried out so far on showing subtle emotional expressions such as deception cues with a humanoid robot.

In the area of virtual humans, facial deception cues have been investigated. Buisine and colleagues [4] present the simulation of blended emotions on different modalities of a virtual character along with the perception of these complex emotions on human observers. In our own former work [5], we found that even subtle expressions of deception can have a negative impact on the users' perception of an agent. To this end, it is not certain whether the observations made for virtual characters apply for humanoid robots as well.

2   Background

The most fundamental and influential work on lies and deception was presented by Ekman and colleagues (e.g., [6,7]). Several modalities of human behavior can be involved while lying. In this paper, facial expressions are further investigated.

According to Ekman and colleagues' studies, there are at least four ways in which facial expressions may vary if they accompany lies: (1) Micro-expressions: A false emotion is displayed but the felt emotion is unconsciously expressed for the fraction of a second. (2) Masks: The felt emotion is intentionally masked by a not corresponding facial expression. (3) Timing: Facial expressions accompanying felt emotions do not last for a very long time. Thus, the longer an expression is shown the more likely it is accompanying a lie. (4) Asymmetry: Voluntarily shown facial expressions tend to be displayed in an asymmetrical way.

In the research literature from the social sciences a real smile (often refered to as Duchenne smile) contains not only lip movements but also movement in the eye region. A so-called faked smile (or Pan-Am smile) vice versa lacks this motion in the eye region, e.g., [6,8].

3   Facial Deception Cues for a Humanoid Robot

For our implementation, we use the *Hanson Robokind* robot Alice[1] which provides a silicon face that can be animated by internal motors. Our facial animations are based on the Facial Action Coding System (FACS) [9] that describes over 40 Action Units (AUs) for a human face. We identified seven of the AUs that can be simulated with the robot's joints: Upper face: *inner brows raiser* (AU 1), *brow lowerer* (AU 4), *upper lid raiser* (AU 5) *eye closure* (AU 43); Lower face: *lip corner puller* (AU 12), *lip corner depressor* (AU 15), and *lip opening* (AU 25).

One facial expression was designed to simulate a real joyful face (Duchenne smile) that serves as a basis for comparison with deceptive smiles. Another facial expression simulates the faked smile (Pan-Am smile) where no movement in the eye region is shown. According to Eckman [9] voluntary produced smiles are often displayed asymmetrically. Following FACS, we created different intensities

---

[1] http://hansonrobokind.com

of asymmetric smiles varying in how far each lip corner is pulled upwards: AB, AC, BC (A=trace, B=clearly visible, C=marked). In masks, different emotions are blended on different parts of the face. Most commonly smiles are used to mask real emotions. For our experiment we blended anger or surprise shown in the eye-region with a smile. Micro expressions and timing were not investigated for reasons such as too slow maximum speed of the joints or audible movements. Figure 1 shows different variations of smiles on the robotic face. Please note, that the motion into these final states is more expressive than the pictures.

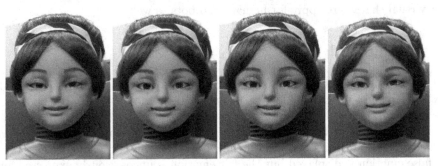

Fig. 1. Different smiles shown on the robotic face. Left: smile with eyes; middle-left: smile without eyes; middle-right: asymmetric smile (AC), right: blended anger.

4   Preliminary Study

In a preliminary perception study we addressed the question whether users react to the subtle deception cues or whether they stay unrecognized. Therefore, seven videos of the animated robotic face were embedded in an online survey, where human observers had to judge how happy Alice seems on a 7-point Likert scale (unhappy to happy): smile with eyes (real or Duchenne smile), smile without eyes (faked or Pan-Am smile), asymmetric smiles (varying in intensities AB, AC, BC), blended surprise, and blended anger. We hypothesize that the *deceptive* smiles are perceived as less happy than the *real* smile (Duchenne smile).

96 participants took part in our study (28 female, 68 male, mean age 22.5). The mean values of their ratings are summarized in Figure 2. We conducted a repeated-measures ANOVA with different facial expressions as within-subjects factor. The test revealed a significant main effect on perceived happiness, $F(6, 90)$ = $30.275, p < .000$. Within-subject contrasts were calculated, comparing each of the deceptive facial expressions with the expression simulating a real smile (smile with eyes). Regarding asymmetrical smiles, we archived significant results ($p < .000$) for the intensities AB and AC, being rated less happy than symmetric smiles independent from their different eye movements. In line with Krumhuber and Manstead [8], who found that the typically mentioned crinkles around the eyes are not a good hint to spot faked smiles, no differences were observed comparing the smile with eyes to the smile without eyes ($p > .05$). Blended emotions (blended anger and blended surprise) did not show the intended results ($p > .05$) and were rated quite similar to the smile with or without eyes. Both

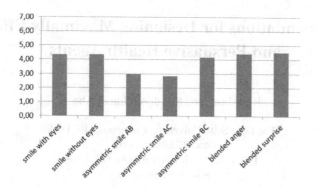

Fig. 2. Mean values of perceived happiness for the different smile conditions

latter results suggest that participants focused on the mouth region more than on the eye region of the robot.

5   Conclusions and Future Work

The present contribution investigates deception cues for a humanoid robotic face and presents a first step towards robots that are able to show subtle emotional cues as indicators of socially expected lies.

As a next step, our findings need to be integrated into a greater scenario, to see whether the solely nonverbal differences investigated in this study apply to a multi-modal setting.

References

1. DePaulo, B.M., Kashy, D.A., Krikendol, S.E., Wyner, M.M., Epstein, J.A.: Lying in everyday life. Journal of Personality and Social Psychology 70(5), 979–995 (1996)
2. Wagner, A.R., Arkin, R.C.: Acting deceptively: Providing robots with the capacity for deception. International Journal of Social Robotics 3(1), 5–26 (2011)
3. Terada, K., Ito, A.: Can a robot deceive humans? In: Proc. of 5th ACM/IEEE Int. Conf. on Human-Robot Interaction (HRI), pp. 191–192 (2010)
4. Buisine, S., Abrilian, S., Niewiadomski, R., Martin, J.-C., Devillers, L., Pelachaud, C.: Perception of blended emotions: From video corpus to expressive agent. In: Gratch, J., Young, M., Aylett, R.S., Ballin, D., Olivier, P. (eds.) IVA 2006. LNCS (LNAI), vol. 4133, pp. 93–106. Springer, Heidelberg (2006)
5. Rehm, M., André, E.: Catch me if you can - exploring lying agents in social settings. In: Int. Conf. on Autonomous Agents and Multiagent Systems, pp. 937–944 (2005)
6. Ekman, P.: Telling Lies - Clues to Deceit in the Marketplace, Politics, and Marriage. Norton & Company, New York (1992)
7. Ekman, P., Friesen, W., O'Sullivan, M.: Smiles when lying. Journal of Personality and Social Psychology 54(3), 414–420 (1988)
8. Krumhuber, E.G., Manstead, A.S.: Can duchenne smiles be feigned? new evidence on felt and false smiles. Emotion 9(6), 807–820 (2009)
9. Ekman, P., Friesen, W.: Facial Action Coding System (1978)

Recommendations for Designing Maximally Effective and Persuasive Health Agents

Jesse Fox[1] and Sun Joo (Grace) Ahn[2]

[1] The Ohio State University, Columbus, OH, USA
fox.775@osu.edu
[2] University of Georgia, Athens, GA, USA
sjahn@uga.edu

Abstract. HCI designers have made significant advancements in the development of health agents. Although these developments are often technologically impressive, social scientific research provides some contraindications. Here, we review relevant social scientific research on tailoring, customization, agency, and realism that provides guidelines on how to design health agents and avatars to maximize persuasive outcomes in health contexts.

Keywords: Agents, avatars, health technology, virtual environments, video games.

1   Introduction

Science fiction often presents a future of synchrony and synthesis between humans and machines, wherein virtual agents and robots are unquestionably accepted as social interactants. In the current era, however, many people remain skeptical about the social role of such technologies. If people do not accept or trust agents, it does not matter how sophisticated their design is, as humans are likely to reject them, especially in a significant, personal area like health care. Social scientific research on human-computer interaction (HCI) and computer-mediated communication (CMC) provides some key insights into how we can best design health agents that people will heed.

2   Tailoring and Customization

One advantage of agents is the ability to customize them to tailor both the source and the message specifically to the user. Health scholars have long touted the advantages of using computers to tailor messages to audiences [1,2]. Recent research has also elaborated how digital technologies can allow us to manipulate the source for maximal effectiveness as well [3,4].

Agent tailoring could manifest in many ways. The visual appearance of a health agent could be tailored to what is most effective for the individual, the message, and the context [5]. The degree of threat present in the message may shift preferences in the appearance of agents [6]. Social cognitive theory also suggests that we are more

T. Bickmore et al. (Eds.): IVA 2014, LNAI 8637, pp. 178–181, 2014.

persuaded by sources that we identify with or feel similar to [1]. A growing body of research demonstrates that photorealistic virtual representations of the self (i.e., virtual doppelgängers) are effective at persuading individuals to engage in health-related behaviors [7,8,9] because users feel high levels of identification with the virtual self, driving feelings of self-efficacy [1]. Further, virtual agents can be manipulated to show the rewards or punishments associated with a health behavior [1]. These virtual selves could show virtual selves tailored to the individual's motivations.

Like other forms of tailoring, virtual health agents may encourage longer-term behavior changes. Virtual selves promoted exercise behavior up to 24 hours following treatment [7]. Augmenting traditional health pamphlets with virtual simulations to promote healthy food choices led to effects that persisted for up to one week [10]. Other studies have studied longer-term interactions for up to six weeks and have found that even small amounts of social interactions between the virtual agent and the user encourages longer-term adherence to the promoted health program [11].

3 Perceived Agency

Human users often engage in their own Turing tests. Although frameworks such as the computers as social actors approach [12] suggest that humans do not distinguish computers and humans, a recent meta-analysis found that when people perceive that they are interacting with a computer that source is less capable of influencing the user than when they believe they are interacting with a human [13].

The model of social influence in virtual environments [14] suggests perceived agency is important because it affects the degree of social presence an individual feels; entities perceived as being controlled by computers (agents) elicit less social presence than those perceived as being controlled by humans (avatars). When greater social presence is experienced, more social influence will occur because users will perceive and interact with the representation like a real person.

In health contexts, users may have negative reactions if they perceive they are interacting with a machine. Perceived caring and interpersonal warmth are among the strongest predictors of satisfaction with health care providers and adherence to prescribed treatments [15]. Although there is limited research on perceptions of agents conducted in actual health settings, research in the area of telemedicine indicates that patients strongly prefer interacting face-to-face compared to video conferencing or interactive virtual environments, which patients find "cold" [16].

When creating health agents, designers may need to reinforce humanness by enabling natural speech, nonverbal behaviors, emotions, flexibility, contingency, context consideration, and other markers of humanness [17,18]. Designers must enable humanness by avoiding highly scripted behaviors, personalizing and tailoring details of the interaction, and even affording disfluencies such as interruptions [18].

4 Realism

Blascovich's [14] model suggests that with increasing behavioral realism, the effect of perceived agency washes out. That is, the more realistic an agent behaves, the more persuasive it becomes. Thus, the end goal for designers should be to create realistic agents that are indistinguishable from humans.

Physical realism is the degree to which something is seen, heard, or experienced as it would in the physical world. This realism is important because it influences perceptions of an agent's credibility [19]. Physical realism would include the work of animators and programmers whose goal is to develop human-like agents that have natural movements, authentic facial expressions, and even a lifelike gleam in their eyes.

Social realism is considerably more complex, and can include nonverbal and verbal behavior. Programmers developing conversational agents and artificial intelligence for interaction must incorporate not only linguistics and logic, but also interpersonal, social, and cultural appropriateness and norms. What social scientific research reveals is that although physical realism can be persuasive in virtual environments, social realism and the resulting social presence is often the more important cue in terms of influence. Indeed, users disclose more to physically unrealistic representations [20], perhaps because they feel less judged.

Designers should also be wary of "not quite real" virtual agents that descend into the uncanny valley and make users uncomfortable [21]. Although theorists expect positive reactions to lifelike entities [14, 21], until we have perfected these technologies, research indicates that near-realism may have drawbacks.

5   Conclusions

In sum, social science provides designers of health agents with some food for thought. Although these guidelines are supported by substantial research and theory, it is crucially important for designers to consider that a one size fits all approach will not work for all health contexts. The need for this information reinforces why it is necessary for HCI designers, medical practitioners, and social scientists to collaborate to optimize the development of health agents.

References

1. Bandura, A.: Health Promotion by Social Cognitive Means. Health Education & Behavior 31, 143–164 (2004)
2. Noar, S.M., Harrington, N.G.: Computer-Tailored Interventions for Improving Health Behaviors. In: Noar, S.M., Harrington, N.G. (eds.) eHealth Applications: Promising Strategies for Behavior Change, pp. 128–146. Routledge, New York (2012)
3. Ahn, S.J., Bailenson, J.N.: Self-Endorsing Versus Other-Endorsing in Virtual Environments: The Effect on Brand Preference. Journal of Advertising 40, 93–106 (2011)
4. Baylor, A.L.: Promoting Motivation with Virtual Agents and Avatars: Role of Visual Presence and Appearance. Philosophical Transactions of the Royal Society B: Biological Sciences 364, 3559–3565 (2009)
5. Fox, J.: Avatars in Health Communication Contexts. In: Noar, S.M., Harrington, N.G. (eds.) eHealth Applications: Promising Strategies for Behavior Change, pp. 96–109. Routledge, New York (2012)

6. Fox, J., Bailenson, J.N.: Manipulating Virtual Representations to Promote Sunscreen Use. Paper presented at the 97th Annual Conference of the National Communication Association, New Orleans, LA (2011)
7. Fox, J., Bailenson, J.N.: Virtual Self-Modeling: The Effects of Vicarious Reinforcement and Identification on Exercise Behaviors. Media Psychology 12, 1–25 (2009)
8. Fox, J., Bailenson, J.N., Binney, J.: Virtual Experiences, Physical Behaviors: The Effect of Presence on Imitation of an Eating Avatar. PRESENCE: Teleoperators & Virtual Environments 18, 294–303 (2009)
9. Fox, J., Bailenson, J.N., Ricciardi, T.: Physiological Responses to Virtual Selves and Virtual Others. Journal of CyberTherapy & Rehabilitation 5, 69–72 (2010)
10. Ahn, S.J.: Incorporating Immersive Virtual Environments in Health Promotion Campaigns: A Construal-Level Theory Approach. Health Communication
11. Bickmore, T., Schulman, D., Yin, L.: Maintaining Engagement in Long-Term Interventions with Relational Agents. International Journal of Applied Artificial Intelligence 24, 648–666 (2010)
12. Fox, J., Ahn, S.J., Janssen, J., Yeykelis, L., Segovia, K.Y., Bailenson, J.N.: A Meta-Analysis Quantifying the Effects of Avatars and Agents on Social Influence. Human-Computer Interaction
13. Blascovich, J., Loomis, J., Beall, A.C., Swinth, K.R., Hoyt, C.L., Bailenson, J.N.: Immersive Virtual Environment Technology as a Methodological Tool for Social Psychology. Psychological Inquiry 13, 103–124 (2002)
14. Nass, C., Moon, Y.: Machines and Mindlessness: Social Responses to Computers. Journal of Social Issues 56, 81–103 (2000)
15. Zolnierek, K.B.H., DiMatteo, M.R.: Physician Communication and Patient Adherence to Treatment: A Meta-Analysis. Medical Care 47, 826 (2009)
16. Buck, S.: Nine Human Factors Contributing to the User Acceptance of Telemedicine Applications: A Cognitive-Emotional Approach. Journal of Telemedicine and Telecare 15, 55–58 (2009)
17. Gratch, J., Marsella, S.: Lessons From Emotion Psychology for the Design of Lifelike Characters. Applied Artificial Intelligence 19, 215–233 (2005)
18. McFarlane, D.C., Latorella, K.A.: The Scope and Importance of Human Interruption in Human-computer Interaction Design. Human-Computer Interaction 17, 1–61 (2002)
19. Nowak, K.L., Rauh, C.: The Influence of the Avatar on Online Perceptions of Anthropomorphism, Androgyny, Credibility, Homophily, and Attraction. Journal of Computer Mediated Communication 11, 153–178 (2005)
20. Bailenson, J.N., Yee, N., Merget, D., Schroeder, R.: The Effect of Behavioral Realism and Form Realism of Real-time Avatar Faces on Verbal Disclosure, Nonverbal Disclosure, Emotion Recognition, and Copresence in Dyadic Interaction. Presence 15, 359–372 (2006)
21. Mori, M.: The Uncanny Valley. Energy 7, 33–35 (1970)

Recorded Speech, Virtual Environments, and the Effectiveness of Embodied Conversational Agents

Ivan Gris, David Novick,
Adriana Camacho, Diego A. Rivera, Mario Gutierrez, and Alex Rayon

Department of Computer Science, The University of Texas at El Paso
500 W. University Ave., El Paso, TX 79912, USA
ivangris4@gmail.com, novick@utep.edu,
{accamacho2,darivera2,mgutierrez19,amrayon2}@miners.utep.edu

Abstract. Development of embodied conversational agents (ECAs) has tended to focus on the character's dialog capabilities, with less research on the design and effect of the agent's voice and of the virtual environments in which the agent exists. For a study of human-ECA rapport, we iteratively developed three versions of a game featuring an ECA, where each version of the game had a different combination of speech generation and virtual environment. Evaluations of the users' interactions with the different versions of the game enabled us to assess the effects of changes in the agent's voice and of changes in the agent's virtual world.

Keywords: Embodied conversational agents, virtual environments, human-agent dialog.

1   Introduction

In this paper, we examine the effect on users' interaction with an embodied conversational agent (ECA) resulting from changes in (1) the ECA's virtual world and (2) the ECA's voice. Specifically, our study compares three versions of an immersive video game in which the user interacts with a life-size ECA. The game we developed is an adventure game, inspired by text-based games such as Zork (Anderson & Galley, 1985) and Colossal Cave (Crowther, Woods & Black, 1976), where the user tries to escape from the castle of an evil vampire king.

The human-ECA interaction reported in this paper took place in a spoken-language adventure game entitled "Escape from the Castle of the Vampire King." The game had a graphical interface with a full-sized ECA that served as the game's narrator, and the player controlled the game through speech commands. The game comprised 26 different rooms, each with its own secret passages, exits, items and clues. Players' interactions occurred in 20-minute sessions on two consecutive days, for a total of approximately 40 minutes per participant. The purpose of the game was to support a study of extroversion-based rapport-building behaviors over time (see Novick & Gris, in press).

T. Bickmore et al. (Eds.): IVA 2014, LNAI 8637, pp. 182–185, 2014.

2   The Agent's Voice

The quality of an agent's speech is measured by the degree to which it replicates a human speaker. While there has been significant progress in this area, users are still unenthusiastic about most synthetic speech (Newell & Edwards, 2008). We hypothesized that increasing voice naturalness would make users less likely to exhibit frustration and interrupt the agent while it speaks.

The first version of our game used Anna, the default voice provided by Microsoft operating systems. Twelve subjects interacted with the agent in two sessions each. After each session, subjects completed a survey that included an optional open question on what would they like to see improved. Subjects indicated that the voice was unclear, hard to understand, robotic, unemotional, unengaged, insensitive, monotone, and broken.

For the second version of the game we used Salli, an American English voice from IVONA. For this version of the system, 22 subjects played the game, again across two sessions each. Most user comments noted a lack of emotion in the voice. In one participant's words, "Even the smallest hint of empathy would greatly improve her demeanor." Systems have been built for emotional synthesized speech (Schröder, 2001). Nevertheless, emotion in synthesized speech in real-time multimodal conversation is still in its infancy, and we were unable to find an emotional synthesized voice that we could satisfactorily adapt for our agent.

For the third version we recorded over 200 different utterances, which were played in place of the synthesized voice. Only 4 out of the 58 participants complained about a lack of emotion. We expect that the residual perception of lack of emotion arose from the use of emotion-neutral phrases that were used in multiple game situations.

3   Increasing Engagement

As the agent's voice improved, other issues of users' engagement with the agent became more apparent, especially with respect to the relatively impoverished nature of the virtual environment in which the agent was presented. In our system, users interacted with first-person perspective rather than the third-person perspective associated with avatars (see Serrels, 2011).

In our experiments across the three versions of the game, we measured gaze away from or toward the agent. We hypothesized that (a) reducing cognitive load would increase the proportion of time that users directed their gaze toward the agent and (b) placing the agent in a virtual world related to the game's story would also increase the proportion of time that users direct their gaze towards the agent.

4   Versions of the Game

Before presenting our results, we review the three versions of the "Escape from the Castle of the Vampire King" game with their respective voices and environments.

- **Version 1.** In the first version of the game, players were given two sheets of paper, one with a printed set of commands and their respective examples and a second with a template for drawing a map to mark the player's progress. This version used the default speech synthesizer provided by the Windows operating system.
- **Version 2.** The second version of the game featured a quick-reference command list in the upper-left corner of the projection and a dynamic map behind the agent. This version of the game used the IVONA Salli speech synthesizer.
- **Version 3.** The third version of the game included 3D scenery, recorded speech, agent movement based on motion-capture, and the quick-reference commands and incremental map display.

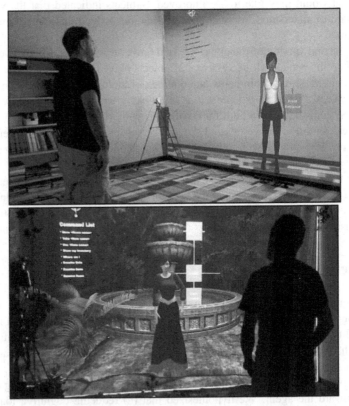

Fig. 1. Top: Version 2 of the game, with quick-reference commands, visible map, and Salli voice. Bottom: Version 3 of the game, with game scene, quick-reference commands, visible map, and recorded voice.

5   Results

In Section 2, we hypothesized that increasing the voice naturalness would make users less likely to interrupt the agent. The data, shown in Table 1, showed a significant ($\chi^2 < 10^{-6}$) reduction in the relative number of times that users interrupted the agent.

In Section 3, we hypothesized that reducing cognitive load would increase the proportion of time that users directed their gaze toward the agent. The data, also shown in Table 1, showed a significant ($\chi^2 < 10^{-6}$) increase in the proportion of time that the users gazed at the agents. We also hypothesized that placing the agent in a virtual world related to the game's story would increase the proportion of time that users directed their gaze towards the agent. The data showed a significant ($\chi^2 < 10^{-6}$) increase in the proportion of time that the users gazed at the agent.

Table 1. Data for analysis of hypotheses

	Version 1	Version 2	Version 3
User interruptions of agent	27	60	14
Agent utterances	871	878	948
Gaze at agent (seconds)	1453.6	3759.9	9603.5
Gaze away (seconds)	5793.8	3616.3	1444.1

Table 2. Gaze shifts away from the agent

	Gaze Shifts Away	Total Time (Seconds)	Average (Seconds/Shift)
V2	742	7376.2	9.94
V3	272	11047.6	40.62

This study was subject to three key limitations. First, the number of subjects varied across the three versions of the game. Second, as similar codings have consistently had high Kappas, we did not calculate interrater reliability. And, third, because the project involved iterative improvements to a system intended for a study of human-agent rapport, the study did not isolate the changes in voice and environment.

References

1. Anderson, T., Galley, S.: The history of Zork. The New Zork Times 4(1-3) (1985)
2. Crowther, W., Woods, D., Black, K.: Colossal cave adventure. Computer Game (1976)
3. Newell, C., Edwards, A.: Place, authenticity time: a framework for synthetic voice acting. International Journal of Performance Arts and Digital Media 4(2-3), 155–180 (2008)
4. Novick, D., Gris, I. (in press). Building rapport between human and ECA: A pilot study. In: HCI International (2014)
5. Schröder, M.: Emotional speech synthesis: a review. In: InterSpeech 2001, pp. 561–564 (September 2001)
6. Serrels, M.: In Real Life: First Or Third Person - What's Your Perspective? (2011), Retrieved from Kotaku: http://www.kotaku.com.au/2011/04/first-or-third-person-whats-your-perspective/

Exploring the Difference of the Impression on Human and Agent Listeners in Active Listening Dialog

Hung-Hsuan Huang*, Natsumi Konishi, Sayumi Shibusawa, and Kyoji Kawagoe

College of Information Science & Engineering, Ritsumeikan University, Japan
hhhuang@acm.org

1 Introduction

Active listening is a communication technique that the listener listens to the speaker carefully and attentively by confirming or asking for more details about what they heard. In order to improve the effect, always-available and trustable conversational partners in enough number are demanded. The ultimate goal of this study is the development of a virtual agent who can engage active listening and maintain a long-term relationship with elderly users. We assume that the task of the active listener (a human volunteer or the agent) is to maintain the speaker's (elderly user) mood in good state. In order to do this, like a human listener, the listener agent has to observe the listener's attitude, has to estimate the listener's mood from the observation, and has to predict the change of listener's mood caused by his / her own behaviors both verbally and non-verbally. On the other hand, the active listener is evaluated by the speaker from his / her impression of the listener's attitude. The hypothesis is, if the impression is good, then the speaker's mood is good. However, virtual agents which are made by computer graphics animations are more limited in expressiveness than human listeners, both in the aspects of quality and communication channels. Therefore, there is a research question that the graphical agent with "reduced expressiveness" can really engage the active listening task at human listeners' level, even if they do the same behaviors, smiles, gestures, or utterances at the same timings. This paper presents our first step of this study, a human-human teleconferencing experiment to foresee whether it is possible to implement an active listener agent.

2 Related Works

Huang et al. [2] developed a rapport agent which analyzes facial expressions, backchannel feedbacks, and eye gazes of the user. The agent is designed to show behaviors which are supposed to elicit rapport. However, it does not try to estimate and react to the user's mood. For example, when the user looks in bad mood, showing the agent's concern on the user by saying "Are you OK?" like human do. The SEMAINE project [3,5] was launched to build a Sensitive Artificial Listener (SAL). SAL is a multimodal dialogue system with the social interaction skills needed for a sustained conversation with the user. They focused on realizing "really natural language processing which aims to allow users to talk with machines as they would talk with another person.

---

* Corresponding author.

T. Bickmore et al. (Eds.): IVA 2014, LNAI 8637, pp. 186–189, 2014.

3 Active Listening Experiment

Modeling of active listening

Two functions of the agent can be considered fundamental: influences the speaker's mood through its attitude, and estimates the speaker's mood from his / her attitude. As the discussion in section 1, we assume that active listening triggers the interaction between the interlocutors' "mood" and gattitudeh in this work. Here, we redefine these two general terms in the following way: *Mood:*someone's internal mental state and is difficult to be directly observed by another person. *Attitude:*someone's mood expressed in the way how he or she behaves toward another person. It is supposed to be able to be observed by another person.

Experiment procedure

Nine pairs of participants with the same gender (five male pairs and four female ones) were recruited as the experiment participants. Due to the difficulty in recruiting elderly participants, and the experiment procedure explained in the following sections may be difficult the elderly, college students (all native Japanese speakers) were recruited in this experiment. Furthermore, we considered the implicit criteria in judging communication partner's attitude to be positive or negative should not vary largely between younger and senior generations. The condition was that they are close friends. This is because close friends were assumed easier to talk with each other in the limited experiment period.

In order to simulate the situation of talking with a 2D graphical agent, the participants of each pair were separated into two rooms and talked with each other via Skype tele-conferencing software. In each session, one participant played the role as the speaker, and the other one played the role as the listener. They were instructed to sit on a chair so that the move of their lower bodies can be controlled within a limited range. Each room was equipped with two video cameras. One was used for recording the participant from the front. The other one was used for logging the Skype window which was duplicated on another monitor. The speaker talked with the listener who was projected on a large screen at around life-size. The height of the projected image was adjusted so that the speaker can see the listener's eyes roughly at the level for eye contact. Natural head movements and eye gazes shifts can be further analyzed.

Each participant pair talked in two sessions. The participants did not change their roles, one of them was assigned as the speaker role in both sessions, and the other one was assigned as the listener role in both sessions. The speaker was instructed to talk with two listeners, one in each session. One of them is a human (his / her friend) listener and the other one is an autonomous agent driven by an artificial intelligence engine. The listener was instructed to do active listening for his / her friend in both sessions in two topics, respectively. However, in one of these two sessions (agent condition), the listener's video was actually substituted by a CG character.

The character animations are created by the software, Poser, and the character with the same gender as the speaker was used. Four kinds of canned animations were prepared: nodding, leaning the head, smiling, and blinking for each character. 15 voice tracks of frequently used feedback utterances [4] in Japanese are prepared in advance with text-to-speech software, AITalk II Plus. Those tracks include back-channeling utterances like "hmm,""yes," as well as wh questions like "who," "where,"etc.

The lip-syncing animations are created by Poser as well. In order to control the two conditions, the possible utterances for the human condition is limited to the same set of utterances. The substitution of listener's video to character was not notified to neither the speaker nor the listener. The agent was operated by one of the experimenter at the listener's room. The experimenter observed the listener's behavior and sent the commands to the animation system which is setup in the speaker's room on the fly. The agent operation interface is designed to minimize the delay, i.e. one or two keys to invoke a specific animation or sound track.

The topics of the conversation were "pleasant experience with family" or "unpleasant experience with family." These topics were chosen because they are common for almost everyone including the young experiment participants and the elderly. Each participant played the role either as the speaker or as the listener. Speaker participant initiates the session and talks to the listener about his / her family. The duration of one session was set to be seven minutes because it is considered long enough for the participants to start to talk something meaningful and keep the whole experiment within a reasonable time period.

Evaluation of attitude and mood

After the end of active listening sessions, the participants were instructed to evaluate the mood and attitude of themselves and their partners by labeling on the recorded video corpus. The video annotation tool, ELAN was used for this purpose. In order to align the granularity and label positions among different coders, the participants were instructed to label their evaluation by following the four rules: (1)The whole time line has to be labeled without blank segments. (2)Starting and ending positions of the label should be aligned to utterance boundaries. (3)One label can include multiple utterances. (4)The maximum length of one individual label is 10 seconds.

Phonetics tool, Praat [1] was used to label the boundaries of participants' utterances, the beginning and ending positions of all utterances 10-second scales are automatically labeled for the participants' easy reference. The following evaluations were conducted with the two participants. Speaker: the mood of himself / herself, how the attitude of himself / herself is supposed to be perceived by the listener, how he / she perceived the listener's attitude. Listener: how the attitude of himself / herself is supposed to be perceived by the speaker, how he / she perceived the speaker's attitude

The mood of the speaker and the attitude of the speaker and the listener were evaluated by the speaker and the listener by following criteria: Mood: evaluated with 7-scale measure from 1 (negative) to 7 (positive). Comfort, intimacy, and sympathy are provided as positive examples in the instruction. Attitude: evaluated with 7-scale measure from 1 (negative) to 7 (positive). Appropriate back-channel feedbacks like nods, questions, silence, agreeing opinions, smiles, or laughs were provided as positive examples in the instruction.

Table 1 shows the results of the evaluation annotation. About the weighted average (according to label lengths) on the attitude of the listeners evaluated by the speaker, there was not significant difference (two-tailed t test, $p=0.66$) in human and agent conditions. This shows generally there is no obvious difference on the impression over agent and human listeners. However, in the group by group results, there can be significant difference of the preference between agent condition and human condition. Especially for female participants, they may had strong preference on the agent listener or the human listener but had no tendency on either of them. Also, the evaluation results from female participants are generally lower than male participants no matter the listener is a human or an agent (2.60:3.75). About the results regarding to session topic and session order, there were no significant differences in these two aspects.

Table 1. Weighted average of evaluation annotation on the attitude of the listener (human and agent condition) by the speaker as well as the results regarding to session topic and order

Pair	Gender	Human	Agent	Pleasant	Unpleasant	1st session	2nd session
1	M	4.43	4.66	4.43	4.66	4.43	4.66
2	F	2.15	3.03	3.03	2.15	2.15	3.03
3	F	2.77	1.11	2.77	1.11	2.77	1.11
4	M	2.77	2.57	2.57	2.77	2.77	2.57
5	M	3.58	3.45	3.58	3.45	3.45	3.58
6	M	3.76	4.31	4.31	3.76	4.31	3.76
7	F	3.55	1.57	1.57	3.55	1.57	3.55
8	M	3.81	4.20	4.20	3.81	4.20	3.81
9	F	2.84	3.80	2.84	3.80	3.80	2.84
Average		3.35	3.11	3.26	3.23	3.27	3.21

4 Conclusion

We conducted an active listing dyadic conversation experiment with two conditions, human-human and human-agent. In human-agent condition, the human listener's video is substituted with a graphical character with the same behaviors. The results showed that generally there were no significant differences between these two conditions. In the future, we would like to increase the corpus size with additional experiments as well as the gaze patterns collected in the experiment. We pan to analyze the low-level signals of listener and how they can be interpreted as the listener's attitude and the listener's strategy in how to react to the speaker's perceived attitude. When the technology becomes matured, we will implement this function to agent and evaluate it with the elderly.

References

1. Boersma, P., Weenink, D.: Praat: doing phonetics by computer (computer software) (2012), Web Site: http://www.praat.org/
2. Huang, L., Morency, L.-P., Gratch, J.: Virtual rapport 2.0. In: Vilhjálmsson, H.H., Kopp, S., Marsella, S., Thórisson, K.R. (eds.) IVA 2011. LNCS, vol. 6895, pp. 68–79. Springer, Heidelberg (2011)
3. McKeown, G., Valstar, M.F., Cowie, R., Pantic, M.: The SEMAINE corpus of emotionally coloured character interactions. In: IEEE International Conference Multimedia and Expo, pp. 1079–1084 (2011)
4. Ohama, R.: The research about turn exchange and bacback-channeling in Japanese. Keisuishya (2006) (in Japanse)
5. Pammi, S., Schro, M.: Annotating meaning of listener vocalizations for speech synthesis. In: 3rd International Conference on Affective Computing and Intelligent Interaction (ACII 2009), pp. 1–6 (2009)

Planning Motions for Virtual Demonstrators

Yazhou Huang and Marcelo Kallmann

University of California, Merced, USA

Abstract. In order to deliver information effectively, virtual human demonstrators must be able to address complex spatial constraints and at the same time replicate motion coordination patterns observed in human-human interactions. We introduce in this paper a whole-body motion planning and synthesis framework that coordinates locomotion, body positioning, action execution and gaze behavior for generic demonstration tasks among obstacles.

Keywords: virtual trainers, motion planning, intelligent virtual humans.

1 Introduction

Virtual humans and embodied conversational agents are promising in the realm of human-computer interaction applications. One central goal in the area is to achieve virtual assistants that can effectively interact, train, and assist people in a wide variety of tasks. The need to demonstrate objects and procedures appears in many situations; however, the underlying motion synthesis problem is complex and has not been specifically addressed before. Simple everyday demonstrations involve a series of coordinated steps that a virtual agent needs to replicate. The agent needs to walk while avoiding obstacles along the way, stop at an appropriate demonstration location with clear view to the target and observer, interact with the object (e.g. point to it and deliver information), and also maintain visual engagement with the observer. This work addresses such harmonious multi-level orchestration of actions and behaviors (see Figure 1).

The proposed model was built from experiments with human subjects where participants were asked to freely approach target objects at different positions and to deliver object information to observers at various locations. These experiments provided ground truth data for defining a coordination model that is able to orchestrate the involved pieces of a demonstration task. The result is a whole-body motion planning

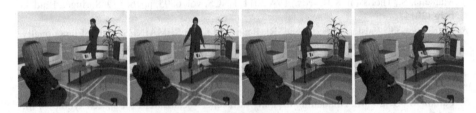

Fig. 1. Our PLACE planner synthesizes whole-body demonstrations for arbitrary targets, observers, obstacles, and visual occluders

T. Bickmore et al. (Eds.): IVA 2014, LNAI 8637, pp. 190–203, 2014.

framework, called PLACE, that addresses the five main pieces of the problem in an unified way:

• Placement: optimal character placement is essential for addressing target and observer visibility, locomotion accessibility, and action execution constraints;

• Locomotion: locomotion synthesis among obstacles and towards precise placements allows the character to position itself in order to perform a demonstration;

• Action: realistic action execution needs to address arbitrary object locations and to avoid nearby obstacles when needed;

• Coordination: coordination is important for well transitioning from locomotion to the upper-body demonstrative action; and

• Engagement: observer engagement is obtained with a gaze behavior that interleaves attention to the observer and the target in order to achieve effective demonstrations.

The realism of the solutions is addressed at two levels. At the behavioral level, placement, coordination and engagement are solved following models extracted from experiments with human subjects. At the motion synthesis level, locomotion and actions are synthesized from collections of motion capture clips organized for efficient synthesis and coordination. The techniques were developed such that solutions can be computed at interactive rates in realistic environments. See Figure 2 for examples.

Contributions: The main contribution of this work is the overall definition, modeling and effective solution of whole-body demonstrative tasks. The proposed techniques are the first to address the overall problem in an integrated fashion.

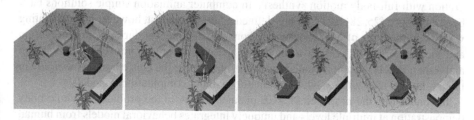

Fig. 2. From left to right: in the first two scenarios the computed demonstrations reasonably face the observer, while in the last two cases a visual occluder (the house plant) leads to solutions with non-trivial placements. The orange and blue lines respectively represent the head and the eye gaze orientations, at the demonstration action stroke point. The resulting gaze always reaches eye contact with the observer.

2   Related Work

Many works have focused on upper-body gesture and action modeling, including stroke-based blending [25], action synthesis with varied spatial constraints [17, 24], motion style control [6, 19], and search in interpolated motion graphs [20]. Our approach for action synthesis relies on available motion interpolation techniques [9, 19] but providing a new collision avoidance mechanism in blending space in order to successfully address realistic scenarios with obstacles.

With respect to data-based locomotion methods, several techniques have been proposed for achieving realistic and controllable locomotion synthesis [7,14–16,26]. While several of these methods can probably be extended to address departures and arrivals with position and orientation constraints, such an extension is not trivial. Our solution is based on a specific organization of locomotion clips that allows for fast locomotion synthesis ensuring such constraints. The locomotion planning problem becomes even more challenging when it has to be coordinated with an upper-body action. Previous work [5, 22] has addressed the combination of arm planning (reaching or grasping) on top of locomotion, however without a coordination model.

When it comes to whole-body motion synthesis that involves the scheduling and synchronization of upper- and lower-body, methods have been developed for splicing upper-body actions from one motion to another [2, 8], and more recently object manipulations have been coordinated with locomotion [1]. However these methods have not addressed a coordination model for transitioning from locomotion into a demonstration action, a specific situation that involves different types of constraints.

The fact that demonstrations have to be performed with respect to an observer also distinguishes our overall motion synthesis problem from previous work. Addressing an observer is important for achieving realistic solutions and as well effective interactions with virtual humans. For instance, it has been shown that visual engagement improves the amount of information memorized by an audience observing robotic storytellers [18] and narrative virtual agents [3]. Although previous work has focused on modeling gaze behavior in great detail [4, 27], little attention has been given to integration with full-body motion synthesis. In computer animation simple solutions have been employed [25,28] based on pre-defined points of interest, however not associating with a complete set of events observed from human subjects during action execution and locomotion. With respect to modeling placement for action execution, Scheflen and Ashcraft [21] present a pioneering work introducing the concept of *territoriality* in human-human interactions, but unfortunately without computational models.

In conclusion, the proposed PLACE planner addresses the problem of whole-body demonstration at multiple levels and uniquely integrates behavioral models from human subjects with realistic data-based motion synthesis.

3   Modeling Demonstrative Tasks

We have modeled the overall problem of synthesizing humanlike demonstrations with the help of experiments with human subjects. Our setup follows the approach in [10], but extending it for extracting complete motion models for demonstration tasks. Four human participants were recruited to perform a variety of pointing tasks with full-body motion capture. Six small target objects T_i, $i \in \{1, \ldots, 6\}$, were placed on a horizontal coarse mesh grid and participants were asked to perform demonstration actions towards each T_i for a human observer O_j standing at five different positions around the targets ($j \in \{1, \ldots, 5\}$). Each action consisted of pointing and delivering a short information about an object. Each configuration $\{T_i, O_j\}$ represented one trial per participant and generated one motion. A total of 30 distinct motions were generated per participant, each motion consisting of a complete pointing action with the associated locomotion

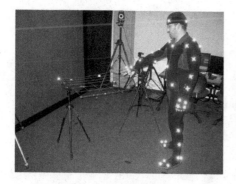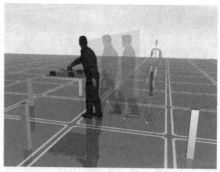

Fig. 3. Left: experiment setup. Right: illustration of one reconstructed motion. The observer location is represented with the green character and the maximum head orientation performed in the direction of the observer is shown with the orange plane.

and gaze behavior. The gaze typically moved several times between T_i and O_j. Each participant started from about 4 feet away from the mesh grid before walking towards the grid to point and describe T_i (see Figure 3). The sequence of target selection was random and the targets were of similar size in order to reduce possible side effects related to their size [23].

The full-body capture data was annotated manually with an annotation tool specifically developed to mark and extract the parameters and timings of all relevant events in each trial. One of the most important behaviors observed was the chosen positioning that each participant used to perform the pointing action. The chosen position ensured that the target and the observer were visible, and that the head rotation needed for eye contact with the observer was feasible. The position also ensured a successful execution of the action and with a fluid transition from locomotion. We now derive a generic placement model based on the observed data.

For each trial in the collected motion data we extracted the corresponding target position p_t, the position of the observer p_o, and the demonstrator position p_d. Position p_d is the position used to perform the demonstration action, and is defined as the position when the locomotion is detected to completely stop, since there is a period when the action execution overlaps with the locomotion. Figure 4 plots locomotion trajectories and their corresponding final demonstration positions. The 5 distinct colors represent the 5 different observer locations. Each color appears 6 times, one for each target T_i. It is possible to observe that the demonstration positions do not show an obvious structure in global coordinates.

A local 2D coordinate system with origin at p_t is then used to derive our model. The coordinate system is illustrated with the XZ frame in Figure 5. The XZ frame can have arbitrary orientation, however it is more intuitive when the Z axis is orthogonal to the table border closest to the target. We can now use angles to locally encode all relevant placement parameters with respect to the target. The used local angles will not model the proximity of the demonstrator to the target, since this is a parameter that is action-dependent and we leave it as a free parameter in our model. For example a pointing motion can be executed with arbitrary distance to the target while this is not

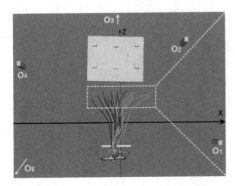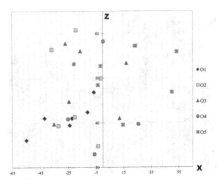

Fig. 4. Locomotion trajectories for each participant (left) and their ending positions in a closer look (right). Motions with the same color are with respect to a same observer.

the case in a manipulation task. The angles considered by our model are the following (see Figure 5): the observer position α with respect to Z, the demonstrator position β with respect to -Z, the demonstrator's body orientation θ with respect to Z, and the maximum head rotation ϕ (in respect to Z) performed towards the observer.

The approach of expressing placement locally with respect to the action target correlates with the *axis concept* used for describing interaction connections [21]. By expressing the collected parameters with respect to our local coordinate system, the plots of their values nicely fit into clusters with good structure. This is shown in Figure 6. Since the proposed placement model shows good structure, we then performed non-linear regressions in order to be able to estimate β, θ and ϕ as a function of an arbitrary input value for α. After smoothing the raw measurements with a least-squares Savitzky-Golay filter, quadratic and cubic polynomial functions were fitted for β, θ and ϕ (see Appendix for details).

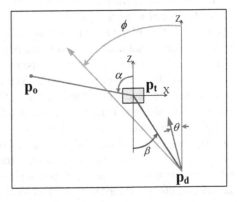

Fig. 5. Local coordinate system of the placement model. Angle α encodes the observer location, β the demonstrator location, θ the body orientation at action start, and ϕ encodes the maximum head rotation towards the observer.

The overall demonstration problem is then modeled as follows: given an upper-body demonstrative action A to be performed, the corresponding target object position p_t, and the position of the observer p_o, the goal of the PLACE planner is to synthesize a full-body motion for approaching the target and performing A with respect to p_t and for the observer located at p_o. The planner solves the problem with the following steps. First, a suitable demonstration position p_d and body orientation q_d are determined by using the placement model and taking into account visual occluders,

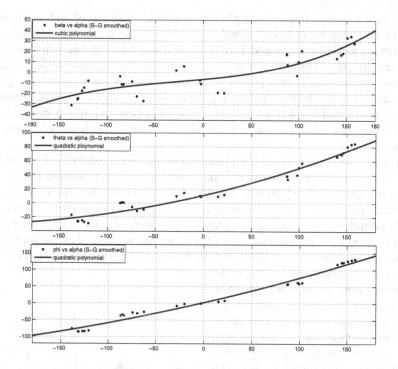

Fig. 6. Parameters of the placement model fitted with non-linear regression on filtered data points. The horizontal axis is the α value and the vertical axis, from top to bottom, represents β, θ, and ϕ respectively. Values are in degrees.

action feasibility and locomotion accessibility. Then, a locomotion sequence $L(\mathbf{p_d}, \mathbf{q_d})$ is synthesized for the character to walk from its current position to the demonstration placement $(\mathbf{p_d}, \mathbf{q_d})$. Action $A(\mathbf{p_t})$ is then synthesized and coordinated with the locomotion L. Finally, the head and eyes are animated to replicate the same gaze behavior patterns observed in the collected motions. These steps represent the five main components of PLACE and they are explained in the following sections.

4   Placement

Given the demonstrative action A, the target object position $\mathbf{p_t}$, and the observer position $\mathbf{p_o}$, the placement module will determine the optimal body position and orientation $(\mathbf{p_d}, \mathbf{q_d})$ for performing A. First, the action synthesis module (described in Section 6) is queried for its preferred distance d_{pref} to execute $A(\mathbf{p_t})$. This distance denotes the preferred Euclidean distance between $\mathbf{p_t}$ and $\mathbf{p_d}$ so that the character will be more likely to succeed in performing the action. The computation of d_{pref} is action-dependent, it may be automatically selected according to reachability constraints if the demonstration has to achieve object contact, or in other cases (like in pointing), it can be a user-specified parameter fixed or dependent on features of the environment (like the size of the target).

The local reference frame of our placement model is then placed with origin at $\mathbf{p_t}$ and with the Z axis set to be orthogonal to the closest edge of the supporting table. At this point our local placement model can be applied in order to estimate a first candidate placement $(\mathbf{p_d^0}, \mathbf{q_d^0})$, where $\mathbf{p_d^0}$ is obtained by combining the estimated angle β with the preferred distance d_{pref}, and $\mathbf{q_d^0}$ represents the orientation estimated by θ in global coordinates. If $\mathbf{p_t}$ lies between $\mathbf{p_o}$ and $\mathbf{p_d^0}$, the Z axis of the local placement coordinate frame is re-oriented towards $\mathbf{p_o}$ and the initial placement $(\mathbf{p_d^0}, \mathbf{q_d^0})$ is re-computed. This will make the initial placement to directly face the observer, a desired property in a placement.

Given a candidate placement, the placement is considered valid if: it does not lead to collisions with the environment, if $A(\mathbf{p_o})$ can be successfully executed from it, and if there is a collision-free path with enough clearance for the character to reach it. If a candidate placement is not valid due a collision, it is tested again a few times with slightly perturbed values and d_{pref} distances, thus increasing the chances of finding valid placements by local adjustment of the generated positions. Several placements may be valid and therefore we will search for the optimal one with respect to visibility, head rotation comfort, and distance to the target.

Starting from $(\mathbf{p_d^0}, \mathbf{q_d^0})$ we determine several valid placements $(\mathbf{p_d^k}, \mathbf{q_d^k})$ by adjusting the Z axis of the local model to new orientations around $\mathbf{p_t}$, for example by rotation increments of five degrees in both directions (see Figure 7). For each new orientation, the respective estimated placement is computed and tested for validity (adjusted if needed) and stored if valid. The search for valid placements may be set to be exhaustive with respect to the used rotation increment or to stop after a certain number of valid samples is found. The result of this phase is a set of

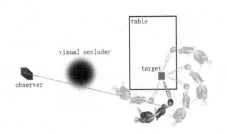

Fig. 7. Valid placements around the target are identified and ranked for selection

K valid placements $(\mathbf{p_d^k}, \mathbf{q_d^k})$, $k \in \{1, \ldots, K\}$. We then sort the placements in this set with respect to the following ranking cost function f_c:

$$f_c = e_{vis} * w_v + e_{neck} * w_n + e_{action} * w_a,$$

where e_{vis} is a measure of how occluded the observer is from the placement, e_{neck} is the amount of neck rotation required for reaching eye contact with the observer, e_{action} is the absolute difference between d_{pref} and the actual distance from $\mathbf{p_d^k}$ to $\mathbf{p_t}$, and the scalar weights are constants used to adjust the relative contributions of each term.

The weights are adjusted such that the contribution of e_{vis} is significant, since uncomfortable (but feasible) placements are preferable to placements with bad visibility. The house plant in the scenarios of Figure 2 is an example of an object modeled with partial occlusion set to $e_{vis} = 50\%$. Candidate placements with zero visibility are discarded, as shown in Figure 7. The result is a sorted list of valid placements that can be used for executing A. The placement with minimum f_c is selected as the target demonstration location $(\mathbf{p_d}, \mathbf{q_d})$ to be used. Since this placement has been already checked for validity, it can be safely passed to the motion synthesis modules described in the next sections. In case simplified validity tests are employed, the motion synthesis may happen to not be successful at some later stage, in which case the next placement in the list can be used as the next alternative.

5 Locomotion Synthesis

The locomotion synthesis module has to be able to address three main requirements:
• To be able to quickly check for locomotion accessibility to candidate placements when queried by the body placement module (Section 4), in order to allow for quick rejection of placements that offer no accessibility;
• To be able to synthesize motions that can navigate through narrow passages and with precise departure and arrival positions and orientations; and
• To produce purposeful motions resembling the ones observed in our experiments with human subjects, which consistently had sharp turnings (with small turning radius) at the departure and arrival locomotion phases.

With respect to the first requirement, accessibility queries are computed with an efficient algorithm for computing paths [12, 13], which is used to determine path feasibility with clearance under a few milliseconds of computation in our scenarios. With respect to the second and third requirements, we adopt a path following approach in order to be able to safely navigate through narrow passages of the environment.

In order to address precise departure and arrival placements, and to achieve the observed behavior of sharp turns during path following, we propose an optimized locomotion synthesis method based on a specific organization of locomotion clips from motion capture. Three specific types of locomotion sequences were collected with a full-body motion capture system: departure motions, arrival motions, and walk cycles. Each motion is then parameterized to cover a small area around its original trajectory, and to depart or arrive with a parameterized orientation at the first or final frame. As a result we obtain parameterized motions that cover all possible required initial and final orientations, and that concatenate into walk cycles during the path following phase. Additional details on the locomotion module are omitted due lack of space, but will be made available from the website of the authors. Figure 8 illustrates one example.

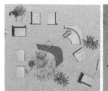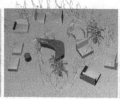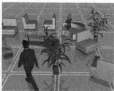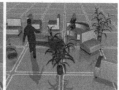

Fig. 8. Illustration of one particular locomotion sequence planned. From left to right: the departure and arrival clips nearby the path to be followed, skeleton trails illustrating the whole motion obtained, and two snapshots of the final result.

6   Action Synthesis

The synthesis of the demonstrative action is performed with blending operations in a cluster of example motions. Given the target position $\mathbf{p_t}$ to be addressed by the end-effector at the stroke point of the action, blending weights are determined by inverse blending optimization [9] in order to address the target precisely. See Figure 9.

Collision avoidance has shown to be important. It not only increases the ability to find solutions in cluttered environments but it also improves the number of successful placements to be considered for action execution. We have developed a collision avoidance method that operates on the blending space of the example motions defining an action. Blending space operations have been employed before in motion planning [11], but here we develop a faster collision avoidance procedure that does not require expensive planning around the obstacles. We create repulsive force fields in 3D and compute a scalar potential of collision P_c that encodes the potential of collision between the agent's end-effector E and the obstacles. Instead of computing the force field in discretized 2D cells [29], we approximate the bounding volume of the nearby obstacles with small spheres S_i (see Figure 9-center), so that $P_c = exp(-\sum distance(E, S_i))$.

Let $\mathbf{p_t}$ be the target object to be addressed by action A. First, blending weights $\mathbf{w_t}$ that generate action $A(\mathbf{p_t})$ are computed by inverse blending. The produced motion can be re-written as a sequence of frames $F_i(\mathbf{w}_i)$, $i \in \{1, \ldots, n\}$, and initialized with $\mathbf{w}_i = \mathbf{w_t}, \forall i \in \{1, \ldots, n\}$. Next, we make a single pass from F_1 to F_n and adjust intermediate frames F_j at a given discretization resolution. The resolution is relative to the distance covered by the end-effector. Given a frame $F_j(\mathbf{w}_j)$ being visited, if its corresponding posture collides or is detected to be too close to an object, $\mathbf{w}_j$ is adjusted by inverse blending in order to minimize P_c at F_j, essentially shifting F_j away from the obstacles. Collisions are checked intermittently at mesh level and the process moves on to F_{j+1} when F_j becomes collision-free. Each time a frame is adjusted, the weights of the nearby frames (according to a smoothness window) are updated so that the overall sequence of weights is smooth, producing a new final motion $A(\mathbf{p_t})$ that smoothly avoids the nearby obstacles.

The method typically solves action synthesis under 300 milliseconds, with most computation time spent on mesh collision checking. The approach is able to control how much deformation is allowed, thus controlling the balance between action motion quality, action adaptation to obstacles, and body placement search time.

7   Locomotion-Action Coordination

The locomotion transition into the action requires special attention in order to generate realistic results. We start by using a transition window of 0.58 seconds that is the average window observed from our studies with human subjects. The window tells how early, before finishing the locomotion, the action should start to be executed. The action will start gradually taking control over the upper-body and will achieve full control when the locomotion stops. An important coordination problem that we address here is to ensure that the resulting arm swing pattern during the transition remains realistic.

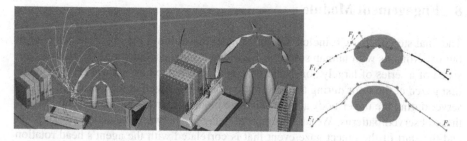

Fig. 9. Left: trajectories of one pointing database with 10 blended motions for one solution marked in red. Center: spheres are used to approximate the nearby objects and to compute P_c. Right: If intermediate frames collide their blending weights are adjusted to remove the collision.

Let S_l^{end} be the arm swing at the end of the locomotion sequence, and S_a be the arm swing direction of the action. In our examples the right arm is used by the action but the presented analysis can be equally employed to both arms. Two main cases may happen: 1) the arm swings can be codirectional, in which case a natural transition is automatically achieved, or 2) the arm swings can be contradirectional, what would cause a sudden change in the arm swing direction during the transition window. Sudden changes in the arm swing were never observed in our experiments with human subjects, who were very good at achieving coherent final steps with clear final arm swings. We therefore fix contradirectional cases in two possible ways. If the final locomotion swing S_l^{end} slightly overlaps into the action arm swing S_a, it is then shortened to match S_a and without having it to return to its target rest position. This is accomplished by repeating the final frames of S_l^{end}, skipping the same amount of initial frames of S_a, then smoothly blending into the latter. If however the final locomotion swing shows a significant overlap, S_l^{end} is then dropped and the previous swing cycle S_l^{prev} is extended to override S_l^{end}, before blending into S_a. We examine the swing velocities generated from both and the one showing better consistency is applied. Figure 10 illustrates the process.

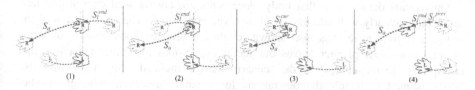

Fig. 10. Overlapping transition of the final arm swing of the locomotion S_l^{end} towards the arm swing direction generated by the action S_a. Codirectional cases can be directly blended (1), however contradirectional cases (2) have to be adjusted either by shortening the final locomotion swing (3) or by overriding it with the previous swing (4).

8   Engagement Module

The final step of PLACE includes a gaze model that follows the observed behavior in our experiments with human subjects. We observed that each demonstration trial consisted of a series of largely consistent gaze and gaze-related events where participants first gazed at the floor during the locomotion, and then gazed at the target and the observer during the upper-body action. Our gaze model generates gaze events that follow these observed patterns. We use a temporal delay Δt between the action stroke point and the start of the object gaze event that is correlated with the agent's head rotation angle ϕ. When the observer is not in the center of the agent's field of view, the gaze towards the observer starts before the action reaches the stroke point, resulting in a negative Δt. The gaze behavior also incorporates gaze durations that decline over time across repeated demonstrations, an observed behavior in our experiments with human subjects. Figure 11 illustrates the main events of the gaze model.

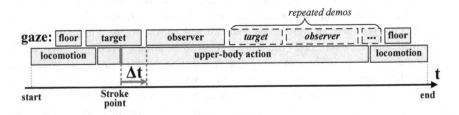

Fig. 11. Synchronization between gaze and motion events

9   Results and Discussion

Results are presented in Figures 1, 2, 12, 13 and 14. Additional results are presented in the accompanying video to this paper, which is available at http://graphics.ucmerced.edu. The planner is capable of synthesizing entire sequences in a range from 100 to 400 milliseconds, depending on the complexity of the environment and the collision avoidance settings.

Our results demonstrate that body placements are always well chosen and lead to positions clearly well addressing all involved constraints. The coordination of the swing arm trajectories has also shown to always produce good results. In terms of limitations, our planner leaves out facial expressions and other behaviors that are specific to the context of the scenario being simulated. Our model was also only designed to handle demonstrations for a single observer, although we believe that multiple observers can be easily incorporated if behavioral data exploring relevant possible configurations is obtained. The collected motion capture actions used in our blending procedures are available from the following project website: http://graphics.ucmerced.edu/software/invbld/.

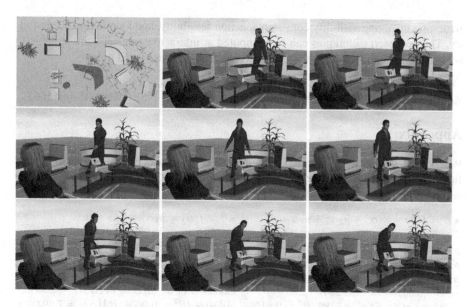

Fig. 12. Example of a solution produced by PLACE. The top-left image shows the planning scenario and the solution placement for execution of the demonstration. The following sequence of snapshots shows the arrival locomotion seamlessly transitioning into the demonstration action pointing at the fax machine with coordinated gaze towards the observer.

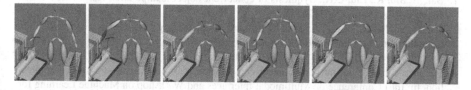

Fig. 13. Short-range solution suitable for pointing and describing the blue bottle

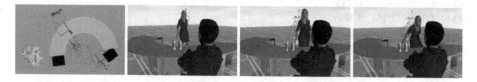

Fig. 14. Action synthesis corrected by force fields in blending space. The left three images show an action that originally produced collisions with obstacles; and the following three images show a collision avoidance solution (along the blue trajectory) for removing the collisions. Without the collision avoidance the action would not be feasible and a new placement would be necessary.

10   Conclusion

We have introduced a new behavioral and motor planning model for solving demonstrative tasks. Our proposed PLACE planner uniquely explores body placement trade-offs involving visibility constraints, action feasibility, and locomotion accessibility. The proposed techniques can be computed at interactive rates and are suitable to several applications relying on interactive virtual humans as virtual trainers.

Acknowledgments. This work was partially supported by NSF Award IIS-0915665.

Appendix

Polynomial (cubic and quadratic) functions were chosen over other types of fitting functions such as Gaussian and Fourier for better extrapolations when $\alpha > 150$ and $\alpha < $ -150. Details are given below.

- $\beta = f(\alpha) = p_1\alpha^3 + p_2\alpha^2 + p_3\alpha + p_4$
Coefficients (with 95% confidence bounds):
$p_1 = 2.392E{-}6({-}6.74E{-}6, 1.152E{-}5)$,
$p_2 = 0.0003056({-}0.0004444, 0.001056)$,
$p_3 = 0.1145({-}0.04067, 0.2697)$,
$p_4 = -6.062({-}15.42, 3.294)$.
Goodness of fit: $SSE = 5386$, $R^2 = 0.6156$,
$Adjusted R^2 = 0.5713$, $RMSE = 14.39$.

- $\phi = f(\alpha) = p_1\alpha^2 + p_2\alpha + p_3$
Coefficients (with 95% confidence bounds):
$p1 = 0.0006673(0.0001145, 0.00122)$,
$p2 = 0.6736(0.6315, 0.7158)$,
$p3 = 2.073({-}5.167, 9.312)$.
Goodness of fit: $SSE : 3381$, $R^2 : 0.9785$,
$Adjusted R^2 : 0.9769$, $RMSE : 11.19$.

- $\theta = f(\alpha) = p_1\alpha^2 + p_2\alpha + p_3$
Coefficients (with 95% confidence bounds):
$p_1 = 0.0006228(0.000262, 0.0009837)$,
$p_2 = 0.3267(0.2991, 0.3542)$,
$p_3 = 11.29(6.564, 16.02)$.
Goodness of fit: $SSE = 1441$, $R^2 = 0.9635$.
$Adjusted R^2 = 0.9608$, $RMSE = 7.304$.

References

1. Bai, Y., Siu, K., Liu, C.K.: Synthesis of concurrent object manipulation tasks. ACM Trans. Graph. 31(6), 156:1–156:9 (2012)
2. van Basten, B.J.H., Egges, A.: Flexible splicing of upper-body motion spaces on locomotion. Computer Graphics Forum 30(7), 1963–1971 (2011)
3. Bee, N., Wagner, J., André, E., Vogt, T., Charles, F., Pizzi, D., Cavazza, M.: Discovering eye gaze behavior during human-agent conversation in an interactive storytelling application. In: Int'l Conference on Multimodal Interfaces and Workshop on Machine Learning for Multimodal Interaction, ICMI-MLMI 2010, pp.9:1–9:8. ACM, New York (2010)
4. Cullen, K.E., Huterer, M., Braidwood, D.A., Sylvestre, P.A.: Time course of vestibuloocular reflex suppression during gaze shifts. Journal of Neurophysiology 92(6), 3408–3422 (2004)
5. Esteves, C., Arechavaleta, G., Pettré, J., Laumond, J.P.: Animation planning for virtual characters cooperation. ACM Trans. Graph. 25(2), 319–339 (2006)
6. Grochow, K., Martin, S., Hertzmann, A., Popović, Z.: Style-based inverse kinematics. ACM Transactions on Graphics (Proceedings of SIGGRAPH) 23(3), 522–531 (2004)
7. Heck, R., Gleicher, M.: Parametric motion graphs. In: Proceedings of the symposium on Interactive 3D Graphics and Games (I3D), pp. 129–136. ACM Press, New York (2007)
8. Heck, R., Kovar, L., Gleicher, M.: Splicing upper-body actions with locomotion. In: Proceedings of Eurographics 2006 (2006)

9. Huang, Y., Kallmann, M.: Motion parameterization with inverse blending. In: Boulic, R., Chrysanthou, Y., Komura, T. (eds.) MIG 2010. LNCS, vol. 6459, pp. 242–253. Springer, Heidelberg (2010)
10. Huang, Y., Matthews, J.L., Matlock, T., Kallmann, M.: Modeling gaze behavior for virtual demonstrators. In: Vilhjálmsson, H.H., Kopp, S., Marsella, S., Thórisson, K.R. (eds.) IVA 2011. LNCS, vol. 6895, pp. 155–161. Springer, Heidelberg (2011)
11. Huang, Y., Mahmudi, M., Kallmann, M.: Planning humanlike actions in blending spaces. In: Proceedings of the IEEE/RSJ International Conference on Intelligent Robots and Systems, IROS (2011)
12. Kallmann, M.: Shortest paths with arbitrary clearance from navigation meshes. In: Proceedings of the Eurographics / SIGGRAPH Symposium on Computer Animation, SCA (2010)
13. Kallmann, M.: Dynamic and robust local clearance triangulations. ACM Transactions on Graphics 33(5) (2014)
14. de Lasa, M., Mordatch, I., Hertzmann, A.: Feature-Based Locomotion Controllers. ACM Transactions on Graphics 29(3) (2010)
15. Lee, Y., Wampler, K., Bernstein, G., Popović, J., Popović, Z.: Motion fields for interactive character locomotion. ACM Trans. Graph. 138, 138:1–138:8 (2010)
16. Levine, S., Wang, J.M., Haraux, A., Popović, Z., Koltun, V.: Continuous character control with low-dimensional embeddings. ACM Trans. Graph. 28, 28:1–28:10 (2012)
17. Mukai, T., Kuriyama, S.: Geostatistical motion interpolation. In: ACM SIGGRAPH, pp. 1062–1070. ACM, New York (2005)
18. Mutlu, B., Hodgins, J.K., Forlizzi, J.: A storytelling robot: Modeling and evaluation of human-like gaze behavior. In: Proceedings of HUMANOIDS 2006, 2006 IEEE-RAS International Conference on Humanoid Robots. IEEE (December 2006)
19. Rose, C., Bodenheimer, B., Cohen, M.F.: Verbs and adverbs: Multidimensional motion interpolation. IEEE Computer Graphics and Applications 18, 32–40 (1998)
20. Safonova, A., Hodgins, J.K.: Construction and optimal search of interpolated motion graphs. ACM Transactions on Graphics (SIGGRAPH 2007) 26(3) (August 2007)
21. Scheflen, A.E., Ashcraft, N.: Human Territories: How We Behave in Space-Time. Prentice-Hall, Englewood Cliffs (1976)
22. Shapiro, A., Kallmann, M., Faloutsos, P.: Interactive motion correction and object manipulation. In: ACM SIGGRAPH Symposium on Interactive 3D Graphics and Games (I3D), Seattle (2007)
23. Soukoreff, R.W., MacKenzie, I.S.: Towards a standard for pointing device evaluation: Perspectives on 27 years of fitts' law research in hci. International Journal of Human-Computer Studies 61, 751–789 (2004)
24. Sumner, R.W., Zwicker, M., Gotsman, C., Popović, J.: Mesh-based inverse kinematics. ACM Trans. Graph. 24(3), 488–495 (2005)
25. Thiebaux, M., Marshall, A., Marsella, S., Kallmann, M.: Smartbody: Behavior realization for embodied conversational agents. In: Seventh International Joint Conference on Autonomous Agents and Multi-Agent Systems, AAMAS (2008)
26. Treuille, A., Lee, Y., Popović, Z.: Near-optimal character animation with continuous control. In: Proceedings of ACM SIGGRAPH. ACM Press (2007)
27. Van Horn, M.R., Sylvestre, P.A., Cullen, K.E.: The brain stem saccadic burst generator encodes gaze in three-dimensional space. J. of Neurophysiology 99(5), 2602–2616 (2008)
28. Yamane, K., Kuffner, J.J., Hodgins, J.K.: Synthesizing animations of human manipulation tasks. ACM Transactions on Graphics (Proceedings of SIGGRAPH) 23(3), 532–539 (2004)
29. Zhang, L., LaValle, S.M., Manocha, D.: Global vector field computation for feedback motion planning. In: Proceedings of the 2009 IEEE International Conference on Robotics and Automation, pp. 3065–3070. IEEE Press, Piscataway (2009)

With Us or Against Us: Simulated Social Touch by Virtual Agents in a Cooperative or Competitive Setting

Gijs Huisman, Jan Kolkmeier, and Dirk Heylen

Human Media Interaction Group, University of Twente, The Netherlands
{gijs.huisman,d.k.j.heylen}@utwente.nl, j.kolkmeier@student.utwente.nl

Abstract. In this paper we examine how simulated social touch by a virtual agent in a cooperative or competitive augmented reality game influences the perceived trustworthiness, warmth and politeness of the agent. Before and after the game, participants interact with two agents whereby one agent touches the participant's arm. Results showed no significant difference in how agents are perceived in the cooperative and competitive situation. However, significant differences between perception of the touching and non-touching agents could be observed for warmth.

Keywords: Simulated social touch, virtual agent, Augmented reality.

1 Introduction

In the field of embodied conversational agents (ECAs), human-to-human communication is approximated through the implementation of various intelligent behaviors inspired by human communication. Verbal or linguistic intelligence in speech synthesis and prosody play a role as well as non-verbal behaviors such as facial expressions, body posture or turn-taking [7]. A modality that is understudied in interactions with ECAs is touch. Handshakes, hugs or pats on the back may occur less frequently during communication than other behaviors, such as smiling or nodding, but social touch is known to have strong effects on subsequent interactions between co-located individuals. It has been shown that co-located social touch can affect compliance to requests [10], can reduce stress [8], and can be used to communicate discrete emotions [16].

Recent studies have indicated that social touch between humans can be mediated by haptic feedback technology (i.e. mediated social touch [11]). Interesting in this regard is that mediated social touch has been found to have effects similar to co-located social touch on compliance to requests [12], perception of the communication partner [13], and the communication of affect [2], or feelings of social presence [3]. Furthermore, early work in which social touch was simulated by an agent with a physical torso and virtual head, showed that social touch by a virtual agent can influence perceptions of this agent [4]. Here, social touch is no longer applied (mediated or otherwise) by a human

T. Bickmore et al. (Eds.): IVA 2014, LNAI 8637, pp. 204–213, 2014.

communication partner, but is simulated by a virtual agent, in sync with other modalities such as speech and gestures.

Though social touch, be it co-located, mediated, or simulated, can have effects on the interaction, such effects may strongly depend on the context in which the touch occurs. One study has found that when co-located social touch was used in a cooperative game setting, later helping behavior in a dictator game increased. However, when the same touch occurred in a competitively framed game, it had an averse effect on helping behavior [5]. In the current paper we conduct a user study to investigate whether simulated social touch by a virtual agent results in different judgements of that agent in a game setting that is either framed cooperatively or competitively.

2 Related Work

There are a number of reasons why adding social touch capabilities to an ECA may be beneficial. Social touch has been found to play a role in a wide range of interpersonal messages, such as the communication of support, appreciation, affection, and others [17]. Furthermore, social touch can positively influence compliance to requests, in a way that the one receiving the touch is more inclined to comply with the request, such as filling out bogus personality questionnaire items [19], or complying to menu item suggestions by a waiter or waitress [10]. Effects of touch that result in a behavioral change in the one receiving the touch may be dependent on the context in which the touch takes place. A study that employed a confederate that touched the participant either in a cooperative or a competitive setting, found that while touches in the collaborative setting had a positive effect on helping behavior, touches in the competitive setting had a negative effect on helping behavior in a dictator game [5].

Social touch can also be simulated by an ECA. One of the few studies investigating simulated social touch used a virtual representation of an agent's head, mounted on top of a physical mannequin [4]. The agent was able to squeeze a participant's hand. It was found that simulated social touch enhanced the perception of the relation with the agent, but only for participants that were comfortable being touched.

3 System Design

We designed a system that places two virtual agents in AR space of a tablet computer. We simulate social touch through a tactile displays worn on both upper arms by the user (see fig. 1(a)) which is actuated in sync with the touch animations of the agents (see fig. 1(b)).

Unity3D[1] with the Qualcomm Vuforia plug-in was used to develop the marker-based Augmented Reality application. As marker, we use a wall covered with printed patterns, as visible in the background of fig. 1(b). The Unity

---

[1] http://unity3d.com/

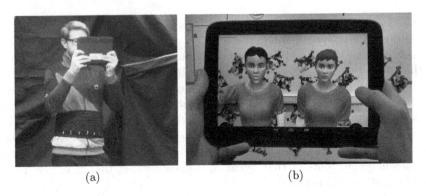

(a)   (b)

Fig. 1. User wearing the vibrotactile displays and holding the tablet (a) and the Agents in AR, as seen by the user on the tablet, during a touch of the left agent (b).

Multipurpose Avatar plug-in was used to generate the two characters seen in fig. 1(b). These can be universally controlled using Unity's *Mecanim* animation system. Speech of the agents is realized with pre-recorded audio clips from speech synthesizers (Microsoft Windows 8 Hazel and Zira). Rudimentary scripts were written to implement amplitude driven lip-syncing and randomized blinking behavior of eyelids. Additional behaviors such as turning, walking, sitting, waving, and touching were implemented. In fig. 1(b), the touching animation is shown as seen by the user.

As tactile display we used the *Elitac Science Suit*[2], a modular system consisting of several eccentric mass vibration motors that can be attached to elastic bands of different sizes using Velcro. The intensity of vibration of each vibration motor can be individually controlled with sixteen levels of vibration intensity. Three actuators, with approximately 10 centimeters spacing between them, were placed in a triangular position, and were attached to each upper arm of the user. An additional six actuators (two rows of three, with approximately 10 centimeter spacing between them vertically, and approximately 20 centimeter spacing between them horizontally) were placed on the participant's abdomen to give general feedback during the game.

4   Experiment Configuration and Game

To investigate the role of touch by a virtual agent in the perception of this agent, as well as the role of a cooperative or competitive context, we designed an experiment (see Section 5). For the experiment, specific scenarios that involve two female virtual agents named Anna and Belle, were scripted using the AR touching virtual agent setup. Variables of the experiment were configured in advance, including the condition (cooperative, competitive), which of the agent was the touching agent, as well as which agent started the interaction on all

---

[2] http://elitac.org/products/sciencesuit.html

occasions. We call the latter, the assertive agent. We hypothesized that the agent that started the interaction could be perceived as more assertive. Assertiveness has been found to influence participant's perceptions of a conversational agent [20]. The flow of the experiment and dialogs is shown in table 1.

As part of the experiment, participants played a game that was framed either cooperatively or competitively. During the game, players (the participant and the two agents) collected virtual coins that were arranged in a three-dimensional grid in AR space (see fourth image in table 1). To collect a coin, the participant pointed the tablet at one of the coins and touched the screen to 'shoot'. Upon hitting the coin, it flew towards the player, increasing a common score in the cooperative condition, or a personal score in the competitive condition. To make the game more interesting, a moving block occluded some of the coins. The game was designed so that it would be impossible to collect all coins during the games duration (40 seconds). The time was shown counting down at the top of the screen. After the time ran out, the participant received feedback about his or her performance compared to the agents. For all participants in both conditions, participants were told that they performed slightly better than both agents. As shown in table 1, the two agents gave different commentary during the game, depending on the condition, and the agent's assertiveness.

5   Experiment

Our first hypothesis was that social touch results in a more positive perception of the agent administering the touch. The second hypothesis was that, while in the cooperatively framed condition, the social touch would have positive effects on the perception of the agent, the effect would be significantly weaker or reversed (i.e. more negative judgements of the agent) in the competitive condition. Finally, we control for participants trait touch receptivity and the assertiveness of the agent. Table 1 provides an overview of the conditions.

Measures. Participants rated the agent on a list of 13 adjectives from [1]. Because of the importance of politeness in communication with ECAs, we decided to add the adjective "polite" (see also [20]), for a total of 14 adjectives. For both agents the participant indicated his or her agreement with statements like "I though Anna was likeable" on a 7-point Likert scale, ranging from "strongly disagree" to "strongly agree". The participant also completed a touch receptivity questionnaire adapted from [4], with two healthcare-specific items removed. Participants indicated their agreement to statements like "I feel uncomfortable when someone casually touches me" on a 7-point Likert scale, ranging from "strongly disagree" to "strongly agree".

Finally, a behavioral measurement was employed. After the final interaction with the participant, the agents both sat down on two of four physical chairs present in the room. The participant was asked to sit down on any of the four chairs. It was hypothesized that participants, on average, would sit next to the touching agent more than next to the non-touching agent.

Table 1. Flow of Experiment. A is the assertive, B the non-assertive agent. Touches happen on lines marked with *, if the respective agent is also the touching agent.

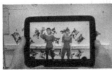

[START]

A: Hi there, I'm [Anne/Belle]. (waving)
B: And my name is [Anne/Belle], hi! (waving)

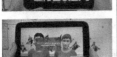

[AGENTS STEP CLOSER]

A: Here, have a look at the game instructions!

[PARTICIPANT READS GAME INSTRUCTIONS]

A: Have you read the instructions?
B: Then lets start!

A: Good luck in the game! *
B: Yes, good luck and have fun! *

[GAME STARTS]

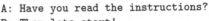

[COMPETITIVE]   [COOPERATIVE]

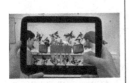

[COMPETITIVE]	[COOPERATIVE]
Only one of us can win	Let's work together
I was quicker than you	Good Job
That one was mine	Nice work
My accuracy is better	Let's collect all
than yours	the coins
These coins are mine	Well done
I will win this	We can do it

[GAME ENDS]

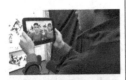

[RESULTS ARE DISPLAYED]

A: You did really well in the game, congrats. *
B: Yes, an impressive performance. Well done! *

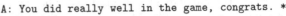

A: We should do this again some time! *
B: Yes, just let us know! *

[AGENTS SIT DOWN]

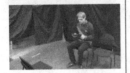

[PARTICIPANT IS PROMPTED TO SIT]

[PARTICIPANT FILLS OUT QUESTIONNAIRE]

Participants. In total 42 people participated in the study. There were 29 male participants and 13 female participants. The average age was 21.5 $(SD = 2.54)$. Participants were all students or employees of the University of Twente.

Procedure. After obtaining written consent, the experimenter explained the study's general procedure. Next, the vibrotactile displays were attached to the participant's body, and the participant received the tablet computer. Instructions on how to hold and use the tablet were given by the experimenter. The principle of the coin-collecting game was introduced for both conditions. Next, the working of the tactile display was tested in a trial version of the game. All further instructions were given on the tablet computer. After completing the game, the participant was asked to sit down on one of the four chairs to fill out the agent perception questionnaire, demographics, and touch receptivity questionnaire using the tablet computer. The touch receptivity questionnaire was given at the end of the session as to not to prime the participant to the agents' touches. After completing all questionnaires the participant was debriefed about the aim of the study. The total duration of the study was approximately 20 minutes.

Results

Data analysis. Data from five participants was removed because they could not correctly identify the touching agent. As it is not possible to confidently attribute these participants' ratings to either the touching or non-touching agents, only the data from the 37 remaining participants was used for all further analysis. A principal component analysis with varimax rotation and Kaiser normalization for the 14 adjectives revealed a three factor structure that explained 59.5% of the total variance. Table 2 shows the factors, items, and factor loadings. The first factor describes the trustworthiness of the agent, which consists of items such as trustworthy, and competent. The second factor, warmth, deals with more affective interpersonal aspects of the agent, such as its friendliness and likeability. Finally, the third factor describes the agent's politeness, with the items polite and modest. The touch receptivity questionnaire had an acceptable internal consistency ($\alpha = .69$). A median split procedure ($Mdn = 4.71$) was used to divide participants into 'touch receptive' ($n = 15$, $M = 5.32$, $SD = 0.38$) and 'non-touch receptive' ($n = 22$, $M = 4.18$, $SD = 0.56$) groups.

Behavioral measure. Overall, the behavioral measure that was employed showed no clear preference for sitting either next to a touching agent (18 participants) or non-touching agent (17 participants)[3]. Furthermore, participants showed no preference for siting next to an assertive (19 participants) or non-asssertive (18 participants) agent. Participants higher in touch receptivity also did not sit next to a touching agent, more than participants who were less touch receptive. These findings are similar for both cooperative and competitive settings.

---

[3] The remainder of the participants chose to sit on a chair occupied by one of the agents in AR.

Table 2. Principal component analysis of 14 adjectives

Factor	Item	Factor loading
Trustworthiness (α = .82)	Honest	.76
	Informed	.75
	Competent	.71
	Trustworthy	.71
	Sincere	.67
	Credible	.62
	Interesting	.48
Warmth (α = .81)	Approachable	.76
	Warm	.74
	Confident	.73
	Friendly	.65
	Likeable	.59
Politeness (α = .69)	Polite	.83
	Modest	.80

Perception of the agents. We ran a repeated measures ANOVA with Greenhouse-Geisser correction, with touch/non-touching agent as the within subjects variable, and agent assertiveness (the agent is assertive or not), touch receptivity (touch receptive and non-touch receptive), and condition (cooperative or competitive) as between subject factors. We found no significant main effects or interaction effects for the between subject factors (all p's >.05). However, we did find a significant main effect of touching/non-touching agent ($F(3.56, 103.13) = 5.96$, p <.001).

Paired-samples tests were used to further explore the within-subject effects. We first compared ratings for trustworthiness, warmth, and politeness between the touching and non-touching agents. Trustworthiness, and politeness did not show a significant difference, however, warmth was rated higher overall for touching agents ($M = 4.90$) compared to non-touching agents ($M = 4.16$)($t(36) = 4.69$, p <.001).

To assess whether the agent's assertiveness influenced participants' perceptions of the agent we ran a paired-samples comparison for the three factors for assertive agents and non-assertive agents. We found a significant difference for trustworthiness between assertive ($M = 4.48$) and non-assertive ($M = 4.23$) agents ($t(36) = 2.31$, p <.05). We found no differences between assertive and non-assertive agents for the other two factors.

To check for the influence of touch receptivity we ran paired-samples comparisons for the three factors, for touch receptive and non-touch receptive participants. For touch receptive participants, warmth, was again rated higher for the touching agent ($M = 5.29$) compared to the non-touching agent ($M = 4.19$)($t(14) = 8.56$, p <.001). For non-touch receptive individuals however, the difference for warmth between the touching ($M = 4.62$) and non-touching agent ($M = 4.16$) was only marginally significant ($t(21) = 2.04$, $p = .054$).

Differences for trustworthiness and politeness were nonsignificant ($p > .05$). Finally, a significant positive correlation ($r = .43$, $p < .01$) between ratings for the touching agent's warmth and touch receptivity, further supports the relation between touch receptivity and perceptions of warmth for the touching agent.

6   Discussion and Conclusions

Overall we found that participants rated the touching virtual agent significantly higher on warmth than the non-touching agent. This effect was more pronounced for touch receptive participants. For non-touch receptive participants the difference for warmth was only marginally significant. Aspects of the agent related to trustworthiness or politeness were not affected by the agent's touch. Our findings suggest that touch by a virtual agent can enhance perceptions of more affective attributes of this agent. Participants who are comfortable with social touch, seem to respond more strongly in this way than participants who are less comfortable with social touch.

We did not find any significant difference in the judgement of assertive or non-assertive agents for warmth or politeness. We did however find a significant difference for trustworthiness between assertive and non-assertive agents. This indicates that the assertive agent, who started the interactions, was seen as a more trustworthy, irrespective of whether the agent applied a social touch or not. However, considering that our manipulation of assertiveness was limited, this conclusion is far from definitive. These findings partially support our initial hypothesis. However, we found that the framing of the context in which the touch by the agent took place, did not affect the participants' judgement of the agent applying the touch. Based on a previous study [5] we expected that social touch by a virtual agent in a cooperative setting would result in more favorable judgements of this agent compared to an agent applying the same touch in a competitive setting. A possible explanation for this difference is that previous research was conducted with co-located social touch occurring between two humans. A reduction in helping behavior was attributed to the participants perceiving the touching confederate in the competitive setting as dominant. It is possible that due to the relatively simple facial animations, and friendly dialog, our touching agent was not perceived as dominant. Thus, no clear negative effect of the touch in the competitive setting occurred. What is more, [5] employed a behavioral measure that involved participants sharing a reward with their competitor (i.e. the confederate). We decided against a behavioral measure similar to [5] because anything valuable to the participant (e.g. a monetary reward) could not reasonably be 'shared' with the virtual agent. Potentially, the lack of a reward contributed to participants in our study not considering the context as 'high stakes', in which a touch by a competitor might be perceived as an expression of dominance. Therefore, the simulated social touch by the agent in the competitive setting did not have a clear negative effect. A stronger manipulation of the cooperativeness or competitiveness of the setting in combination with an agent's simulated social touch would be an interesting direct for future research.

In our study we did not find such an overall effect of touch receptivity on the perception of the touching agents. The lack of a more clear distinction between touch receptive and non-touch receptive participants in our study can be attributed to a number of factors. First, the touches applied in our study were more casual in nature, with the interaction less focussed on the touch per se. This might have negated any clear negative effect of the touch that non-touch receptive participants might have experienced. Second, the distinction between touch receptive and non-touch receptive participants was more pronounced in [4], compared to participants in our study. Finally, our touch receptivity measure was taken after the experiment as to not to prime participants to the agent's touches. However, the experiment itself might have primed participants to think of themselves as more touch receptive individuals.

To conclude, our study indicates that simulated social touch by a virtual agent enhances the perception of more affective aspects (i.e. warmth) of this agent. This effect occurred more strongly for individuals who were comfortable with social touch. Neither the assertiveness of the agent, nor the context in which the touch occurred had an influence on this effect in our study. Our findings suggest that touch might be a useful modality in the communication with virtual agents, specifically where the communication of affect is concerned. Simulated social touch by a virtual agent might be used in therapy settings, where the agent shows support or empathy [4]. Furthermore, touch by an ECA may be employed in settings where an ECA assists a user with a task, such as an information search task, to make the agent seem more warm irrespective of it's actual performance. Finally, a touching agent could be used in entertainment or gaming scenarios to enhance feelings of warmth between the player and a virtual character in the game. Ultimately, simulated social touch might be used to forge stronger affective bonds between agents and their human communication partners.

Acknowledgements. This publication was supported by the Dutch national program COMMIT.

References

1. Bailenson, J.N., Yee, N., Patel, K., Beall, A.C.: Detecting digital chameleons. Computers in Human Behavior 24(1), 66–87 (2008)
2. Bailenson, J., Yee, N., Brave, S., Merget, D., Koslow, D.: Virtual interpersonal touch: Expressing and recognizing emotions through haptic devices. Human-Computer Interaction 22(3), 325–353 (2007)
3. Beelen, T., Blaauboer, R., Bovenmars, N., Loos, B., Zielonka, L., van Delden, R., Huisman, G., Reidsma, D.: The art of tug of war: Investigating the influence of remote touch on social presence in a distributed rope pulling game. In: Reidsma, D., Katayose, H., Nijholt, A. (eds.) ACE 2013. LNCS, vol. 8253, pp. 246–257. Springer, Heidelberg (2013)
4. Bickmore, T.W., Fernando, R., Ring, L., Schulman, D.: Empathic Touch by Relational Agents. IEEE Transactions on Affective Computing 1(1), 60–71 (2010)

5. Camps, J., Tuteleers, C., Stouten, J., Nelissen, J.: A situational touch: How touch affects people's decision behavior. Social Influence 8(4), 237–250 (2013)
6. Cramer, H., Kemper, N., Amin, A., Wielinga, B., Evers, V.: give me a hug: the effects of touch and autonomy on people's responses to embodied social agents. Computer Animation and Virtual Worlds 20(2-3), 437–445 (2009)
7. Dehn, D., Van Mulken, S.: The impact of animated interface agents: a review of empirical research. International Journal of Human-Computer Studies 52(1), 1–22 (2000)
8. Ditzen, B., Neumann, I.D., Bodenmann, G., von Dawans, B., Turner, R.A., Ehlert, U., Heinrichs, M.: Effects of different kinds of couple interaction on cortisol and heart rate responses to stress in women. Psychoneuroendocrinology 32(5), 565–574 (2007)
9. Drescher, V.M., Gantt, W.H., Whitehead, W.E.: Heart rate response to touch. Psychosomatic Medicine 42(6), 559–565 (1980)
10. Guéguen, N., Jacob, C., Boulbry, G.: The effect of touch on compliance with a restaurant's employee suggestion. International Journal of Hospitality Management 26(4), 1019–1023 (2007)
11. Haans, A., IJsselsteijn, W.A.: Mediated social touch: a review of current research and future directions. Virtual Reality 9(2-3), 149–159 (2006)
12. Haans, A., IJsselsteijn, W.A.: The Virtual Midas Touch: Helping Behavior After a Mediated Social Touch. IEEE Transactions on Haptics 2(3), 136–140 (2009)
13. Haans, A., de Nood, C., IJsselsteijn, W.A.: Investigating response similarities between real and mediated social touch: a first test. In: Proceedings of CHI 2007, pp. 2405–2410. ACM (2007)
14. Henricson, M., Ersson, A., Määttä, S., Segesten, K., Berglund, A.L.: The outcome of tactile touch on stress parameters in intensive care: a randomized controlled trial. Complementary Therapies in Clinical Practice 14(4), 244–254 (2008)
15. Hertenstein, M.J., Keltner, D., App, B., Bulleit, B.A., Jaskolka, A.R.: Touch communicates distinct emotions. Emotion 6(3), 528–533 (2006)
16. Hertenstein, M.J., Verkamp, J.M., Kerestes, A.M., Holmes, R.M.: The communicative functions of touch in humans, nonhuman primates, and rats: A review and synthesis of the empirical research. Genetic, Social, and General Psychology Monographs 132(1), 5–94 (2006)
17. Jones, S.E., Yarbrough, A.E.: A naturalistic study of the meanings of touch. Communication Monographs 52(1), 19–56 (1985)
18. Nakagawa, K., Shiomi, M., Shinozawa, K., Matsumura, R., Ishiguro, H., Hagita, N.: Effect of robot's active touch on people's motivation. In: HRI 2011, pp. 465–472. ACM (2011)
19. Patterson, M.L., Powell, J.L., Lenihan, M.G.: Touch, compliance, and interpersonal affect. Journal of Nonverbal Behavior 10(1), 41–50 (1986)
20. ter Maat, M., Truong, K.P., Heylen, D.: How turn-taking strategies influence users' impressions of an agent. In: Allbeck, J., Badler, N., Bickmore, T., Pelachaud, C., Safonova, A. (eds.) IVA 2010. LNCS, vol. 6356, pp. 441–453. Springer, Heidelberg (2010)
21. Whitcher, S.J., Fisher, J.D.: Multidimensional reaction to therapeutic touch in a hospital setting. Journal of Personality and Social Psychology 37(1), 87–96 (1979)

A Step towards Modelling Group Behaviour in Autonomous Synthetic Characters

Naziya Hussaini and Ruth Aylett

School of Mathematical and Computer Sciences, Heriot-Watt University, Edinburgh,
EH14 4AS, United Kingdom
{nh4,R.S.Aylett}@hw.ac.uk

Abstract. This paper discusses the ability of IVAs to show group behaviour and act as a team, increasing their 'believability' as groups. We discuss the modelling of group behaviour based on the theory of interpersonal relations given by Schutz in IVAs by using FAtiMA-PSI architecture. A test scenario has been created and the next step is to test the implemented model on this.

Keywords: IVAs, Autonomous Synthetic Characters, FAtiMA-PSI, Group Dynamics.

1   Introduction

Research in virtual agents has produced IVAs that can plan and execute their own actions and react to users and other characters affectively [1]. However, much of this work focuses on characters as individuals. We focus on group dynamics for collections of autonomous characters. In a group, it is important that agents should be able to come together with their respective priorities or individualities and interact comfortably with each other [1]. Agents that have individual preferences for contextual emotions and can continuously learn from their past behaviour can, if synced with group dynamics become significantly more believable.

This paper explores how interaction among group members can be made believable and reasonable by applying social theories to the autonomous synthetic characters based on the FAtiMA-PSI architecture [2].

2   Background

Work is going on to improve the believability of IVAs through different perspectives, such as *emotions* [4], *culture* [5], etc. However we explore how *social interaction* can be included in the behaviour of IVAs. We use the FAtiMA-PSI architecture, to support characters that interact with each other and work in groups without losing their autonomy. We argue this produce a more social interactions and thus increase believability.

T. Bickmore et al. (Eds.): IVA 2014, LNAI 8637, pp. 214–217, 2014.

2.1   Group Dynamics

Group dynamics deals with the study of the various stages of a group i.e., from the formation of a group until the its termination. It includes the study of the behaviour of individuals, interaction between the members within the group (intergroup interactions) and also between the groups (intragroup interactions) [1].

William Schutz studied group behaviour and developed a theory based on interpersonal relations. His theory seems a very relevant one in relation to virtual characters, as this theory is widely used in group-training [1] and is based on drives; and is thus compatible with existing models such as FAtiMA-PSI that is also based on drives.

2.2   Fundamental Interpersonal Relations Orientation (FIRO)

Schutz's theory of interpersonal relations is known as Fundamental Interpersonal Relations Orientation (or FIRO, rhyming with 'Cairo') [1]. According to the theory, interaction in a group mainly depends on the three dimensions of interpersonal relation: inclusion, control, and affection [1].

Inclusion. According to Schutz, "the interpersonal need for inclusion is defined behaviourally as the need to establish and maintain a satisfactory relation with people with respect to interaction and association" [pp.18, 3].   The drive to satisfy the interpersonal need for inclusion results in generating inclusion behaviour.

Inclusion is mainly concerned with the formation of groups based on interpersonal relations.   It generally deals with the problem of being in or out of the group.

Control. Schutz defined control as the need to establish and maintain a satisfactory relation with other people with respect to control and power [pp.18, 3]. Control is normally required during decision-making processes.

Control and affection (considered next) are concerned with the relations that already exist at the previous stage of need for inclusion.   These normally deal with the problem of being at the top or bottom position in the group.

Affection. The interpersonal need for affection is defined behaviourally as the need to establish and maintain a satisfactory relation with others with respect to love and affection [pp.20, 3]. Affection behaviour relates to how an individual is attached emotionally to the other. Negative affection would result in hate, hostility, and rejection. It could be a cause of termination of the group. The type of affection generated would depend upon the action taken by an individual to satisfy their need for inclusion and control. Affection concerns the feeling of being close or distant.

2.3   The Postulate of Group Development

According to Schutz, any interpersonal relation between two or more people always follows the same sequence from formation to termination, starting with inclusion, followed by control and finally by affection [1]. This cycle may repeat itself. At the termination stage, this cycle may reverses.

$$I - C - A - I - C - A - I - C - A.........A - C - I$$

(Where, I = Inclusion, C = Control, and A = Affection)

3   Group Dynamics Based Agent Model

In the FAtiMA-PSI architecture, goals are guided by the five basic drives: Energy, Integrity, Affiliation, Certainty, and Competence [2, 6]. In order to model group behaviour in IVAs, we argue that if we introduce drives relating to interpersonal needs into the FAtiMA-PSI architecture, and if these drives further help in improving the goal selection mechanism then they can produce group behaviour. For this, a mapping is required between the interpersonal need drives (or we can say, group dimensions) and the drives of the motivation part. The value of motivational drives would affect the value of the group dimensions thus generating the need for inclusion, control, and affection. These needs are the basis for starting interaction between group members and thus forming a strong interpersonal relationship.

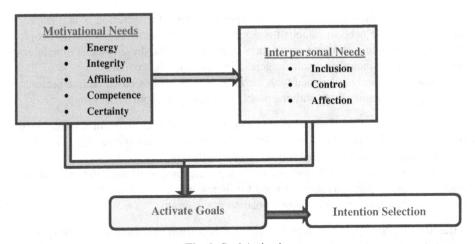

Fig. 1. Goal Activation

Each agent has a set of initial values for their motivational drives and a list of goals that they have to perform under various circumstances. Apart from these, each goal contains the information as to what extent it satisfies the drives of the agent, if that goal succeeds. The values of the group dimensions depend upon the values of the motivational drives. Before activating any goal the agent checks for the values of group dimensions. If the need for interpersonal relations arises then the agent would activate the goal that simultaneously satisfies its motivational needs along with its interpersonal needs. Thus it would activate a goal that would involve it in group activities, otherwise it would activate a goal that the agent would perform individually.

In our model, the value of the inclusion dimension depends upon the values of the affiliation, competence, and certainty drives; the value of the control dimension depends upon the value of competence and certainty; while the value of the affiliation drive impacts the value of the affection dimension. [1]

Let us consider a scenario with three children characters: John, James and Harry, to explain its functionality. Suppose James and Harry were playing a game of hide-and-seek. John was watching them play for some time. Since his need for inclusion is low, he does not want to play with them. But later on, he get interested in the game and does want to play with them. Thus the need for affiliation would become high which in turn raises the need for inclusion that would force him to go and ask for their permission to play with them. If the existing group members grant him the permission then his need would be satisfied thus resulting in him-included-in-the-group.

Once the need for inclusion is satisfied and the agent is involved in group interactions then the need for control arises in order to maintain discipline and to avoid conflicts in the group and help them to focus on their purpose. Depending upon the time they spend with each other, and how much they enjoy each other's company, emotions would be generated. If they enjoy each other's company, positive emotions are generated, otherwise negative emotions. This will lead to affection or negative affection respectively. For affection, the relationship might develop and they might become good friends. For negative affection, they may go their separate ways until another opportunity arises for their interaction that provides them with another chance to develop affection.

4   Summary

In this paper, we have briefly introduce theoretical background to model group behaviour in FAtiMA-PSI agents, which results in increasing their interaction capability and thus helps them to attain social believability. It would further helps in improving the authoring mechanisms in FAtiMA-PSI model to perform tasks at group level.

References

1. Hussaini, N., Aylett, R.: An Idea for Modelling Group Dynamics in Autonomous Synthetic Characters. In: AISB (2013)
2. Lim, M.Y., Aylett, R., Dias, J., Paiva, A.: Creating Adaptive Affective Autonomous NPCs 24(2), 287–311 (2012)
3. Schutz, W.: The Interpersonal Underworld, Science & Behavior Books, 577 College Avenue, Palo Alto, California (1966)
4. Bates, J.: The role of emotion in believable agents. Communications of the ACM 37(7), 122–125 (1994)
5. Aylett, R., Paiva, A.: Computational Modelling of Culture and Affect. Emotion Review (2011)
6. Dörner, D.: The mathematics of emotions. In: Frank Detje, D.D., Schaub, H. (eds.) Proceedings of the Fifth International Conference on Cognitive Modeling, Bamberg, Germany, pp. 75–79 (2003)

Dynamical Systems to Account for Turn-Taking in Spoken Interactions

Mathieu Jégou[1,2], Pierre Chevaillier[1], and Pierre De Loor[1]

[1] ENIB–UEB; Lab-STICC; F29200 Brest, France
{pierre.chevaillier,pierre.deloor}@enib.fr
[2] Technologic Research Institute b<>com; F29200 Brest, France
mathieu.jegou@b-com.com

1   Introduction

Turn management is considered as essential for an Embodied Conversational Agent (ECA) to increase user's engagement with it [2]. This article presents a dynamical model for turn management in dyadic interactions. The model is a system of differential equations that mixes two models from the cognitive sciences, the Drift Diffusion Model, and the Behavioral Dynamics. Decision-making and the control of actions are two coupled processes that modulate continuously the behavior of the interacting agent. This conceptual model accounts for the emergence of smooth transitions without using neither prediction nor planning of the agent's behavior. The objective was not to obtain a fully realistic behavior, but to show how the model could account for the main qualitative properties of turn management, such as interrupting the current speaker, signaling its willingness to go on speaking, or yielding the turn to the next speaker.

2   Conceptual Model for Turn Management

2.1   Turn-Taking without Prediction

In their seminal work, Sacks et al. made a fundamental observation: participants exchange turns in a smooth way, most of the time without overlaps nor too long pauses [4]. To explain that, they proposed that listeners predict the end of a turn constructional unit to identify Transition Relevant Places (TRP). They do it by integrating a set of non verbal and verbal cues to identify when a TRP will occur [1]. Nevertheless the active role that listeners play in the emergence of turn transition [6] and the importance of signal variations for a transition to take place [1], make us claim that the occurrence of transitions is a self-organized, co-creative process, emerging from the interaction between participants. Based on some authors' works (see [1] for a review), we hypothesized that a conversational agent can rely mainly on non verbal signals to manage smooth turns.

T. Bickmore et al. (Eds.): IVA 2014, LNAI 8637, pp. 218–221, 2014.

2.2   Behavioral Architecture

Fig. 1 summarizes the principles of our behavioral architecture. First, the agent has an intrinsic motivation to be the speaker or the listener, depending on the conversational context. This communicative intention is under the control of the dialogue manager that generates some communicative intentions, captured here by the variable I (not controlled by our model). This intention depends on the conversational context (what the agent has to say), its personality or its mental state. Moreover, the agent will act to become the next speaker (or the next listener), or to keep its current role, depending on the non verbal cues it can get from the other participant's behavior. Acting means here producing verbal and non verbal signals. The loose coupling between the production of signals, the agent's own intention, and its perception of the other's behavior creates a complex relationship between the tendency to act on its own, and to be influenced by the other participant's behavior. As a result, turn management is emergent: no particular agent controls the occurrence of turn transitions, nor the duration of the transitions.

In our model, the agents continuously produce signals, following the principles of the behavioral dynamics elaborated by Warren [5]. In his view, behavior is self-organized, emerging from the interaction between the agent and its environment. The agent does not control entirely its behavior, but explores the global dynamics of the interaction, and adjusts its action to reach its goal. Besides, agents may have to make a decision (eg. to yield the turn or not) based on uncertain, if not contradicting, information about the intention of the opposite agent. The process of integrating evidence about the other agent's intention is controlled by the Drift Diffusion Model (DDM) [3]. The variable γ is the resulting confidence the agent holds about the intention of the other agent.

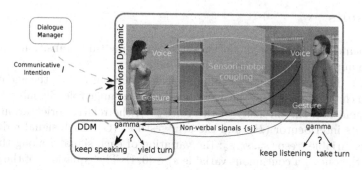

Fig. 1. Illustration of the role of the DDM and of the behavioral dynamic

Decision-Making. The DDM accounts for human decision-making when an agent has to choose between two alternatives [3]. It assumes that agents continuously integrate over time the difference in the noisy information favoring each alternative they get and choose the most favorable alternative when this accumulated value reaches a given threshold. We implemented the DDM as follows:

$$d\gamma = \alpha dt + \sigma d\epsilon \quad ; \quad \alpha(t) = \sum_{j=1}^{n_s} \alpha_j \Big(s_j(t), \dot{s}_j(t) \Big) \tag{1}$$

The model computes γ by integrating a set of signals $\{s_j\}$ produced by the other agent. It defines two thresholds $t_\gamma^+ = 1$, and $t_\gamma^- = -1$. When γ raises up t_γ^+, the agent considers that the other is willing to change its role, when γ falls down below t_γ^-, the agent considers that the other is not willing to change role. When γ is between the two thresholds, the agent is more or less confident about one or the other alternative. The drift coefficient α sums the accumulation of evidence corresponding to each signal j.

Sensory-motor coupling. For each non verbal signal s_j, the agent varies its production according to Warren's general equation:

$$\ddot{s}_j = -b\dot{s}_j - f_{\dot{s}_j}(s_j, \gamma, I) \tag{2}$$

The specific shapes of non verbal actions are defined by Eq. 3:

$$f_{\dot{s}_j}(s_j, \gamma, I) = \underbrace{t_\gamma^+ k_1(s_j - c_1)}_{a1} + \underbrace{t_\gamma^- k_2(s_j - c_2)}_{a2} + \underbrace{(1 - t_\gamma^+)(1 - t_\gamma^-)f'_{\dot{s}_j}(s_j, \gamma, I)}_{a3} \tag{3}$$

where: $t_\gamma^+ = 1$, if $\gamma \geq t_\gamma^+$ (0 otherwise) and $t_\gamma^- = 1$ if $\gamma \leq t_\gamma^-$ (0 otherwise).

Depending on the result of the accumulation process, one particular action, i.e. one of the terms a1, a2 or a3 is executed. a1 is executed when the agent has accumulated enough evidence about option 1 ($\gamma = 1$), and a2 is executed when evidence are against this option ($\gamma = -1$). a3 is applied when $\gamma \in [t_\gamma^-, t_\gamma^+]$.

3   Results

The implementation of the model produced emerging turn transitions that satisfied the qualitative properties of human behavior.

$I \in [0, 1]$ denotes the agent's communicative intention: $I < .5$, the agent is not willing to change role, $I > .5$ the agent is willing to change role. Signals produced by the agent are: the intensity of the voice (V), the relative orientation of the agent to its interlocutor (B), and the arm gestures (G). Each signal reduces to one state variable, resp. s_v, s_b, s_g: the variation of each signal j along the time matches the one of a continuous variable $s_j \in [0, 1]$. The equations of the signals were devised to account for the following behaviors. V_S: the speaker lowers its voice to yield the turn, and speaks louder when it does not want to yield the floor whilst the other wants to take it. V_L: The agent starts speaking when it is confident about the willingness of the current speaker to yield the turn, G: the listener makes gestures to indicate it wants to take the turn, B: the higher the agent's intention to change role, the faster it faces its interlocutor.

Different scenarios, corresponding to different communicative intentions, have been simulated. Fig. 2 shows two examples of agent-agent interactions. It shows

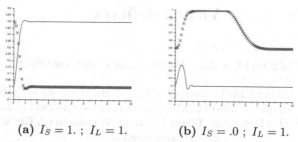

(a) $I_S = 1.$; $I_L = 1.$ (b) $I_S = .0$; $I_L = 1.$

I_S: speaker's intention to give the turn; I_L: listener's intention to take it.

Fig. 2. Time series of the voice intensity of the Speaker V_S (crosses) and the Listener V_L (plain) in two scenarios.

that the model reproduces different patterns depending on the scenario: Fig. 2a, shows two agents that are strongly willing to change turns and Fig 2b, a speaker that strongly wants to keep the floor and a listener that strongly wants to take the turn. In the first case, the turn actually occurs, not in the second one.

4   Conclusion

Simulations of agent-agent interactions show that our model reproduces the richness of turn management behavior. This is the first step towards a realistic agent. Our next goal is now to define the equations that could produce realistic behaviors, and to evaluate the realism of our agent by confronting it to users.

Acknowledgments. This work was supported in part by a grant from the ANR (Corvette project ANR-10-CORD-012).

References

1. Gravano, A., Hirschberg, J.: Turn-taking cues in task-oriented dialogue. Computer Speech & Language 25(3), 601–634 (2011)
2. ter Maat, M.: Response selection and turn-taking for a sensitive artificial listening agent. Ph.D. thesis, University of Twente [Host], Enschede (2011)
3. Ratcliff, R.: A note on modeling accumulation of information when the rate of accumulation change over time. J. of Mathematical Psychology 21, 178–184 (1980)
4. Sacks, H., Schegloff, E.A., Jefferson, G.A.: A simplest systematics for the organisation of turn-taking in conversation. Language 50, 696–735 (1974)
5. Warren, W.H.: The dynamics of perception and action. Psychological Review 113(2), 358–389 (2006)
6. Wilson, M., Wilson, T.P.: An oscillator model of the timing of turn-taking. Psychonomic Bulletin & Review 12(6), 957–968 (2005)

Virtual Reflexes

Catholijn M. Jonker[1], Joost Broekens[1], and Aske Plaat[2]

[1] Interactive Intelligence, Delft University of Technology, Mekelweg 4, The Netherlands
c.m.jonker@tudelft.nl, joost.broekens@gmail.com
[2] Tilburg School of Humanities, Tilburg University, Warandelaan 2, The Netherlands
aske.plaat@gmail.com

Abstract. Virtual Reality is used successfully to treat people for regular phobias. A new challenge is to develop Virtual Reality Exposure Training for social skills. Virtual actors in such systems have to show appropriate social behavior including emotions, gaze, and keeping distance. The behavior must be realistic and real-time. Current approaches are usually based on heavy information processing in terms of behavior planning, scripting of behavior and use of predefined animations. We believe this limits the directness of human bodily reflexes and causes unrealistic responses and delay. We propose to investigate *virtual reflexes* as concurrent sensory-motor processes to control individual parts of the virtual actor's skeleton with a body integrity model that keeps the effects coherent. We explain how emotion and cognitive modulation could be embedded, and give an example description of the interplay between emotion and a reflex.

1 Introduction

The idea of using virtual reality to treat regular phobia—such as fear of heights, or flying—relies on the success with which we can immerse the patient in a virtual situation. Patients should have an experience corresponding to a real life situation. For training *social* skills, the VR setting has to be such that the emotions and intentions that trainees would attribute to a real person are now attributed to a Virtual Character (VC).

To produce appropriate social virtual character behavior, typically heavy processing is involved in deciding based on sensory input generated by the trainee what responses need to be generated at the skeleton level of the VC. In particular, pattern recognition, reasoning and behavior planning, and virtual character animations need to be addressed. In contrast to this processing intensive approach, in this paper we propose a low-level approach based on the idea of virtual reflexes, in which observations directly cause VC muscle actuations *with limited intermediate processing*. Based on various primitive inputs, the muscle actuations are immediate and create bodily reactions. This generates fluent and fast responses in the VC. Perceived emotions emerge out of the interaction between sensory and motor information. Although no cognitive intermediate processing takes place, cognition and affect do modulate the sensory motor loops. As happens in the human body, various virtual reflexes can occur simultaneously and operate as concurrent subsystems.

T. Bickmore et al. (Eds.): IVA 2014, LNAI 8637, pp. 222–231, 2014.

The idea that social signals emerge from virtual reflexes is motivated intuitively, practically and theoretically. First, when engaging in day-to-day activities, people do whatever it is they are doing, in unthinking response to the "moment-to-moment local forces acting upon them" [41, p. 263]. This is closer to a reflex-based approach than to a reasoning-based one. Second, virtual reflexes provide the speed necessary for realistic social interaction [26]. Third, reflex-based control corresponds to theories on embodied cognition and affect [42, 43]. The contributions of this paper are as follows:

- We introduce an architecture for virtual reflexes.
- We link the architecture to neuropsychological theories on emotion & cognition.
- We formalize part of the reflexes in a virtual aggression training case study.

2   Related Work

Virtual reality techniques have been shown to have significant therapeutic value, and in particular, VR stress inoculation training works well in various settings [36]. Virtual reality exposure therapy [11, 23, 33] has been shown to be as effective as in vivo (real-world) exposure therapy [33]. Popovic et al [32] present a Stress Inoculation system using an interactive VR system. Virtual reality systems have yielded positive training results [7, 16, 30, 38, 3, 22], and can also be used for personality assessment [39].

The real-time aspect of emotion modeling has been addressed in, e.g., the work on autonomous real-time sensitive artificial listeners [10, 35, 40], the work on backchannel communication [5, 17, 37], to create "rapport" between virtual agents and humans [15, 18, 13], and in computational models of coping [27] and synthetic emotion generation for games [31]. The challenge of generating real-time behavior has motivated [4] to develop the subsumption architecture. Our architecture is inspired by Brooks' work in the sense that it consists of multiple subsystems running concurrently. Key novelty in our approach compared to other Virtual Character control architectures is that particular sensory inputs have immediate influences on particular parts of the VC skeleton. The overall research question is thus to what extend it is possible to generate plausible social behaviors without explicit coordination of sensory – motor loops, except coordination enforced by the VC's body integrity.

3   Virtual Reflex Architecture

The basis of our architecture is the uncoupling of various sensor-actuator channels. Behavior is generated by reflex nodes that dynamically couple sensory input and motor output. To cope with high-level influences on behavior, such as training scenarios, activity of these nodes is modulated by cognitive and emotional factors (see figure 1). Each reflex node can be seen as a small control node that influences body parts. Its output is based on whether its sensory input deviates from a preset baseline, much like drives would need to be met in a homeostatic approach [6]. Upon deviation, three things happen concurrently. First, the deviation triggers activation of the body parts coupled to the reflex node. Second, the deviation has an effect on the emotional state. We envision a Pleasure–Arousal–Dominance (PAD) representation [28] of the emotional state (Emotion, in figure 1). Third, the deviation is available for cognition to reason upon. The emotional state is simply a correlate of the aggregated deviations from the drives, and as such "setting" the emotional state will also bias the drives towards a different baseline. This provides a natural and behaviorally grounded mechanism to model the influence of emotion on behavior, and also the emergence of emotion out of behavior and reflexes [6]. The cognitive model operates on sensory-motor primitives, as the information it gets is not the raw sensory information but the deviation and drive-based control effect following from the sensory information. In our architecture, cognition is grounded in sensory-motor representations, which is in line with embodied cognition approaches [42]. Cognition influences behavior by modulating the virtual reflex decision node activities and parameters, just like emotion does. Emotion and cognition thus follow from and operate on reflexes in similar ways. In our approach the emotional state is simply a different representation of the emergent pattern of reflex activities, while cognition can hold any processing mechanism, as long as it takes as input reflex-node activity and it outputs reflex-node biases. The link from the body of the virtual character to the proprioceptive part of the perception system is in line with the body loop of Damasio [8]. It allows the virtual character to perceive, and respond to, its own actions.

The virtual character's immediate responses are controlled by the virtual reflex-loop, while the agent's high-level decisions are modeled as cognitive biases to the virtual reflex decision nodes. In this way the architecture also allows emotional coping [14] by means of influencing the reflexive behaviors, which, in turn, influence the

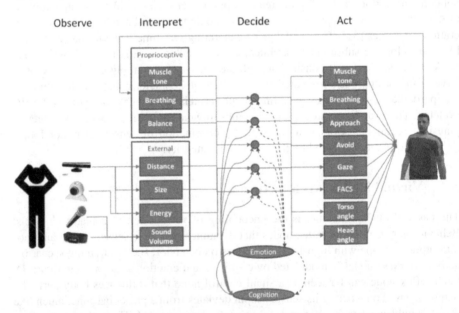

Fig. 1. Virtual Reflex architecture showing examples of reflex nodes for different sensor-subsystem. Nodes process the signals and yield appropriate responses in parallel. Note that Virtual Reflexes are modulated by cognition and emotion.

emotional state. This is a natural way of modeling coping, as this grounds the coping process in the actual "physiology" of the virtual character instead of simply influencing the representation of the emotional state.

We assume that the VC has a body integrity model allowing it to, e.g., propagate a head nod to the torso. Candidate solutions are physics based models [12] and inverse kinematics modeling how effects of body parts propagate through the complete body.

4   Neuropsychological Basis

In our approach behavior generation is the cognitive (and affective) modulation of automatic reflex processes [2]. Our approach is compatible with embodied cognition theory [42, 43], where the basic premise is that thought is tightly coupled to behavior and the representations used for behavior.

Note that the idea of multiple levels of increasingly complex processing involved in affective responses is not new. For example, LeDoux [24, 25] describes a high and a low route to emotion processing. The low route is "quick and dirty" and evaluates stimuli in a fast but inaccurate way, while the high route is cortical and evaluates stimuli in a slow but detailed way. Scherer [34] also considers appraisal as a process of multi-level sequential checking with lower levels triggering activity at higher levels. Each level typically involves more complex information processing, and is only activated to the full extent when that is needed based on simpler appraisals. For example, appraising stimulus relevance is done first based on suddenness, a simple stimulus-based appraisal, and when relevance is high this triggers implication-related appraisals such as goal-conduciveness, a more cognitive-based appraisal. This model of appraisal can be computationally integrated with other models that assume appraisal is layered from simple to complex processing [3].

The ideas of thinking fast and slow [19] contain the same basic idea, i.e., that there are multiple concurrent processes for different aspects of behavior and reasoning. The fastest behaviors we have are reflex behaviors, developed early in our evolution, and essential for survival. Body language is an important part of social interaction [1, 21], and is recognized as expressions of emotions. Mimicry is an essential part of the human social repertoire that is inexorably bound up to basic social processes of empathy, bonding, and in-group formation [20]. In contrast, higher order cognitive appraisal processes take more time, e.g., [29], and explain how we appraise our progress with respect to our social and personal goals.

Our approach is also inspired by Damasio's somatic marker hypothesis [8]. Somatic markers are the affective counterparts of situational representations in terms of sensory-motor activity. Such markers get triggered by activities and thoughts, and can bias behavior and thought at the same time (for example, during decision making). Our emotional state emerges from the activity of the reflex nodes; it is grounded in sensory-motor activity. The state itself influences these nodes, as the relation between emotion and reflex is bidirectional. If the agent is in a high arousal state, this biases the reflexes towards high energy. This, in turn, biases cognition to trigger those associations that are related to high energetic reflex behavior, closing the loop from emotion to cognition through sensory-motor representations. In our approach, "feelings are mental experiences of body states" [9].

5   Case: Aggression De-escalation

As an example case we explain how the Virtual Reflex architecture can form the basis for a Virtual Reality training system for coping with verbal aggressive situations. The system confronts a trainee in virtual reality with a verbal aggressor. During the training a virtual character confronts the human trainee with verbal aggressive behavior and subsequently reacts in real-time to the actions and behaviors of the human trainee. In this paper we focus on the VC behavior generation component by means of a virtual reflex architecture, not on the scenario or verbal behavior.

5.1   Behavior Generation and Virtual Reflex-Loops Example

We now explain how the architecture presented in Section 2 is used for behavior generation in virtual aggression training. The complete system will contain parallel channels for bodily reflexes including nodes that control torso-, and head-posture, muscle tone, blush, breathing, gaze, and eyes openness. These nodes react to sensors focused on the trainee, but also on virtual sensors of the VC such as muscle tone, breathing in balance. The virtual balance sensor will impact the architecture when the VC is getting out of balance, in which case the appropriate nodes and then actuators are triggered to restore balance (e.g, by taking a step). In the case study, we focus on torso-movement only and assume postures are described using pitch, roll and yaw. We focus on the decision node for torso-pitch. Torso-pitch is influenced by the bodily movements of the trainee, but also by the VC's emotion. Furthermore, we show that in an indirect way, the Virtual Reflex-loops influence emotion. One of the modeling concept for torso-pitch is social distance as modulated by emotion (feeling of Dominance of the VC, to be precise). In this example we describe how the torso-pitch changes throughout a scenario. We propose the following rough formalization of the dynamics of torso-pitch (tp) behavior as follows:

$$tp_{t+1} = C_{sd}*(tpp_t - tpp_{t-1}) + \beta * tp_t$$
$$m_t = C_{sd}*(sd_{target} - d_t)$$
$$sd_{target} = (1-D)*sd_{default} + CD$$
$$C_{sd} = (A+1)/2$$

Here, $C_{sd} \in [0,1]$ is the social distance inertia factor, tpp_t is the torso-pitch of the player at time t, d_t is the physical distance at time t. The factor $\beta \in [0,1]$ ensures that over time, if the player does not change his torso pitch, the torso pitch of the VC will return to normal (0). The intended move at time t is denoted by m_t. Note that physics (such as the counter in the case study) might (partially) prohibit the execution of m. D is Dominance [-1,1] and relates to social stance, perceived control, and self-efficacy. Dominance moderates the default target distance. High dominant Virtual Characters will have a closer preferred social distance, and vice versa. A is Arousal [-1,1] and relates to energy. Energy thus defines the speed with which the torso angle changes. CD is defined as cultural distance. The closer two individuals are with respect to their cultural background, the smaller CD is. CD should be calibrated based on existing social science findings. $Sd_{default}$ is defined as the Virtual Character's personal preferred social distance. This factor is needed to model individual differences in preferred social distance as this varies from person to person. The parameter is set in the cognition model. Similarly, the PAD emotion values are set by the emotion model, thus modeling the effect of emotion on the Virtual Reflex-loop.

Conversely, each of the Virtual Reflex-loops potentially influences emotion and cognition (dotted lines from decision nodes to the emotion component, figure 1). In the case study, the values computed in the torso-pitch decision node are passed to the emotion component. For example, forward torso pitch can induce anxiety or aggression (depending on the VC's personality and the current affective state). Similarly, the cognitive component receives input from the sensors, the decision nodes and the emotion component. For now we focus on the input from the decision nodes that send information on the body state of the VC. The VC's cognition component plans on overall and longer term changes in behavior, e.g., changes in posture, dialogue, etc. We assume (and this is part of the open questions) that the VC's body integrity model ensures that movements caused by different Virtual Reflex-loops result in physically coherent behavior.

5.2   Virtual Reflex-Based Scenario Formalization

In this section we describe how torso pitch changes throughout an example scenario in a social welfare office (see picture below). The scenario time labels refers to moments of change. In this way every reaction triggers a new number.

Event	Informal description	Formalisation
0	Behind the social welfare office counter is Barney (not depicted). Barney is new in his job and feels uncertain. The man in the T-shirt (the VC) is frustrated and angry as his allowance has been canceled. He came to demand his money.	tp_0: 0 /* torso-pitch of VC neutral */ tpp_0: 0 /* torso-pitch Barney neutral */ $PAD_{default}$=(0, 0, -0.5) /* VC's personality */ PAD = (-1, 1, 1), β = 0.95 /* not changed during the scenario */
1	VC is at the counter and scowls.	tp_1: 0 /* torso-pitch of VC neutral */ tpp_1: 0 /* torso-pitch Barney neutral */ $face_1$: scowl
2	Barney stretches his arms against the counter, thus pushing his torso backward.	tp_2: 0 /* torso-pitch of VC neutral */ tpp_2: -0.1 /* torso-pitch Barney backwards */
3	The torso pitch of the VC reflexively comes forward in response to Barney's movement.	C_{sd}=(A+1)/2=1 tp_3 =C_{sd}*(tpp_1-tpp_2) + β*tp_2 = 1*(0 - -0.1)+0=0.1 tpp_3 = -0.1

4	VC slams his hand on the counter and shouts "I demand my money!".	tp_4: $C_{sd}*(tpp_2-tpp_3) + \beta*tp_3 = 1*0+0.95*0.1 = 0.095$ tpp_4: -0.1
5	Barney, jerks back for a moment.	tp_5: $C_{sd}*(tpp_3-tpp_4) + \beta*tp_4 = 1*0+0.95*0.095 = 0.09$ tpp_5: -0.2
6	VC leans in.	tp_6: $C_{sd}*(tpp_4-tpp_5) + \beta*tp_5 = 1*(-0.1- -0.2)+0.95*0.09 = 0.185$ 0.09 tpp_6: -0.2
7	However, Barney relaxes his muscles, thus neutralizes his torso-pitch, and stays polite.	tp_7: $C_{sd}*(tpp_5-tpp_6) + \beta*tp_6 = 1*(-0.2- -0.2)+0.95*0.185 = 0 + 0.176$ tpp_7: 0
8	VC stops leaning on the counter by a backward torso movement.	tp_8: $C_{sd}*(tpp_6-tpp_7) + \beta*tp_7 = 1*(-0.2- -0)+0.95*0.176 = -0.2 + 0.167$ -0.03 tpp_8: 0

As Barney keeps a neutral torso-pitch, after a while, also the torso-pitch of VC returns to neutral.

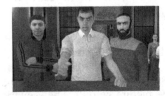

Fig. 2. Case study: VC demands his money from a social welfare officer. The trainee (officer) is not in the picture. The VC described in the example wears the T-shirt.

This short example shows how behavior can be generated by reflex nodes, and how this behavior can be modulated with emotion. It does not show how emotion emerges from the reflex nodes. However, the system of equations should be interpreted as a dynamic system. The VC's Dominance results from interaction with the virtual character as well, simply by the fact that the system settles only at a particular close social distance if dominance is high. (Note the bidirectional nature of the reflex nodes and the emotional state.). So, if the trainee (Barney) is able to calm down the VC (e.g., by keeping distance and staying calm so that the PAD state will decay to $PAD_{default}$, i.e., the personality of the VC), dominance and arousal drop due to calm sensory input that modulates C_{sd} and increases sd_{target} (not taken into account in the example). Both changes would further stabilize the situation.

9	VC's arousal drops due to calm sensory input	$PAD_9 = PAD_{default} = (0, 0, -0.5)$ $C_{sd}=(A+1)/2=0.5$ tp_9: $C_{sd}*(tpp_6-tpp_7) + \beta*tp_7 = 0.5*(0 - 0)+0.95*-0.03 = -0.028$ tpp_9: 0

6   Conclusions

The purpose of our work is to achieve immersive and realistic virtual environments for social skill training. To realize this, we propose a computational model for virtual character behavior based on parallel virtual reflexes that involve limited processing and operate directly on parts of the VC skeleton based on sensory input. Emotions emerge out of this interaction between sensory and motor information. Cognition is envisioned to modulate the sensory-motor loop. Virtual reflexes can occur simultaneously. Current limitations (we consider to be open questions) to our approach are (a) the ability of the body integrity model to enforce coherence, (b) the ability to generate scenario-relevant modulations of behavior solely based on cognitive modulation of parallel sensory motor loops, and (c) uncertainty about the emotion dynamics induced by a bidirectional relation between emotion and sensory-motor activation.

Acknowledgements. We gratefully acknowledge the support of Guntur Sandino, Arnaud Wirschell, Fred Schrijber, Ron Knaap, Otto Adang, Ron Boelsma, Willem-Paul Brinkman, Koen Hindriks, and Birna van Riemsdijk, and Jaap van den Herik.

References

1. Argyle, M.: Social Interaction. Transaction Publishers Rutgers, New Jersey (2009)
2. Berthoz, A.: The brains sense of movement. Harvard Univ. Press (2002)
3. Broekens, J., Harbers, M., Brinkman, W.-P., Jonker, C.M., Van den Bosch, K., Meyer, J.-J.: Virtual Reality Negotiation Training Increases Negotiation Knowledge and Skill. In: Nakano, Y., Neff, M., Paiva, A., Walker, M. (eds.) IVA 2012. LNCS, vol. 7502, pp. 218–230. Springer, Heidelberg (2012)
4. Brooks, R.A.: Cambrian intelligence: the early history of the new AI. MIT Press (1999)
5. Cafaro, A., Vilhjálmsson, H.H., Bickmore, T., Heylen, D., Jóhannsdóttir, K.R., Valgarðsson, G.S.: First Impressions: Users' Judgments of Virtual Agents' Personality and Interpersonal Attitude in First Encounters. In: Nakano, Y., Neff, M., Paiva, A., Walker, M. (eds.) IVA 2012. LNCS, vol. 7502, pp. 67–80. Springer, Heidelberg (2012)
6. Cañamero, L.: Designing Emotional Artifacts for Social Interaction: Challenges and Perspectives. In: Cañamero, L., Aylett, R. (eds.) Animating Expressive Characters for Social Interaction. Adv. in Consciousness Research (2005)
7. Core, M., Traum, D., Lane, H.C., Swartout, W., Gratch, J., van Lent, M.: Teaching Negotiation Skills through Practice and Reflection with Virtual Humans. Simulation 82(11), 685–701 (2006)
8. Damasio, A.: The Feeling of What Happens: Body and Emotion in the Making of Consciousness, Harcourt (1999)
9. Damasio, A., Carvalho, G.B.: The nature of feelings: evolutionary and neurobiological origins. Nature Reviews Neuroscience 14, 143–152 (2013); PubMed
10. D'Mello, S., Picard, R.W., Graesser, A.: Toward an Affect-Sensitive AutoTutor. 22, 53–61 (2007)
11. Emmelkamp, P.M.G., Bruynzeel, M., Drost, L., van der Mast, C.A.P.G.: Virtual reality treatment in acrophobia: a comparison with exposure in vivo. Cyber Psychology & Behavior 4(3), 335–339 (2001)

12. Faloutsos, P., van de Panne, M., Terzopoulos, D.: Composable controllers for physics-based character animation. Paper Presented at the Proceedings of the 28th Annual Conference on Computer Graphics and Interactive Techniques (2001)
13. Ogan, A., Finkelstein, S., Walker, E., Carlson, R., Cassell, J.: Rudeness and rapport: Insults and learning gains in peer tutoring. In: Cerri, S.A., Clancey, W.J., Papadourakis, G., Panourgia, K. (eds.) ITS 2012. LNCS, vol. 7315, pp. 11–21. Springer, Heidelberg (2012)
14. Folkman, S., Lazarus, R.S.: Coping and emotion. In: Stein, N.L., Leventhal, B., Trabasso, T. (eds.) Psych. and Bio Appr. Emo., pp. 313–332. Erlbaum, Hillsdale (1990)
15. Gratch, J., Wang, N., Gerten, J., Fast, E., Duffy, R.: Creating Rapport with Virtual Agents. In: Pelachaud, C., Martin, J.-C., André, E., Chollet, G., Karpouzis, K., Pelé, D. (eds.) IVA 2007. LNCS (LNAI), vol. 4722, pp. 125–138. Springer, Heidelberg (2007)
16. Hays, M.J., Ogan, A., Lane, H.C.: The Evolution of Assessment: Learning about Culture from a Serious Game. In: Lynch, C., Ashley, K.D., Mitrovic, T., Dimitrova, V., Pinkwart, N., Aleven, V. (eds.) IllDef 2010, pp. 37–44 (2010)
17. Heylen, D., Nijholt, A., op den Akker, R.: Affect in tutoring dialogues. Applied Artificial Intelligence: An International Journal 19(3), 287–311 (2005)
18. Huang, L., Morency, L.-P., Gratch, J.: Virtual Rapport 2.0. In: Vilhjálmsson, H.H., Kopp, S., Marsella, S., Thórisson, K.R. (eds.) IVA 2011. LNCS, vol. 6895, pp. 68–79. Springer, Heidelberg (2011)
19. Kahnemann, D.: Thinking, fast and slow. Penguin Books (2011)
20. Kavanagh, L., Bakhtiari, G., Suhler, C., Churchland, P.S., Holland, R.W., Winkielman, P.: Nuanced Social Inferences about Trustworthiness from Observation of Mimicry. In: Knauff, M., Pauen, M., Sebanz, N., Wachsmuth, I. (eds.) Proceedings of the 35th Annual Conference of the Cognitive Science Society, pp. 734–739. Cognitive Science Society, Berlin (2013)
21. Kendon, A.: Conducting interaction. Studies in Interactional Sociolinguistics, vol. 7. Cambridge University Press (1990)
22. Kim, J.M., Hill, J.R.W., Durlach, P.J., Lane, H.C., Forbell, E., Core, M., et al.: BiLAT: A Game-Based Environment for Practicing Negotiation in a Cultural Context. International Journal of Artificial Intelligence in Education 19(3), 289–308 (2009)
23. Krijn, M., Emmelkamp, P.M.G., Olafsson, R.P., Biemond, R.: Virtual reality exposure therapy of anxiety disorders: A review. Clinical Psych Review 24(3), 259–281 (2004)
24. LeDoux, J.: The Emotional Brain. Simon and Shuster, New York (1996)
25. LeDoux, J.E.: Emotion: Clues from the brain. Ann. Rev. Psy. 46(1), 209–235 (1995)
26. Magnenat-Thalmann, N., Thalmann, D.: Virtual humans: thirty years of research, what next? The Visual Computer 21, 997–1015 (2005)
27. Marsella, S., Gratch, J., Ning, W., Stankovic, B.: Assessing the validity of a computational model of emotional coping. In: Affective Computing and Intelligent Interaction and Workshops, ACII 2009 (2009)
28. Mehrabian, A.: Basic Dimensions for a General Psychological Theory. OG&H (1980)
29. Ortony, A., Clore, G.L., Collins, A.: The Cognitive Structure of Emotions. Cambridge University Press (1988)
30. Parsons, S., Mitchell, P.: The potential of virtual reality in social skills training for people with autistic spectrum disorders. J. Intell. Disability Research 46(5), 430–443 (2002)
31. Popescu, A., Broekens, J., van Someren, M.: GAMYGDALA: An Emotion Engine for Games. IEEE Transactions on Affective Computing 5(1), 32–44 (2014)
32. Popović, S., Horvat, M., Kukolja, D., Dropuljić, B., Cosić, K.: Stress inoculation training supported by physiology-driven adaptive virtual reality stimulation. Stud. Health Technol. Inform. 144, 50–54 (2009)

33. Powers, M.B., Emmelkamp, P.M.G.: Virtual reality exposure therapy for anxiety disorders: A meta-analysis. Journal of Anxiety Disorders 22(3), 561–569 (2008)
34. Scherer, K.R.: Appraisal considered as a process of multilevel sequential checking. In: Scherer, K.R., Schorr, A., Johnstone, T. (eds.) Appraisal Processes in Emotion: Theory, Methods, Research, pp. 92–120 (2001)
35. Schroder, M., Bevacqua, E., Cowie, R., Eyben, F., Gunes, H., Heylen, D., et al.: Building Autonomous Sensitive Artificial Listeners. IEEE Aff. Computing 3(2), 165–183 (2012)
36. Serino, S., Triberti, S., Villani, D., Cipresso, P., Gaggioli, A., Riva, G.: Toward a validation of cyber-interventions for stress disorders based on stress inoculation training: a systematic review. Virtual Reality, 1–15 (2013)
37. de Sevin, E., Hyniewska, S.J., Pelachaud, C.: Influence of Personality Traits on Backchannel Selection. In: Allbeck, J., Badler, N., Bickmore, T., Pelachaud, C., Safonova, A. (eds.) IVA 2010. LNCS, vol. 6356, pp. 187–193. Springer, Heidelberg (2010)
38. Van der Spek, E.: Experiments in Serious Game Design. University of Utrecht (2011)
39. Tekofsky, S., Spronck, P., Plaat, A., Van den Herik, J., Broersen, J.: Psyops: Personality assessment through gaming behavior. Paper Presented at the Proceedings of the International Conference on the Foundations of Digital Games (2013)
40. Thiebaux, M., Marsella, S., Marshall, A.N., Kallmann, M.: Smartbody: Behavior realization for embodied conversational agents. In: Proceedings of the 7th Conf. Autonomous Agents and Multiagent Systems, vol. 1, pp. 151–158. IFAAMS (2008)
41. Wakefield, J.C., Dreyfus, H.L.: Intentionality and the phenomenology of action. In: Lepore, Gulick (eds.) John Searle and His Critics. Blackwell, Cambridge (1991)
42. Wilson, M.: Six views of embodied cognition. Psych. Bull. & Rev. 9(4), 625–636 (2002)
43. Ziemke, T.: What's that thing called embodiment. In: Proceedings of the 25th Annual Conference of the Cognitive Science Society. Erlbaum, Mahwah (2003)

Ascribed Gender and Characteristics of a Visually Androgynous Teachable Agent

Camilla Kirkegaard[1], Betty Tärning[2], Magnus Haake[2],
Agneta Gulz[1], and Annika Silvervarg[1]

[1] Dept. of Computer and Information Science, Linköping University, Linköping, Sweden
{camilla.kirkegaard,agneta.gulz,annika.silvervarg}@liu.se
[2] Cognitive Science, Lund University, Kungshuset, Lundagård, Lund, Sweden
{betty.tarning,magnus.haake}@lucs.lu.se

1   Introduction

This paper explores how users ascribe gender to a visually androgynous teachable agent, and if and how the ascribed gender can influence the perceived personality characteristics of the agent. Previous studies have shown positive effects of using agents with more neutral or androgynous appearances, for instance, a more gender neutral agent evoked more positive attitudes on females than did a more stereotypical female agent [1] and androgynous agents were less abused than female agents [2]. Another study showed that even though an agent was visually androgynous, the user typically ascribed a gender to it [3].

We wanted to further explore the use of visually androgynous agents when the user can choose to ascribe them a gender and how the ascribed gender affects how the agents are perceived. A pilot study was conducted in a Swedish primary school with 11-year olds, 21 girls and 16 boys. The agent used in this study was a *teachable agent* (TA), acting as a tutee in an educational software for learning history. The TA, portrayed as a time elf (see Fig 1.), needs help to learn about history in order to succeed as the new "Guardian of Time". The students can teach the TA using different teaching activities as well as asking the TA to take tests in order to receive feedback on how well they have taught their TA.

2   Study

The study consisted of two 30 minutes sessions. During these sessions, the participants were instructed to teach their TA to help it pass some tests in the learning environment. After completing the second session, the students were given a questionnaire regarding their experience with the digital learning environment and how they perceived the time elf (their TA). One questionnaire item addressed the perceived gender of the TA with the following five answer options: *absolutely like a girl, a little like a girl, neither girl nor boy, a little like a boy, absolutely like a boy*. The questionnaire also contained a list of personality related words (adjectives) where the students were asked to mark the words they found applicable to the time elf (TA). The list of words

T. Bickmore et al. (Eds.): IVA 2014, LNAI 8637, pp. 232–235, 2014.

was created by including words from the TIPI test, a 10-item measure of the Big Five (or Five-Factor Model) dimensions [4] together with words related to intelligence, politeness, and naturalness. Half of the adjectives were positive words (friendly, dependable, self-disciplined, curious, caring, funny, sympathetic, warm, self-confident, intelligent, clever, natural); the other half of the adjectives were negative ones (shy, forgetful, disorganized, quarrelsome, critical, timid, stupid, easy-to-fool, mean, unkind, selfish, unnatural).

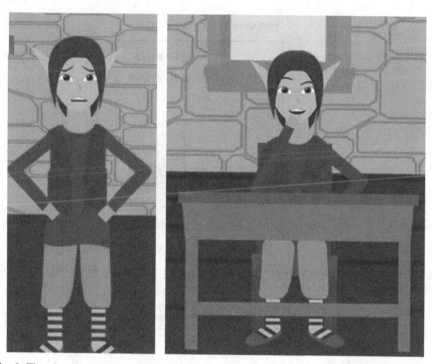

Fig. 1. The visually androgynous teachable agent in two different emotional states, unhappy to the left and eager to learn to the right

Our intention was to explore whether or not we would find a characteristics bias based on the ascribed gender. The previous mentioned study by Gulz and Haake [1] showed, for example, that a female agent typically was described with less positive words than the male version. However, this study used agents with visually stereotypical attributes. Would a visually androgynous agent generate the same response based on the genders ascribed by the students themselves?

The number of participants in this pilot study were quite few and were therefore allocated into two main groups: one group where the TA was perceived as "absolutely like a girl" or "a little like a girl" ($N = 9$) and another group where the TA was perceived as "absolutely like a boy" or "a little like a boy" ($N = 21$).

An overall observation was that in the entire group, 69% (153 out of 220) of the characteristics ascribed to the TA (disregarding ascribed gender) were positive. What is more interesting, however, is that when the TA was perceived as a boy the students seem to describe it with more positive words (with a mean of 5.6 for positive words and a mean of 2.0 for negative words) compared to when it was perceived as a girl (with a mean of 4.0 for positive words and a mean of 2.8 for negative words), see Fig. 2. A Chi-square test on the chosen words indicated a significant difference between the characteristics given to the TA when it was perceived as a boy compared to when it was perceived as a girl ($X^2(1, N = 220) = 4.42, p < .05$).

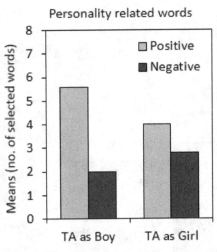

Fig. 2. Agents perceived as male are described with more positive and fewer negative words than agents perceived as female

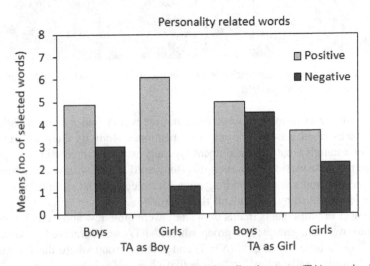

Fig. 3. The difference in personality words used to describe the agent (TA) perceived as male versus female differ for female students compared to male students, especially when the agent was perceived as male

Looking more closely at the differences of the distributions of the personality words, a Chi-square test suggested a significant difference between the distribution of positive and negative words with regard to ascribed gender of the TA in relation to the gender of the students ($X^2(1, N = 220) = 11.4$, $p < .01$). Furthermore, the TA perceived as a boy received a mean of 6.1 for positive words together with a mean of 1.3 for negative words from the girls, while it received a mean of 4.9 for positive words and a mean of 3.0 for negative words from the boys. For the agent perceived as a girl the corresponding numbers were a mean of 3.7 for positive words together with a mean of 2.3 for negative words from the girls and a mean of 5.0 for positive words together with a mean of 4.5 for negative words from the boys, see Fig. 3.

3   Conclusion and Discussion

Previous studies have shown that an agent's appearance can influence how it is perceived and that female agents typically are subjected to more negative descriptions as well as abuse [2, 5]. In this pilot study we found the same pattern, namely that the TA perceived as a girl received fewer positive words and more negative words than the very same TA perceived as a boy. We are aware that the number of students in this study is small and we intend to follow up with a large scale study looking deeper into this question and also relating it to how well the agent actually performs in the learning environment. We will also revise the appearance of the agent to make it more androgynous since there was a tendency to more often ascribe a male gender to the agent.

References

1. Gulz, A., Haake, M.: Challenging Gender Stereotypes Using Virtual Pedagogical Characters. In: Goodman, S., Booth, S., Kirkup, G. (eds.) Gender Issues in Learning and Working with IT: Social Constructs and Cultural Contexts, pp. 113–132. IGI Global, Hershey (2010)
2. Silvervarg, A., Raukola, K., Haake, M., Gulz, A.: The Effect of Visual Gender on Abuse in Conversation with ECAs. In: Nakano, Y., Neff, M., Paiva, A., Walker, M. (eds.) IVA 2012. LNCS, vol. 7502, pp. 153–160. Springer, Heidelberg (2012)
3. Silvervarg, A., Haake, M., Gulz, A.: Educational Potentials in Visually Androgynous Pedagogical Agents. In: Lane, H.C., Yacef, K., Mostow, J., Pavlik, P. (eds.) AIED 2013. LNCS, vol. 7926, pp. 599–602. Springer, Heidelberg (2013)
4. Gosling, S.D., Rentfrow, P.D., Swann Jr., W.B.: A very brief measure of the big five personality domains. Journal of Research in Personality 37, 504–528 (2003)
5. Veletsianos, G., Scharber, C., Doering, A.: When Sex, Drugs, and Violence Enter the Classroom: Conversations Between Adolescent Social Studies Students and a Female Pedagogical Agent. Interact. Compu. 20(3), 292–301 (2008)

Full Body Interaction with Virtual Characters in an Interactive Storytelling Scenario

Felix Kistler, Birgit Endrass, and Elisabeth André

Human Centered Multimedia, Augsburg University,
Universitätsstr. 6a, 86159 Augsburg, Germany
{kistler,endrass,andre}@hcm-lab.de

Abstract. This paper presents a full body interaction approach developed for Traveller, an intercultural training game for young adults based on an interactive storytelling scenario. Traveller involves virtual characters interacting with the users on a large display screen. The users interact with a Kinect, performing full body gestures and controlling a freehand swipe menu to trigger navigation and dialogue actions in the game. A first evaluation proved the recognition capabilities of our system and the comparison with a mouse interface in terms of usability and user experience showed higher positive affect with the Kinect, but a tendency for higher usability and flow with the mouse.

Keywords: full body interaction, intercultural training, freehand, Kinect.

1   Introduction

To support experiential learning in simulation environments, technologies are required that allow for intuitive and natural forms of interaction. Frequently, such simulation environments are inhabited by virtual characters. To provide basic interaction with the characters, users need to be able to move towards the characters (navigation) and communicate with them (dialogue). Traditionally, navigation and dialogue have been controlled with keyboard, mouse or joystick input often accompanied by a graphical interface [9]. However, this does not allow for human-like interaction styles and may affect the user experience. Better options are speech [3,5] or gesture input [6,1] that emulate human-human conversation in a more direct manner. While there is empirical evidence that bodily interaction contributes to a greater sense of presence, some studies also revealed usability issues that negatively affected user experience. For example, Dow and colleagues [3] revealed that interaction in Augmented Reality contributed to an enhanced sense of presence, but the increased immersion also interfered with the players engagement. Aylett and colleagues [1] found that users enjoyed interaction using the dance pad and the WiiMote. However, they also realized that the interaction hampered the users activities and demanded considerable effort and concentration. To provide immersive interaction, we employ full body gestures and a swipe menu in our interactive storytelling scenario. We further apply a user-centerd design process to create an intuitive gesture set. The details of our approach are described in the following section.

T. Bickmore et al. (Eds.): IVA 2014, LNAI 8637, pp. 236–239, 2014.

2   Full Body Interaction in Traveller

Traveller aims to provide intercultural training for 18-25 year olds. The users learn by participating actively in the narrative and interacting with virtual characters simulated by FAtiMA [2] and representing different synthetic cultures defined in Hofstedes dimensions [4]. The users start a journey through three different countries and in each country, they have to interact with locals in so-called critical incidents (CIs) to progress. The appropriate interaction is dependent on the agents synthetic culture.

By default, actions in Traveller are taken by performing a related full body gesture. Figure 1 on the left-hand side depicts a user performing an informal greeting represented by a waving gesture. An iterative user-centred design approach for user-defined gestures was used with Traveller to create intuitive gestures. More details on this can be found in [7]. For integrating the gestures in our application we use the full body interaction framework (FUBI) of which an earlier version was presented in [8]. To assist the users in performing the gestures we label the possible actions and display symbols that visualise how the gestures for these actions should be performed. In Figure 1, two such symbols can be seen in the left-hand image in cyan color.

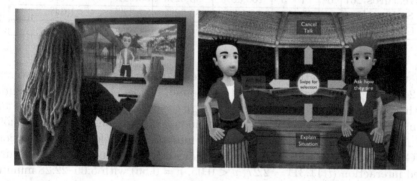

Fig. 1. *Left image:* User performing a greeting gesture. *Right image:* The swipe menu.

At certain points, we further integrate a graphical menu that includes additional dialogue options as shown in Figure 1 on the right-hand side. Within the menu, interaction options are arranged around a middle circle. For selecting an option, users first have to stretch out their hand to the front, wait until the menu gets activated, and then perform a swiping gesture in the direction of the option they would like to select. This enables us to have as many and as complex actions as we want without worrying about how all of them could be represented by unambiguous gestures. However, the two interaction types are similar enough to provide a fluent user experience.

In a single walk through the complete story, an average user selects about 50 different actions (40 by gestures and 10 by swipes) and further has to perform 36 swipes for selecting "continue".

3   Preliminary Evaluation

In a first evaluation study, we had two groups of participants: one interacting with the actual full body interaction interface, and the other one interacting with a traditional mouse interface. In the latter case, participants selected the in-game actions by clicking on them with a mouse, however, we only displayed the action labels, but omitted the gesture symbols.

The full body interaction group consisted of twelve participants (two females, average age 24.3), all with German cultural background and right-handed. Regarding recognition, we counted true positives ($= TP$), false positives ($= FP$), false negatives ($= FN$), and gestures obviously wrongly performed by the participants (user errors $= UE$). We further calculated precision, accuracy, recall and user error-rate. The results are shown in Table 1. A Pearson's chi-square test further indicated significantly less recognition errors ($FP + FN$) for the gestures in comparison to the swipes, $\chi^2(1) = 28.48$, $p < 0.001$.

Table 1. Accuracy measures for the recognition of our full body gestures and swipes

	TP	FP	FN	UE	Precision	Accuracy	Recall	User Error-Rate
Gestures	267	0	14	5	100,00%	95,02%	95,02%	1,75%
Swipes	241	24	35	5	90,94%	80,33%	87,32%	1,64%
Overall	508	24	49	10	95,49%	87,44%	91,20%	1,69%

In the mouse interaction group, we had ten participants (two females, average age 24.6), all with German cultural background, one left-handed. We measured the time it took the participants to go through the evaluated part of the story and the number of actions they selected. With mouse interaction, they needed 5:50–7:42 minutes (AVG 6:30 minutes, SD 0:37 minutes) and selected 25–39 actions (AVG 31.4, SD 3.69), while they spent significantly more time with the gesture-based interaction ($t(11.31) = 2.27$, $p < 0.05$, $r = 0.56$) with 5:06–22:28 minutes (AVG 10:16 minutes, SD 5:43 minutes) and they selected 26–40 actions (AVG 32.4, SD 4.58). Questionnaires revealed a tendency for higher usability ($t(20) = 2.00$, $p = 0.059$, $r = 0.41$) and higher flow ($t(16.40) = 1.98$, $p = 0.065$, $r = 0.44$) with the mouse in comparison to the Kinect, similar to Dow and colleagues [3]. However, in our case, this effect was less pronounced. Furthermore, we measured a significantly higher positive affect ($t(20) = 2.12$, $p < 0.05$, $r = 0.43$) with the Kinect in comparison to the mouse. Apparently, participants enjoyed playing with the Kinect more than with the mouse although the interaction might have been slightly more difficult and sometimes distracted them from the application.

4   Conclusion and Future Work

We presented a gameplay approach incorporating full body user interaction with virtual characters, which was developed for the intercultural training scenario

Traveller. We implemented two interaction types: symbolic full body gestures and a circular menu with freehand swiping gestures. Both types received high recognition rates, however, only the gesture interaction reached our goal of 90% recognition accuracy, while the swipe interaction stayed slightly below it. In comparison with the mouse interface, participants spend significantly more time in the game when using full body interaction. However, the novel interaction did not necessarily slow down the participants, as the fastest participants actually were using this interaction modality. Furthermore, our results indicate higher usability and flow with the mouse, but higher positive affect with the Kinect. While full body interaction might be more complicated to use, it still has the potential to increase the enjoyment in interaction.

Although we did not receive significant differences regarding immersion or spatial presence, the full body interaction might get higher scores when using it in a virtual reality setup. In addition, we plan to include further methods to help the user during the interaction such as automatic feedback why a gesture has not been recognised, and step-wise instructions for more complex gestures.

Acknowledgments. This work was partially funded by the European Commission within FP7 under grant agreement eCute (FP7-ICT-257666).

References

1. Aylett, R., Vannini, N., Andre, E., Paiva, A., Enz, S., Hall, L.: But that was in another country: Agents and intercultural empathy. In: Proc. AAMAS 2009, pp. 329–336. IFAAMAS (2009)
2. Dias, J., Mascarenhas, S., Paiva, A.: Fatima modular: Towards an agent architecture with a generic appraisal framework. In: Proc. Workshop on Standards for Emotion Modeling (2011)
3. Dow, S., Mehta, M., Harmon, E., MacIntyre, B., Mateas, M.: Presence and engagement in an interactive drama. In: Proc. CHI 2007, pp. 1475–1484. ACM, New York (2007)
4. Hofstede, G.J.: Role playing with synthetic cultures: the evasive rules of the game. Experimental Interactive Learning in Industrial Management: New approaches to Learning, Studying and Teaching p. 49 (2005)
5. Janowski, K., Kistler, F., André, E.: Gestures or speech? comparing modality selection for different interaction tasks in a virtual environment. In: Proc. Tilburg Gesture Research Meeting 2013 (2013), http://tiger.uvt.nl
6. Kadobayashi, R., Nishimoto, K., Mase, K.: Design and evaluation of gesture interface of an immersive walk-through application for exploring cyberspace. In: Proc. Automatic Face and Gesture Recognition, pp. 534–539 (1998)
7. Kistler, F., André, E.: User-defined body gestures for an interactive storytelling scenario. In: Kotzé, P., Marsden, G., Lindgaard, G., Wesson, J., Winckler, M. (eds.) INTERACT 2013, Part II. LNCS, vol. 8118, pp. 264–281. Springer, Heidelberg (2013)
8. Kistler, F., Endrass, B., Damian, I., Dang, C., André, E.: Natural interaction with culturally adaptive virtual characters. Journal on Multimodal User Interfaces 6, 39–47 (2012); 10.1007/s12193-011-0087-z
9. Raybourn, E.M., Deagle, M.E., Mendini, K., Heneghan, J.: Adaptive thinking & leadership simulation game training for special forces officers. In: Proc. I/ITSEC 2005. NTSA (2005)

Effects of an Agent's Displaying Self-adaptors during a Serious Conversation

Tomoko Koda and Yuko Mori

Department of Information Science and Technology, Osaka Institute of Technology,
1-79-1 Kitayama, Hirakata-shi, Osaka, 573-0196 Japan
koda@is.oit.ac.jp

Abstract. Self-adaptors are bodily behaviors that often involve self-touch. In our previous research, perceived friendliness of an agent that displays self-adaptors did not decrease over multiple interactions. This research evaluated interactions with agents that exhibit either relaxed self-adaptors or stressful self-adaptors in a desert survival task. The result suggests the need to tailor non-verbal behavior of virtual agents according to conversational contents between an agent and a human.

Keywords: Intelligent virtual agents, self-adapter, gesture, evaluation.

1 Introduction

Intelligent virtual agents (IVAs) that interact face-to-face with humans are beginning to spread to general users, and IVA research is being actively pursued. IVAs require both verbal and nonverbal communication abilities. Among those non-verbal communications, Ekman classifies gestures into five categories: emblems, illustrators, affect displays, adapters, and regulators [1]. Self-adaptors are non-signaling gestures that are not intended to convey a particular meaning [2]. They are exhibited as hand movements where one part of the body is applied to another part of the body, such as scratching one's head and face, or tapping the foot. Many self-adaptors are considered taboo in public, and individuals with low emotional stability perform more self-adaptors, and the number of self-adaptors increases with psychological discomfort or anxiety [2, 3, 4]. According to Caso et al. self-adaptor gestures were used more often when telling the truth than when lying [5].

Because of its non-relevance to conversational content, there has not been much IVA research done on self-adaptors, compared with nonverbal communication with high message content, such as facial expressions and gazes. Among few research that has dealt with an IVA with self-adaptors, Neff et al. reported that an agent performing self-adaptors (repetitive quick motion with a combination of scratching its face and head, touching its body, and rubbing its head, etc.) were perceived as having low emotional stability [6]. Although showing emotional unstableness might not be appropriate in some social interactions, their finding suggests the importance of self-adaptors in conveying a personality of an agent.

T. Bickmore et al. (Eds.): IVA 2014, LNAI 8637, pp. 240–249, 2014.

However, self-adaptors are not always the sign of emotional unstableness or stress. Blacking states self-adaptors also occur in casual conversations, where conversant are very relaxed [7]. If those relaxed self-adaptors occur with a conversant that one feels friendliness, one can be induced to feel friendliness toward a conversant that displays self-adaptors. We apply this to the case of agent conversant, and hypothesized that users can be induced to feel friendliness toward the agent that performs self-adaptors.

We focused on the self-adaptors performed in a casual conversation in our previous study [8]. Based on the results of video analysis of the conversations between friends in a Japanese university, we found the following three types of self-adaptors occurred most frequently in most pairs: "touching hair," "touching chin," and "touching nose." Each stroke occurred once as a slow movement. The timing was either at the beginning or at the end of an utterance. The self-adaptors implemented for the agents in [6] were repetitive quick hand scratches, rubbing, tapping, etc., as we see when the human conversant is nervous (We call them as "stressful self-adaptors" in this paper). We did not find those stressful self-adaptors during the casual conversations in the video recordings.

We evaluated continual interactions with an agent that exhibited self-adaptors which are seen to be friendly actions, such as "hair-touching", "chin-touching", and "nose-touching" (we call them as "relaxed self-adaptors" in this paper). The results showed agents that exhibited relaxed self-adaptors were more likely to prevent any deterioration in the perceived friendliness with the agents than agents that have no self-adaptors [8]. In addition, people with higher social skills harbor a higher perceived friendliness with agents that exhibited relaxed self-adaptors than people with lower social skills. Thus, we expect that it would be possible to improve humanness and friendliness of agents by implementing self-adaptors in them. We take the view that impressions of self-adaptors in human-agent interactions are formed through multiple interactions. Thus, we do not evaluate impressions after one trial, but instead conduct multiple trials and evaluations.

We set a hypothesis from the research of IVAs with self-adaptors, one with stressful adaptors [6] and relaxed self-adaptors [8] as follows: "agents that exhibited relaxed self-adaptors are evaluated to give a better impression than agents that exhibited stressful self-adaptors, which improves the perceived friendliness of the agents in continual interactions". In the previous research, the interactions with agents were either one-sided utterances from the agents [6] or selective interactions done in casual conversation such as favorite food, hobbies, etc [8]. In this research, we verify the effects of self-adaptors on task-oriented interactions using a desert survival task [9], by users cooperating with agents to solve problems in continual interactions.

2   Development of the Agent

2.1   Agent Design

We used a female 3D model using Poser 7 (http://poser.smithmicro.com/poser.html) for the agent's appearance and created animations with three sets of conditions:

"agents that exhibit relaxed self-adaptors", "agents that exhibit no self-adaptors", and "agents that exhibit stressful self-adaptors". The self-adaptors implemented for the "agents that exhibit relaxed self-adaptors" are the three types that were implemented in [8]: "hair-touching", "chin-touching", and "nose-touching". A relaxed self-adaptor is a one-off action with a narrow range of hand movements, such as touching the nose or flicking the hair. The self-adaptors implemented for the "agents that exhibit stressful self-adaptors" are three of the self-adaptors used in [6]: "head-scratching", "neck-scratching", and "chin-scratching". A stressful self-adaptor is a scratching action which occurs a number of times over a wider range of hand movements than a relaxed self-adaptor. Agents exhibiting relaxed self-adaptors are shown in Fig. 1 and agents exhibiting stressful self-adaptors are shown in Fig. 2.

Since self-adaptors in conversations between people often start at the beginning and end of utterances from our video analysis of conversation between human friends [8], we implemented the self-adaptors of the agents at the beginning of utterances. Separate from these self-adaptors, we implemented gestures in all the agents such as "head-tilting" at the end of questions and "raising hand to chest" when indicating themselves, in order to ensure that the self-adaptors alone were not too obvious.

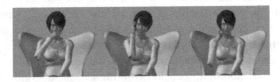

Fig. 1. Agents Exhibiting Relaxed Self-adaptors

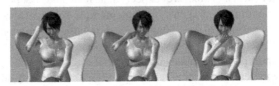

Fig. 2. Agents Exhibiting Stressful Self-adaptors

2.2   Agent Interaction Method

The agent's conversation system was developed in C++ using Microsoft Visual Studio 2008. The agent's voice was synthesized in a woman's voice using the Japanese voice synthesis package AITalk (http://www.ai-j.jp/). The contents of the conversations were casual (the route to school, residential area, and favorite food, etc.) for the first and second sessions, and desert survival task from third to fifth sessions. The interaction between the agent and a participant was restricted as a pseudo conversation. The reason we adopted the pseudo-conversation method was to eliminate the effect of the accuracy of speech recognition of the users' spoken answers, which would otherwise be used, on the participants' impression of the agent.

Conversation scenarios, composed of questions from the agent and response choices, were created beforehand. The interactions between the agent and a participant were conducted as follows: 1) The agent always asks a question to the participant. 2)

Possible answers were displayed on the screen with the agent. 3) The participant se-lects one answer from the selection from a keyboard. 4) The agent makes remarks and asks the next question based on the user's answer. The scenarios are similar regard-less of the answers from the participant. 5) The agent performs three different self-adaptors at the beginning of three utterances in any session. The average session time was about 5 minutes.

3   Evaluation Experiments

3.1   Experimental Design and Conversational Scenarios

We divided the experiment participants between three conditions: "agents that exhibit relaxed self-adaptors", "agents that exhibit no self-adaptors", and "agents that exhibit stressful self-adaptors", and conducted experiments as between subjects design. Each participant interacted with the agent five times. They were asked to answer a questionnaire about the impression of agents and interactions after each session. There was one interaction with an agent per day, and the type of agent in the interactions was the same for all the five experiment sessions. For example, the participants who are assigned the "relaxed- self-adaptor" condition keep interacting with the agent with relaxed self-adaptor throughout the five sessions.

The conversational scenarios differ for each session of the experiment. The first and second sessions are used as a social relationship building phase involving everyday conversation such as favorite food and hobbies. The third to fifth sessions are used as a brainstorming phase that try to solve a desert survival task by exchanging different opinions between a participant and the agent. The sequence of interactive scenarios in the experiment sessions is the same, irrespective of the agent condition A desert survival task is a challenge in which the participants select and prioritize objects necessary for survival from multiple items, in a situation in which an aircraft has crash-landed in the desert [9]. In this experiments, we use a simplified desert survival task, in which asked the participants to select three items out of eight that they thought would be necessary after a desert crash. At the start of the interaction, the agent queries an item selected by the participant and recommends a different item from the participant's selection. There were three item-selection reasons: "for sustaining life", "for calling for help", and "for getting oneself moving". If, for example, a participant selects "water" in the "for sustaining life" category, the agent recommends a "mirror" in the "for calling for help" category. We made the conversational scenarios to repeat that interaction for all three items.

We conduct experiments between subjects in the three conditions, for the type of agent (with relaxed self-adaptors, no self-adaptors, or stressful self-adaptors) and the experiment session number (1-5 session). The only differences in the agents were the presence/absence of self-adaptors and their types. The physical appearance, voice, and timing of performing self-adaptors and other gestures are the same in all conditions as well as the number of sessions and the conversation scenarios.

The participants were 38 university students between the ages of 20 and 23 (27 males and 11 females). The numbers of participants for each condition was 13 for the relaxed self-adaptor condition, 13 for the no self-adaptor condition, and 12 for the stressful self-adaptor condition.

3.2   Experimental Procedure and Questionnaires

The participants were asked to answer a questionnaire after each session. The questionnaire consisted of questions regarding perceived friendliness, empathy, intentionality, and shyness of the agent and interaction likeability and interaction stress with respect to the interaction with the agent. For a total of 21 questions were rated using a 7-point Likert scale (7: high– 1: low). A post-experiment questionnaire was conducted after the end of the fifth session in order to evaluate factors such as recognition of the agents' actions and impressions of the perceived intelligence level of the agents during the desert survival task, on a 7-point Likert scale.

The experimental procedure for the social relationship building phase and the cooperative task phase are as follows:

- First and second experiment sessions: social relationship building phase

    (1) Interact with agent (everyday conversation)
    (2) Answer to the impression evaluation questionnaire

- Third to fifth experiment sessions: cooperative task phase

    (3) Engage in desert survival task
    (4) Interact with agent (opinion switching)
    (5) At the end of the interaction, engage in the desert survival task again (rethink opinions given in (3)
    (6) Answer to the impression evaluation questionnaire
- After the end of all experiments: Answer to the post-experiment questionnaire

4   Results

4.1   Analysis of Impression Evaluation Questionnaire

We performed two-way ANOVA with repeated measurements on the results of the impression evaluation questionnaire in two factors, with self-adaptor (relaxed, none, stressful) and experiment session number (1-5 sessions). We verify whether there are differences in the impressions of the agents and impressions of the interactions according to the types and presence/absence of self-adaptor as well as experiment session number and phase of interaction.

Firstly, for the results of the impressions of the agents, the results of two-way ANOVA for "friendliness towards agent", "empathy with the agent", "intentionality of agent", and "shyness of agent" indicated the following: concerning friendliness, empathy, purpose, and humanness, main effects of the self-adaptor factor (friendliness: $F = 7.435$, $p = 0.001$; empathy: $F = 3.517$, $p = 0.035$; purpose: $F = 3.779$, $p = 0.027$), main effects of the experiment session number factor (friendliness:

$F = 5.345$, $p = 0.001$; empathy: $F = 9.433$, $p < 0.001$; purpose: $F = 4.887$, $p = 0.001$), and mutual-interaction (friendliness: $F = 3.378$, $p = 0.001$; empathy: $F = 3.125$, $p = 0.002$; purpose: $F = 2.135$, $p = 0.040$) were seen. We also conducted multiple comparisons on shyness, since there are main effects of the experiment session number factor ($F = 9.954$, $p < 0.001$) and mutual-interaction ($F = 2.260$, $p = 0.033$). The results of the multiple comparisons of impressions of the agent for the self-adaptor factor are shown in Fig. 3, those for the experiment session number factor are shown in Fig. 4, and the comparison of perceived friendliness for the adaptor and session number factors are shown in Fig. 5.

From Fig. 3, there is no significant difference between relaxed self-adaptors and stressful self-adaptors in the multiple comparison results of the self-adaptor factor with respect to impressions of the agents. However, from the results of friendliness towards the agents, agents without self-adaptors were evaluated significantly higher than those of agents with relaxed self-adaptors or stressful self-adaptors ($p \leqq 0.01$). In addition, from the results for empathy and intentionality, agents with no self-adaptors were evaluated significantly higher than those with relaxed self-adaptors ($p \leqq 0.05$), and the same tendency was observed for those with stressful self-adaptors. From Fig. 4, which shows multiple comparison results of experiment session number factor with respect to impressions of the agents, the agents in the cooperative task phase (from the third to fifth sessions) were evaluated significantly lower for agent's perceived empathy and shyness ($p \leqq 0.01$), and significantly higher for agent's intentionality than those in the social relationship building phase (the first and second session) ($p \leqq 0.01$). In terms of perceived friendliness of the agents, agents in the second session were rated more friendly than that of the first session ($p \leqq 0.01$), and agents in the fourth session were rated more friendly than that of the third session ($p \leqq 0.05$). From Fig.5, there are interactions between the self-adaptor and experiment session number factors in the perceived friendliness of the agent. Despite there being no difference in the perceived friendliness of agents between self-adaptor factors in the social relationship building phase, in the cooperative task phase, agents with no self-adaptors had significant differences ($p \leqq 0.01$) indicating higher evaluations of friendliness than both types of agent having self-adaptors.

Secondly, for the impression of the interactions, we performed two-way ANOVA on "interaction smoothness", "interaction likeability", and "interaction stress" in the questionnaire. The results of evaluations of the interactions showed there were no main effects of the self-adaptor factor (smoothness: $F = 2.383$, $p = 0.099$, likeability rating: $F = 2.792$, $p = 0.066$, stress: $F = 2.092$, $p = 0.128$) or main effects of experiment session number factor (smoothness: $F = 0.991$, $p = 0.412$, likeability rating: $F = 1.623$, $p = 0.176$, stress: $F = 0.437$, $p = 0.769$), but there was mutual-interaction with interaction likeability rating and interaction stress (smoothness: $F = 1.201$, $p = 0.298$, likeability rating: $F = 2.136$, $p = 0.040$, stress: $F = 3.016$, $p = 0.003$). Further multiple comparison results of the interaction likeability and interaction stress rating with the experiment session number as factor showed the following: there was no significant difference between the numbers of sessions for relaxed self-adaptors and stressful self-adaptors, but there was a significant difference ($p \leqq 0.05$).

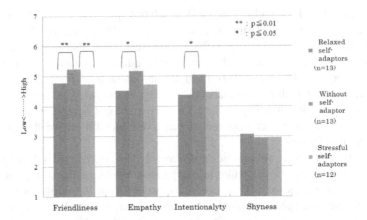

Fig. 3. Comparison of the Impression of the Agent for the Self-adaptor Factor

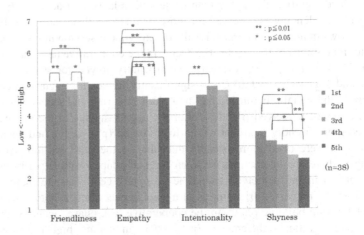

Fig. 4. Comparisons of the Impression of the Agent for the Experiment Session Number Factor

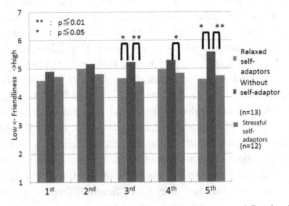

Fig. 5. Comparison of Perceived Friendliness for Adaptor and Session Factors

indicating that the interaction likeability rating was higher (1: low − 7: high, 1st = 5.1, 2nd = 4.9, 3rd = 5.5, 4th = 5.5, 5th = 5.4) and the stress was lower (1: low − 7: high, 1st = 2.2, 2nd = 2.6, 3rd = 2.2, 4th = 2.1, 5th = 1.8) in the third to fifth sessions of the cooperative task phase than in the second session of the social relationship building phase, for agents with no self-adaptors.

4.2   Analysis of Post-experiment Questionnaire

In the post-experiment questionnaire, we asked the participants about the perceived intelligence of the agent in the desert survival task, and naturalness and bothered-ness of the agents behaviors. There was a significant difference indicating a higher evaluation for agents with no self-adaptors than those with relaxed self-adaptors (1: low − 7: high, relaxed = 3.8, without = 5.5, $p \leq 0.01$) in terms of agent's perceived knowledge about the desert survival task. There was a significant difference indicating that users rated the agents with stressful self-adaptors as less natural (relaxed = 3.9, without = 3.1, stressful = 5.0, $p \leq 0.05$) and more bothering (relaxed = 3.7, without = 2.6, stressful = 4.1, $p \leq 0.05$) than those with no self-adaptors. The rating for the agents with relaxed self-adaptors had similar tendency to those of the stressful self-adaptors but the differences in rating were not significant.

5   Discussion

5.1   Discussion of Impression Evaluation of the Agents and Interactions

In the impression evaluations of the agents for each type of self-adaptor factor, shown in Fig. 3, agents that did not exhibit self-adaptors had significant differences indicating they were evaluated more highly for friendliness, empathy, and intentionality than both types of agent that exhibited self-adaptors, or there was a tendency towards that. In other words, the exhibiting of self-adaptors is thought to affect a deterioration in the user's impressions of the agents. These results are the same as reported in [2, 3, 4] for humans and [6] for agents.

In the impression evaluations of agents for each experiment session number factor, shown in Fig. 4, there were significant differences indicating that perceived empathy and shyness were evaluated lower and intentionality was evaluated higher during the cooperative task phase, in comparison with the social relationship building phase. In the cooperative task phase, the agents offered opinions that were different from the replies given by the users in the desert survival task. That is thought to be why perceived empathy and shyness of the agents deteriorates and perceived intentionality is improved in the cooperative task phase. Perceived friendliness increased significantly during each of the two phase (friendliness in the second session was significantly higher than those of the first, fourth was significantly higher than the third) but dropped between the social relationship building phase and the cooperative task phase.

There are interactions in the cooperative task phase indicating that agents that did not exhibit self-adaptors were evaluated more highly for friendliness than agents that exhibited any kind of self-adaptors. In interactions that require exchanging serious opinions and logical reasoning, such as in this desert survival task, we could say that the exhibiting self-adaptors causes a deterioration in the impressions of the agents as reported in [2, 3, 4, 6]. However, interesting results are that there are not significant differences in the friendliness ratings in the social relationship building phase where everyday conversation was conducted. This result during the social relationship building phase confirm the results in [8], in which showed that the exhibiting of relaxed self-adaptors in informal everyday conversation prevented any deterioration in friendliness.

The above leads to the result that the hypothesis is not supported, with no difference in impression evaluation being seen between relaxed self-adaptors and stressful self-adaptors. However, we found the dichotomy of the user's impression on the agents with self-adaptor and without with contrast to conversational contents. In other words, users unconsciously expect agents to behave in a manner that is appropriate to the topic of conversation as we do with humans. That suggests the non-verbal behavior of agents must adapt to the conversational topics.

The impression evaluations of the interactions with the agents indicate that agents that did not exhibit self-adaptors had a higher interaction likeability rating and lower interaction stress in the cooperative task phase than in the social relationship building phase. In other words, we could say that impressions of the interactions themselves are improved by having agents that do not exhibit self-adaptors during the execution of the cooperative tasks. In the experiment overall, there were no main effects of the self-adaptor factor and experiment session number factor in impression evaluations of the agents. The results suggest that impressions of the interactions are not formed by the self-adaptors of the agents or the conversational content, but rather mutual-interactions between the self-adaptors and the conversational content affect the impressions of the interactions with the agents.

5.2   Discussion of Post-experiment Questionnaire Analysis Results

The post questionnaire results showed agents without self-adaptors have higher evaluations concerning their perceived intelligence level than agents that exhibited self-adaptors. In conversations that call for agreement of opinions or situations intended to persuade changes in opinions, the agents impressions deteriorate in the presence of self-adaptors, making it difficult to achieve agreement or persuasion. In addition, the answers to the questions to the agents perceived intelligence, annoyance and naturalness level of the agents actions, showed there was an overall tendency for stressful self-adaptors to be better than relaxed self-adaptors. Since the conversational contents were a serious topic, the agent's exhibiting relaxed self-adaptors gave impressions that seriousness was lacking. This suggests not only we regard agents displaying self-adaptors as less friendly and empathetic, but also we expect agents to "behave" appropriately according the conversational content.

6   Conclusions

From the results of impression of the agents, we found that the exhibiting of self-adaptors in interactions that exchange serious opinions, such as a desert survival task, caused deterioration in the agents perceived friendliness and empathy, although such deterioration does not occur during a casual conversation with the agent displays self-adaptors. This leads to the result that the hypothesis in this research is not supported, with no difference in impression evaluation being seen between relaxed self-adaptors and stressful self-adaptors. Users unconsciously expect agents to behave in a manner that is appropriate to the topic of conversation as we do with humans. That suggests that the non-verbal behavior of agents must adapt to the conversational topics. Taken together with the results of previous research, the results shows that it will be necessary to make the non-verbal behavior of an agent, at least, self-adaptors, adapt to the social skills of the other person in an interaction, and to the conversational content. We believe these results would lead to the development of IVAs that adapt to users and conversational context in continual interactions.

Acknowledgement. This research is partially supported by a Grant-in-Aid for Scientific Research (C) 23500266 (2011-2013) and 26330236 (2014-2016) from the JSPS.

References

1. Ekman, P.: Three classes of nonverbal behavior. In: Aspects of Nonverbal Communication. Swets and Zeitlinger (1980)
2. Waxer, P.: Nonverbal cues for anxiety: An examination of emotional leakage. Journal of Abnormal Psychology 86(3), 306–314 (1988)
3. Ekman, P., Friesen, W.V.: Hand movements. Journal of Communication 22, 353–374 (1972)
4. Argyle, M.: Bodily communication. Taylor & Francis (1988)
5. Caso, L., Maricchiolo, F., Bonaiuto, M., Vrij, A., Mann, S.: The Impact of Deception and Suspicion on Different Hand Movements. Journal of Nonverbal Behavior 30(1), 1–19 (2006)
6. Neff, M., Toothman, N., Bowmani, R., Fox Tree, J.E., Walker, M.: Don't Scratch! Self-adaptors Reflect Emotional Stability. In: Vilhjálmsson, H.H., Kopp, S., Marsella, S., Thórisson, K.R. (eds.) IVA 2011. LNCS, vol. 6895, pp. 398–411. Springer, Heidelberg (2011)
7. Blacking, J. (ed.): The Anthropology of the Body. Academic Press (1977)
8. Koda, T., Higashino, H.: Importance of Considering User's Social Skills in Human-agent Interactions. In: Proc. of the 6th International Conference on Agents and Artifcial Intelligence (ICAART 2014), pp. 115–122 (2014)
9. Lafferty, J.C., Eady, P.M.: The Desert Survival Problem. Experimental Learning Methods, Plymouth (1974)

Let's Be Serious and Have a Laugh: Can Humor Support Cooperation with a Virtual Agent?

Philipp Kulms[1], Stefan Kopp[1], and Nicole C. Krämer[2]

[1] Sociable Agents Group, Center of Excellence 'Cognitive Interaction Technology' (CITEC), Faculty of Technology, Bielefeld University, Germany
{pkulms,skopp}@techfak.uni-bielefeld.de
[2] Department of Social Psychology: Media and Communication, University of Duisburg-Essen, Germany
nicole.kraemer@uni-due.de

Abstract. A crucial goal within human-computer interaction is to establish cooperation. There is evidence that among the tools being available, humor might be a promising and not uncommon choice. The appeal of humor is supported by its fundamentality for human-human interaction and the variety of functions humor serves, for it can achieve much more than making the user smile. In the present experiment, we sought to further investigate the potential effects of humor for virtual agents. Subjects played the iterated prisoner's dilemma with a virtual agent that was intended to be funny or not. Additionally, we manipulated cooperativeness of the agent. First, although humor did not increase cooperation among subjects, our results indicate that humor modulates how cooperation is perceived in an agent. Second, humor facilitated the interaction with respect to enjoyment and rapport. Third, although increased enjoyment and overall affective reactions were both measured subjectively, the results were not in line with each other.

Keywords: Virtual agent, Humor, Cooperation, Prisoner's dilemma.

1 Introduction

Humor is the source of pleasure and entertainment, of distress relief, and the experience of teaching and discovering [1]. It stands for delight and positive emotions. We may attribute these desirable aspects to a communicator we find humorous. Humor makes it easier to connect with others. Experiencing humor at a given occasion leads to the desire to repeat the experience. In interpersonal communication, a speaker is evaluated more favorably when she displays humor. If a person is believed to have a sense of humor, this assumption automatically creates a halo effect with regard to other desirable personality traits such as friendliness, pleasantness, and creativeness [2]. However, from the viewpoint of human-computer interaction (HCI), humor has received only little attention. In scenarios where humans and lifelike artificial characters need to cooperate or negotiate a task, the use of humor may serve a variety of

T. Bickmore et al. (Eds.): IVA 2014, LNAI 8637, pp. 250–259, 2014.

goals. It could make the interaction more natural and meaningful and even affect the outcome. Humor is a form of cognitive play, leading to a considerable amount of pleasure and motivation.

We review the role of humor for social interactions and how it has been applied to HCI. In interpersonal communication, humor is one of the most important facilitators and an important social skill. Humor can be used to promote social influence and cooperation, in a completely playful manner. It is, however, not easy to channel this potential. Our aim was to create a funny agent in order to analyze experimentally how its humorousness and cooperativeness influence human partners in a social dilemma.

2   Theoretical Background

Humor in Social Interactions. Humor is an important tool to shape social interactions and influence others [5]. It plays a role for rapport, cooperation, and person perception. Understanding humor and laughter as social skills that people need to learn, control, and regularly practice [6] indicates how difficult it is to implement it into technology. The richest source of humor lies within natural and spontaneous everyday interactions [3]. Accordingly, within everyday conversation, humor serves as social facilitator that can be deployed in a variety of different contexts such as negotiating requests and building group solidarity [4]. Humor is an antecedent of rapport; it fosters a positive and friendly environment [7] and connects people with each other [8]. But humor may also interfere with involvement and thus with rapport, because joking requires recipients to ignore the obvious meaning and find interpretations that are funny [9]. If listeners fail to understand a humorous remark or feel that it is rather inappropriate, specific facilitative functions of humor are disrupted. On the other hand, if listeners participate in the joking and appreciate it, experiences and attitudes are shared, rapport is promoted, and politeness is conveyed [10]. Humor influences person perception. Evidence from social psychology provides support for effects on liking [11] and credibility [12]. In line with this, sense of humor is very often used as social category [13]. According to [2], having sense of humor is associated with being more friendly, pleasant, interesting, cooperative, imaginative, creative, clever, and less cold and passive. Finally, experimental studies successfully manipulated the experience of humor in the context of interpersonal interaction and showed the effect on outcome variables. [14] showed that in a fictional bargaining situation, conversational humor ("Well, my final offer is $7,000 and I'll throw in my pet frog") leads to social influence to the extent that subjects agreed to pay a significantly higher price for a painting. Subjects laughed more, reported more amusement, and were more likely to agree that their partner was a fun person.

Humor in Human-Computer Interaction. It is argued that social cues relying on human cognitive and affective processes lead to more meaningful interactions with artificial entities and more user appreciation [15, 16]. It was proposed to implement humorous behavior into human-agent interactions in order to tease out the potential of humor for establishing social relationships [16]. An experimental study by [18] revealed that a virtual exercise advisor displaying a set of relational behaviors including social dialogue, empathy, and humor led to increased liking, trust, and higher self-reported desire to continue working with it. Until today, experimental approaches placing detailed scrutiny on humor have remained scarce.

[17] found evidence for why humor could fit into task settings. In two different experiments, the authors had subjects chat and solve the Desert Survival Problem with a humorous or non-humorous computer. In both experiments the computer made pre-programmed comments, but in study 1 subjects were led to believe they were interacting with another person. In the humor conditions subjects received a number of funny comments, for instance: "The mirror is probably too small to be used as a signaling device to alert rescue teams to your location. Rank it lower. (On the other hand, it offers endless opportunity for self-reflection)". In the no-humor conditions, the computer/partner would leave out the funny remark. Subjects who knew they communicated with a computer (study 2) responded less sociable and showed less mirth. Nevertheless, when isolating study 2, some important effects remained. Subjects in the humor condition liked the computer more, showed more mirth responses, made more sociable comments, and joked back more. The study showed that it is possible to create humorous computers, even with preprogrammed text-based jokes. A similar experiment focused on the effect of virtual agent humor on social influence [19]. Social influence was conceptualized as rating similarity in the Lunar Survival Scenario. Again, participants were asked to engage in text-based communication with a virtual entity and again, the computer's reasoning about the items' relative relevance was subject to the humor manipulation (e.g. "We can use the FM receiver to communicate with another ship, or we can pass time with some fun music on the radio"). This time participants were presented a chat interface that showed a picture of their partner, a male virtual agent named Bradley. The interaction was no longer pre-scripted as the agent had the ability to answer questions. Differences between initial and post-chat item rankings reflected the extent to which the agent was able to influence its partner toward the ideal item rankings. When Bradley was perceived as funny, he was more effective at influencing the participants. Moreover, for participants in the humor condition, a positive correlation between perceived humorousness and influence on their rankings emerged. Strikingly, the manipulation check for perceived humorousness of the agent was not successful. Instead, there was a considerable fraction of no-humor participants who judged the agent as funny.

Taken together, humor may play a crucial role for establishing relationships with virtual agents [20] but there are not enough studies on the potentials and pitfalls. For instance, more experimental investigations are needed to explore potential research directions for task-related settings. We present such an investigation.

Hypotheses. We expect an agent that makes conversational and situation-specific jokes to be judged as funnier compared to an agent that does not joke (H1; manipulation check). This manipulation check is important because there were "misperceptions" of an agent's funniness in the past [19]. Cooperation determines a large fraction of the appeal of interacting with computers. The question to what extent users cooperate with computers in social dilemmas has gained some attention in the past [21, 22]. Humorous (non-animated) virtual agents can foster cooperation [19], but none of the previous studies varied the degree of cooperation. We therefore combined manipulations of humor and cooperation. We hypothesize that in a social dilemma, the cooperative agent is judged as more cooperative than the competitive agent (H2; manipulation check). According to the norm of reciprocity [23], we expect that the agent's observable behavior will evoke similar reactions by the subjects. Thus there will be more cooperation when playing with the cooperative agent (H3). Given the meaning of humor for social interactions and social influence, we expect the funny agent to elicit more cooperation than the unfunny version (H4). Furthermore, a funny agent will evoke more positive affective reactions (H5) and lead to increased rapport (H6).

3   Method

Experimental Design and Subjects. We conducted an experiment in which subjects played the iterated Prisoner's Dilemma Game (PDG) with a virtual agent. The study was based on a 2 (*Agent humor:* humor vs. no humor) x 2 (*Agent behavior:* cooperative vs. selfish) between-subjects design. Eighty (80) subjects participated in the experiment (44 females, 36 males). Their age ranged between 19 and 34 years ($M = 24.91$, $SD = 3.06$). Subjects were randomly assigned to one of the four conditions.

Table 1. Payoff matrix in the iterated prisoner's dilemma (investment game version)

	Project green	Project blue
Project green	Subject: 5€ Agent: 5€	Subject: 3€ Agent: 7€
Project blue	Subject: 7€ Agent: 3€	Subject: 4€ Agent: 4€

Materials. In the social sciences, the PDG is a widely used and well-elaborated method to explore determinants of cooperation and altruism. The fictional scenario puts subjects in the role of an arrested convict. Since their partner was also arrested, the convicts can either remain silent (cooperate) or testify against the partner (defect). The combination of both decisions determines the punishment for both convicts. Recently the PDG was also used to investigate cooperation with virtual agents capable of facial emotional displays [21].

In the present study, subjects did not know how many rounds were left but were given a hint when half of the turns were over. There was no display on played rounds, rounds left, or elapsed time. Since in the iterated version it does not make sense instructing subjects to either remain silent or testify multiple times in a row, the iterated PDG was cast into an investment game [e.g. 22]. In this version, subjects are asked to choose between two projects, Project Green and Project Blue. The payoff matrix does not change, Project Green is the cooperative option and Project Blue is the selfish choice (see Table 1). The utility-maximizing choice for both players is to play selfishly in each round. However, both players' payoff is higher for mutual cooperation than for mutual selfishness, thus the resulting dilemma. Two windows were

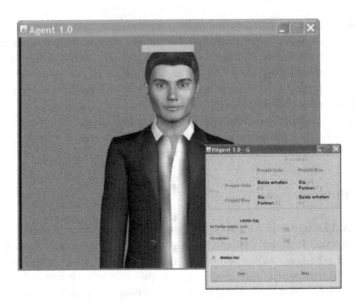

Fig. 1. Agent and PDG window with arranged overlap

presented, one for the agent and one for the PDG (see Fig. 1). The game window showed the payoff matrix and the game statistics, consisting of both players' last choices, the last and the total payoff.

The agent was created with the CharAT avatar editor, a proprietary toolkit (Copyright by Charamel GmbH, 2008-2010). It chose between the two options and gave occasional task-related feedback on the previous turns (see Table 2). Decisions were random-based with a bias for one of the two choices, depending on the behavior condition. While the agent was able to speak, it was not allowed to directly negotiate with the player.

Procedure. Upon arrival, subjects were told that they are about to play an investment game with a virtual counterpart and were asked to rate the interaction subsequently. They were told that their goal would be to maximize their own outcome. The more points they earned the higher their chance to win a 25€ voucher. Each round would be initiated by the agent. After each round both players' decisions and their individual payoff were revealed. The detailed overview of the game was explained by the virtual partner. After the investigator's introduction the agent explained the rationale behind the game and introduced the possible outcomes, depending on both players' investment choices. The instructions were adopted from [22]. After the game was finished, subjects rated their interaction with the agent using the post-questionnaire. They were debriefed and thanked for their participation. Each session lasted approximately 40 minutes.

Manipulations. We manipulated the agent's decision policy and its humorousness. In the humor condition the agent teases, baffles, and engages the player in a playful way. Since the PDG itself only features minimal interactive cues, it was assumed that even trivial jokes would facilitate the interaction. A simple time-based rule was implemented to add enough variety into the decision about when the agent should make a joke or say something trivial and unfunny instead. First we tracked how long the subject took for her turns. On this time series we performed exponential smoothing to compute naïve predictions about future turn times of this subject. We used the predicted values for future turns as threshold and checked if the subsequent turn time was above or below this threshold. If it was below, indicating that the subject was quicker than expected, the agent performed a joke. If it was above, indicating that the subject took longer than expected, the agent made a normal comment. As a result, the agent quasi-regularly switched between funny and unfunny comments and adapted to the subject. The content was held identical in terms of (ostensibly) personal information the agent disclosed. Table 2 provides examples of jokes and control comments by the agent. The sets of jokes and control comments each contained 22 utterances for the agent to choose from. While the agent did say something after each round, it did not always make a joke (control comment). Instead, when the requirement for a joke was not given, the agent either said "Now it's my turn again" or "OK, now it's my turn". The agent cooperated (played selfishly) 66% of the time. The exact decision order was random-based with the exception of the first five rounds. Here the agent played the following sequence: (project) green, green, blue, blue, green. The fixed sequence was implemented to avoid too many identical choices in a row at session beginning, making it harder for the subjects to guess the agent's gaming behavior [21]. Based on pre-evaluations and the joke collection size, the round limit was set to 38 rounds.

Table 2. Examples of conversational jokes and control comments by the agent

Humor	No humor
Please press start if you wish to begin. Age before beauty, so it's my turn first.	Please press start if you wish to begin.
You are better than the last player. With him I could not even play Uno.	You are better than the last player, he was indeed very unlucky.
Maybe I should have another look at the rules, with my reading glasses.	Maybe I should have another look at the rules.
I hope you haven't found any software errors yet. Do you have any idea how difficult it is to find good staff nowadays?	I hope you haven't found any software errors yet. It surely shouldn't be too hard to write error-free software.
Don't let yourself get distracted by me. Attention, behind you!	Don't let yourself get distracted by me.
You can read the Matrix like no other.	You understand the game like no other.
Here's something I'd like to know. When you see me like this, do you think I'm wearing pants?	Here's something I'd like to know. When you see me like this, do you ask yourself why I'm dressed like this?

Dependent Measures. Humorousness of the agent was assessed with five items [17] ('funny', 'witty', 'entertaining', 'creative', 'playful'; Cronbach's $\alpha = .84$). Subjects were asked to indicate how much they had to smile and laugh. Two statements were used: "My partner made me laugh" and "I sometimes had to smile" (correlation: r = .65, p < .001). Perceived cooperation of the agent was measured with two statements: "My partner predominantly chose Project Green" and "My Partner predominantly chose Project Blue" (reverse coded). Both statements correlated highly with each other (r = .70, p < .001). Affective reactions were assessed using the Positive and Negative Affect Schedule [24]. The scale consists of 20 items divided into the 10-items subscales positive (e.g. active, strong, proud; α = .88) and negative affect (e.g. 'afraid', 'nervous', 'angry'; α = .77). Perceptions of rapport were assessed using the items [25] derived from [26, 27]. For this subjects were asked to rate themselves in the interaction (11 items, e.g. 'comfortable', 'involved') and to rate the interaction itself (18 items, e.g. 'harmonious', 'awkward'). For the first set, varimax rotated principal component analyses revealed the factor 'Positivity' (29.11% explained variance, α = .83), indicating whether subjects perceived themselves as positive during the interaction. For the second set, the factors 'Intense' (17.10%, α = .78), 'Well-coordinated' (16.45%, α = .80), 'Awkward' (14.68%, α = .75), and 'Boring' (12.97%, α = .75) emerged. Cooperation was measured counting each time subjects chose project green (maximum: 38 times). All items and statements were rated on 5-point Likert scales.

4   Results

The humor manipulation was successful (H1), a two-way MANOVA revealed a main effect of humor on humorousness of the agent: the funny agent (M = 3.29, SD = .13) was perceived as funnier than the non-funny agent (M = 2.64, SD = .13), F(1, 76) = 13.18, p < .01, η_p^2 = .15. In line with this, there was a significant main effect of humor on smiling and laughter: when interacting with the funny agent (M = 3.58, SD = .18), subjects indicated to express more smiling and laughter than when interacting with the non-funny agent (M = 2.68, SD = .18), F(1, 76) = 12.37, p < .01, η_p^2 = .14. There also was a significant correlation between self-reported smiling and laughter and humorousness of the agent (r = .52, p < .001). The behavior manipulation was also successful (H2). There was a significant main effect of behavior on perceived cooperation of the agent: the cooperative agent (M = 3.52, SD = .11) was perceived as more cooperative than the selfish agent (M = 2.47, SD = .11), F(1, 76) = 46.67, p < .001, η_p^2 = .38. Unexpectedly, there was a significant main effect of humor on perceived cooperation of the agent. The funny agent (M = 2.84, SD = .11) was perceived as less cooperative than the non-funny agent (M = 3.15, SD = .11), F(1, 76) = 4.05, p < .05, η_p^2 = .05. H3 was supported as there was a significant main effect of agent behavior on cooperation. Subjects cooperated more with the cooperative agent (M = 12.19, SD = 1.08) than with the selfish agent (M = 9.18, SD = 1.06), F(1, 76) = 3.95, p = .05, ηp^2 = .05. However, two-way ANOVA results on subjects' cooperation show that the main effect of humor on cooperation was not significant (F(1, 76) < .001, p = .99). H4 was not supported. Two-way MANOVA results showed that interacting with the funny agent did not significantly enhance affective reactions. Neither positive (F(1, 76) = 1.65, p = .20) nor negative affective reactions (F(1, 76) = 1.53, p = .22) were influenced by agent humor (H5 not supported). Further analysis revealed that positive affective reactions correlate significantly with perceived humorousness of the agent ($r = .42$, $p < .001$) but not with self-reported smiling and laughter ($r = .16$, $p > .05$). Two significant effects were observed for rapport. First, there was a significant main effect of humor: interacting with the funny agent ($M = -.33$, $SD = .15$) led to less experiences of awkwardness compared with the non-funny agent ($M = .34$, $SD = .15$), $F(1, 76) = 9.56$, $p < .01$, $\eta p^2 = .12$ (H6 supported). Second, there was also a significant main effect of behavior on rapport such that interacting with the cooperative agent ($M = .25$, $SD = .16$) led to more positivity than the selfish agent ($M = -.24$, $SD = .15$), $F(1, 76) = 4.88$, $p < .05$, $\eta p^2 = .06$.

5   Discussion

Using a social dilemma, we evaluated under which circumstances people cooperate with a virtual counterpart. Leading to social influence in past HCI research, humor was implemented as a tool to support cooperation. Although we succeeded in designing a funny agent for a task-related environment that made subjects smile and laugh, subject cooperation was not affected by humor. This result should be discussed considering the funny agent was perceived as less cooperative. The attributions subjects drew as a result of this impression may explain to a certain degree why they did not cooperate more with the funny agent. Agent humor may have contributed to the impression that it did not take the task seriously enough. While it is unclear if this affected perceived task difficulty, subjects probably demanded a partner who takes the game and themselves more seriously. Since it did not, they may have associated its behavior with a tendency toward the selfish choice.

Cooperation of the agent determined whether subjects also cooperated. In task situations, designing cooperative agent behavior is thus useful to facilitate cooperation among humans. Although the selfish choice promised a better outcome, subjects chose to cooperate occasionally. The display of the agent's choices within the game was minimal and did not include any social cues whatsoever. While the effect of such minimal cues on subject cooperation is encouraging, it might be further improved by trust-relevant nonverbal cues [28] and the display of moral emotions [21]. Furthermore, subjects correctly identified the agent in the cooperative condition as a cooperative actor. Thus it may be speculated whether they followed specific intentions, such as returning the favor and, conversely, punishing the agent for selfishness in the other condition, reflecting the inherent concern for fairness within social decision making [29]. However, the punishment explanation must take into account that in the selfish condition, the rational option to avoid losing the game is to play selfishly as well.

Our results show that in conflicting and ambiguous situations, virtual agent humor can enhance the flow of interaction. Agent cooperation had a similar effect as subjects indicated more positivity toward the agent. On the other hand, the role of affective reactions in this study is surprising in that they correlated with perceived humorousness of the agent, yet they were not enhanced by virtual agent humor. It is also unclear why positive affective reactions did not correlate with self-reported smiling and laughter. Since subjects reported increased smiling and laughter in the humor condition and thus showed clear signs of enjoyment, it can be ruled out that negative contextual aspects such as goal obstruction became more salient. It can also be ruled out that subjects merely recognized the agent's attempts at humor and simply played along by smiling and laughing. This explanation, although it fits well with the application of social norms, is incoherent to the increased humorousness ratings. Since the subjective measuring of affective reactions may have been confounded by contextual elements, it can be speculated that the higher humor ratings of the funny agent did in fact reflect enhanced positive affect: "Funniness ratings presumably reflect the degree to which each stimulus elicited mirth in the participants" [13, p. 182]. In future experiments, psychophysiological measures could resolve this issue.

Although we could not support the positive relation between humor and cooperation in HCI, we were able to show how humor may influence the perception of virtual agents on supposedly non-related levels, for instance cooperativeness. As a social tool, humor can facilitate the interaction with a virtual agent, yet we need to know which forms of humor are most appreciated in a given situation (sarcasm, irony, wordplay, classic jokes). Researchers should be motivated to approach humor in HCI by asking how humor affects the user understanding of the situation, given that it is surprising and may require cognitive effort. Users do not share the same appreciation for humor, nor do they react to and use humor in the same way, a funny virtual agent thus needs to adapt to user preferences.

Acknowledgements. This research was supported by the German Federal Ministry of Education and Research (BMBF) within the Leading-Edge Cluster 'it's OWL', managed by the Project Management Agency Karlsruhe (PTKA), as well as by the Deutsche Forschungsgemeinschaft (DFG) within the Center of Excellence 277 'Cognitive Interaction Technology' (CITEC).

References

1. Fry, W.F.: Humor and paradox. American Behavioral Scientist 30(3), 42–71 (1987)
2. Cann, A., Calhoun, L.G.: Perceived personality associations with differences in sense of humor: Stereotypes of hypothetical others with high or low senses of humor. Humor 14(2), 117–130 (2001)
3. Martin, R.A., Kuiper, N.A.: Daily occurrence of laughter: Relationships with age, gender, and Type A personality. Humor 12(4), 355–384 (1999)
4. Norrick, N.R.: Conversational Joking: Humor in Everyday Life. Indiana University Press, Bloomington (1993)
5. Kane, T., Suls, J., Tedeschi, J.: Humour as a tool of social influence. In: Chapman, A.J., Foot, H.C. (eds.) It's a Funny Thing, Humour, pp. 13–16. Pergamon Press, Oxford (1977)
6. Hargie, O.D.W.: Communication as skilled performance. In: Hargie, O.D.W. (ed.) The Handbook of Communication Skills, 2nd edn., pp. 7–28. Routledge, London (1997)
7. Granitz, N.A., Koernig, S.K., Harich, K.R.: Now it's personal: Antecedents and outcomes of rapport between business faculty and their students. Journal of Marketing Education 31(1), 52–65 (2008)
8. Gremler, D.D., Gwinner, K.P.: Rapport-building behaviors used by retail employees. Journal of Retailing 84(3), 308–324 (2008)
9. Norrick, N.R.: Involvement and joking in conversation. Journal of Pragmatics 22(3-4), 409–430 (1994)

10. Norrick, N.R.: Issues in conversational joking. Journal of Pragmatics 35(9), 1333–1359 (2003)
11. Mettee, D.R., Hrelec, E.S., Wilkens, P.C.: Humor as an interpersonal asset and liability. The Journal of Social Psychology 85(1), 51–64 (1971)
12. Wrench, J.S., Booth-Butterfield, M.: Increasing patient satisfaction and compliance: An examination of physician humor orientation, compliance-gaining strategies, and perceived credibility. Communication Quarterly 51(4), 482–503 (2003)
13. Martin, R.A.: The Psychology of Humor: An Integrative Approach. Elsevier Academic Press, Burlington (2007)
14. O'Quin, K., Aronoff, J.: Humor as a technique of social influence. Social Psychology Quarterly 44(4), 349–357 (1981)
15. Krämer, N.C.: Theory of mind as a theoretical prerequisite to model communication with virtual humans. In: Wachsmuth, I., Knoblich, G. (eds.) ZiF Research Group International Workshop. LNCS (LNAI), vol. 4930, pp. 222–240. Springer, Heidelberg (2008)
16. Nijholt, A.: Where computers disappear, virtual humans appear. Computers & Graphics 28(4), 467–476 (2004)
17. Morkes, J., Kernal, H., Nass, C.: Effects of humor in task-oriented human-computer interaction and computer-mediated communication: A direct test of SRCT theory. Human-Computer Interaction 14(4), 395–435 (1999)
18. Bickmore, T.W., Picard, R.W.: Establishing and maintaining long-term human-computer relationships. ACM Transactions on Computer-Human Interaction 12(2), 293–327 (2005)
19. Khooshabeh, P., McCall, C., Gandhe, S., Gratch, J., Blascovich, J.: Does it matter if a computer jokes? In: CHI Conference on Human Factors in Computing Systems, pp. 77–86. ACM (2011)
20. Nijholt, A.: Embodied conversational agents: "A little humor too". IEEE Intelligent Systems 21(2), 62–64 (2006)
21. de Melo, C.M., Carnevale, P., Gratch, J.: The influence of emotions in embodied agents on human decision-making. In: Allbeck, J., Badler, N., Bickmore, T., Pelachaud, C., Safonova, A. (eds.) IVA 2010. LNCS, vol. 6356, pp. 357–370. Springer, Heidelberg (2010)
22. Kiesler, S., Sproull, L., Waters, K.: A prisoner's dilemma experiment on cooperation with people and human-like computers. Journal of Personality and Social Psychology 70(1), 47–65 (1996)
23. Gouldner, A.W.: The norm of reciprocity: A preliminary statement. American Sociological Review 25(2), 161–178 (1960)
24. Watson, D., Clark, L.A., Tellegen, A.: Development and validation of brief measures of positive and negative affect: the PANAS scales. Journal of Personality and Social Psychology 54(6), 1063–1070 (1988)
25. Bernieri, F., Gillis, J.S.: The judgment of rapport: A cross-cultural comparison between Americans and Greeks. Journal of Nonverbal Behavior 19(2), 115–130 (1995)
26. Tickle-Degnen, L., Rosenthal, R.: Group rapport and nonverbal behavior. Review of Personality and Social Psychology 9, 113–136 (1987)
27. Tickle-Degnen, L., Rosenthal, R.: The nature of rapport and its nonverbal correlates. Psychological Inquiry 1, 285–293 (1990)
28. DeSteno, D., Breazeal, C., Frank, R.H., Pizarro, D., Baumann, J., Dickens, L., Lee, J.J.: Detecting the trustworthiness of novel partners in economic exchange. Psychological Science 23(12), 1549–1556 (2012)
29. Lee, D.: Game theory and neural basis of social decision making. Nature Neuroscience 11(4), 404–409 (2008)

Towards Realistic Female Avatar Creation
A Tool for Virtual Actor Design and Player Choice

James Lee and Stefan Rank

Drexel University, Philadelphia, USA
stefan.rank @ drexel.edu

Abstract. Female gamer numbers are on the rise, but females have been disproportionately underrepresented and inaccurately portrayed in video games. Recent findings also reveal many negative effects misrepresentation can have on women's self esteem and body image. Based on a review of the literature on media effects, and using available anthropometric data, we propose a more realistic and responsive character creation tool for the designers of virtual agents and as a basis for researchers to assess the impact of female character models on the enjoyment and self-concept of the players. We first report on studies regarding media effects on women as well as the current situation regarding female player avatars as well as NPCs in games, followed by our approach towards more realistic avatar creation.

Keywords: Virtual actor design, social impact, character modeling.

1   Introduction

The portrayal of female body proportions in various media has been a heavily debated topic for years. While there have been many studies done on the sexualization and mistreatment of women in games [1] [2] [3] [4], studies that examine the body proportions of female game models regarding realism are still rare [5]. Sexualization of a character may sometimes be a subjective argument. However, offering realistic proportions of a female body to gamers should be a choice that is more widely available in all genres of games. Currently, there is a distinct disparity between video game character body proportions and real life measurements and, if left unaddressed, this disparity is likely to lead to serious negative effects in gamers' perceptions of gaming and self-concept [1] [6] [7] [8].

Research suggests the image of the body often becomes paramount to women's sense of personal identity and self worth [9]. Furthermore, research shows that media plays a significant role and becomes a source of comparison through which women and men form gender expectations and norms of females. The constant conflict that women have between the media's portrayal of the female body and their own body is an issue that may last until old age. The idealized body images found in media can lead to body image dissatisfaction in women [10] [11] [12]. Young girls briefly exposed to idealized female body images developed lower self-esteem about their own

T. Bickmore et al. (Eds.): IVA 2014, LNAI 8637, pp. 260–263, 2014.
© Springer International Publishing Switzerland 2014

bodies [13]. Exposure to idealized media images predicted bulimia, anorexia, and body dissatisfaction in middle and high school female students [14].

There are many varieties of *3D character creation tools* in video games. Different genres of video games such as action, shooter, or adventure all have distinct features regarding character creation. Not only do gamers create their avatars using these character creation tools, game developers often use the same toolset to create NPCs that populate the game as intelligent virtual agents.

In the popular MMORPG *World of Warcraft*, the character creation process involves choosing between gender, race, and cosmetic options such as hair color. However, changes to the individual body parts and proportions are not available. In the online world *Second Life*, the character creation process also allows choosing between genders and even allows players to choose options such as becoming animals, robots, or even vehicles. While the Second Life tools offer premade templates for players to choose from, full customization of the body parts is only available if players choose to upload their own models or purchase them from other players. While *EVE Online* is a persistent-world MMORPG and the game's focus is on spaceships and galactic economy, EVE Online also boasts one of the most robust and intricate avatar creation systems. Even though players spend the majority of the game without their avatars on screen, the level of detail customizable with the creation tool is similar to that of a 3D modeling/sculpting tool. In the latest iteration of the second best selling shooter franchise Battlefield, *Battlefield 4*, the character creation process is also limited to cosmetic changes such as weapon/gear textures, skin tone, and hairstyles. There are also options to choose between male and female, but the models are largely covered up by uniforms and have no options to change body proportions. In *Call of Duty: Ghosts*, the most recent release of the best selling shooter franchise, female character models are introduced for the first time. However, female character models utilize the same model sizes as the male models, to ensure fairness of the characters' "hitbox" in game. The character creation options are again limited to cosmetic changes to the skin, hair, and gear. No changes to the body proportions are available.

2   Realistic Avatar Creation

The use of a more realistic and responsive character creation tool, both in-game and for game designers, is a step towards assessing the impact of female characters' models on the enjoyment and self-concept of players. As a first step towards such a tool, we created appropriate models and a character creation tools based on the above literature review. It is intended as a proof-of-concept for such a tool and preliminary qualitative evaluation has shown interest in such a tool among game designers.

We created the "Realistic Avatar Creation" (RAC) tool for the game engine Unity based on the toolset of Unity Multipurpose Avatar (UMA). In its final incarnation, the RAC tool will have six realistic model templates based on anthropometric data sets from the U.S. Army Anthropometric surveys, the Center for Disease Control and cross-referenced with data from ANSUR and ASTM, see Fig.1. RAC also includes extensive options for body part customization, including the width and girth of chest, stomach, waists, buttocks, arms, and legs. As part of the responsive feedback for users of the tool, the tool indicates where the current choices fall on the standard deviation based on the database chosen.

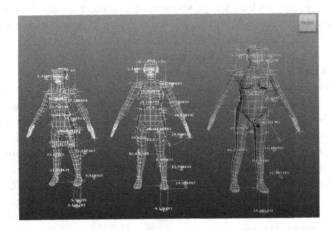

Fig. 1. 3D models based on anthropometric data

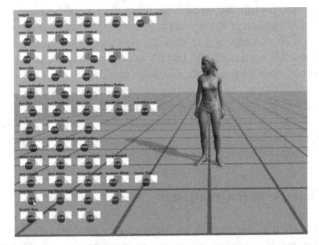

Fig. 2. Variation for displaying standard deviations in the RAC tool

The tool includes realistic model templates with body proportions based on the data sources. The goal is to recreate models that are completely proportionately accurate representations according to NSRDEC anthropometric surveys from 2007 - 2010. Based on the database from CDC and NSRDEC, the user is able to see the standard deviation displayed behind the input elements that control different body parts. This standard deviation is tied with the specific demographics requested by the user, for example, the 20 year-old female civilian CDC data. RAC also incorporates a display option that allows users to view their avatars from the side, top, front, and perspective view simultaneously. This allows users to assess their avatar's body proportions from multiple angles. To achieve usable options in the interface, models utilizes at least 20 measurements from the data sets to reproduce models of the first, fiftieth, and ninety-ninth percentile of the NSRDEC or CDC data sets respectively.

Throughout the development of the RAC tool, feedback is collected from game developers, the UMA community, and gender studies researchers to evaluate how RAC can help studying video game's effects on body image and self-efficacy. In future work, we plan to extend RAC to help game designers and gender studies researchers understand player choice regarding 3D character body proportions. Methods from game telemetry can be used as an element to document choices that users make when designing virtual agents, providing feedback for game designers on choices for the various body parts as well as the amount of time spent on each option.

References

1. Behm-Morawitz, E., Mastro, D.: The Effects of Sexualization of Female Video Game Characters on Gender Stereotyping and Female Self-Concept. Sex Roles (2009)
2. Burgess, M.: Sex, Lies, and Video Games: The Portrayal of Male and Female Characters on Video Game Covers. Sex Roles 57, 419–433 (2007)
3. Dill, K.E., Kathryn, P.T.: Video Game Characters and the Socialization of Gender Roles: Young People's Perceptions Mirror Sexist Media Depictions. Sex Roles 57, 851–864 (2007)
4. Beasley, B., Standley, T.: Shirts vs. Skins: Clothing as an Indicator of Gender Role Stereotyping in Video Games 5, 279–293 (2002)
5. Rachel, M.: Female And Male Preference. In: The Body Proportions Of Customizable Female Video Game Characters (Master's thesis, Southern Methodist University) (2011)
6. Bessenoff, G.R.: Can the media affect us: Social comparison,self-discrepancy, and the thin ideal. Psychology of Women Quarterly 30, 239–251 (2006)
7. Clay, D., Vignoles, V.L., Dittmar, H.: Body image and self-esteem among adolescent girls: Testing the influence of sociocultural factors. Journal of Research on Adolescence 15, 451–477 (2005)
8. Hawkins, N., Richards, P.S., Granley, H.M., Stein, D.M.: The impact of exposure to the thin-ideal media image on women. Eating Disorders 12, 35–50 (2004)
9. Ussher, J.M.: The Psychology of the Female Body. Routledge, New York (1989)
10. Altabe, M.N., Thompson, J.K.: Body image: A cognitive self-schema construct? Cognitive Therapy and Research 20, 171–193 (1996)
11. Heinberg, L.J., Thompson, J.K.: Body image and televised images of thinness and attractiveness: A controlled laboratory investigation. Journal of Social and Clinical Psychology 14(4), 325–338 (1995)
12. Fallon, A.: Culture in the mirror: Sociocultural determinants of body image. Body images: Development, deviance and change 21, 80–109 (1990)
13. Murnen, S.K., Smolak, L., Mills, J.A., Good, L.: Thin, sexy women and strong, muscular men: Grade-school children's responses to objectified images of women and men. Sex Roles 49(9-10), 427–437 (2003)
14. Harrison, K.: Television viewing, fat stereotyping, body shape standards, and eating disorder symptomatology in grade school children. Communication Research 27, 617–641 (2000)

Metaphoric Gestures: Towards Grounded Mental Spaces

Margot Lhommet and Stacy Marsella

Northeastern University,
360 Huntington Avenue - Boston, MA, USA
{m.lhommet,s.marsella}@neu.edu

Abstract. Gestures are related to the mental states and unfolding processes of thought, reasoning and verbal language production. This is especially apparent in the case of metaphors and metaphoric gestures. For example, talking about the importance of an idea by calling it a big idea and gesturing to indicate that large size is a manifestation of the use of metaphors in language and gesture. We propose a computational model of the influence of conceptual metaphors on gestures that maps from mental state representations of ideas to their expression in concrete, physical metaphoric gestures. This model relies on conceptual primary metaphors to map the abstract elements of the mental space to concrete physical elements that can be conveyed with gestures.

Keywords: Nonverbal behavior, gesture, metaphor, embodied cognition, embodied conversational agent.

1 Introduction

Gestures play a powerful and diverse role in face-to-face interaction. They are meaningfully related to the structure of mental states and unfolding processes of thought.

Our work focuses on a generative model of gesturing that allows virtual humans to communicate by using multimodal behaviors including speech, gesture and other nonverbal behaviors such as gaze, posture shifts or facial expressions.

When studying the relation between mental state and gestures, a key challenge arises: gestures' form and meaning are largely improvised and understood in context. *Emblems* have highly conventionalized meaning (such as the "thumb-up" gesture that means "okay" [9]). *Iconic* gestures detail the mental image conveyed by the speaker by depicting properties or actions taken on objects, such as their size or mimicking their movement. *Deictics* consist in pointing at world locations and are particularly useful to disambiguate references to objects and locations. Gestures can also be physical manifestations of abstract concepts, showing the size of ideas to represent their importance or locating events on a time line as if they were objects in space. Once materialized, physical actions can be taken on these objects such as rejecting an idea by a sideways flip of

T. Bickmore et al. (Eds.): IVA 2014, LNAI 8637, pp. 264–274, 2014.
© Springer International Publishing Switzerland 2014

the hand [2]. These gestures are called *metaphoric* since they consider abstract objects "as-if" they were concrete objects.

Gestures' meaning is manifold and context dependent. In their realization, however, gestures are physical actions in the speaker's immediate physical environment, inherently described in physical terms such as size, location or path.

Our long-term research aims to generate verbal and nonverbal behavior that realize specific communicative intentions from a speaker's mental space. In this paper, we focus on the generation of metaphorical gestures[1]. How can physically constrained gestures express such a wide range of mental states?

Indeed, speech and gesture don't reflect the entirety of ongoing thoughts. A speaker's discourse follows a flow of ideas, combining speech and nonverbal behaviors to convey certain intentions and facilitate a listener's understanding. What is actually expressed is a specific part of the mental state, a *mental space*, a "partial and temporary structure which speakers construct when thinking or talking about a perceived, imagined, past, present or future situation."[8, p.3][2]. How this mental space is built and what it contains depends on the context and on the communicative intentions of the speaker.

Our model draws inspiration from embodied cognition that suggests that we use the same set of sensory and motor representation to make sense of our world. Cognitive linguists proposed the Conceptual Metaphor Theory according to which we understand abstract concepts by mapping them to concrete elements by using *conceptual metaphors* (sometimes called *image schemas*) [12]. For example, we make sense of a "big idea" by mapping the importance of an idea (an abstract property of an abstract object) to the size of a concrete object.

We propose that, to be expressed with gestures, the mental space has first to be conceptually grounded, i.e. mapped to concrete elements from which they inherit physical properties. These properties are then combined into gestures that convey the desired communicative intentions. Such a model supports a generative model of gesturing that:

1. allows for a large space of mental representations to be mapped to a comparatively small space of metaphoric gestures,
2. can convey complex communicative intentions via composition over this small set of gestures,
3. guides how properties in abstract propositions (such as "important idea") can be conveyed by manipulations of the gestures (big gesture).

After describing the components of our model, we detail its current implementation and illustrate it with examples. Finally, we comment on the implementation and discuss future work.

---

[1] See the discussion for an account of the generation of multimodal behavior.
[2] A mental space is similar to McNeill's Growth Point, "a minimal unit of dialectic in which imagery and linguistic content are combined."[18, p.18]

2   Related Work

Researchers have explored several techniques to automate the generation of virtual humans' nonverbal behaviors that realize communicative intentions.

Most approaches take speech as input to generate appropriate nonverbal behavior, but they differ on how the models were developed, the degree of automation in the generation process itself and the particular classes of nonverbal behaviors that are handled. Specifically, some systems use annotated text that specifies what information has to be conveyed nonverbally (e.g. [11]). Such approach is cumbersome since it requires manual annotations of the utterance's text. Data-driven techniques can automate the generation of specific classes of nonverbal behaviors from specific input. For example, prosody has been used to generate gestures [16] and text has been mapped to head movements [14] and gesturing style [10,19]. Another approach consists in analyzing the speech to infer the underlying communicative intentions. BEAT infers rheme and theme from the text to generate intonation and emphasis [3]. NVBG detects communicative functions in the text (e.g. affirmation, emphasis, disfluencies) based on a keywords mapping [15]. Cerebella integrates acoustic, syntactic and semantic analyses to infer communicative intentions and elements of the mental state (emotional state, energy, emphasis,...) [17]. The common critique is that while deeper and more elaborate analyses allow inferring and conveying the communicative intentions present in the speech, the nonverbal behavior generated is limited in the range of what can be inferred from the speech utterance only.

This can be overcome by integrating deeper cognitive processes that co-generate speech and gesture. [1] study the co-production and coordination of speech and gesture production under linguistic and cognitive constraints. In particular they show how the conceptualization of path, motion and manner constrain speech and iconic gesture production. [13] formalize the relation of gesture and speech with a logical form of multimodal discourse, in particular between a discourse's spatial elements and deictic gestures.

Our goal is the co-generation of speech and gesture based on a common representation of the communicative intentions. Therefore, our work investigates the content of this underlying common representation (the mental space) and the processes that map it to speech, gestures and nonverbal behaviors. In particular, we propose to explicitly represent the mental space and its grounded counterparts, that allows to combine its expression through multiple channels as well as representing sequences of actions taken on existing elements. In this paper, we investigate the generation of metaphorical gestures.

3   Model

The Figure 1 presents the elements involved in our model. To generate a gesture plan according to a mental space, we propose to ground this mental space in concrete domains by using primary metaphors. Primary metaphors are conventional mappings that associate elements from abstract domains to elements

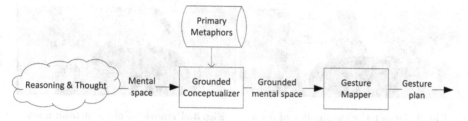

Fig. 1. Elements and processes of the model.

in the concrete domain [12,8]. "There are hundreds of such primary conceptual metaphors, most of them learned unconsciously and automatically in childhood simply by functioning in the everyday world with a human body and brain. There are primary metaphors for time, causation, events, morality, emotions, and other domains that are central to human thought" [12, p.257].

Mental Space. What the processes of thought and reasoning look like, what the content of the mental space is, are open questions that we do not claim to answer in their entirety. We define a mental space as a structure that reflects communicative intentions: it contains the information to express, as well as information regarding how to express it or modify something previously said.

Grounded Conceptualizer. The Grounded Conceptualizer maps the abstract elements of a mental space to concrete physical elements. This mapping consists in a systematic projection of the objects, properties and relations from one domain to another and is based on primary metaphors. Once grounded, the abstract elements of the mental space have concrete counterparts that can be expressed with gestures and the communicative intention is mapped into actions on these concrete objects.

Gesture Mapper. Gestures are physical actions on the speaker's immediate physical environment. Therefore, gestures are inherently described in physical terms such as size, location, path... The Gesture Mapper generates a gesture plan by combining the concrete elements of the grounded mental space according to the communicative intention.

4   Implementation

In this paper, we formalize the relation between an abstract idea and a concrete object, and a set and a container, respectively following the metaphors AB-STRACT OBJECT IS CONCRETE OBJECT and SET IS A CONTAINER). These two metaphors seem to be the root elements involved in many primary metaphors [12,8]. Indeed, the concrete domains used in metaphorical mappings can be more elaborated but in this paper we explore the range of metaphors and metaphorical gestures that we can reach with these two.

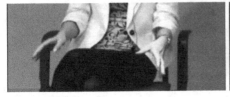   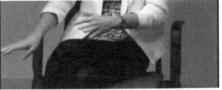

Fig. 2. Depict the cardinality of a set   **Fig. 3.** Remove an element from a set

In this section, we detail the current implementation of our model. We use an example that comes from a role-play conversation between a clinician (the speaker) and an actress pretending to suffer from PTSD (Figures 2-6).

4.1 Mental Space

The two main concepts used in this paper are *elements* and *sets*. Elements represent abstract concepts. they have a type, some properties and can be associated to other elements via predicates. Sets are structures that group elements sharing a similar property. Mental spaces are described using OpenCyc[3].

In this paper, we demonstrate the implementation of three communicative intentions:

- Depict a property of an element: *depict_property(e p)*
- Manipulate an existing set[4] to add or remove elements: *add(e s) remove(e s)*.
- Contrast the difference of value between a property of two elements[5]: *contrast(p e1 e2)*

As stated above, the content of the mental space is driven by what information is required to convey a specific intention with metaphoric gestures. The information required for these communicative intentions is given below.

Depict a property

```
(operation depict_property(s p))
(isa s set)
(p s value)
```

Remove an element

```
(operation remove(s e))
(isa e element)
(isa s set)
(contains s e)
```

Contrast two elements

```
(operation contrast(p e1 e2))
(isa p property)
(isa e1 element)
(isa e2 element)
(f e1 value1)
(f e2 value2)
```

---

[3] OpenCyc is a large ontology-like knowledge base. Collections are hierarchically organized and properties can be inherited. http://www.cyc.com

[4] The grounded elements of the mental space are persistent over time.

[5] For clarity we only show a contrast between two elements, but the notation could be extended to consider more of them.

Example. The clinician asks: "(1) Is there anything, (2) besides what he wants, anything you want to work on?" On the first part of the sentence (1), she offers to discuss any thing and depicts the cardinality of a large set that contains all the possible discussion topics (see Figure 2). On the second part of the sentence (2), she realizes that there is a topic included in this set that she does not want to discuss ("what your husband wants") so she removes it from the set, generating a similar action on the container created earlier (see Figure 3). These mental spaces are described below.

Depict cardinality	*Remove an element*
```(operation depict_property(s cardinality))```	
```(isa s set)```	```(operation remove(s e))```
```(cardinality s count(s contains t))```	```(isa e element)```
```(forall t```	```(isa s set)```
``` (and (isa t element)```	```(contains s e)```
``` (type t discussionTopics)```	```(type e discussionTopics)```
``` (contains s t)))```	```(wants husband e)```

4.2   Grounded Conceptualizer

The Grounded Conceptualizer maps the abstract elements of the mental space to physical properties that convey the same meaning. As mentioned above, we particularly study the domains of *Object* and *Container*. An *Object* has physical properties such as a size, a weight, a location . . . A *Container* is an object that contains other objects.

A set of rules, based on primary metaphors, maps the content of the mental space to physical objects and properties. The following rules state that an element is mapped to an object and a set to a container.

```
(type e element) --> (type e' object)
(type e set) --> (type e' container)
```

OpenCyc uses a large hierarchy of collections to represent concrete elements such as Location, Path, Shape. . . that we use to represent the physical properties of objects and containers. Once the mapping space is grounded, the physical knowledge is leveraged by rules that represent the logics of the physical world. These objects are created in a specific micro-theory inside OpenCyc to control the inferences that are made. For example, the rule below associates a container's location to the objects it contains.

```
(type c container) (location c loc) (contains c obj) --> (location obj loc)
```

Example. To illustrate this grounding process, we show how the first part of the sentence cited earlier is grounded and what information is elaborated. The set of possible topics is mapped to a container that contains all topics objects. The operation consisting in depicting the cardinality of the set is mapped to an operation depicting the size of the bound container. A physical inference is made: the size of a container depends on what it contains; here, the whole set of topic objects, and is therefore big.

```
(type s' container)                    (operation depict_property(s' size))
(contains s' (all (type  t' object)))  (size s' big)
```

4.3   Gesture Mapper

Generic gesture rules combine the physical properties of the grounded mental space according to the desired communicative function. They are explained below and illustrated on the previous examples.

Depict a Property. Because they are grounded, all abstract properties (such as the importance or the cardinality of a set) are mapped to physical elements (for example, size, location, shape, weight,...). The physical properties of objects are retrieved to generate a gesture. In particular, the salient property to express (p) and its value val are added to the gesture specification. Other physical properties are also added to further refine the gesture, but they are optional. For example, the first part of the clinician sentence (i.e. "Is there anything you want to talk about ?") is transformed into the following structure:

```
<goal=depict id=Container01 type=container size=big/>
```

Add or Remove an Element from a Set. This communicative intention implies that the set (and the bound container) already exist in the mental space (as well as in the physical gesture space, i.e. they have a location). The gesture rule to remove an element from a container is:

```
(operation remove(s o)), (isa s container), (location s loc)
--> <goal=remove source_location=loc target=not(location)/>
```

4.4   Other examples

To show the range of metaphorical gestures that our model can generate, let's study how the general representation and processes we just defined can be used to express an enumeration and a contrast.

Enumerating a Set. An enumeration is a rhetorical structure that consists in denoting each element of a set. The elements are grounded as objects inside a container and the enumeration operation consists in depicting the "contains" property of the container. This creates a unit with one discourse root whose goal is to enumerate each elements. Each element inside the container is then sequentially depicted at the container's location.

```
(operation (depict_property(c contains)))
--> <goals goal=enumerate type=container id=GenId() location=(location c)/>
    for each element (contains c e):
      <goal=depict location=(location c) type=object/>
    </goals>
```

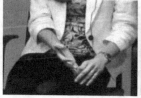 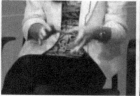 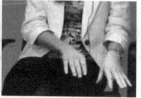

Fig. 4. Enumeration   **Fig. 5.** Contrast now   **Fig. 6.** Contrast past

Example. At the beginning of the conversation, the clinician counts on her left-hand fingers the specific facts mentioned by the patient's husband. (see Figure 4).

Contrast. A contrast shows the difference of value between a property of two elements. For example, we compare the size of two persons or the duration of two movies.

When applied to the concept, the property returns a scalar value that is grounded as a location on an axis (horizontal, vertical or frontal axis). Most of the properties returning a scalar value use the vertical axis (following the metaphor MORE IS UP). Properties associated to time points use the horizontal axis when the speaker is not actively involved (PROGRESSION IS A WRITING LINE), and the frontal line when she is (PROGRESSION IS MOVING FORWARD) [2].

Example. When the clinician says: "You and him feel a little bit distant compared to how it used to be in the past.", she contrasts the situation now and how it was. Her mental space is described on the first column above.

To ground this mental space, the Grounded Conceptualizer first retrieves the axis associated to the *time* property (*horizontal axis*). Then, the abstract values (*now* and *past*) returned by the p*time* roperty are mapped to locations on the axis; the primary metaphors PAST IS LEFT and PRESENT IS CENTER are used. Finally, the communicative intention is mapped to depicting the two locations, leading to a sequence of gestures that locates each object (see Figures 5 and 6).

Mental Space	*Grounded Mental Space*
`(type s1 Situation)`	
`(actors s1 (patient husband))`	
`(time s1 now)`	`(operation depict_property(location s1 s2))`
`(type s2 Situation)`	`(type isa Object)`
`(actors s2 (patient husband))`	`(location s1 horizontal:center)`
`(time s2 past)`	`(type s2 Object)`
`(operation contrast(time s1 s2))`	`(location s2 horizontal:left)`

5 Discussion

In this paper, we showed that our model can transform various different mental spaces into gestures specifications by grounding their elements in a physical context. We particularly detailed the conceptual mapping from *abstract object* and *set* to *concrete object* and *container*. We showed how properties in abstract propositions can be conveyed by physical properties of gestures and presented how a relatively small set of operations can combine the physical components of the grounded mental spaces to convey a speaker's more elaborated communicative intention such as an enumeration or a contrast over time.

Even though the model presented in this paper focuses on the generation of metaphorical gestures, we believe that it is generic enough to take into account other kinds of gestures, namely *iconics* and *deictics*. Since *Iconics* consist in depicting one physical property of an object, the mental space is already grounded and the gesture can be directed specified. *Deictics* require information about the objects location in the physical space so pointing gestures can be appropriately generated. Therefore, integrating these other gestures in this framework seem, *a priori*, feasible.

Another question regards the generation of multimodal performances that would go beyond gestures. Two options can be considered. First, this model could be coupled to a behavior planner that generates nonverbal behaviors using either a natural language generator capable of also generating communicative intentions along with the utterance, or an inference process that would derive the underlying mental space from the utterance text and audio (in a process similar to inference-based behavior planners like Cerebella [17]). Generating nonverbal behaviors based on what is expressed in the speech confines the gesture performance as an illustration of the speech. The other -preferred- option consists in integrating this model in an architecture that generates speech and gesture. One lead is the model of [5] because it supports an arbitrary granularity of semantics that would allow us to align the natural language generation to the granularity of our mental space representation.

A key issue with the current implementation concerns selecting between alternative metaphors. For example, to convey that one idea is important, the grounding conceptualizer detects that "idea" and "importance" are abstract concepts and try to map them to concrete objects and properties. Therefore, it has to select which property is appropriate to represent the abstract notion of importance. By using primary metaphors, either the size or the weight could convey the desired intent[6]. Currently, we randomly pick one candidate mapping. Other options would be to internally evaluate the performances resulting from all candidate mappings. Because conflicts may arise downstream, such as incompatible grounded spaces or the absence of an appropriate gesture in the virtual human repertoire, the generated performance might not actually convey the speaker's intentions. Preferences could be propagated backwards to decide which mapping to use in this specific context.

A preferable option would be to have a deeper model of what influences this choice. Several researchers have focused on this question. For example, the

---

[6] Much more information about which salient property to express is required to guide the grounding process and address the subtle distinction that a "heavy" decision has negative outcomes if one is wrong.

Structure Mapping Theory computes similarity by detecting a similar structure in source and target elements [7]. Since primary metaphors are not based on any objective similarity, they cannot be detected or generated by similarity-based model.

More fundamentally, this problem arises because we currently separate the reasoning and thought process from the conceptual grounding process. In a more radical view of embodied cognition, they could be treated as a combined process and the mental spaces would be inherently grounded. The grounding conceptualizer would not be a process in itself, but an underlying process on top of which our whole thinking and reasoning system is based. Creating such a model would require to understand -and computationally model- the whole range and dynamics of thought and reasoning, which still seems quite unrealistic.

Instead, we propose to keep on incrementally leveraging the mental space representation and its relation to gesture, speech and nonverbal behaviors. We will study what information is salient in speech, other kinds of gestures and nonverbal behaviors, and how these modalities relate to each other. Each one can embellish, substitute for and even contradict the information conveyed by the others [6]. For example, the same communicative intention can be expressed by co-occurrent yet different metaphors in speech and gesture [4]. This raises a number of issues concerning whether each modality can have its own grounded space, what determines what part is conveyed by each modality and how these modalities are synchronized.

Beyond providing virtual humans with better communication skills, addressing such questions will inform both the representation of the mental space and the dynamic processes resulting from thought and reasoning, from a perspective that merges cognitive linguistics and gesture studies.

References

1. Bergmann, K., Kahl, S., Kopp, S.: Modeling the semantic coordination of speech and gesture under cognitive and linguistic constraints. In: Aylett, R., Krenn, B., Pelachaud, C., Shimodaira, H. (eds.) IVA 2013. LNCS, vol. 8108, pp. 203–216. Springer, Heidelberg (2013)
2. Calbris, G.: From left to right: Coverbal gestures and their symbolic use of space. Metaphor and Gesture, 27–53 (2008)
3. Cassell, J., Vilhjálmsson, H.H., Bickmore, T.: BEAT: the behavior expression animation toolkit. In: Proc.of the 28th Conference on Computer Graphics and Interactive Techniques, SIGGRAPH 2001, pp. 477–486. ACM, New York (2001)
4. Cienki, A., Müller, C.: Metaphor and gesture. John Benjamins Pub. Co. (2008)
5. DeVault, D., Traum, D., Artstein, R.: Practical grammar-based NLG from examples. In: Proc. of the 5th International Natural Language Generation Conference, pp. 77–85. Asso. for Computational Linguistics (2008)
6. Ekman, P., Friesen, W.V.: Nonverbal leakage and clues to deception. Psychiatry: Journal for the Study of Interpersonal Processes 32(1), 88–106 (1969)
7. Gentner, D.: Structure-Mapping: a theoretical framework for analogy. Cognitive Science 7(2), 155–170 (1983)

8. Grady, J., Oakley, T., Coulson, S.: Blending and metaphor. Metaphor in Cognitive Linguistics, 101–124 (1999)
9. Kendon, A.: Language and gesture. In: McNeill, D. (ed.) Language and Gesture. No. 2 in Language, culture & cognition, pp. 47–63. Cambridge Univ. P. (2000)
10. Kopp, S., Bergmann, K.: Individualized gesture production in embodied conversational agents. In: Human-Computer Interaction, pp. 287–301 (2012)
11. Kopp, S., Wachsmuth, I.: Model-based animation of co-verbal gesture. In: Proceedings of Computer Animation, pp. 252–257 (2002)
12. Lakoff, G., Johnson, M.: Metaphors we live by. Univ. of Chicago Press (1980)
13. Lascarides, A., Stone, M.: A formal semantic analysis of gesture. Journal of Semantics 26(4), 393–449 (2009)
14. Lee, J., Marsella, S.: Learning a model of speaker head nods using gesture corpora. In: Conference on Autonomous Agents and Multiagent Systems, pp. 289–296 (2009)
15. Lee, J., Marsella, S.C.: Nonverbal behavior generator for embodied conversational agents. In: Gratch, J., Young, M., Aylett, R.S., Ballin, D., Olivier, P. (eds.) IVA 2006. LNCS (LNAI), vol. 4133, pp. 243–255. Springer, Heidelberg (2006)
16. Levine, S., Krähenbühl, P., Thrun, S., Koltun, V.: Gesture controllers. ACM Trans. Graph. 29(4), 1–124 (2010)
17. Lhommet, M., Marsella, S.C.: Gesture with meaning. In: Aylett, R., Krenn, B., Pelachaud, C., Shimodaira, H. (eds.) IVA 2013. LNCS, vol. 8108, pp. 303–312. Springer, Heidelberg (2013)
18. McNeill, D.: Gesture and thought. Univ. of Chicago Press (2005)
19. Neff, M., Kipp, M., Albrecht, I., Seidel, H.-P.: Gesture modeling and animation based on a probabilistic recreation of speaker style. ACM Transactions on Graphics 27(1), 5 (2008)

From Data to Storytelling Agents

Boyang Li, Mohini Thakkar, Yijie Wang, and and Mark O. Riedl

School of Interactive Computing, Georgia Institute of Technology,
Atlanta, GA 30332, USA
{boyangli,mthakkar,yijiewang,riedl}@gatech.edu

Abstract. The ability to craft, tell, and understand stories is important for virtual agents that wish to communicate with human users and simulate human capabilities. We provide an overview of an end-to-end storytelling system named SCHEHERAZADE, which learns domain-specific narrative knowledge from crowdsourced stories, generates stories and discourses, and presents stories in natural language with diverse personal styles and sentiments. Extending previous work, this paper addresses discourse planning and text generation. Discourse planning selectively omits events using typicality of events derived from graph structures. Text generation considers language features computed directly from large-scale data sets such as the Google N-Gram Corpus and Project Gutenberg books. Learning from these data sets instills virtual agents with linguistic and social behavioral knowledge.

1   Introduction

Storytelling is considered a hallmark of human intelligence and an effective method to build interpersonal bonding. As a result, storytelling can be used by virtual characters to communicate effectively with human users. Bickmore, Schulman, and Yin [2] describe a study where virtual healthcare agents were equipped with the ability to gossip about the lives they supposedly have lived when not interacting with a human. The agents are shown to engage human users, leading to prolonged periods of interaction. For storytelling agents that intend to interact with human users over the long term, such as in chronic patient care, the traditional technique of manual scripting all stories becomes impractical. Automated story generation techniques, on the other hand, requires substantial amount of knowledge in order to produce coherent and interesting stories. Most current story generation systems are manually set up to operate in only a few micro-worlds at a time.

Open Story Generation systems (e.g. [5,7,11]) can learn the needed knowledge for story generation and storytelling without *a priori* knowledge engineering about a particular domain. This paper extends prior work [4,5] to address the problem of *telling* the story with different personal styles and sentiments from virtual characters.

Our system is an end-to-end storytelling system whereas other Open Story Generation systems tend to focus on selected aspects of storytelling. The SayAnything system [11] generates stories from snippets of natural language mined from

T. Bickmore et al. (Eds.): IVA 2014, LNAI 8637, pp. 275–278, 2014.

blogs. However, it requires human intervention to maintain story coherence. McIntyre and Lapata [7] learn plot graphs containing temporal precedences in the domain of fairy tales and use a genetic algorithm to maximize the coherence of generated stories. They do not explicitly model discourse or generate stories with different linguistic styles and sentiments.

Several systems generate speech for virtual characters in storytelling applications. Rowe *et al.* [10] rely on manual-authored knowledge but use probabilistic unification grammar to improve robustness. The PERSONAGE system [6] maps the introversion / extraversion psychological dimension to a large number of linguistic parameters and has been used to generate text for stories [9]. Instead of generating from a symbolic representation, we select from existing sentences and consider an additional parameter, fictionality.

2   The SCHEHERAZADE System

The SCHEHERAZADE system [4, 5] learns the structure of events in a given situation from crowdsourced exemplar stories describing that situation. The system architecture is shown in Figure 1. SCHEHERAZADE is a just-in-time learner; if the system does not know the structure of a situation when it is called for, it attempts to learn what it needs to know from a crowd of people on the Web. This results in a script-like knowledge structure, called a *plot graph*. The graph contains events that can be expected to occur, temporal precedences between events, and mutual exclusions between events that create branching alternatives.

After acquiring a number of crowdsourced exemplar stories for a particular social or procedural situation from Amazon Mechanical Turk (AMT), the learning of the plot graph proceeds in four steps. First, we cluster sentences with similar semantic meaning from exemplar stories, each cluster becoming one event in the plot graph. In order to reduce the difficulty in natural language processing, we have asked crowd workers from AMT to use simple language, i.e., using one sentence with a single verb to describe one event, avoiding pronouns, etc. In the second step, we identify temporal precedences between the events by formulating a constrained integer optimization problem. We compute the confidence for each possible temporal precedence by performing a hypothesis testing based on the binomial distribution. Precedence relations with confidence lower than 50% are excluded. The optimization preserves as many precedence relations as possible while avoiding cycles in the plot graph. The third step learns mutual exclusion relations using mutual information. Two events involved in the same mutual exclusion relation cannot both happen in the same story. The final step identifies certain events as optional, so that it is possible for each event to appear in at least one generated story.

Story generation in SCHEHERAZADE is the process of generating a linear sequence of events while respecting the constraints posed by the temporal precedences, mutual exclusion relations, and event optionality. This linear sequence contains all events that are presumed to have happened in the virtual world, which may be told as a story. A user study shows the stories generated to be of good coherence [5].

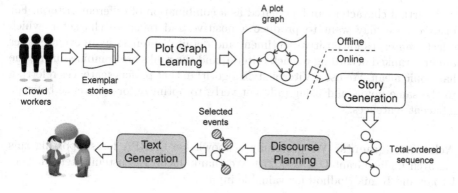

Fig. 1. The system pipeline

This paper addresses two later stages in Figure 1: discourse planning and text generation. Discourse planning is the process of selecting a subset of events from all events presumed to have happened. Though a story can contain every event that happened, there are probably trivial and uninteresting events that we want to avoid in an interesting story. We propose that an interesting story should contain some events very typical to a situation to establish and communicate this situation, as well as events that are relatively rare to make the story interesting. An event's typicality is computed from the connectivity in the plot graph, using an algorithm based on Personalized Page Rank [3], incorporating bias for events frequently appearing in the corpus and penalties for mutual exclusivity.

Text generation depicts a given event sequence in a verbal format. SCHEHERA-ZADE selects sentences from the exemplar stories to describe each event and creates the desired style of the virtual character in terms of the level of detail, fictional language, and sentiments. We model the amount of details as the probability of a sentence in English, as Information Theory suggests a less likely sentence should contain more information. The probability of a sentence is computed using the bag-of-word model, where the probability of each English word is its frequency in the Google N-Gram corpus [8]. We further model the *fictionality* of a sentence, or how much its language resembles fictional novels. The language used in fictions has distinctive word choice as fictions tend to accurately describe actions (e.g. "snatch" instead of "take"), emotions, and make less use of formal words (e.g. facility, presentation). The fictionality of a word is the ratio between its frequencies in Google N-Gram's "English Fiction 2012" corpus and the "English 2012" corpus. The fictionality of a sentence is a weighted average of the words it contains. In modeling the sentiments of sentences, we improve SentiWordNet (SWN) [1], a sentiment dictionary, to reduce erroneous values and expand its coverage. Sentiment values from SWN are used as seeds. New sentiments for words are computed by smoothing seed values over a corpus containing 9108 English fiction books from Project Gutenberg (www.gutenberg.org), based on the intuition that neighboring words should have similar sentiments.

A virtual character can be created as a combination of different criteria. For instance, we may want to produce a positive and talkative character, which selects sentences for positive sentiment and detail. Sentences in an event cluster are first ranked according to each criteria, and the ranks are combined using the harmonic mean. We use a Viterbi-style algorithm that prefers sentences referring to the same nouns and using different verbs to optimize for coherence between adjacent sentences.

Acknowledgments. We gratefully acknowledge DARPA for supporting this research under Grant D11AP00270. We thank Jacob Eisenstein, Stephen Lee-Urban and Rania Hodhod for valuable inputs.

References

1. Baccianella, S., Esuli, A., Sebastani, F.: SENTIWORDNET 3.0: An enhanced lexical resource for sentiment analysis and opinion mining. In: The 7th Conference on International Language Resources and Evaluation (2010)
2. Bickmore, T., Schulman, D., Yin, L.: Engagement vs. Deceit: Virtual humans with human autobiographies. In: Ruttkay, Z., Kipp, M., Nijholt, A., Vilhjálmsson, H.H. (eds.) IVA 2009. LNCS, vol. 5773, pp. 6–19. Springer, Heidelberg (2009)
3. Haveliwala, T.H.: Topic-sensitive PageRank. In: The 11th International World Wide Web Conference (2002)
4. Li, B., Lee-Urban, S., Appling, D.S., Riedl, M.O.: Crowdsourcing narrative intelligence. Advances in Cognitive Systems 2 (2012)
5. Li, B., Lee-Urban, S., Johnston, G., Riedl, M.O.: Story generation with crowd-sourced plot graphs. In: The 27th AAAI Conference on Artificial Intelligence (2013)
6. Mairesse, F., Walker, M.A.: PERSONAGE: Personality generation for dialogue. In: The 45th Annual Meeting of the Association for Computational Linguistics (2007)
7. McIntyre, N., Lapata, M.: Plot induction and evolutionary search for story generation. In: The 48th Annual Meeting of the Association for Computational Linguistics, pp. 1562–1572 (2010)
8. Michel, J.B., Shen, Y., Aiden, A., Veres, A., Gray, M., Brockman, W., Pickett, J., Hoiberg, D., Clancy, D., Norvig, P., Orwant, J., Pinker, S., Nowak, M., Aiden, E.: Quantitative analysis of culture using millions of digitized books. Science 331, 176–182 (2011)
9. Rishes, E., Lukin, S.M., Elson, D.K., Walker, M.A.: Generating different story tellings from semantic representations of narrative. In: Koenitz, H., Sezen, T.I., Ferri, G., Haahr, M., Sezen, D., Çatak, G. (eds.) ICIDS 2013. LNCS, vol. 8230, pp. 192–204. Springer, Heidelberg (2013)
10. Rowe, J.P., Ha, E.Y., Lester, J.C.: Archetype-driven character dialogue generation for interactive narrative. In: Prendinger, H., Lester, J.C., Ishizuka, M. (eds.) IVA 2008. LNCS (LNAI), vol. 5208, pp. 45–58. Springer, Heidelberg (2008)
11. Swanson, R., Gordon, A.: Say anything: Using textual case-based reasoning to enable open-domain interactive storytelling. ACM Transactions on Interactive Intelligent Systems 2, 1–35 (2012)

Building Community and Commitment with a Virtual Coach in Mobile Wellness Programs

Stephanie M. Lukin[1], G. Michael Youngblood[2],
Honglu Du[2], and Marilyn Walker[1]

[1] Natural Language and Dialogue Systems Lab,
University of California Santa Cruz, Santa Cruz, CA, USA
{slukin,maw}@soe.ucsc.edu
[2] Interactive Intelligence Area,
PARC, a Xerox Company, Palo Alto, CA, USA
{michael.youngblood,honglu.du}@parc.com

Abstract. FittleBot is virtual coach provided as part of a mobile application named Fittle that aims to provide users with social support and motivation for achieving the user's health and wellness goals. Fittle's wellness challenges are based around teams, where each team has its own FittleBot to provide personalized recommendations, support team building and provide information or tips. Here we present a quantitative analysis from a 2-week field study where we test new FittleBot strategies to increase FittleBot's effectiveness in building team community. Participants using the enhanced FittleBot improved compliance over the two weeks by 8.8% and increased their sense of community by 4%.

Keywords: Virtual Agents, Health, Wellness, Conversation, Social.

1 Introduction

Personalization is a critical feature of natural interaction and there is growing evidence that virtual agents that deliver personalized interaction are more effective. For example, virtual agents that match the user's personality have been shown to help the user spend more time doing their exercises [1], or are judged as more competent at the task [2,3]. Our work aims to build social capital [4,5] in teams of users through the use of an *in-situ* virtual agent called FittleBot in the conversation feed of the Fittle mobile, social wellness-related application [6]. FittleBot participates in the team by developing and exerting its own social influence [7] within the team. Our belief is that an artificial agent can increase the overall level of engagement in the system through interventions in the activity space of an application.

The Fittle platform is highly team oriented. We want the participants to feel connected to their team mates whom they may not know, but share a desire to take care of their health, as in other related work [8,9]. There exists a temptation to defect in these social systems [10]. Group performance in Fittle is important, and if one individual doesn't perform well, the overall performance

T. Bickmore et al. (Eds.): IVA 2014, LNAI 8637, pp. 279–284, 2014.

goes down. Building social accountability and leveraging social influence have been shown to help counteract defections, but more work is needed in this area especially with regard to using team-based social agents to maintain and improve engagement. This paper aims to better understand how virtual agents can participate effectively in a social teams oriented to achieving particular health and wellness goals.

2   Design and Empirical Evaluation

We present a 2-week field study comparing the enhanced Fittlebot2 with Fittlebot-Basic [6]. FittleBot2 has new interaction strategies intended to foster a sense of community, increase social accountability and decrease defection. Fittlebot2 attempts to engage users unobtrusively and naturally by prompting team members with self reflective comments and conversation starters. We hypothesize that an increase in trust needs to happen early on in the challenge before the team can begin to support each others' goals. We believe that this also applies to groups who do know each other in person, but may not be as close or are not sure how to interact with each other through Fittle. FittleBot2 support strategies include asking questions in a generic way and allowing users to answer concisely (Fig. 1). FittleBot2 also encourages users to reflect about self progress and provides information and shares knowledge with the team to develop a sense of comradery and shared goals.

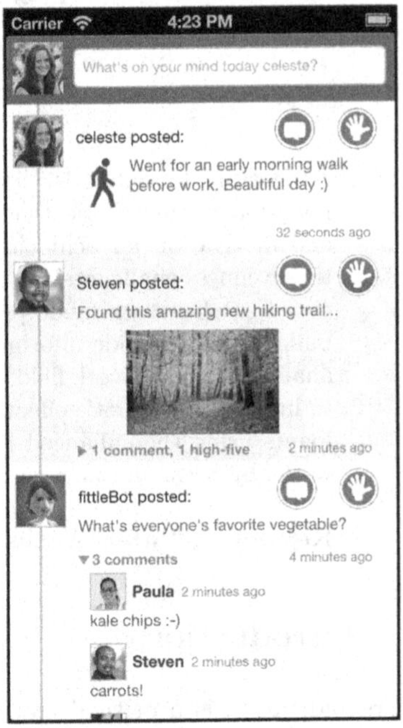

Fig. 1. Fittle mobile application team-based social activity feed

The study uses the Presidential Activity Lifestyle Award Challenge (PALA+). PALA+ is a loosely detailed routine with room for adaptability and preference selection. Every day, participants perform a physical activity for 30 minutes and work towards incorporating a new healthy eating habit each week. All the instructions are adapted directly from the PALA+ website or prepared by certified trainers from a third party.

We collected information about the participants' personality, and demographic information of age, gender, and ethnicity. Pre-test and post-test surveys assess participants general attitudes towards nutrition and physical activities. After the experiment, a post survey asked questions about participants general attitudes towards the FittleBot and their team. We measure "attitudes towards FittleBot" with a 3-item, 7-point scale, "perceived social support" with an adapted 9-item,

7-point scale from [11], and "sense of community" with an adapted 8-item, 7-point scale from [12] detailed in the next section.

3   Experimental Results

Participants in this study were volunteers from a research center on the west coast of the U.S. The participants were required to read English and be age 18 or older and were not compensated in any manner. Fourteen people signed up for the study. The average age of the participants is 44 years old (SD=8), ranging from 31 to 60 years of age. Seven of the participants are White; 6 Asian; and 1 Hispanic. We split the participants into 2 teams of 7 people each. Teams were distributed across gender and previous Fittle experience, so that 3 experienced Fittle users were present on both teams.

Both teams participated in the two-week PALA+ challenge. One team was given FittleBot-Basic, and the other team was assigned to FittleBot2. None of the team members knew each other prior to the study. This created an ideal environment for testing pre and post study sense of community. Two experienced Fittle individuals on each team were asked to be team leaders.

Table 1. Groups in the study and average compliance rate; Mean (Standard Deviation)

	FittleBot2 Team	FittleBot-Basic Team
Participants (M/F)	7 (2/5)	7 (3/4)
Week 1 Compliance (%)	69.4 (31.3)	79.6 (30.4)
Week 2 Compliance (%)	73.5 (19.2)	45.6 (33.5)
Average 2-week Compliance (%)	71.4 (24.7)	62.6 (26.7)

Table 1 shows the distribution of the participants' compliance in the challenge, and shows that the FittleBot2 team has a higher overall compliance. Furthermore, the compliance rate actually improves for the FittleBot2 team while it drops drastically for the FittleBot-Basic team ($t(12) = 0.62$, $p = 0.54$ for week 1; $t(10) = 0.01$, $p = 0.08$ for week 2; $t(12) = 0.64$, $p = 0.53$ for average 2-weeks). The FittleBot-Basic team started off strong, but exhibits the typical Law of Attrition drop off rates from the first to second weeks. Interestingly, the FittleBot2 team starts off less strong, and increases compliance in the second week. Next, we explore the impact of specific elements of FittleBot2 and analyze the results of the post surveys

Conversation starters. Conversation starters were posted by FittleBot2 once a day if there seemed to be little activity within the team, to try to encourage members to log on and share. Five of the 7 team members of the FittleBot2 team responded to "What's everyone's favorite vegetable?" with a variety of responses: "yellow beets!!", "Tough choice...Asparagus and broccoli are a close first...Spinach cooked or salad...", "Raw: peppers; cooked, with oil and garlic and ginger: eggplant. But heritage tomatoes are pretty darn good too. And broccoli with cheese", "Large pea leaf sprouts", "Brussels sprouts—sauteed so they carmelize". FittleBot2 also provided self reflection questions like "What are you hoping to gain from this challenge?" Some team responses included "I'll be going on a canoe trip next summer and I want to get into a routine that improves my upper body strength so I will enjoy the trip more," and "Positive and healthier lifestyle changes." Two other team members supported their teammates' answers with a *High Five* (the Fittle app equivalent of a *Like*).

Attitudes towards FittleBot. We looked at how each team felt about their own team and the way that FittleBot paid attention to them as an individual and a team. Across teams, the FittleBot2 team felt stronger about FittleBot ($t(21) = 2.57$, $p < 0.01$, Cohen's $d = 0.95$; means 4.6 and 3.5 respectively). Across teams, there was no different between the FittleBot2 team and FittleBot-Basic team's attitudes towards their team ($t(22) = 0.98$, $p = 0.37$, Cohen's $d = 0.37$; means 5.6 and 5.2 respectively). Within each team, the FittleBot-Basic team feels stronger about their own team ($t(22) = 3.8$, $p < 0.005$, Cohen's $d = 1.39$; means 5.2 and 3.5 respectively) and the FittleBot2 team surprising show no difference in their attitudes towards the team and FittleBot ($t(20) = 2.6$, $p = 0.013$, Cohen's $d = 0.9$; means 4.5 and 5.6 respectively). This suggests that the FittleBot2 team perceives their own team and FittleBot similarly in terms attention paid to them.

Sense of community. The Sense of Community scale represents the dimensions of needs fulfillment, group membership, influence, and shared emotional connection, which were found to be "correlated as expected with community participation, psychological empowerment, mental health, and depression." Table 2 shows the measured means for each subscale for each team. For each of the four subscales, the FittleBot2 team reported higher scores ("fulfillment" $t(10) = 0.65$, $p = 0.53$; "membership" $t(9) = 2.2$, $p < 0.05$; "influence" $t(7) = 0.98$, $p = 0.35$; "emotional connection" $t(10) = 0.1.3$, $p = 0.2$). Note that there is a wider spread of "influence" and "emotional connectedness" on the FittleBot2 team than the Fittlebot-Basic team. This suggests that people on the FittleBot2 team had a diverse level of sense of community with FittleBot2.

Table 2. Sense of Community among teams; Mean (Standard Deviation)

	FittleBot2 Team	FittleBot-Basic Team
Fulfillment	8.2 (1.5)	7.8 (1.1)
Membership	10 (1.5)	8.4 (1.5)
Influence	8.9 (1.7)	8.2 (0.44)
Emotional Connectedness	9.4 (2.0)	8.2 (1.1)
Total	36.5	32.6

Perceived social support. Perceived social support refers to one's personal appraisal of his or her available support [11], which is is more important than actually receiving that support [13]. The *Perceived Social Support Scale* measures one's perceived level of support towards friends, family (which we interpreted as team) and a significant other. We excluded measuring significant others in our study. Examples of questions include, "My team really tries to help me" for

Table 3. Perceived Social Support among teams; Mean (Standard Deviation)

	FittleBot2 Team	FittleBot-Basic Team
Team/Family	16.6 (2.1)	15.2 (1.3)
Friends	3.4 (1.1)	3.8 (0.45)
Total	20	19

the family subscale, "I can count on my friends when things go wrong" for the friends subscale. Higher scores indicate higher social support ("team" $t(10) = 1.37$, $p = 0.2$; "friends" $t(8) = 0.78$, $p = 0.45$).

Table 3 shows the measured means for each subscale for each team. While the FittleBot2 team found a greater perceived support from their team, they found a lower perceived support from the individuals on that team. Again, note the wider spread of scores on the FittleBot2 team. This suggests that people on the FittleBot2 team had a diverse level of perceived support possibly speaking to individual preferences for FittleBot2's new strategies.

4   Conclusions and Future Work

This paper presents a field study of Fittlebot2, a virtual agent in the Fittle app, that aims to foster a sense of community with conversation starters. We see a trend towards an increase in compliance for the FittleBot2 team, and observe that conversation starters seem to engage teammates of the Fittlebot2 team. We measure a greater sense of community amongst the FittleBot2 team members than the FittleBot-Basic team members. The FittleBot2 team also saw its own team on the same level as FittleBot2, whereas there was a significant difference in how the FittleBot-Basic team saw its team and FittleBot-Basic.

References

1. Tapus, A., Mataric, M.: Socially assistive robots: The link between personality, empathy, physiological signals, and task performance. In: AAAI Spring Symposium (2008)
2. Cassell, J., Bickmore, T.: Negotiated collusion: Modeling social language and its relationship effects in intelligent agents. User Modeling and User-Adapted Interaction 13, 89–132 (2003)
3. Isbister, K., Nass, C.: Consistency of personality in interactive characters: verbal cues, non-verbal cues, and user characteristics. International Journal of Human-Computer Studies 53, 251–267 (2000)
4. Putnam, R.: Bowling Alone: The Collapse and Revival of American Community. Simpn and Schuster (2000)
5. Homans, G.C.: Social behavior as exchange. American Journal of Sociology (1958)
6. Du, H., Youngblood, G.M., Pirolli, P.: Efficacy of a Smartphone System to Support Groups in Behavior Change Programs programs. Wireless Health (2014) (in review)
7. Kelman, H.C.: Compliance, identification, and internalization: Three processes of attitude change. Journal of Conflict Resolution, 51–60 (1958)

8. Rogers, Y., Brignull, H.: Subtle ice-breaking: encouraging socializing and interaction around a large public display. In: Workshop on Public, Community and Situated Displays (2002)
9. Borovoy, R., Martin, F., Vemuri, S., Resnick, M., Silverman, B., Hancock, C.: Meme tags and community mirrors: moving from conferences to collaboration. In: Proceedings of the 1998 ACM Conference on Computer Supported Cooperative Work, pp. 159–168. ACM (1998)
10. Rocco, E.: Trust breaks down in electronic contexts but can be repaired by some initial face-to-face contact. In: Proceedings of the SIGCHI Conference on Human Factors in Computing Systems, pp. 496–502. ACM Press/Addison-Wesley Publishing Co. (1998)
11. Zimet, G.D., Dahlem, N.W., Zimet, S.G., Farley, G.K.: The multidimensional scale of perceived social support. Journal of Personality Assessment 52, 30–41 (1988)
12. Peterson, N.A., Speer, P.W., McMillan, D.W.: Validation of a brief sense of community scale: Confirmation of the principal theory of sense of community. Journal of Community Psychology 36, 61–73 (2008)
13. Day, A.L., Livingstone, H.A.: Gender differences in perceptions of stressors and utilization of social support among university students. Canadian Journal of Behavioural Science (2003)

Look on the Bright Side: A Model of Cognitive Change in Virtual Agents

Juan Martínez-Miranda, Adrián Bresó, and Juan Miguel García-Gómez

ITACA Institute, Biomedical Informatics Group, Universitat Politècnica de València,
Camino de Vera s/n Valencia, Spain
{juama25,adbregua,juanmig}@upv.es

Abstract. The modelling of empathic reactions in virtual agents has been recognised as a key aspect to improve agent-user relationship. Empathy is particularly important in a virtual agent used in computer-based psychotherapy applications. From a clinical perspective, it is more useful to produce *therapeutic-empathy* responses in the agent and not only *natural* empathic reactions as response to patient's inputs. Based on Gross's theory of emotion regulation, this paper presents a model of cognitive change used to reappraise with a more positive perspective those negative situations reported by the user and provide an adequate emotional reaction during the interaction. An initial evaluation of the model is also presented and the further work is described.

Keywords: affective process modelling, emotion regulation, reappraisal.

1 Introduction

The development of applications for computer-based psychotherapy has been increased in last years due to the multiple advantages they offer, including reduction of costs, logistics of scheduling, stigma, or availability of therapists among others [6]. The use and benefits of virtual agents as enhanced interfaces for this type of applications have been explored to support people with different mental health related conditions (see e.g. [17], [18]). The key idea behind the use of virtual agents in psychotherapy is to create improved relationships between the users and the agent. If patients builds a rapport with their agents, they are more likely to use the system, more motivated to complete longer sessions, which in turn facilitate a better adherence to support the treatment process [1].

A key characteristic that believable virtual agents should have for their use in clinical psychiatry is the generation of *adequate* emotional responses that convey *empathy* during the interaction with the user [2]. This is something not new in psychotherapy where empathy is considered a fundamental aspect in promoting therapeutic change when providing counseling and psychotherapeutic interventions [19]. The modelling of empathic responses in synthetic characters as virtual assistants to support the treatment of mental health disorders faces some challenges that need to be carefully addressed. For example, in the treatment of major depression, an interactive virtual agent must not display a *pure*

T. Bickmore et al. (Eds.): IVA 2014, LNAI 8637, pp. 285–294, 2014.

emotional empathic behaviours by adopting the same typically negative mood of the patient. The disadvantage is that these behaviours can be interpreted as sympathetic expressions of condolence that may imply a sense of unintended agreement with the patients (negative) views [7]. What is most beneficial from a clinical perspective is not to produce *only* natural empathic reactions as response to the patient's input, but to convey *therapeutic-empathy* responses.

Thus, it is important to distinguish *natural empathy* (experienced by people in everyday situations) from *therapeutic empathy* in order to provide the patients with useful feedback for their particular condition [20]. One of the key differences between natural and therapeutic empathy is the *"addition of the cognitive perspective-taking component to the emotional one; the cognitive component helps the therapist to conceptualize the client's distress in cognitive terms"* ([20], pp. 594). In other words, a therapist should *"assume both the role of an emotional involvement in an interview with a patient and an emotional detachment that allows for a more objective appraisal"* ([7], pp. 102) in order to avoid a wrong empathic attitude generated when the therapist does not to some degree maintain an emotional distance from the patient.

In this paper, we describe a model of this *perspective-taking component* aimed to produce in a virtual agent the required emotional detachment or emotional distance at specific stages of the interaction with particular users e.g. those under treatment of major depression. The theoretical basis of the proposed model lies in J. J. Gross' process model of emotion regulation [9]. We particulary describe the modelling of *cognitive change*, one of the strategies of emotion regulation proposed by Gross. The implementation of the model have been developed as an extension of the FAtiMA (appraisal-based) computational architecture of emotions [8]. The main aim of this extension is to create a mechanism that *down-regulates* those negative emotions that would be elicited in the virtual agent as a consequence of a negative event produced in the agent's world.

2   Related Work

There are currently just few works that have implemented a computational model of emotion regulation. One of these works is the developed in the group of Bosse and colleagues which have also used Gross's emotion regulation model as the theoretical basis. In this work, the four antecedent-focused emotion regulation strategies defined in Gross's work [10] have been formally modelled and incorporated in synthetic characters as participants in a virtual storytelling [4].

In a subsequent work, Bosse and colleagues constructed virtual agents not only with the capacity of regulate their emotions, but also with the ability of *reasoning* about the emotion regulation processes of other agents [3]. This model has been called CoMERG (the Cognitive Model for Emotion Regulation based on Gross) and it formalizes Gross model through a set of difference equations and rules to simulate the dynamics of Gross' emotion-regulation strategies [5]. The modelling and simulation of the different emotion regulation strategies is the main aim of CoMERG, but the underlying appraisal and affect derivation mechanisms required to generate specific emotions according to the observed world-state are not explicitly addressed. In a more recent work [12] the integration of CoMERG with other two computational models of emotions EMA [14] and I-PEFIC^{ADM} [11] is proposed to cover the complete process of emotion generation, regulation and action responses in virtual agents.

The FAtiMA architecture [8] also applies its own strategy (which is based on [13]) for changing world interpretation and lowering strong negative emotions. This mechanism is part of the FAtiMA deliberative layer which implements two types of coping to deal with changes in the environment. The problem-focused coping acts on the agent's world to deal with the situation and consists of a set of actions to be executed to achieve the desired state of the world. The emotional focused coping is used to change the agent's interpretation of circumstances. When a specific plan or action fails in the intention to achieve or maintain a desired goal, a mental disengagement is applied. Mental disengagement works by reducing the importance of the goal, which in turn reduces the intensity of the negative emotions triggered when a goal fails [8].

In a virtual agent used to support the treatment and recovery of people with major depression, what is still needed is a mechanism to re-interpret (i.e. reappraise) a situation that is detected as adverse to the patient's condition and that could lead to the triggering of a negative emotion in the agent. While the current emotion-focused coping of FAtiMA is concentrated in the achievement/maintenance, or not, of the agent's internal goals and the reduction of the intensity in the negative OCC prospect based emotions [16], we need an emotional regulation module that down-regulates the intensity of the negative affective state produced by a situation derived from those negative events in the patient's status. Thus, the verbal and nonverbal feedback provided to the patient based on the VA's affective state would contribute to a better therapeutic empathy communication during the course of the interactive session.

3 A Model of Cognitive Change

3.1 Theoretical Roots

An important research work that proposes a theory about the generative process of emotion regulation is the model proposed by J. J. Gross [9], [10] which refers to *the heterogeneous set of processes by which emotions are themselves regulated.* His proposed model covers the conscious and unconscious strategies used to increase, maintain, or decrease one or more components of an emotional response. Gross identifies and defines five families of emotion regulation processes: *situation selection, situation modification, attentional deployment, cognitive change* and *response modulation.*

Situation selection is described as when an individual takes the necessary actions to be in a situation the individual expects will raise a certain desirable emotion. *Situation modification* refers to the efforts employed by the individual to directly modify the actual situation to alter its emotional impact. The third family, *attentional deployment,* refers to how individuals direct their attention within the current situation in order to influence their emotions. The *Cognitive change* family is described as when the individual changes how the actual situation is appraised to alter its emotional significance, either by changing how the individual thinks about the situation or the capacity to manage it. Finally, the *response modulation* family refers when the individual influences the physiological, experiential, or behavioural responses to the situation.

Each family of emotion regulation processes occurs at different points in the emotion generation process and there are substantial differences between them (see details in [10]). An important aspect to consider is that the first four emotion regulation families occur before any appraisal produces the full emotional response (antecedent-focused), while the last family (response modulation) occurs after response tendencies have been initiated (response-focused). One particular strategy studied in [9] as a type of cognitive change (antecedent-focused) is *reappraisal*. According to Gross, reappraisal occurs early in the emotion generation process and it involves cognitively neutralizing a potentially emotion-eliciting situation. The model described in the following section uses the reappraisal strategy as the core mechanism to generate a cognitive change in the agent once a particular situation is detected.

3.2   The Modelling of Reappraisal as Cognitive Change

Based on Gross theory, we have designed a mechanism to reappraise those events susceptible to triggering negative emotions in the agent. Using the concepts of Gross theory, we represent a **situation** composed by the **event** or events produced in the agent's **environment** (see Fig. 1). In our scenario, the events occur during the interaction with the user and most of them are related with the actual detected or reported condition of the user. The actual situation meaning can be changed using a pre-defined set of **situation meanings** which in turn are formed by the different events that are used during the reappraisal process. The reappraisal is triggered only when the target (negative) emotion exceeds a predefined threshold which represents the maximum intensity allowed in the target emotion. Reappraisal can produce a different -positive- emotion or the same negative emotion with a decreased -*down-regulated*- intensity. The diagram in Fig. 1 represents the concepts and the flow of the reappraisal process.

According to Gross's theory, the cognitive change is an antecedent-focused strategy of emotion regulation, which means that it occurs before appraisals give rise to full-blown emotional response tendencies [10]. Thus, our reappraisal mechanism is activated when a new event is received from the agent's environment. A **prospective appraisal** is executed to assess if the event derives from a desirable or undesirable (in terms of the agent's goals) situation related to the patient's condition. The result of this prospective appraisal is the projection of the potential emotional state produced by this event. In other words, our model "simulates" the appraisal and affect derivation processes to analyse the emotional consequences of the current situation, but without producing the full-blown emotional responses.

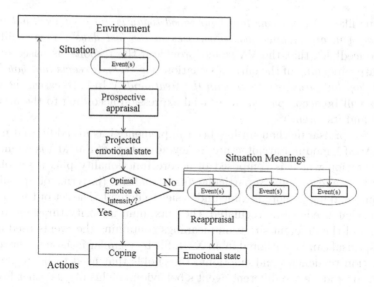

Fig. 1. Cognitive change model diagram

If the **projected emotional state** involves the activation of a positive emotion -no emotion regulation is required- then the same event is used to execute the *real* appraisal and generates the corresponding responses in the agent. On the other hand, if the projected emotional state includes the activation of a negative emotion with an intensity greater than the pre-defined maximum threshold, the corresponding pre-defined alternative event(s) is selected for reappraisal which would construct a more positive meaning of the original situation. If the emotional state produced by the reappraisal is better (i.e. produces a positive emotion or the same negative emotion but with a reduced intensity) than the simulated situation, the reactive and deliberative responses -i.e. the **coping** process- are executed continuing with the next interaction cycle.

To exemplify this process consider an interactive session where the agent administers a standardised questionnaire to daily collect information about the patient's wellbeing. One specific question is to get information about the mood of the user. If the patient is reporting a *low mood,* the agent can appraise this event as highly undesirable for the patient's condition, generating a strong negative emotion. Using the cognitive change strategy of emotion regulation, the agent can change the meaning of this situation using an alternative view. In the example, the agent can consult the responses obtained to this question during previous sessions which is stored in a model of the patient. Using a linear regression approach, those previous responses are analysed to check whether those values shows a positive tendency in the patient's mood. If this positive tendency is found, the original event would be reappraised as "not much undesirable" to the patient (thought the current level of mood reported is not the optimal).

The reappraisal process can change the emotional state or the emotion's intensity in the VA which is reflected in the feedback provided to the patient, something like "*Ok, it seems that your mood today is not very good, but in general terms you are making good progresses in the last days*". This is different from the feedback that the VA would provide if the response is based only on the negative meaning of the current situation (e.g. "*Ok, it seems that you have a difficult day, but please continue with the treatment*"). In both cases, the verbal feedback will be accompanied by a facial expression according to the activated emotion and its intensity.

This reappraisal mechanism has been implemented as an additional module of the FAtiMA modular architecture. A key advantage of FAtiMA is its modular implementation which is composed of a core functionality plus a set of components that add or remove particular functionalities (in terms of appraisal or behaviour) making it more flexible and easier to extend. The set of the targeted emotions that needs to be regulated, the maximum intensity threshold of each emotion and the different situation meanings containing the events used during the reappraisal can be authored in an XML file in a similar fashion as the agent's goals, action tendencies and emotional thresholds that need to be authored in FAtiMA to produce the different agent's behaviours. This file, as other FAtiMA setting files is loaded when the agents and their scenario are started. An example of the file used in the cognitive change model is as follows:

```
<EmotionRegulation>
  <!--Targeted emotions for regulation-->
  <EmotionalDesiredIntensities>
    <EmotionalDesiredIntensity emotion="Distress" desiredIntensity="3">
    <EmotionalDesiredIntensity emotion="Pity" desiredIntensity="3">
    ...
  </EmotionalDesiredIntensities>

  <!--Situation meanings used for reappraisal-->
  <SituationMeanings>
    <Situation name="High_Depression_Score">
      <ElicitingEmotion type="Distress" minIntensity="6">
        <CauseEvent subject="User" action="High_Score_PHQ-9">
      </ElicitingEmotion>
      </EventForReappraisal subject="[SELF]" action="getPreviousDepressionScore"
                            target="User" parameters="2">
    <Situation>

    <Situation name="Low_Mood">
      <ElicitingEmotion type="Distress" minIntensity="6">
        <CauseEvent subject="User" action="Low_Score_DailyMoodCheck">
      </ElicitingEmotion>
      </EventForReappraisal subject="[SELF]" action="getPreviousMood" target="User"
                            parameters="5">
    <Situation>
  </SituationMeanings>
</EmotionRegulation>
```

The content of the file is divided into two main parts: the first part under the <EmotionalDesiredIntensities> tag defines the targeted emotions that need to be regulated (in our scenario, at the moment we are concentrating only on negative emotions). The file sets the *desiredIntensity* of each *emotion* representing the maximum intensity allowed for that emotion. When a new event is appraised and the prospective emotion is elicited with a higher intensity than the value defined in this parameter, the reappraisal process is triggered. The second part of the content under the `<SituationMeanings>` tag defines the set of situations that are candidates to be reappraised with a more *positive* perspective. Each situation contains the event (`<CauseEvent>`) that would elicit the *negative* emotion (`<ElicitingEmotion>`) and the definition of the event used for the reappraisal (`<EventForReappraisal>`) process. The event used during the reappraisal is composed by four parameters following the same definition of an event used in FAtiMA [8]: the *subject* who performs the action; the *action* to perform; the *target* of the action; and a list of parameters with additional information.

The mechanism to select the specific situation in the emotion regulation component is also based on the activation of action tendencies of FAtiMA. When executing the prospective appraisal using the event defined in the `<CauseEvent>` tag, if the projected emotional state activates the emotion type with an intensity equal or greater than the *minIntensity* value, then the event defined in `<EventForReappraisal>` is selected to execute the reappraisal process. This event contains the action that will be executed to get an alternative meaning of the current situation (e.g. in the *Low_Mood* situation of the XML example, the virtual agent gets the scores of the mood reported by the patient in the past 5 days to detect if the mean of the previous values is high or if there is a positive tendency in the mood of the patient).

It is important to consider that the result of the reappraisal does not necessarily change a negative situation. Continuing with our example, the result of the previous values in the patient's mood state could indicate a negative tendency in the evolution of his/her wellbeing. In these cases, the resultant emotional state could even increase the intensity of the negative emotion. As a requirement of our scenario is not to convey strong negative emotional responses during the interaction, the *response modulation* strategy is applied as an alternative to the cognitive change strategy (not described here for lack of space but details are presented in [15]).

4   Initial Evaluation

The presented model is part of the mechanism that generates the behaviour of a virtual agent developed in the context of the EC-FP7 Help4Mood research initiative (www.help4mood.info). The main aim of Help4Mood is to support the treatment of people who are recovering from major depressive disorder in the community. The complete Help4Mood system is composed of three main components: the virtual agent which acts as the main interface with the user; a Decision Support System (DSS) which manages, analyses and summarises the users daily sessions; and the Personal Monitoring System (PMS) in the form of sensor devices used to collect patterns of physical activity and sleep.

The virtual agent has been designed to facilitate the collection of relevant data including subjective measures (by applying standardised questionnaires and guided interviews), and neuropsychomotor measures (by offering tasks for speech input) which are designed to complement the objective measures obtained from the PMS. The collection of the patient data is carried out through daily sessions

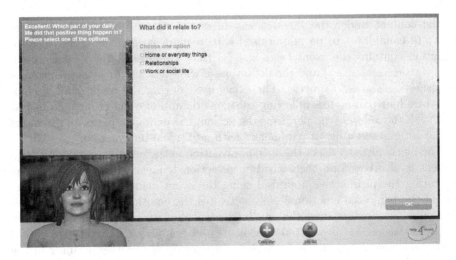

Fig. 2. The Help4Mood GUI

where the content of each session varies, with some tasks being carried out every day and some others executed weekly (see Fig. 2).

A first evaluation of the proposed model has been performed configuring two different scenarios. In **scenario I**, the cognitive change model is not included in the virtual agent. For this case, when something *bad* is detected in the wellbeing condition of the patient (inferred in the DSS from the PMS data or from patients self-reports), a neutral attitude (i.e. no emotion) is adopted by the agent which is reflected in the feedback dialogue and in its facial expressions. In **scenario II**, the cognitive change model has been included allowing the elicitation of negative (but regulated) emotions in the agent during the interaction with the user. Enrolled participants were individuals with major depressive disorder as a primary diagnosis with a mild to moderate range; aged between 18 and 64 inclusive; and living at home.

A total of 8 participants were enrolled in the pilot, 5 of them (two male and three females) were assigned to scenario I and 3 (all of them females) to scenario II. The participants used the Help4Mood system for 2 weeks followed by an exit interview containing questions to assess the acceptability of the system's components. The method to assess the emotional behaviour of the agent included two Likert-based scale questions Q1: *"The virtual agent behaves cold and aloof"* and Q2:*"I am comfortable with the emotional responses of the VA"*. While in the first scenario only 1 of the 5 participants noted the emotional reactions in the VA, the participants in the second scenario noted better the emotional behaviour of the agent. In concrete, two of the three participants in scenario II rated Q1 as *disagree* stating that they did not consider the VA behaves cold and aloof. Similar results were obtained for Q2: 2 participants were *agree* and 1 *disagree* regarding the emotional responses provided by the agent.

Although this initial feedback is interesting, the small number of participants in the first pilot is not relevant to get definite conclusions. These initial results will be complemented with the final pilot of the project involving a minimum of 15 participants using the system during 4 weeks and which is already started. Nevertheless, what is interesting from the initial evaluation is that with the inclusion of the emotion regulation model, the participants in scenario II noted better the emotional reactions from the VA than the participants in scenario I. This suggests that the inclusion of negative (but regulated) emotional reactions in the VA to the reported adverse events in patient's wellbeing contributes to better convey *adequate* empathic reactions.

5 Conclusions and Further Work

The modelling of a reappraisal process as an strategy of emotion regulation has been presented as the mechanism to produce more varied and adequate emotional responses in a virtual agent used to interact with individuals recovering from major depression. In particular, the emotional reactions of the VA in front of *adverse situations*, related with the detected wellbeing of the user, have been improved and facilitates the provision of a more empathic feedback according to the detected events. Initial tests have been performed to analyse the different reactions and feedback produced during the reappraisal of some negative events. These new emotional reactions has facilitated the inclusion of more specific dialogues during the session which in turn would facilitate a better level of acceptability in the users. Nevertheless, the significant evaluation of the model is expected during at the end of the final pilot where the feedback from a greater number of participants will be collected.

An additional interesting further work is to investigate whether the regulation of negative emotions is enough to produce useful therapeutic empathy responses. At the moment, and following clinicians recommendations, we have concentrated on the regulation of negative emotions. Depending on the results collected from the final pilot, we would assess if there would be situations where even when the user is reporting a good input to a specific question, the agent should also regulate its positive emotional responses reflecting on a more general assessments of current patient's condition.

Acknowledgements. This paper reflects only the authors views. The European Community is not liable for any use that may be made of the information contained herein. This research is carried out within the EU-FP7 Project "Help4Mood: A Computational Distributed System to Support the Treatment of Patients with Major Depression" (ICT-248765).

References

1. Bickmore, T., Mauer, D.: Modalities for building relationships with handheld computer agents. ACM Press, New York (April 2006)
2. Bickmore, T., Gruber, A.: Relational agents in clinical psychiatry. Harvard Review of Psychiatry 18(2), 119–130 (2010)

3. Bosse, T., de Lange, F.P.J.: Development of Virtual Agents with a Theory of Emotion Regulation. In: Proc. of IEEE/WIC/ACM International Conference on Web Intelligence and Intelligent Agent Technology, WI-IAT 2008, vol. 2, pp. 461–468 (2008)
4. Bosse, T., Pontier, M., Siddiqui, G.F., Treur, J.: Incorporating Emotion Regulation into Virtual Stories. In: Pelachaud, C., Martin, J.-C., André, E., Chollet, G., Karpouzis, K., Pelé, D. (eds.) IVA 2007. LNCS (LNAI), vol. 4722, pp. 339–347. Springer, Heidelberg (2007)
5. Bosse, T., Pontier, M., Treur, J.: A computational model based on Gross' emotion regulation theory. Cognitive Systems Research 11, 211–230 (2010)
6. Cartreine, J.A., Ahern, D.K., Locke, S.E.: A roadmap to computer-based psychotherapy in the United States. Harvard Review of Psychiatry 18(2), 80–95 (2010)
7. Clark, A.J.: Empathy in Counseling and Psychotherapy. Perspectives and Practices. Lawrence Erlbaum Associates (2007)
8. Dias, J., Paiva, A.: Feeling and Reasoning: A Computational Model for Emotional Characters. In: Bento, C., Cardoso, A., Dias, G. (eds.) EPIA 2005. LNCS (LNAI), vol. 3808, pp. 127–140. Springer, Heidelberg (2005)
9. Gross, J.J.: Emotion Regulation in Adulthood: Timing is Everything. Current Directions in Psychological Science 10(6), 214–219 (2001)
10. Gross, J.J., Thompson, R.A.: Emotion Regulation: Conceptual Foundations. In: Gross, J.J. (ed.) Handbook of Emotion Regulation, pp. 3–24. Guilford Press (2007)
11. Hoorn, J.F., Pontier, M., Siddiqui, G.F.: When the user is instrumental to robot goals. First try: Agent uses agent. In: Proc. of IEEE/WIC/ACM Web Intelligence and Intelligent Agent Technology WI-IAT 2008, vol. 2, pp. 296–301 (2008)
12. Hoorn, J.F., Pontier, M., Siddiqui, G.F.: Coppélius' concoction: Similarity and complementarity among three affect-related agent models. Cognitive Systems Research 15-16, 33–49 (2012)
13. Marsella, S., Gratch, J.: Modeling Coping Behavior in Virtual Humans Don't Worry, Be Happy. In: Proc. of the 2nd Int. Joint Conf. on Autonomous Agents and Multiagent Systems - AAMAS (2003)
14. Marsella, S., Gratch, J. E.: A model of emotional dynamics. Cognitive Systems Research 10(1), 70–90 (2009)
15. Martínez-Miranda, J., Bresó, A., García-Gómez, J.M.: Modelling Two Emotion Regulation Strategies as Key Features of Therapeutic Empathy. Under Review (2014)
16. Ortony, A., Clore, G., Collins, A.: The Cognitive Structure of Emotions. Cambridge University Press (1988)
17. Puskar, K., Schlenk, E., Callan, J., Bickmore, T., Sereika, S.: Relational Agents as an Adjunct in Treating Schizophrenia: Case Studies. Journal of Psychosocial Nursing and Mental Health Services 49(8), 22–29 (2012)
18. Rizzo, A., Forbell, E., Lange, B., Buckwalter, J.G., Williams, J., Sagae, K., Traum, D.: SimCoach: An Online Intelligent Virtual Agent System for Breaking Down Barriers to Care for Service Members and Veterans. In: Healing War Trauma: A Handbook of Creative Approaches. Routledge (2012)
19. Rogers, C.R.: On Becoming a Person: a therapist's view of psychotherapy. Constable and Company, London (1967)
20. Thwaites, R., Bennett-Levy, J.: Conceptualizing Empathy in Cognitive Behaviour Therapy: Making the Implicit Explicit. Behavioural and Cognitive Psychotherapy 35, 291–612 (2007)

Naturalistic Pain Synthesis for Virtual Patients

Maryam Moosaei, Michael J. Gonzales, and Laurel D. Riek

Department of Computer Science and Engineering,
University of Notre Dame, Notre Dame, IN, 46556, USA
{mmoosaei,mgonza14,lriek}@nd.edu

Abstract. Within the clinical education community, there is a desire to improve learners' pain observation skills. Virtual patients can be used as a training tool for this purpose. In this paper, we present a pioneering approach for synthesizing naturalistic pain on virtual patients. Using the UNBC-McMaster pain archive and a CLM-based face tracker, we performed naturalistic pain synthesis. We conducted an experiment to validate our synthesis approach and compared it to manual methods that use FACS-trained animators. Our results suggest that our approach was effective, and yielded higher pain labeling accuracies compared to manually animated painful faces. This research offers a new tool to both the virtual patient and clinical education communities.

Keywords: Virtual patients, pain synthesis, facial expression synthesis, healthcare simulation, patient simulation.

1 Introduction

Many researchers in the fields of affective computing and clinical education are interested in patient simulation (c.f., [1–4]). Simulated patients provide safe experiences for clinical trainees, where they can practice communication, assessment, and intervention skills, without fear of harming a real patient. (See Fig. 1). Although this technology is in widespread use today, commercial patient simulators lack sufficient realism. They have static faces with no capability to convey facial expressions, despite the vital importance of these non-verbal expressivity cues in how clinicians assess and treat patients [5, 6].

This is a critical omission, because almost all areas of health care involve face-to-face interaction [7]. Furthermore, there is overwhelming evidence that providers who are skilled at decoding communication cues are better healthcare providers: they have improved patient outcomes, higher patient compliance and satisfaction, greater patient safety, and experience fewer malpractice lawsuits [6, 8, 9]. In fact, communication errors are the leading cause of avoidable patient harm: they are the root cause of 70% of sentinel events, 75% of which lead to a patient's death [10].

In studying how individuals, teams, and operators interact with inexpressive simulators, our work suggests that commercially available systems are inadequate for the task of training students due to their complete inability to provide human communication cues [11–14]. In particular, these simulators cannot

T. Bickmore et al. (Eds.): IVA 2014, LNAI 8637, pp. 295–309, 2014.

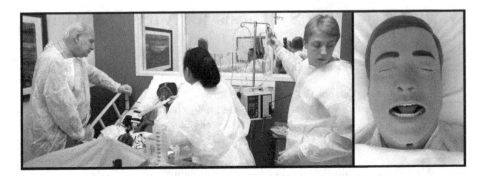

Fig. 1. Left: A team of clinicians treat a simulated patient, who is conscious during the simulation, but has no capability for facial expression. Right: A commonly used inexpressive mannequin head.

convey visual signals of pain to medical trainees even though perceiving a patient's nonverbal pain cues is an exceptionally important factor in how clinicians make decisions. Existing systems may be preventing students from picking up on patients' pain signals, possibly inculcating poor safety habits due to a lack of realism in the simulation [15, 16].

Our work focuses on making patient simulators more realistic by enabling them to convey realistic, patient-driven facial expressions to clinical trainees. We are designing a new type of physical patient simulator with a wider range of expressivity, including the ability to express pain and other pathologies in its face [4]. This paper presents one aspect of this project, which includes research questions surrounding synthesizing naturalistic[1] painful faces on a virtual avatar and evaluating how they are perceived.

This research fills a gap in the virtual patient problem domain, because although there is a growing body of literature on automatic pain recognition [18–20], there is little published work on automatic pain synthesis, particularly using naturalistic data. This work also will enable medical educators improve their face-to-face communication skills and pain recognition skills, which, according to the literature, are both in need of attention [5, 6, 21].

1.1 Our Work and Contribution

In this paper, we describe a technique for naturalistic pain synthesis on virtual patients, and report on several perceptual studies to validate the quality of the synthesis. For synthesis, we used a constrained local model (CLM)-based facial feature tracker applied to examples from the UNBC-McMaster Pain Archive [22].

We modeled our perceptual experiment on work by Riva et al. [23], where participants classified videos of three types of synthesized facial expressions: pain, anger, and disgust, across three genders - male, female, and androgynous. Riva et al. considered anger and disgust as reasonable expressions for comparison

---

[1] Here, *naturalistic* refers to non-acted, real-world data obtained "in the wild". c.f. [17].

because of their "negative valence and threat-relevant nature". They explored avatar gender variations, because previous work in the field suggested a relationship between actor gender and pain detection accuracy [24]. In their work, the facial expressions were manually created by an animator using FaceGen 3.1, and reviewed by experts trained in the Facial Action Coding System (FACS).

Riva et al. [23] had two findings of note. First, they found participants were less accurate in decoding expressions of pain compared to anger and disgust (similar to other work, c.f. [25–27]). Second, regardless of gender, participants had better pain detection accuracy for male avatars. Given a naturalistic approach to synthesis, we wondered if the findings by Riva et al. [23] would hold, and, thus, replicated their experiment.

We have two main research questions. First, are participants able to distinguish expressions of pain from anger and disgust, and how do their accuracies differ? Based on findings by Riva et al. [23], we predict that overall, participants will be more accurate at detecting disgust compared with pain, and more accurate at detecting anger compared with disgust.

Second, how does an avatar's gender affect pain detection accuracy? In addition to being curious if we can replicate findings by Riva et al. [23], we also would like evidence-based insights into how to design our physical robotic patient. We eventually will need to make decisions about the apparent gender of the robot, and this will require careful weighing of our findings. Based on findings by Riva et al. [23], we predicted that pain detection accuracy will be lower overall when expressed on a female avatar compared to a male avatar[2].

Our methodology, described in Section 2, addresses these research questions through a 3x3 online study in which subjects labeled videos of male, female, and androgynous avatars displaying pain, anger, and disgust.

Our results, discussed in Section 3, showed that participants were able to distinguish facial expressions of pain from anger and disgust by performing naturalistic synthesis, and were less accurate in decoding disgust compared to pain and anger. Furthermore, we did not find support for the avatar gender finding by Riva et al.; in our data avatar gender did not have significant effect on pain detection accuracy. Finally, our results suggest that naturalistic pain synthesis on virtual avatars is comparable to manual pain synthesis, and arithmetically, may be better. We discuss the implications of our findings for the community in Section 4.

2 Methodology

2.1 Background

Similar to other expressions of emotion, facial expressions of pain are an important non-verbal communication signal, particularly in healthcare [30, 31]. Until

---

[2] In this work we did not explore the effect of participant gender. The reason is that despite findings about how it affects accuracy in detecting some aspects of expressivity (e.g., arousal and valence) [28, 29], there is no evidence to suggest it affects overall categorization.

recently, self-reporting and clinical observations were the primary ways used to detect pain. However, these methods have several issues. For example, self-report cannot be used for children or patients with communication challenges (e.g. cognitive impairments, unstable states of consciousness or lucidity, etc.). Moreover, there are differences between how clinician and how patients conceptualize pain, which can lead to problems [18, 19, 31, 32].

Psychologists propose that pain is expressed by certain facial movements. While there is some research suggesting pain can be idiosyncratic [33, 34], we approach our research with respect to the Facial Action Coding System (FACS) which states pain can be interpreted universally from face. FACS uses 46 action units (AUs) as its building blocks to code facial expressions. This system was developed initially by Ekman [35] to code basic emotions based on facial muscle activities, and later was applied to pain, notably by Prkachin [19] and Craig [36].

To date, several research groups have worked on techniques for automatic pain detection, a process that involves automatic facial feature extraction and training of classifiers to detect pain. For example, Ashraf et al. [18] classified videos from the UNBC-McMaster Shoulder Pain Expression Archive Database [22] into pain/no pain categories using machine learning approaches. Their feature extraction was based on Active Appearance Models (AAM), which we describe in more detail in Section 2.4. The researchers decoupled shape and appearance parameters from facial images and used Support Vector Machines (SVM) for classification. Others have also explored automatic pain recognition, c.f. Prkachin et al., Monwar and Rezaei, and Hammal et al. [20, 37, 38]

Despite the aforementioned work on automatic pain detection, there is little work on automatic pain synthesis. In our work we studied features that were used in the literature for pain facial expression detection and instead employed them to synthesize facial expression of pain.

2.2   Overview of Our Work

We employed performance-driven synthesis of pain, anger, and disgust on three virtual avatar faces (female, male, and androgynous) to answer the aforementioned research questions. Performance-driven synthesis is a commonly used animation technique that tracks motions from either a live or recorded actor and maps them to an embodied agent, such as a virtual avatar or physical robot [39, 40]. This technique has been used in the literature to synthesize a wide range of naturalistic facial expressions [41, 42], but not pain.

In our work, the source videos we used for pain synthesis came from the UNBC-McMaster Pain Archive [22] and the source videos for anger and disgust from the MMI database [43]. We used ten source videos for each expression type. Our stimuli creation process included four steps. First, we used a Constrained Local Model (CLM) based tracker to extract 68 feature points frame-by-frame from each source video. Next, we mapped the extracted feature points to the virtual character control points for animation in Steam Source SDK. Then, we animated three different virtual characters (female, male, androgynous) per each expression type, resulting in 90 stimuli videos. Finally, we ran several pilot studies to label both gender and expression, and to establish which videos to include in our main study. This resulted in 27 stimuli videos.

2.3 Source Video Acquisition

For the source videos depicting painful expressions, we used the UNBC-McMaster Shoulder Pain Expression Archive Database [22]. This is a fully labeled, naturalistic data set of 200 video sequences from 25 participants suffering from shoulder pain (52% female). Participants performed range-of-motion tests on both their affected and unaffected limbs under the instruction of a physiotherapist. At the frame level, each frame was coded using the facial action coding scheme (FACS), and contained 66-point AAM landmarks. Each frame also received a pain score ranging from 0 to 12. At the sequence level, each video has both self-report and observer ratings of pain, the latter ranging from zero to five.

In our study we only included videos in which pain was present. Similar to Ashraf et al., [22] we considered pain to be present in a sequence if its observer rating was three or greater, and pain to be absent if its observer rating was zero.

For the source videos depicting anger and disgust, we used the MMI database [43]. This is a database of posed expressions from 19 participants (44% female) who were instructed by a FACS expert to express six basic emotions (surprise, fear, happiness, sadness, anger and disgust). Each video begins with a neutral expression and then transitions into the target expression.

We included source videos from these two databases that were determined by two human judges to be accurately tracked by our face tracker. Judges watched the source videos with the CLM mesh drawn on the face and rated all videos on a scale from one to four, depending on how well the mesh aligned with the face throughout the video. We only included videos in which both judges gave the video a tracking score of one. This resulted in 10 source videos from each expression category (pain, anger, disgust). Figure 3 (top) shows some sample frames from these databases.

2.4 Feature Extraction

For tracking facial features, we used Constrained Local Models (CLMs), which are a shape-based tracking technique similar to Active Appearance models (AAM). AAMs are statistical methods for matching the model of a user's face to an unseen face. A CLM-based approach is similar to an AAM-based approach, except it is person-independent, and does not require any manual labeling of an actor's face [44–46].

To our knowledge, CLM-based models have been mostly used in the literature for face tracking, or expression detection, not for synthesis [44, 45]. In our work we use this technique to synthesize facial expressions of pain, anger, and disgust.

In a CLM-based method, the shape of the face is estimated by labeling some feature points on several facial images in the training set [47]. There are also several extensions of CLM-based tracking approaches [46]. For example, Baltrusitus et al. [44] introduced a 3D Constrained Local Model (CLM-Z) method

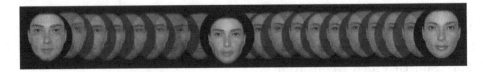

Fig. 2. The spectrum of avatar genders we created, with the final three highlighted. From right to left: male, androgynous, female.

for detecting facial features and tracking them using a depth camera, such as a Kinect. This method is robust to light variations and head-pose rotations, and is thus an improvement over the traditional CLM method.

For our work, we were able to create our stimuli based on a wide range of source videos using the CLM-Z tracker [44]. However, because our source videos were pre-recorded and did not contain depth information, we were not able to take full advantage of the CLM-Z tracker. In the future when we transition to performing real-time facial synthesis on an android robot, we will employ depth information to increase synthesis validity.

2.5 Avatar Model Creation

We used three avatar models in this work: female, male, and androgynous. When creating the avatar models, we aimed to remove any effects of age and ethnicity. In order to generate our avatars, we extracted avatars from the video game Half-life 2 from the Steam Source SDK. We used the program GCFscape to extract our textures from the video game files, and used a program called VTFEdit to convert the textures to modifiable TARGA files (a raster graphics file format).

For the purposes of this experiment, we used the character ("Alyx") [48] as the base for our virtual avatars to ensure consistency of ethinicity and age. Within Adobe Photoshop, certain areas were darkened or lightened to exhibit qualities normally attributed to male or female characteristics. For example, we enlarged the jaw-line, cheekbones, and chin during the creation of male-looking avatars. Similarly, androgynous textures also employed similar changes, but to a smaller degree. We also changed other areas of the face to create variation among these textures.

We created a total of twenty different texture variations employing these changes for our pilot to determine our androgynous, female, and male avatars. Similar to the stimuli created by Riva et al. [23], we cropped the face to remove any neck, clothing, or hair visibility to avoid any unintentional conveyance of gender cues.

We ran a pilot study to establish ground truth gender labels for each avatars' gender, following the methodology of Riva et al. [23]. The goal of this pilot was to select three avatar models as distinctly female, male, and androgynous out of the 20 models we made. We had 16 American participants, 11 female, mean age 44.5 years old. Participants were recruited using Amazon MTurk.

Participants viewed 20 still images of the avatars in a random order and labeled their gender using an 11-point Discrete Visual Analogue Scale (DVAS). A zero on the scale corresponded to "completely masculine" and ten to "completely feminine". We used these results to select our female, male, and androgynous avatar models. We chose the female model with score of 9.13, the male model with a score of 1.81, and the androgynous model with a score of 4.88. See Figure 2 for the final three avatar models.

The average score for each of the three chosen avatars ensured us that we could use these three avatar models as female, male, and androgynous in our main experiment. The next step was to animate each of these three avatars using the 30 source videos.

2.6   Stimuli Creation and Labeling

We initially created 90 stimuli videos. We had three avatar models (female, male, androgynous), three expression types (pain, anger, and disgust), and ten samples of each expression. We tracked 68 facial feature points frame-by-frame from each of our 30 source videos. We removed rotation, translation, and scaling based on eye corner positions. We measured movement of each point in relation to a normalized frame that was calculated during runtime.

We then measured the movement of each point. In order to map our facial points to our avatars, we generated source files that the Source SDK is capable of understanding. To do this, we ran the CLM tracker twice on each video. In the first run, we calculated the maximum movement of each point on the face. This was done to have a maximum scale factor for Source SDK to have as a reference point. In the second run we computed the movement of each feature point in relation to this maximum scale factor. To do this, we divided the movement measured in the second run by the maximum movement for the same point measured in calculation step. This gave us a ratio value between zero and one (zero being neutral, and one being the maximum amount a given point can move) for use with the featuring mapping in Source SDK.

We recorded each of the three avatar types enacting the expressions. The playback duration for each expression was manually adjusted to be 0.3 times slower to compensate for slight variations in how some of the source videos were tracked. After generating the recordings using CamStudio [49], we cropped the stimuli videos to be three to five seconds long to ensure consistency. Figure 3 shows example frames of the created stimuli videos.

We ran a second pilot study to decide which stimuli videos would be included in our main study, and to establish their ground expression truth labels. Each video was modified before being used in the pilot. A black screen with a white crosshair was added to the beginning of each video and appeared for exactly 2.5 seconds to prepare participants for the stimulus video. Then, a facial expression on a virtual character was presented for 2-4 seconds, followed by a black screen. We hosted the videos on Vimeo, and used an HTML 5 video player to remove all logos or player options. The pilot was conducted on SurveyMonkey.

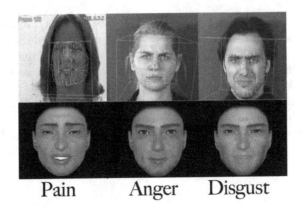

Pain   Anger   Disgust

Fig. 3. Sample frames from the stimuli videos and their corresponding source videos, with CLM meshes. The pain source videos are from the UNBC-McMaster pain archive [22]; the others are from the MMI database [43].

The source and stimuli videos had slightly different lengths due to the fact that source videos of pain came from a different database than the videos of disgust and anger. We cut these videos to be nearly equal in length without removing informative frames from each video.

20 participants were recruited using Amazon MTurk, 11 female and 9 Male. All participants were American, and their ages ranged from 22-58 years old with mean age of 38.05 years old. Participants who participated in our previous pilot were excluded from this pilot. Participants were only allowed to view each video once and were allowed two 30 second breaks where a nature video was shown. Participants watched the 90 stimuli videos in a random order and labeled the avatar's gender and expression.

For gender labeling, we used the same scale as in Pilot 1 (an 11-point DVAS). We aimed to ensure that gender classification was the same as the first pilot when expressions were actually animated on the avatars. We found this was the case: Cronbach's $\alpha = 0.961$, indicating high inter-rater reliability on gender labeling.

Expression labels were fixed choice - anger, disgust, pain, and none of the above. This labeling approach was based on work by Tottenham et al. [50], who found a semi-forced choice method was less strict than a forced choice method (to which Russell [51] objects), while being more easy to interpret findings from than a free-choice method.

We calculated the accuracy of each of our videos across our participants, and chose the three best videos of each expression that had the highest average accuracy across our three genders. We had average accuracies of 80%, 75%, and 63.33% for pain, 80%, 71.67%, and 63.33% for anger, and 33.33%, 31.67%, and 28.33% for disgust[3].

---

[3] We were not surprised by the low detection accuracies for disgust, since it is known to be a poorly distinguishable facial expression in the literature [26, 27].

Table 1. Frequencies and percentages of hits and errors in the main study

	Overall	Female	Male	Androgynous
Pain				
Total number of responses	450	150	150	150
Correct answers	303(67.33%)	100(66.67%)	98(65.33%)	105 (70%)
Judged as anger	2 (0.44%)	0 (0%)	1 (0.67%)	1(0.67%)
Judged as disgust	31(6.89%)	10 (6.67%)	7 (4.67%)	14 (9.33%)
Judged as none of the above	114 (25.33%)	40 (26.67%)	44 (29.33%)	30 (20%)
Anger				
Total number of responses	450	150	150	150
Correct answers	292(64.89%)	101(67.33%)	95(63.33%)	96(64%)
Judged as disgust	84(18.67%)	30(20%)	25(16.67%)	29(19.33%)
Judged as pain	44(9.78%)	10(6.67%)	20(13.33%)	14(9.33%)
Judged as none of the above	30(6.67%)	9(6%)	10(6.67%)	11(7.33%)
Disgust				
Total number of responses	450	150	150	150
Correct answers	133(29.56%)	47(31.33%)	43(28.67%)	43(28.67%)
Judged as anger	120(26.67%)	40 (26.67%)	42(28%)	38(25.33%)
Judged as pain	91(20.22%)	26(17.33%)	34(22.67%)	31(20.67%)
Judged as none of the above	106(23.56%)	37(24.67%)	31(20.67%)	38(25.33%)

Main experiment: Following the pilot, we selected three videos of each expression with the highest accuracy across our three avatar genders to use in our main experiment, resulting in 27 videos. Videos were prepared and presented in the same format as our previous pilot and randomized accordingly.

We recruited 50 participants using Amazon MTurk. Again, participants were eligible only if they did not participate in our previous studies. Participant ages ranged from 20-57 (mean age = 38.6 years). Participants were of mixed heritage, and had each lived in the United States at least 17 years.

Participants were asked to label the avatar's expression in each of the 27 videos. The results from the main experiment are described in the subsequent sections. We measured accuracy (correct or incorrect) across our two independent variables (gender and expression type). We describe the statistical details of our analysis below, but first present a brief summary.

3 Results

3.1 Summary of Key Findings

Our first research question was to explore if participants are able to distinguish pain from expressions of anger and disgust. Table 3 shows that expression is a significant predictor for accuracy. Therefore, we found participants were able to distinguish these three expressions. The results further showed that participants were more accurate in detecting pain than two other expressions. Thus, we did not find the same accuracy ordering as Riva et al. [23]; i.e., disgust > pain > anger.

Table 2. Omnibus Tests of Model Coefficients. $\chi^2(4) = 165.646$, $p < .001$.

		Chi-square	df	Sig.
	Step	165.646	4	0.000
Step 1	Block	165.646	4	0.000
	Model	165.646	4	0.000

Our second research question concerned the effect of the avatar's gender on pain detection accuracy. As seen in Table 3, gender is not a significant predictor for accuracy as the p-values for all the three genders are greater than .05. This suggests that there is no significant relation between an avatar's gender and pain detection accuracy. Thus, we were not able to replicate findings by Riva et al. [23] suggesting that people are more accurate at detecting pain when it is expressed on a male face.

3.2   Regression Method

We had one dependent variable and two independent variables. The dependent variable derived from the expression classification task was accuracy (i.e. classification of the expressions as pain, anger, or disgust). Accuracy is based on the ground truth that we gained from our pilot studies. We had two categorical independent variables. The independent variables were expression with three levels (pain, anger, and disgust) and gender with three levels (androgynous, male, and female).

The dependent variable was analyzed using an appropriate within-subjects binary logistic regression since the only dependent variable is binary (1: accurate, 0: inaccurate). In the following analyses, significant effects are those with p-values < .05.

Table 1 shows the details regarding the exact number of errors each participant made in the classification of 27 videos. In this classification, we considered an answer correct if participant's label matched with the source video label. The percentage of correct classifications was computed across each of the three expressions types within each of the three genders. 3 *(Expression: pain, anger, or disgust)* × 3 *(Gender: androgynous, male, and female)*.

Table 1 indicates the details of errors for each expression and each gender. Participants' answers were classified as either accurate or inaccurate. Overall, participants labeled 622 videos incorrectly, representing 46.07% of our responses.

The independent variables (gender and expression) were significant predictors for the dependent variable (see Table 2). We compared the full model with two predictors (gender and expression) with the restricted model with just a constant factor. The results of the analysis of the full model with two predictors (independent variables) suggest a significant effect of the set of predictors on the correct identification rate as the dependent variable.

The Wald test in Table 3 shows the degree to which each expression affected accuracy. While the chi-square value in Table 2 shows that predictors together

Table 3. Variables in the regression equation

	B	S.E	Wald	df	Sig.	Exp(B)	95% C.I.for EXP(B)	
							Lower	Upper
Pain			151.609	2	0.000			
Disgust	-0.109	0.141	0.600	1	0.438	0.897	0.680	1.182
Anger	-1.593	0.144	122.017	1	0.000	0.203	0.153	0.270
Step 1 Androgynous	0.759	2		0.684				
Male	0.041	0.143	0.082	1	0.775	1.042	0.787	1.378
Female	-0.081	0.142	0.324	1	0.569	0.922	0.697	1.219
Constant	0.737	0.130	32.118	1	0.000	2.090		

have significant effect on the model, the Wald test is the significant test for each individual predictor separated. Table 3 shows the effect of each individual independent variable on the classification rate. The standardized *Beta* value represents the weight that each predictor has in the final model. Negative weight shows a negative relation. Since the regression was run with pain as the reference value, it does not have a *Beta* value[4].

The results of the Wald test suggest that disgust and three genders can be dropped from the model for accuracy prediction. The Wald test suggests that pain by itself is a significant predictor for accuracy, $W = 151.609$, $p <.001$. Disgust by itself is not a significant predictor for the accuracy, $W = .600$, $p >.05$. Anger by itself is a significant predictor for accuracy, $W = 122.017$, $p <.001$. None of the three genders are significant predictors for accuracy. Pain has the largest effect on accuracy prediction followed by anger.

4   Discussion

Participants were able to distinguish pain from anger and disgust in virtual patients created using automatic naturalistic synthesis. Thus, we found support for our first research question (RQ1). Our results support Riva et al.'s findings that participants are able to detect pain from anger and disgust when being expressed by a virtual avatar face.

Our results do not support the claim by Riva et al. [23] that participants are less accurate in decoding the facial expression of pain compared to anger and disgust. Our results instead reflect the opposite - participants are more accurate in decoding facial expressions of pain compared with anger and disgust. Also, participants are more accurate at detecting anger compared to disgust.

We have also found support that naturally driven pain synthesis is comparable to FACS-animated pain synthesis. To the best of our knowledge, this is the first work on naturally performance-driven pain synthesis. Riva et al. [23] manually synthesized facial expressions on a virtual avatar, and found 60.4% as the overall pain labeling accuracy rate. Our pain labeling accuracy rate was

---

[4] SPSS considers pain as the base expression and androgynous as the base gender. Thus, these columns are empty for these two predictors.

67.33%. While we cannot statistically compare these results due to variability in the two experiments, arithmetically they are encouraging.

These findings suggest that our method may be used for automatic pain expression synthesis without requiring a FACS-trained animator to manually synthesize painful expressions. For practitioners and researchers in the clinical education community without such resources, this may prove beneficial.

Our results do not support the previous findings by Riva et al. [23] that pain expression recognition is a function of the gender of the avatar displaying it. We did not find any significant relation between the avatar's gender and the participants' accuracy in detecting pain, anger, or disgust. This further lends support to the idea that automatic pain expression synthesis from naturalistic sources may, in some cases, be preferable to FACS/animator-generated synthesis.

One limitation of our work was that the avatar model from the Source SDK had neither wrinkles nor control points around the nose area. Therefore, we could not map AU9, which is important in expressing disgust and pain [37]. Adding this action unit could help improve the detection accuracy for both disgust and pain. Another limitation was that the source videos for pain came from a naturalistic dataset, whereas the anger and disgust videos were acted and exaggerated. At the time this paper was published, we were not aware of any naturalistic databases for these expressions, but in the future this would be good to explore.

Similar to Riva et al. [23], we ran our experiments with lay participants. The literature suggests that the expressions of pain can be clearly recognized and discriminated by lay participants [36]. However, in the future, we are also interested to see how different populations perceive painful facial expressions, for example, if clinicians at different stages of training perceive an avatar's pain differently. Prkachin et al. [31] showed that clinical experience with patients results in underestimating patients' pain. It would be exciting to test this hypothesis more thoroughly with our avatars and explore if interventions can be designed.

Acknowledgement. This material is based upon work supported by the National Science Foundation under Grant No. IIS-1253935.

References

1. Kenny, P., Parsons, T.D., Gratch, J., Leuski, A., Rizzo, A.A.: Virtual patients for clinical therapist skills training. In: Pelachaud, C., Martin, J.-C., André, E., Chollet, G., Karpouzis, K., Pelé, D. (eds.) IVA 2007. LNCS (LNAI), vol. 4722, pp. 197–210. Springer, Heidelberg (2007)
2. Benjamin, L.: Shader lamps virtual patients: the physical manifestation of virtual patients. In: Medicine Meets Virtual Reality 19: NextMed, vol. 173 (2012)
3. Mitchell, S.E., et al.: Developing virtual patient advocate technology for shared decision making. In: 34th Annual Meeting of the Society for Medical Decision Making (2012)
4. Gonzales, M.J., Moosaei, M., Riek, L.D.: A novel method for synthesizing naturalistic pain on virtual patients. In: Simulation in Healthcare (2013)

5. Ryan, K.F.: Human simulation for medicine. In: Human Simulation for Nursing and Health Professions (2011)
6. Henry, S.G., Fuhrel-Forbis, A., Rogers, M.A., Eggly, S.: Association between non-verbal communication during clinical interactions and outcomes: A systematic review and meta-analysis. Patient Education and Counseling 86(3) (2012)
7. Martin, L.R., Friedman, H.S.: Nonverbal communication and health care. In: Applications of Nonverbal Communication (2005)
8. Back, A.L., et al.: Efficacy of communication skills training for giving bad news and discussing transitions to palliative care. Arch. Intern. Med. 167(5) (2007)
9. Brown, J.: How clinical communication has become a core part of medical education in the UK. Medical Education 42(3) (2008)
10. Leonard, M.: The human factor: the critical importance of effective teamwork and communication in providing safe care. Qual. Saf. Health Care 13 (2004)
11. Huus, A., Riek, L.D.: An Expressive Robotic Patient to Improve Clinical Communication. In: 7th ACM International Conference on Human-Robot Interaction (HRI), Pioneers Workshop (2012)
12. Martin, T.J., Rzepczynski, A.P., Riek, L.D.: Ask, inform, or act: communication with a robotic patient before haptic action. In: Proceedings of the International Conference on Human-Robot Interaction, HRI (2012)
13. Rzepcynski, A., Martin, T., Riek, L.: Communication and awareness: the building blocks of a successful clinical environment. In: Proceedings of the International Conference on Clinical Communication (2012)
14. Janiw, A., Woodrick, L., Riek, L.D.: Patient situational awareness support appears to fall with advancing levels of nursing student education. In: Simulation in Healthcare (2013)
15. Rzepcynski, A., Martin, T., Riek, L.: Informed consent and haptic actions in interdisciplinary simulation training. In: Proceedings of the American Public Health Association, APHA (2012)
16. Henneman, E.A., Roche, J.P., Fisher, D.L., Cunningham, H., Reilly, C.A., Nathanson, B.H., Henneman, P.L.: Error identification and recovery by student nurses using human patient simulation: Opportunity to improve patient safety. Appl. Nurs. Res. 23(1) (2010)
17. Douglas-Cowie, E., Cowie, R., Sneddon, I., Cox, C., Lowry, O., Mcrorie, M., Martin, J.-C., Devillers, L., Abrilian, S., Batliner, A., et al.: The humaine database: addressing the collection and annotation of naturalistic and induced emotional data. In: Affective Computing and Intelligent Interaction, pp. 488–500. Springer, Heidelberg (2007)
18. Ashraf, A.B., Lucey, S., Cohn, J.F., et al.: The painful face: pain expression recognition using active appearance models. ACM ICMI (2007)
19. Lucey, P., et al.: Automatically detecting pain using facial actions. In: 3rd Int'l Conference on Affective Computing and Intelligent Interaction, ACII (2009)
20. Hammal, Z., Cohn, J.F.: Automatic detection of pain intensity. In: ICMI (2012)
21. Coll, M.-P., Grégoire, M., Latimer, M., Eugène, F., Jackson, P.L.: Perception of pain in others: implication for caregivers. Pain Management 1(3), 257–265 (2011)
22. Lucey, P., Cohn, J.F., Prkachin, K.M., Solomon, P.E., Matthews, I.: Painful data: The unbc-mcmaster shoulder pain expression archive database. In: IEEE International Conference on Automatic Face & Gesture Recognition (2011)
23. Riva, P., Sacchi, S., Montali, L., Frigerio, A.: Gender effects in pain detection: Speed and accuracy in decoding female and male pain expressions. Eur. J. Pain (2011)

24. Hirsh, A.T., Alqudah, A.F., Stutts, L.A., Robinson, M.E.: Virtual human technology: Capturing sex, race, and age influences in individual pain decision policies. Pain 140(1) (2008)
25. Kappesser, J.,, A.C., de C. Williams, A.C.: Pain and negative emotions in the face: judgements by health care professionals. Pain 99(1) (2002)
26. Bazo, D., Vaidyanathan, R., Lentz, A., Melhuish, C.: Design and testing of a hybrid expressive face for a humanoid robot. IEEE (IROS) (2010)
27. Berns, K., Hirth, J.: Control of facial expressions of the humanoid robot head roman. In: IEEE/RSJ IROS (2006)
28. Bernardes, S.F., Lima, M.L.: On the contextual nature of sex-related biases in pain judgments: The effects of pain duration, patient's distress and judge's sex. Eur. J. Pain 15(9) (2011)
29. Simon, D., Craig, K.D., Miltner, W.H., Rainville, P.: Brain responses to dynamic facial expressions of pain. Pain 126(1) (2006)
30. Hadjistavropoulos, T., Craig, K.D., Fuchs-Lacelle, S.: Social influences and the communication of pain. Pain: Psychological Perspectives (2004)
31. Prkachin, K.M., Craig, K.D.: Expressing pain: The communication and interpretation of facial pain signals. J. Nonverbal Behav. 19(4) (1995)
32. de C. Williams, A.C., Davies, H.T.O., Chadury, Y.: Simple pain rating scales hide complex idiosyncratic meanings. Pain 85(3) (2000)
33. Aung, M., Romera-Paredes, B., Singh, A., Lim, S., Kanakam, N., de C. Williams, A., Bianchi-Berthouze, N.: Getting rid of pain-related behaviour to improve social and self perception: a technology-based perspective. In: 14th International Workshop on Image Analysis for Multimedia Interactive Services, WIAMIS (2013)
34. Romera-Paredes, B., et al.: Transfer learning to account for idiosyncrasy in face and body expressions. IEEE Face and Gesture (2013)
35. Ekman, P., Rosenberg, E.L.: What the face reveals: Basic and applied studies of spontaneous expression using the Facial Action Coding System, Oxford (1997)
36. Simon, D., Craig, K.D., et al.: Recognition and discrimination of prototypical dynamic expressions of pain and emotions. Pain 135 (2008)
37. Prkachin, K.M., Berzins, S., Mercer, S.R.: Encoding and decoding of pain expressions: a judgement study. Pain 58(2) (1994)
38. Monwar, M.M., Rezaei, S.: Pain recognition using artificial neural network. In: IEEE Symposium on Signal Processing and Information Technology (2006)
39. Williams, L.: Performance-driven facial animation. ACM SIGGRAPH Computer Graphics 24(4) (1990)
40. Wan, X., Jin, X.: Data-driven facial expression synthesis via laplacian deformation. Multimedia Tools and Applications 58(1) (2012)
41. Beeler, T., et al.: High-quality passive facial performance capture using anchor frames. ACM T. Graphic 30 (2011)
42. Bickel, B., et al.: Physical face cloning. ACM T. Graphic. 31 (2012)
43. Pantic, M., Valstar, M., Rademaker, R., Maat, L.: Web-based database for facial expression analysis. In: IEEE Int'l Conf. on Multimedia and Expo, ICME (2005)
44. Baltrusaitis, T., Robinson, P., Morency, L.: 3d constrained local model for rigid and non-rigid facial tracking. In: CVPR (2012)
45. Chew, S.W., Lucey, P., Lucey, S., Saragih, J., Cohn, J.F., Sridharan, S.: Person-independent facial expression detection using constrained local models. In: IEEE Int'l Conf. on Automatic Face and Gesture Recognition, FG (2011)

46. Cristinacce, D., Cootes, T.: Feature detection and tracking with constrained local models. Proceedings of British Machine Vision Conference 3 (2006)
47. Abboud, B., Davoine, F., Dang, M.: Facial expression recognition and synthesis based on an appearance model. Signal Process-Image 19(8) (2004)
48. Valve Software: Source SDK, http://source.valvesoftware.com/sourcesdk.php
49. Camstudio: Open source streaming video software, http://camstudio.org
50. Tottenham, N., et al.: The nimstim set of facial expressions: judgments from untrained research participants. Psychiatry Research 168(3) (2009)
51. Russell, J.A.: Is there universal recognition of emotion from facial expressions? a review of the cross-cultural studies. Psychological Bulletin 115(1) (1994)

Generative Models of Cultural Decision Making for Virtual Agents Based on User's Reported Values

Elnaz Nouri[1,2] and David Traum[1,2]

[1] Institute for Creative Technologies,
12015 Waterfront Dr, Playa Vista, CA 90094, USA
[2] Computer Science Department,
University of Southern California, Los Angeles, CA 90007, USA

Abstract. Building computational models of cultural decision making for virtual agents based on behavioral data is a challenge because finding a reasonable mapping between the statistical data and the computational model is a difficult task. This paper shows how the weights on a multi attribute utility based decision making model can be set according to the values held by people elicited through a survey. If survey data from different cultures is available then this can be done to simulate cultural decision making behavior. We used the survey data of two sets of players from US and India playing the Dictator Game and the Ultimatum Game on-line. Analyzing their reported values in the survey enabled us to set up our model's parameters based on their culture and simulate their behavior in the Ultimatum Game.

Keywords: Cultural Decision Making Models, Dictator Game, Prediction Models.

1 Introduction

In this paper we address one of the major challenges in building behavioral models of culture through data driven approaches which is the task of finding an appropriate mapping from statistical behavior data onto computational models. This paper shows how the reported values of people can be used for building generative models for cultural decision making. The model is a multi attribute decision making model that takes into account several valuation functions such as the utility for self, the utility for the others in the interaction, the competitiveness and etc. This model can be used by virtual humans to make a wide variety of decisions in different contexts, including interacting with both other virtual agents or humans [1].

2 Background

2.1 The Multi Attribute Relational Value Decision Making Model

We briefly introduce the MARV framework (Multi Attribute Relational Value). (for more details you can refer to [2]). In [1] cultural decision models based on

T. Bickmore et al. (Eds.): IVA 2014, LNAI 8637, pp. 310–315, 2014.

this framework were built by setting the weights on the attributes based on the Hofstede's dimensional scores [3] but our goal here is to find these weights on the attributes based on the survey reports. The framework considers a number of different metrics for evaluating a given situation. The metrics considered include:

{Self Interest (the agent's own utility), Other Interest (the utility of another), Total Utility (sum of individual utilities of all participants), Average Utility (may not be derivable from Total Utility when the number of participants is variable), Relative Utilities (viewed in several ways, such as self/total, self/other, self-other, self/average), Minimum Utility, Uncertainty (variation among possible outcomes)}

Each of these metrics can be given one or more valuations, choosing an optimum point and scale. Each individual agent has a vector of weights, one per valuation, indicating the relative importance of that valuation. The total value for each choice is the sum of the product of values and weights for each valuation, as shown below in Formula 1:

$$Utility(choice_i) = \Sigma(W_j * V_j) \tag{1}$$

For every decision, the agent calculates the utility of all of its possible choices and selects the one that has the highest overall valuation (according to the agent's knowledge and ability to calculate or estimate these values).

2.2 Self Reported Values in Games with MARV Survey

Based on the set of attributes in MARV model, [4] made a survey of 8 questions for eliciting the values of people after they make their decisions.[4] used the survey to collect the values of people playing the Ultimatum and the Dictator game over a 100 points. The effect of culture on offers and values was investigated by recruiting people from US and India. 101 and 107 people from each country were recruited using Amazon Mechanical Turk to play the Ultimatum Game and the Dictator game respectively. In the Dictator game the players is asked to split a 100 points between themselves and the other player. The Ultimatum game is played similarly but the other player gets to decide whether he accepts the offer or not. If he accepts they split the points accordingly, if he rejects, they both end up with zero points.

Participants were asked to report how much they cared about each of the values (shown in Table 1.), on a scale from -5 to 5.

3   Mapping the Reported Survey Values to Utility Valuation Functions

Step 1: Calculate Basic Valuation Functions for the Choices. We first defined a set of simple mathematical functions (F) capturing the meaning of each survey question. These functions are called "valuation functions". Table 1

Table 1. MARV Value Survey

Survey Value	Description	Valuation Function
V_{self}	Getting a lot of points	$f_{self} = 100 - offer$
V_{other}	The other player getting a lot of points	$f_{other} = offer$
$V_{compete}$	Getting more points than the other player	$f_{compete} = \lvert f_{self} - f_{other}\rvert = \lvert(100 - offer) - offer\rvert)$
V_{equal}	Having the same number of points as the other player	$f_{equal} = 50/(50 - \lvert f_{self} - f_{other}\rvert = 50/(50 - \lvert(100 - offer) - offer\rvert)$
V_{joint}	Making sure that added together we got as many points as possible	$f_{joint} = 100$
V_{rawls}	The player with fewest points gets as many as possible [5]	$f_{rawls} = min\{f_{self}, f_{other}\} = min\{offer, 100 - offer\}$
$V_{lowerbound}$	Making sure to get some points (even if not as many as possible)	$f_{lower-bound} = min\{f_{self}, f_{other}\} = min\{offer, 100 - offer\}$
V_{chance}	The chance to get a lot of points (even if there's also a chance not to get any points)	$f_{chance} = 100 - offer$

shows the definition of the functions. The definition of f_{self} and f_{other} functions are based on the structure of the game.[1]

The utility of each choice is calculated based on a linear combination of the valuation functions (f_j) and appropriate weights (W_j) on them. The reported importance for each value (R_j) is used as contributing factors to the weights on these valuation functions. The weight (W_j) on each valuation functions is defined as $W_j = S_j * R_j$ so the formula is:

$$Utility(c_i \in C) = \sum_{f_j \in F}(Wj * f_j) = \sum_{f_j \in F}(S_j * R_j * f_j) \qquad (2)$$

In Formula 2, f_j refers to the valuation functions. R_j is the corresponding weight reported by the player and $Scale_j$ is a parameter in the model that is set according to the dataset.

Example: When the proposed offer is 20 then split is (80 self ,20 other). The valuation functions for this offer (choice) are calculated according to the formulas in the table 1.[2] Utility equation of choice 'offer 20' for the proposer in the Dictator Game:

$Utility(choice_{offer20}) = (80*W_{self}) + (20*W_{other}) + (80/20*W_{compete}) + (50/50 - abs(80 - 20) * W_{fairness}) + (100 * W_{joint}) + (20 * W_{rawls}) + (20 * W_{lowerbound}) + (80 * W_{chance})$

Step 2: Find Appropriate Scales for the Model based on the Culture.
For the scales S_j in Formula 2 on the valuation functions. This is done by search-

---

[1] Note that these valuation functions can be generalized to other games based on the definition of the f_{self} and f_{other} functions. (for example in the case of the Dictator Game being played over 100 points $f_{self} + f_{other} = 100$). Their interpretation depends on the definition of the game but the other functions can be computed based on these two basic functions.

[2] Note that if the offer is rejected in the Ultimatum Game the $f_{self} = 0$ and $f_{other} = 0$ according to the rules of the game but the remaining valuation functions can be calculated like the previous cases.

ing the space of different possible values for each of the scale variables (All possible combinations of the scales drawn from the range of $s \in S = \{-10^3 to 10^3\}$ were tried for finding the culture specific scales on each attribute in our simulations.), calculating the utilities and comparing the square distance of the generated behavior for the set of training observations to that of the actual cultural data. The combination of the scales that result in the minimum distance from the cultural data are selected as the scales on the valuation function for the members of that culture.

Step 3: Calculate Prior Probability of Choices based on the Culture. With appropriate scales found for each culture the model can be used for deterministic calculation of the utility of each choice based on each player's value profile. However, our agent uses the notion of Expected Utility (Equation 3) in order to asses the desirability of the choice. At time t in the game, the Expected Utility of each choice (c_t) is calculated by:

$$E(Utility(c_t)) = Utility(c_t)^\alpha * P(c_t)^\beta \qquad (3)$$

Variations in the decisions of the individuals within a culture by calculating the probability of the offers based on his value profile and the Bayesian likelihood of choosing each offer amount based on the offers made by people holding similar values with the culture of the player. For each value ($v_j \in V$) the distribution of offers for each possible answers determined.

$$\forall c_i \in C, \forall v_j \in V : P(c_i \mid v_j) = \frac{P(v_j \mid c_i)P(c_i)}{P(v_j)} = \frac{P(c_i \cap v_j)}{P(v_j)} \qquad (4)$$

The general formula for calculating the probability of offer c_t when the player has reported a profile $v_{self}, v_{other}, \ldots$ of importance on the survey questions is calculated as:

$$P(c_t \mid \bigcap_{v_j \in V} v_j) = \prod_{v_j \in V} \frac{P(c_t \cap v_j)}{P(v_j)} \qquad (5)$$

These probabilities are based on the reports and offers made among players from the cultural group that the the player belongs to.

Step 4: Select the Choice. This is the final step in the algorithm, the $Decision_t$ is made from the set of possible choices (C) by selecting the choice associated with highest expected utility (previously shown in formula 3).[3]

4   Evaluation

We use the algorithm to generate behavior for agents representing US and India. We use the ten-fold cross validation paradigm for splitting our dataset into the training and test segments. We use two methods for evaluating our model:

---

[3] It is possible to define other selection functions at this step. For example one can use a selection function enabling the agent to make decisions as soon as a minimum threshold is met on a specific value. We discuss this in future work section.

Table 2. KL Divergence Distance of the Simulated Behavior to Human Behavior

Game	Model	US	India
Dictator Game	Selfish Model	1.64	1.40
	Majority Model	0.76	1.11
	Our Model	0.26	0.39
Ultimatum Game	Selfish Model	2.42	2.88
	Majority Model	0.87	0.50
	Our Model	0.81	0.30

Table 3. Accuracy of the Prediction of the Offers

Game	Model	US	India
Dictator Game	Selfish Model	12%	20%
	Majority Model	52%	20%
	Our Model	56%	28%
Ultimatum Game	Selfish Model	0%	4%
	Majority Model	52%	56%
	Our Model	48%	64%

Comparing the Model's Output with the Actual Data. The distribution of the offers made by the model were compared against the actual offers and two based lines:

- Selfish baseline: This model chooses the decisions that maximize self-utility.
- Majority baseline: This model chooses the most common decision made by the members of the culture. For both US and Indian in the Dictator Game and the Ultimatum Game this was an offer of 50 (the equal split).

In Table 2 the distribution of offers made by our model and the baseline models are compared to the actual data by using the KL divergence distance metric.[4] Our model is performing significantly better for US and Indian players playing both games.

Predicting Future Offers of Players based on their Values. In Table 3 we compare the performance of our model versus the "Selfish model" and the "Majority model" in predicting the future offers of the players when provided with their values.

Our model outperforms the other models in the prediction task in all conditions except for the US players playing the Ultimatum Game.

5   Conclusions and Future Work

In this paper we provided an algorithm for effectively mapping people's reported values to the utility calculation component of the agent. The cultural variations

---

[4] To measure the difference between the distributions of offers we use Kullback-Leibler divergence measure between two probability distributions.

in behavior are captured by adjusting the weights of the attributes in the model according to the data and calculating the Bayesian probabilities of occurrences of the decisions in the culture group. We compared the performance of our model to human behavioral data by using two well-known games of the Dictator Game and the Ultimatum Game which are widely used by researchers for studying decision making among different groups of people.One of the advantage of using this approach is that its based on a short 8-question survey and doesn't rely on other culture models. We acknowledge that there are other possible mapping functions for this purpose. We address these mappings in future work.

References

1. Nouri, E., Traum, D.: A cultural decision-making model for virtual agents playing negotiation games. In: Proceedings of the International Workshop on Culturally Motivated Virtual Characters, 11th International Conference on Intelligent Virtual Agents (2011)
2. Nouri, E., Georgila, K., Traum, D.: Culture-specific models of negotiation for virtual characters: multi-attribute decision-making based on culture-specific values. Journal of AI and Society 1(1), 87–111 (2014)
3. Hofstede, G., Hofstede, G.J., Minkov, M.: Cultures and organizations: software of the mind, 3rd edn. McGraw-Hill Professional (2010)
4. Nouri, E., Traum, D.: Prediction of game behavior based on culture factors. In: Proceedings of Group Decision and Negotiation Conference (2013)
5. Rawls, J.: Some reasons for the maximin criterion. The American Economic Review 64(2), 141–146 (1974)

Mapping Personality to the Appearance of Virtual Characters Using Interactive Genetic Algorithms

Fabrizio Nunnari[1] and Alexis Heloir[2]

[1] DFKI / MMCI, Germany
fabrizio.nunnari@dfki.de
http://www.dfki.de/~fanu01/
[2] DFKI / MMCI / LAMIH-UMR CNRS 8201, Germany
alexis.heloir@dfki.de
http://slsi.dfki.de

Abstract. We present an architecture for the generation of believable virtual characters from their personality traits. Using a crowd-based approach, we infer how people's beliefs relate personality profile to physical appearance. The method we propose uses interactive genetic algorithms. Combined with natural language processing and sentiment analysis, it has the potential to drive the generation of new virtual characters from written description. In video games and online virtual worlds, it might replace traditional slider-based character personalization approaches by more creative, story-driven ones.

Keywords: Character generation, genetic algorithms, avatar, virtual character, personality traits, OCEAN model.

1 Introduction

Character design is a complex process that involves a number of different professionals: starting from a textual description, sketches and concept drawings, the character is later modelled, textured, rigged, integrated into the scenes, animated, and rendered. The artists involved in the pipeline account for the believability of the resulting character. However, such production pipeline is normally employed in big productions (movies or AAA-class videogames), but cannot be afforded in application domains like avatars for independent video games, shared virtual environments, conversational agents for education and customer care.

A consistent character gathers an outer appearance, a life story and an inner personality. For such a character, believability does not only depend on behavior and motion style [1,2], it also depends on appearance [3]. Our research question is thus "how to build a mapping between two symbolic representations: personality profile and character appearance (morphological and aesthetic features)." In our view, the best way to create a mapping satisfying people expectations is to involve users themselves using crowdsourcing [4].

T. Bickmore et al. (Eds.): IVA 2014, LNAI 8637, pp. 316–319, 2014.
© Springer International Publishing Switzerland 2014

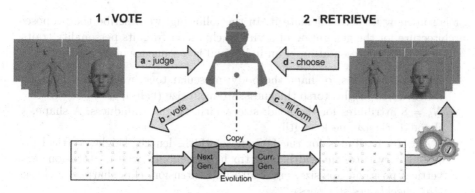

Fig. 1. The workflow of the proposed approach. Voting (left): contributing users assess the individuals of a new forming generation. Evolution (bottom): from time to time, the new generation will replace the current one. Retrieval (right): the user input a personality profile and the system proposes a set of best matching individuals.

To achieve this, we propose an evolutionary approach using Interactive Genetic Algorithms. We start from a set of randomly generated virtual characters that people will assess, or score, along the OCEAN [5] personality traits. After collecting enough votes, the set of individuals will evolve to a new generation that should better represent people expectations. Participants act as calculators of the *fitness function* of the genetic algorithm. Once the repository of individuals reaches a sufficient evolutionary level, it can be used to retrieve a believable character corresponding to a personality profile. Figure 1 depicts the approach introduced above.

2   Mapping Personality to Appearance

Solving a problem with genetic algorithms requires the definition of a *genetic representation* and a *fitness function*. The former is used to univocally represent the characteristics of an individual, the latter, applied to an individual, gives an evaluation of "how good" it is with respect to a desired target solution. A set of individuals in a given moment is called *generation*. The first generation is generally randomly generated. Further generations are calculated, mimicking real-world phenomena like *election, mutation* and *cross-over*.

Ideally, the more generations are calculated, the better are the individuals in it, whose average fitness function value has increased. The computation of new generations ends when a satisfying fitness function value has been reached for an individual, or when a maximum allowed computation time has elapsed. However, for some problems a fitness function cannot be identified, or might be related to tasks that only humans can accomplish (like evaluating the quality of a picture). This led to the introduction of Interactive Genetic Algorithms (IGAs): in this approach genetic algorithms are run by asking humans to perform an evaluation for each individual of a generation. The evaluation is directly used as fitness value or is somehow used to calculate it. In the following, we describe the proposed architecture for the generation of a virtual character from its personality traits.

The genetic representation of an individual is a sequence of 32 attributes:

- $N_b = 8$ attributes to shape the body: muscular tone, weight, height, torso width, torso height, torso thickness, stomach size (belly),
- $N_h = 8$ attributes for the head: size, width, height, roundness, A shape, V shape, neck size, neck length,
- $N_f = 16$ attributes for the face: nose width, length, height, vertical position, curvature, tip width, and tip height; mouth width, extrusion, and vertical position, lips size, jaw width and extrusion, chin sharpness, cheeks size, cheekbones sharpness.

In the voting phase, users contribute in calculating the fitness function value of individuals by describing them according to the OCEAN model. This model describes the personality of a character through 5 dimensions whose values lie in a continuous range $[-1, 1]$. The five dimensions are: Openness, Conscientiousness, Extraversion, Agreeableness, and Neuroticism.

Users will vote through an on-line form that shows a full body picture and a face close up of the individual. Below the pictures there are 5 lines of check boxes, one for each of the Big Five traits. Each trait presents 7 check boxes. Each checkbox corresponds to a discrete qualification of the trait. For example, for the Extraversion/Introversion trait, users can check one or more of the following: Very Extravert, Somewhat Extravert, Slightly Extravert, Neutral (Neither Extravert nor Introvert), Slightly Introvert, Somewhat Introvert, Very Introvert. This yields to a total of 35 checkable *slots*.

Each slot corresponds to a counter. Each counter is incremented when a voting user checks the slot. Before calculating the fitness function, the counters will be normalised in the range $[0, 1]$, separately for each dimension. For example, an individual collecting, in the Extraversion trait, Neutral=2, Slightly Extravert=2, and Somewhat Extravert=6, will be normalised to the vector $[0.0, 0.0, 0.0, 0.2, 0.2, 0.4, 0.0]$. The same is done in each trait.

Given an individual x, let's denote with $C_t^i(x)$ the function retrieving the normalised score (in the range $[0, 1]$) for a segment i (from 1 to 7) in the personality trait t (one among the Big Five: O,C,E,A,N). The fitness function is defined as the maximum among all normalised counters:

$$\max\{C_t^i(x)\}, 1 \leq i \leq 7, t \in \{o, c, e, a, n\}$$

In the retrieval phase, the system takes as input a personality vector $\bar{P} = (P_o, P_c, P_e, P_a, P_n)$, where the range of values is normalised so that: $P_t \in [-1, 1]$ for each trait $t \in \{o, c, e, a, n\}$. Then, the value of each personality trait is discretised to an integer value in the range $[1, 7]$, like in the creation of the voting form. Hence, a new vector is defined: $\bar{P}' = (P_o', P_c', P_e', P_a', P_n')$, where $1 \leq P_t' \leq 7$ for each trait $t \in \{o, c, e, a, n\}$. In other words the vector $\bar{P}'$ identifies a combination of one segment for each of the 5 personalities (7^5 possible values). The retrieval of an individual can then be formulated as a maximisation problem. Given a set of individuals in a generation X, and a discretised personality vector $\bar{P}'$, we want to retrieve the individual whose normalised counter of each dimension have the highest value in the identified segments:

$$\arg\max_{x\in X}\{C_t^i(x)/i = P_t'(x)\}, t \in \{o, c, e, a, n\}$$

The system will present to the user a set of alternatives, not only the best candidate. Possibly, candidates might be scattered across the solution space, as they represents different views that people have of the same personality.

The system has been tested by 5 subjects for 5 days. Then a survey form has been filled. Since there are not enough contributions for meaningful retrieving, only the voting task has been evaluated. The comments are overall positive, with 4 out of 5 users able to understand and fulfill the task without the need of any additional help.

3   Conclusions and Future Work

If successful, we believe that our approach might provide a valuable tool for game designers and virtual story-tellers. A tool that would help them creating believable characters with regard to the story being told. The platform is implemented and in beta test stage. Once it will be publicly available, our aim will be to gather enough data to guarantee convergence towards a stable mapping between appearance features and personality traits.

According to the results of our preliminary study, the users were more inclined to use the platform for a longer time per day (6 votes instead of 3) but less frequently (once a week instead of once per day). This is in our opinion suggesting that the task is rather interesting, appealing, and people prefer to dig into the task rather than occasionally contributing. To make the voting task lighter we plan to develop a voting system based on a side-to-side comparison of two individuals. There the voters will be asked to simply select which of the two characters look, for example, more Extrovert, or Closed. This approach will be more faster-paced for the users, favouring casual, sporadic, contributions.

References

1. Thomas, F., Johnston, O.: The illusion of life: Disney animation. Hyperion, New York (1995)
2. Bates, J.: The role of emotion in believable agents. Communications of the ACM 37(7), 122–125 (1994)
3. Lee, S., Heeter, C.: Computer science and communication perspectives on character believability in games. In: Annual Meeting of the International Communication Association, Montreal, Quebec, Canada (May 2008)
4. Howe, J.: The rise of crowdsourcing. Wired 6(14) (June 2006)
5. McCrae, R.R., John, O.P.: An introduction to the five-factor model and its applications. Journal of Personality 60(2), 175–215 (1992)

Towards a Computational Architecture of Dyadic Rapport Management for Virtual Agents

Alexandros Papangelis, Ran Zhao, and Justine Cassell

ArticuLab, Carnegie Mellon University, 5000 Forbes Ave, Pittsburgh, PA, USA

Abstract. Rapport has been identified as an important factor in human task performance. Motivated by the proliferation of virtual agents that assist humans on various tasks, we propose a computational architecture for virtual agents, building on our own work on a dyadic model of rapport between humans and virtual agents. We show how such a system can be trained in order to build, maintain and destroy rapport.

1 Introduction and Related Work

While rapport, or feeling "in sync" with a partner, has sound theoretical foundations and demonstrated benefits in a variety of contexts, little success has been achieved in long-term rapport between a human and virtual agent / embodied conversational agent (ECA). To fill this gap, we analyzed existing social science literature, as well as our own data, and proposed a theoretical framework and computational model of rapport for human to virtual agent interaction (published in this same volume) [11]. Building on that work, we here propose a computational architecture that treats rapport as a dyadic phenomenon, and allows the virtual agent to manage it in real-time with human users. We argue that the proposed architecture enables the system to build, maintain and even destroy rapport, over multiple interactions with the same user. Our contribution, therefore, in this work is a computational architecture for real-time rapport management in human agent interaction, built on the dyadic model proposed in [11].

Some relational agents are designed for building long term social companionship, for example [1, 5, 6]. [3, 9] inter alia, propose agents that interact through verbal and non-verbal signals. [4] propose an architecture for generating social behavior in human to robot interactions, [12] takes achievement of synchrony into account, but the only other demonstration of rapport management comes from the VH Toolkit [2], which focuses only on non-verbal behavior, and only for "instant rapport." Our work improves on prior approaches by relying on strong theoretical foundations in the social sciences, as well as an analysis of peer tutoring data, which together allow us to construct a dyadic framework based on actual conversational strategies which are carried by specific behaviors and which achieve specific rapport goals.

T. Bickmore et al. (Eds.): IVA 2014, LNAI 8637, pp. 320–324, 2014.
© Springer International Publishing Switzerland 2014

2 Towards a Computational Architecture of Rapport

The dyadic nature of our architecture means that updates and grounding are achieved by taking into account both user and system state. More specifically, we follow [11] who define rapport-management strategies whose effect cannot be grounded until we observe the user's reaction. To achieve this it is necessary to represent a dyadic state that models what has been grounded; a model of the user representing the system's beliefs about the user; and a putative ECA state inside that user model, representing the system's beliefs of how the user perceives it. The proposed architecture is presented in Figure 1, where we extend a generic ECA architecture. Clear components denote generic modules, while shaded components denote our contribution to the overall architecture, where Intention Understanding interprets and then maps the intentions behind the user's actions to our model of rapport, the Friendship Classifier implements [10], Rapport carries out updates to the rapport state, and the Conversation Manager plans verbal and non-verbal output.

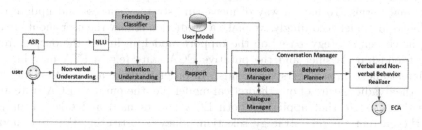

Fig. 1. The proposed VA architecture, incorporating our model of rapport

The most important data structures in our architecture, derived from our model, include the *dyadic state* representing the current state of rapport and a *user model* containing information acquired during the interaction. More specifically, the *dyadic state* comprises the following: 1) The System's goals, represented as a tree and split into task-oriented and social; 2) Rapport State, containing information about coordination, mutual attentiveness [8] and face [7]; 3) a behavioral model representing sociocultural and interpersonal norms (i.e. the ECA's behavioral expectations); 4) Friendship status, as a binary variable; and 5) History, containing information user act intentions, an estimate of the whether rapport is increasing or not, etc. The *user model*, contains information about the user's goals, shared knowledge, which may either be short-term (i.e. relevant to the current interaction only) or long-term, and a task model representing the user's progress regarding the task. In the *user model* we also represent a putative ECA state – an estimate of how the user perceives the system and comprising a rapport state, friendship status, shared knowledge and action intentions of the ECA.

In order to manipulate rapport a set of strategies have been defined, following [11], that allow the ECA to build, maintain and destroy rapport. For each strategy, a set of available system actions (or dialogue moves) $A_s \subset A$ can be defined, where A is the set of all (non-)verbal system actions; it is up to the Dialogue Manager (DM) to select the most appropriate ones. Rapport strategy selection is facilitated by taking into account the *dyadic state* and the *user model*. The selected strategy is then forwarded to the DM, responsible for selecting a set of appropriate actions, by taking into account the *dialogue state* which contains task- and interaction-related information. To assess rapport and update the *rapport state*, we estimate the user's intentions and, mapping these to the model, we update the *rapport state* accordingly[1]. Reinforcement Learning (RL) is a good candidate for learning which strategy and action to follow, paired with good feature selection methods. The behavioral model and dialogue policies, initialized to reflect general sociocultural norms for behavior in the particular context, are updated after each user action, according to how well the system's goals were met. As system and user interact, the strategy and dialogue policies gradually shift to reflect the increasingly interpersonal norms they follow. The policies, therefore, can be thought of as the facilitators of the rapport model, as they select strategies and actions based on the rapport state and current interpersonal norms. To have a way of measuring strategy success and update the behavioral model accordingly, we make a prediction of how the user should react to the chosen strategy, based on the rapport model, including the output from the friendship classifier and the putative ECA state (e.g. a FTA may have a different effect on strangers vs. friends). In order to make a prediction, we utilize the dyadic nature of our theoretical model (i.e. the putative ECA state and the *dyadic state* that applies to both ECA and human) and take advantage of the current (learnt) strategy selection policy, substituting the user model with the putative ECA state.

There are two phases where the Rapport module is used: rapport generation and rapport assessment. In the generation phase, we decide which rapport strategy to follow, based on the current *dyadic state* and the *user model*, while in the assessment phase, we assess the impact of the chosen strategy on the *dyadic state*, according to our model. During the rapport assessment phase, we observe the user's action and infer the intentions behind it, again according to our model, and use these inferred intentions to update the rapport state. It should be noted here that the dimensions of the rapport state pertaining to the Tickle-Degnen & Rosenthal [8] model, reflect an overall assessment of the system's and user's respective attentiveness and coordination. The system's face as well as the user's face are updated separately, immediately after performing a system or user action.

3   Concluding Remarks

Aiming to reduce complexity and improve tractability, it may be a reasonable first approximation to assume that task goals are independent of social goals and social features (*dyadic state* and *user model* separated from task model). Simplifying further, we assume that the overall strategy can be decomposed into

---

[1] http://tinyurl.com/dyadic-rapport

task-related and social-interaction-related moves. Thus, instead of learning an overall dialogue policy that achieves all the goals, we can now learn a task-related dialogue policy and a social-interaction-related policy. The selected strategy is forwarded to the DM, where action selection occurs by taking both dialogue policies into account. This, however, raises many interesting challenges such as dealing with competing strategies or incompatible actions (w.r.t task and social interaction), or including a module to aggregate the two strategies into one single strategy where possible. A complete treatment of this issue is kept for future work. We plan to train the system using our peer tutoring data and data from a Wizard of Oz study we plan to conduct, to train a simulated user that will interact with the system. To achieve this, we will apply inverse RL to estimate a good reward function and then direct sparse RL methods to train the simulator, and allow it to replicate and generalize from the data. Initially, competing goals will be addressed by the DM or the behavior planner.

As we increasingly refine the computational model presented in [11], we will incrementally implement our computational architecture, starting with a virtual peer reciprocal tutoring application for algebra. Foreseeable challenges include recognition of the human users' rapport strategies (which may span several dialogue turns or interleave with other strategies) in order to correctly update our model as well as react in the appropriate fashion, and training our learning modules before deployment for evaluation to ensure that our rapport strategies achieve the rapport management they are designed to convey.

Acknowledgments. The authors would like to thank Zhou Yu for her contribution to this work, as well as the other students and staff of the Articu-Lab. This work was partially supported by the R.K. Mellon Foundation, and NSF IIS.

References

1. Bickmore, T.W., Caruso, L., Clough-Gorr, K., Heeren, T.: "It's just like you talk to a friend" relational agents for older adults. Interacting with Computers 17(6), 711–735 (2005)
2. Hartholt, A., Traum, D., Marsella, S.C., Shapiro, A., Stratou, G., Leuski, A., Morency, L.-P., Gratch, J.: All together now: Introducing the virtual human toolkit. In: Aylett, R., Krenn, B., Pelachaud, C., Shimodaira, H. (eds.) IVA 2013. LNCS, vol. 8108, pp. 368–381. Springer, Heidelberg (2013)
3. Hoque, M.E., Courgeon, M., Martin, J.-C., Mutlu, B., Picard, R.W.: Mach: My automated conversation coach (2013)
4. Huang, C.-M., Mutlu, B.: Robot behavior toolkit: generating effective social behaviors for robots. In: Proc. of the 7th ACM/IEEE Int. Conf. on Human-Robot Interaction, pp. 25–32. ACM (2012)
5. Khosla, R., Chu, M.-T., Kachouie, R., Yamada, K., Yamaguchi, T.: Embodying care in matilda: an affective communication robot for the elderly in australia (2012)
6. Sidner, C.: Engagement: Looking and not looking as evidence for disengagement. In: Workshop at HRI, vol. 12 (2012)

7. Spencer-Oatey, H.: (im) politeness, face and perceptions of rapport: unpackaging their bases and interrelationships (2005)
8. Tickle-Degnen, L., Rosenthal, R.: The nature of rapport and its nonverbal correlates. Psychological Inquiry 1(4), 285–293 (1990)
9. Wilks, Y., Jasiewicz, J.: Calonis: An artificial companion for the care of cognitively impaired patients. In: MEMCA-14. This Proc. (2014)
10. Yu, Z., Gerritsen, D., Ogan, A., Black, A., Cassell, J.: Automatic prediction of friendship via multi-model dyadic features (August 2013)
11. Zhao, R., Papangelis, A., Cassell, J.: Towards a dyadic computational model of rapport management for human-virtual agent interaction. In: Bickmore, T., Marsella, S., Sidner, C. (eds.) IVA 2014. LNCS (LNAI), vol. 8637, pp. 514–527. Springer, Heidelberg (2014)
12. Zwiers, J., van Welbergen, H., Reidsma, D.: Continuous interaction within the saiba framework. In: Vilhjálmsson, H.H., Kopp, S., Marsella, S., Thórisson, K.R. (eds.) IVA 2011. LNCS, vol. 6895, pp. 324–330. Springer, Heidelberg (2011)

A Cognitive Model of Social Relations
for Artificial Companions

Florian Pecune, Magalie Ochs, and Catherine Pelachaud

CNRS-LTCI, Telecom ParisTech, France
{pecune,ochs,pelachaud}@telecom-paristech.fr

Abstract. Artificial companions are made to establish and maintain long-term relationships with users. In order to model the companion's social relations and to capture its dynamics, we propose a neural network model based on a formal representation of social relations. Based on psychological theories, we characterize social relations over two dimensions, namely liking and dominance. These two dimensions are formally described as a combination of beliefs and goals of the agent's mental state. Such a model allows us to automatically compute the social relation of a virtual agent towards its interlocutor depending on its beliefs and goals.

Keywords: Virtual agents, artificial companions, social relations, social dynamics.

1   Introduction

According to [1], a companion can be defined as *"a robot or a virtual conversational agent that possesses a certain level of intelligence and autonomy as well as social skills that allow it to establish and maintain long-term relationships with users"*. Our research work aims at developing virtual companions endowed with a cognitive model of social relations that allows them to (1) compute their social relations towards the user, (2) determine how this social relation evolves depending on the interaction and (3) influence their decision making. Indeed, a companion playing the role of a teacher should have a different behaviour than another one embodied as a play friend. In this paper, as a first step, we focus on the first problematic, that is how to compute the social relation of a virtual companion towards the user given the context of the interaction. More precisely, we propose a cognitive model in which the social relation of the companion is represented and initialized based on its goals and beliefs. The cognitive model is coupled with a neural network to represent the dynamics of the relation. From this model combining a formal representation and a neural network representation, several strategies emerge that enables a companion to determine how to modify its own relation towards the user.

2   Related Work

In the domain of virtual agents, social relations are often represented by a dimensional representation. Among these agents, some try to model the social

T. Bickmore et al. (Eds.): IVA 2014, LNAI 8637, pp. 325–328, 2014.

relations and more precisely their dynamics during interactions. *Laura* [2], for example, encourages users to exercise on a daily basis. Laura's behaviour evolves over everyday interactions, through pre-scripted dialogues. The relationship is based on a stage model, which could be related to the dimension of intimacy.

One approach to model the dynamics of social relations is based on logical concepts. In [3], the authors try to team up humans with a group of synthetic characters, using a formal representation of liking and dominance. The evolution of these two dimensions rely on the content of the interactions between the agents. Finally, in [4], the author formalizes the five bases of power described by Raven [5] with four different categories. The author also models the agent's decisions, knowing the power relations in which it is involved.

Although most of the models above focused on the dynamics of social relations, few of them initialize these relations in a formal way. Indeed, the initial values of the social relations are generally fixed intuitively depending on the context of the interaction. In this paper, we propose a model to formally compute the social relation of a virtual agent considering the two dimensions of dominance and liking.

3   A Cognitive Model of Social Relations

In our research, we consider cognitive agents with an explicit representation of beliefs and goals that allow them to reason about their environments. As in [6], our cognitive agents have beliefs about the other agents, constituting a theory of mind (*ToM*). Therefore, the relation between an agent A and an agent B will change whenever A updates its beliefs about B. To capture the dynamics of the relation, the cognitive model is combined with a neural network representation. Each goal and belief of the agent is represented by a neuron. The importance accorded to these beliefs and goals by the agent is represented by the weights of the links of the neural network: the more important they are for the agent, the higher the influence on dominance and liking will be.

3.1   Liking

In our work, the formal representation of the liking dimension is based on Heider's Balance Theory [7]. This theory can be represented as a triangular schema between an agent A as the focus of the analysis, another agent B and an impersonal entity C, which could be a physical object, an idea or an event. Since the Balance Theory assumes that people tend to seek balanced states, two scenarios can be defined: (1) if A believes that both A and B share the same appreciation about a concept C, then A's liking towards B will increase. (2) On the other hand, if A believes that A and B have contradictory appreciations about the same concept C, then A's liking towards B will decrease.

To model the liking between an agent A and an agent B, we first need to represent each concept of agent A's world and its appreciation degree towards these concepts. In our model, each concept is represented by a neuron. The activation of this neuron represents the degree of appreciation of the concept. Then, considering a theory of mind, we introduce A's beliefs about B's appreciations concerning these concepts, and we compute the values of agreement or disagreement. These values will eventually influence the final liking value, depending on the importance accorded by A to each concept. The more important A considers a concept, the more agreeing or disagreeing with B will influence its liking.

Since A's liking value towards B is based on beliefs and a theory of mind of the agent B, the agent A might like B, but B might dislike A. This is consistent with the work presented in [3] claiming that liking is not necessary mutual.

3.2 Dominance

The theoretical background for our formal model of dominance is based on the work of Emerson [8], and more particularly on his definition of dependence. For Emerson, the dependence of an agent A upon another agent B is "(1) directly proportional to A's motivational investment in goals mediated by B and (2) inversely proportional to the availability of those goals to A outside of the A-B relation". The motivational investment corresponds to the importance accorded by an agent A to a goal G for which another agent B has an influence (positive or negative). The availability of the goal, in the definition of Emerson, corresponds to the number of agents D different from B that also have a positive influence on the same goal G.

Our work differs from Castelfranchi's dependence theory [9] in the sense that our dependence is subjective: if the agent A does not believe that B can influence one of its goal, it will not be dependent. Another difference with this theory is that the agent B can, not only be helpful, but also threatening to one of A's goals. An agent B is said helpful if it can do an action that helps A to achieve its goal. On the contrary, an agent B is said threatening if it can do an action that prevents A to achieve its goal.

To model the dominance of an agent A towards an agent B, we first need to represent *A's dependence upon B*. For each goal of the agent A, we define two cases, represented by two neurons: B can be helpful or threatening. Then, considering a theory of mind, we represent A's beliefs about B's actions and their influence (which could be positive or negative) on A's goals. The more A considers its goals as important, the more A will be dependent upon B. We also introduce the number of potential helpers, inhibiting the dependence value. The second step is to model A's belief about B dependence. This can be done by modelling A's belief about B's goals and A's actions.

In his work, Emerson [8] defines the power of an agent A over an agent B as a potential influence depending on A's dependence upon B and B's dependence upon A. In our model, an agent A is dominant towards an agent B if A believes that B is more dependent towards A than A is towards B. Thus, the value of dominance is set as the difference between A's dependence towards B and A's belief about B dependence.

4 Conclusion

In this work, we introduced a cognitive model for artificial companions. The social relation between two agents is represented by two different dimensions: dominance and liking. Dominance can be defined by the degree of influence on the intentions of the agent's interlocutor. It also depends on the degree of dependence upon this same agent. The value of liking indicates the degree of like-mindedness between the two agents; an agent will like another agent if it believes that they share the same feelings (positive or negative) about particular concepts. We also introduced a neural network to model the dynamics of these dimensions. Agents may use different strategies to change their own mental state or try to influence other agent's relations.

Acknowledgement. This research has been supported by the ANR Project MoCA.

References

1. Lim, M.Y.: Memory models for intelligent social companions. In: Zacarias, M., de Oliveira, J.V. (eds.) Human-Computer Interaction. SCI, vol. 396, pp. 241–262. Springer, Heidelberg (2012)
2. Bickmore, T., Picard, R.: Establishing and maintaining long-term human-computer relationships. ACM Transactions on Computer-Human Interaction (TOCHI) 12(2), 293–327 (2005)
3. Prada, R., Paiva, A.: Teaming up humans with autonomous synthetic characters. Artificial Intelligence 173(1), 80–103 (2009)
4. Pereira, G., Prada, R., Santos, P.A.: Conceptualizing Social Power for Agents. In: Aylett, R., Krenn, B., Pelachaud, C., Shimodaira, H. (eds.) IVA 2013. LNCS, vol. 8108, pp. 313–324. Springer, Heidelberg (2013)
5. Raven, B.: The bases of power and the power/interaction model of interpersonal influence. Analyses of Social Issues and Public Policy 8(1), 1–22 (2008)
6. Marsella, S.C., Pynadath, D.V., Read, S.J.: Psychsim: Agent-based modeling of social interactions and influence. In: Proceedings of the International Conference on Cognitive Modeling, pp. 243–248. Citeseer (2004)
7. Heider, F.: The Psychology of Interpersonal Relations. Lawrence Erlbaum Associates Inc. (1958)
8. Emerson, R.: Power-dependence relations. American Sociological Review 27(1), 31–41 (1962)
9. Castlefranchi, C., Miceli, M., Cesta, A.: Dependence relations among autonomous agents. ACM SIGOIS Bulletin 13(3), 14 (1992)

An Eye Tracking Evaluation of a Virtual Pediatric Patient Training System for Nurses

Toni B. Pence[1], Lauren C. Dukes[1] Larry F. Hodges[1],
Nancy K. Meehan[1], and Arlene Johnson[2]

[1] Clemson University,
100 McAdams Hall, Clemson SC 29634, USA
tbloodw@g.clemson.edu
[2] The College of Saint Scholastica,
1200 Kenwood Avenue, Duluth, Minnesota, 55811, USA

Abstract. We report an eye tracking experiment conducted on a virtual pediatric patient system to determine the effect of different visual interface layouts on the amount of visual interaction of student nurses with a virtual mother-child dyad. The results of this experiment provide insight into the tradeoffs between using animated or non-animated virtual patients and relative advantages/disadvantages of interacting with the system though a tablet interface.

Keywords: Virtual Characters, Virtual Environment, Virtual Patients, Simulation Training, Eye Tracking.

1 Introduction

Nursing students have limited opportunities for interaction with real patients, especially with pediatric patients, and often do not receive immediate and impartial feedback on their performance during their patient interaction. We created a virtual pediatric patient system for nursing students in order to provide an alternative educational method to practice their interviewing skills, with guidance, feedback and consistent experiences for all students. Experiential learning through simulation may help students develop the skills necessary for clinical practice and help develop the self-efficacy and critical thinking skills they need to provide the safest care possible. Since children are a vulnerable population, nurses must develop appropriate pediatric skills necessary to provide safe care to infants, children, and teens.

During the development and previous usability evaluations of our system, we realized the importance of determining what type of interface layout would give nursing students the most realistic experience. In our previous publiciation, we found that our current interface layout afforded the achievement of positive learning outcomes [1], but we were also interested in the importance of eye contact between nurses and their patients. In order to investigate this we first needed to determine how often users looked at our virtual patients and the surrounding visual interface. In this paper, we discuss an eye tracking evaluation

T. Bickmore et al. (Eds.): IVA 2014, LNAI 8637, pp. 329–338, 2014.

conducted on our virtual pediatric patient training system in which we compared three different system layouts.

2   Related Work

2.1   Simulation Learning and Training

The Institute of Medicine has recommended the use of simulation training as a method to improve health care delivery [2]. Simulation training is an effective strategy to help promote safe clinical practices [3] and impacts the development of self-efficacy and judgment skills for nurses that are essential to provide the safest and most effective care possible [4]. Simulation learning that mimics real world scenarios is beneficial to nursing students and will provide standardized experiences in which students can practice problem solving techniques and clinical decision making abilities [4].

One of the current simulation exercises in the Clemson University School of Nursing involves students acting out written scenarios, where one student acts as the patient while the other acts as the nurse. Our virtual pediatric patient system can replace the student patient with a virtual patient. Researchers have used virtual patients to teach communications skills to medical students, and students have rated the virtual patient experience as being as effective as a standardized patient (actor) [4]. Medical students have also used virtual patients to help practice patient interviewing skills with a high level of immersion. Results indicate that using life-size virtual characters with speech recognition is useful in their education [5]. Adult virtual patients are fairly common, but virtual pediatric patients are rare. The use of virtual pediatric patients was first addressed in [6], but the technology for creating virtual childrens behaviors was lacking, therefore the realism needed for this project was not available.

2.2   Communication and Interaction

The dynamics related to the nurse-family-child relationship are extensive due to the many factors that enter into this relationship, including ethnicity, age, culture, and illness. During an assessment, the nurse must obtain information (verbal and nonverbal) from the parent(s) and child, and observe any interactions between them [4]. Studies by pediatric experts have shown that the nurse-family-child relationship is heavily dependent upon effective communication, which is a skill that is developed through interaction with different kinds of pediatric patients and families [7]. Student nurses must be aware of the interactions that may negatively or positively affect their communication skills, therefore affecting the relationship [7].

Effective communication is widely accepted by the nursing community as a key factor in patient satisfaction, recovery and compliance [8]. A study done by Johnson et al. showed that virtual patient systems using natural interaction methods will facilitate effective teaching and training of communication skills with medical students [9]. Stevens et al. reports on the development and initial testing of a virtual patient system that incorporates an interactive virtual clinic scenario and virtual instructor to teach history-taking skills [2]. In this study, students were able to interact with the virtual patient and virtual instructor via speech recognition software, which gave the student a more natural method of interacting with the virtual patient.

Studies have shown that using virtual environments for simulation training can be effective [10] and that using life-like animated virtual characters can increase the level of realism of the training simulation [11]. The study done by Johnson et al. also showed that virtual patient systems with highly detailed human models create a more realistic experience [9]. Gulz et al. finds that the most established effect of animated agents in educational systems is the potential they provide to make the experience more engaging for the student [12].

2.3 Eye Tracking

Eye tracking is a technique where a person's eye movements are measured so that a researcher knows where a person is looking for a given amount of time and the sequence of how their eyes shift [13]. A wide variety of disciplines use eye tracking techniques, such as human factors, virtual reality, vehicle simulation, and medical research. Eye tracking has become prevalent in usability research and human computer interaction. Researchers use eye tracking evaluations to make informed interface design descisions [14]. For instance, eye trackers have been used to evaluate the design of cockpit controls in an airplane [15], improve doctor's performance in a virtual laparoscopic surgery training environment [16], and improving a radiologist performance in detecting breast cancer during a mammogram [17].

3   System Description

The SIDNIE (Scaffolded Interviews Developed by Nurses in Education) system is designed to teach nursing students pediatric patient interview techniques by providing interview practice with guidance and feedback from a virtual agent named Sidnie. Sidnie is a male nurse that serves as our virtual nurse educator, who guides the user through several scaffolded practice opportunities and provides feedback on user choices. The user conducts an interview with a five year old virtual patient and her mother by selecting questions from a preset list of questions developed by our nursing collaborators. Then the virtual patient-parent dyad responds appropriately by performing speech and animations based on the question selected.

One of SIDNIEs novel aspects is that it provides criteria-based scoring on questions that students ask. Currently, SIDNIE scores student questions on two aspects: *age appropriateness*, which means that if the question is addressed to the child, it uses words that the child will understand, or if the question requires more difficult phrases, it is directed towards the parent, and *unbiasedness*, which means that the question does not imply a certain answer or assume something to be true that the patient has not confirmed. During a requirements analysis meeting with our nursing collaborators, they identified these attributes as important characteristics for questions in a successful pediatric patient interview. Each question choice presented to the student is scored within our database on the basis of these two criteria, allowing SIDNIE to give automated feedback and scoring on each question the student selects. Figure 1 shows what the user sees when interacting with the system.

The application either runs on a standard desktop computer or tablet and a large screen TV, and the user interacts with the system using either a mouse or touch. We used an off-the-shelf high performance eye tracker by Gazepoint, called the GP3 Eye Tracker [18] . For a more detailed description of SIDNIE including scenario development, system design, scaffolded level descriptions, database contents (questions, answers and animations) and system implementation please refer to [19].

4   Experiments

4.1   Experimental Description

Here we report on an eye tracking experiment conducted on SIDNIE in which we compared three different visual interface layouts. Each layout presented the same scenario: a mother with her five year old daughter, who has an earache.

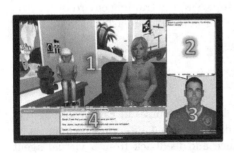
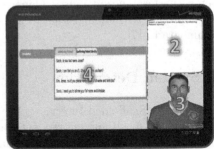

(a) TV Layout   (b) Tablet Layout

Fig. 1. (a) shows the interface layout for *Condition 0* and *Condition 1*, as shown on a large screen tv. (b) shows the interface layout for the tablet used in *Condition 2* where **Section 1** is displayed on a large screen tv.

The visual interface layouts are divided into four sections. **Section 1** houses the virtual pediatric office with the virtual patient-mother dyad present, **Section 2** is a response bubble that provides appropriate feedback to the participant, **Section 3** is Sidnie, the nursing assistant, and **Section 4** contains the available bank of questions related to the scenario (Figure 1(a)).

In *Condition 0*, the visual layout is presented to the user on a large screen TV with **Section 1** containing non-animated virtual characters (Figure 1(a)). In *Condition 1*, the visual layout is displayed to the user on a large screen TV with **Section 1** containing animated virtual characters with lip syncing (Figure 1(a)). In *Condition 2*, the visual layout is displayed on a tablet (Figure 1(b)), except for **Section 1**, which is displayed on a large screen TV and contained animated virtual characters with lip syncing.

Our primary *goal* of the research study was to determine if virtual characters containing life-like animations would affect how often users looked at the virtual patient-mother dyad (**Section 1**). We *hypothesized* that the amount of time spent looking at **Section 1** would be higher in *Condition 1* than in *Condition 0*. Another *goal* was to determine whether or not displaying **Sections 2, 3** and **4** on a tablet while **Section 1** was displayed on a large screen tv would have an effect on how often the users looked at the virtual patient and her mother (**Section 1**). Our *hypothesis* was that the amount of time spent looking at **Section 1** would be higher in *Condition 2* than in *Condition 1* or *Condition 0*. In relation to *Condition 0* and *Condition 1*, we were also interested in determing the amount of time participants spent in each of the four sections, regardless of condition. We *hypothesized* that participants would spend most of their time looking at the virtual patients section, followed by the bank of questions, then the response bubble, and lastly they would spend the least amount of time looking at Sidnie.

4.2   Experimental Procedures

In all three conditions, the participants read and signed an informed consent and completed a qualification questionnaire modified from the screener questionnaire outlined by the Nielsen Norman Group [20] . If the participant passed the qualification questionnaire, we then asked the participant to complete a demographics questionnaire, including questions about previous computer usage, experience in health care, and exposure to virtual environments or eye tracking.

Next we seated the participant at a desktop computer and started the 5 point calibration process for the eye tracker, which was provided with the Gazepoint GP3 software. Next, we started recording the eye tracking data, which consisted of a gaze replay video (gaze plot and heat map) and a csv file of fixation related data (such as coordinates, timestamps, validity, left and right eye). We recorded eye tracking data from the beginning of the tutorial until the end of the interaction with the system.

Next, we began the SIDNIE system by taking the participant through tutorial screens on how to use the system. Then, we asked the participant to conduct an interview with the patients to the best of their ability. The SIDNIE system required that the nursing student ask a correct (both age appropriate and unbiased) question from each of the 15 categories. Sidnie gave feedback on each question selected. At the end of the scenario, participants received feedback on their overall performance in chart form, with a line for each question the participant asked during the interview that contained its scoring information for the criteria.

After the participant completed the interview, we asked them to fill out the interview post-questionnaire. Then the participant completed the System Usability Scale (SUS) [21] and was given the opportunity to provide written feedback. The participant was also given a questionnaire on co-presence adapted from the Slater co-presence questionnaire found in [22]. Finally, the participant completed a debriefing interview with the experimenter, where we asked questions about his or her opinion of the system.

4.3   Participants

Fifty-two students participated in the eye tracking evaluation of SIDNIE, with 17 participants in *Condition 0*, 16 participants in *Condition 1*, and 19 participants in *Condition 2*. All 52 participants were freshman undergraduate nursing students (19-20 years old). Two participants were male, while 50 participants were female. For all pre-questionniare questions the scale went from 1=none to 5=a great deal. Participants reported a high amount of daily computer use (mean=4.46, sd=0.64), a medium level of experience working with children (mean=3.76, sd=1.05), a low level of exposure to virtual humans (mean=1.19, sd=0.44), and a low level of exposure to eye tracking (mean=1.03, sd=0.19). There were no significant demographic differences between conditions.

5   Results

5.1   Eye Tracking

To analyze the eye tracking data we gathered from the Gazepoint GP3 Eye Tracker software, we used an Area-of-Interest (AOI) Identification algorithm as described by Salvucci and Goldberg [23]. For each participant we were interested in the data collected between the first question the participant asked the virtual patients and the last question the participants asked the virtual patients, so we excluded all eye tracking points outside of this range.

The AOI algorithm starts by associating all data points to specific target areas. We identified five target areas, where Area 0 represents all points recorded off the screen, and the other four areas (Areas 1-4) relate to the sections described in Figure 1(a) and Figure 1(b). Next, we collapsed all consecutive fixation points for the same target area into fixation groups. For each fixation group, we mapped that group to a single fixation point located at the centroid of its points. We then analyzed that filtered set of fixations.

Several participants were excluded due to system failure, eye tracker failure, or failure to pass the screening qualification questionnaire (due to reasons such as glaucoma, screen reader assistance, glasses or contacts). This yielded 12 participants in the no animation, large screen tv condition (*Condition 0*), 13 participants in the animation, large screen tv condition (*Condition 1*), and 12 participants in the animation, tablet condition (*Condition 2*).

We conducted One-way ANOVAs using the condition as the independent variables to determine if there were any significant differences in the amount of time

Table 1. Eye tracking results for each of the five areas and total time. We do not have eye tracking data for Areas 2,3, and 4 in Condition 2, because those areas were displayed on a tablet not being tracked.

Area	Condition	Mean (%)	Standard Deviation	Condition Effects F-Test	P-Value
Area 0: Off the screen	0	2.55	1.70	$F(2,36) =$ 77.4973	<0.001*
	1	6.18	5.07		
	2	70.85	26.15		
Area 1: Virtual Patients in Section 1	0	37.42	40.66	$F(2,36)=$ 0.4373	0.6493
	1	26.09	24.48		
	2	29.14	26.15		
Area 2: Response Bubble in Section 2	0	3.99	9.10	$F(1,24)=$ 0.0052	0.9429
	1	4.21	5.52		
Area 3: Sidnie in Section 3	0	0.18	0.29	$F(1,24)=$ 0.9152	0.3487
	1	1.04	3.10		
Area 4: Question Bank in Section 4	0	55.84	41.19	$F(1,24)=$ 0.2308	0.6355
	1	62.45	26.70		

Area	Condition	Mean	Standard Deviation	Condition Effects F-Test	P-Value
Total Time: Entire Interaction	0	3105.02	1676.29	$F(2,36)=$ 10.0379	0.0004*
	1	3421.28	2007.84		
	2	752.00	894.33		

spent in each of the five areas as shown in Table 1. For Area 0, we found a significant difference in the amount of fixations that were identified as being off the screen, between all three conditions. Doing a comparison for all pairs using Tukey's, we found a significant difference between *Condition 0* and *Condition 2* (p-value <0.0001) and a significant difference between *Condition 1* and *Condition 2* (p-value <0.0001). Over 70% of the valid fixations recorded in *Condition 2* were classified to Area 0. This result is indicitive of the head movements required to look down at the tablet and then back to the large screen tv in *Condition 2*. This may also indicate that our virtual environment lacks the amount of stimuli needed to entice the user to spend longer amounts of time looking at the virtual patient and her mother.

Furthermore, we wanted to compare the amount of time spent looking at **Section 2**, **Section 3**, and **Section 4**, between *Condition 0* and *Condition 1*. In Table 1, you will see that we did not find any significant differences in those three areas. In comparing *Condition 0* to *Condition 1*, it is important to notice that in *Condition 0*, over 55% of the user's eye tracking fixations were focused on **Section 4** and in *Condition 1*, over 62% of the user's time was spent looking at the bank of questions (**Section 4**). This may be indicative of the fact that our participants were freshman nursing students with little experience interviewing patients. Students in *Condition 0* and *Condition 1* spent the least amount of time looking at Sidnie, which may indicate that a visual representation of Sidnie is not needed and we can allot more space to the virtual environment section.

We also conducted a One-way ANOVA to determine if there was an effect on the total amount of time participants spent interacting with the system. We found a significant difference in the total amount of time participants spent using the system. Doing a comparison for all pairs using Tukey's, we found a significant difference between *Condition 0* and *Condition 2* (p-value = 0.0006) and a significant difference between *Condition 1* and *Condition 2* (p-value = 0.0006). From Table 1, you can see that participants in *Condition 2* spent less time using the system than the participants in *Condition 0* and *Condition 1*. This may be due to the fact that participants in *Condition 2* spent most of their time interacting with the tablet and that by the time they looked up to the large screen tv, the virtual characters were already finished with their animations.

For *Condition 0* and *Condition 1*, we were interested in determing if there was a significant difference between the four areas displayed on the large screen tv, regardless of condition. We conducted a t-test to compare means across all areas and found significant differences for each area. Participants spent significantly more time looking at **Section 1** (the virtual characters) than **Section 2** (p-value = 0.0003) and **Section 3**(p-value = 0.0001). Participants spent significantly more time looking at **Section 4** (bank of questions) than they did **Section 1** (p-value = 0.0236), **Section 2** (p-value = <0.0001), or **Section 3** (p-value = <0.0001). Also participants spent significantly less time looking at **Section 3** (Sidnie) then they did **Section 2** (p-value = 0.0191).

5.2   Qualitative Feedback

Although we had to exclude some participants' data in the eye tracking results, we included all 52 participants in the analysis of the qualitative feedback. Overall, our system scored high on the System Usability Scale, with individual overall scores ranging from 55% to 97.5%, with an average score of 80% (sd=8.24) for *Condition 0*, an average score of 83.75% (sd=7.85) for *Condtion 1*, and an average score of 81.05% (sd=9.32) for *Condition 2*. In our post-questionnaire we found significance when we asked about the presence of an eye tracker. For the prompt "How frequent did you look at the eye tracker?", we found a significant difference between *Condition 1* and *Condtion 2* (p-value = 0.04). Participants in *Condtion 2* reported looking at the eye tracker more frequently than the other conditions, which may be indicative of how often participants looked between the tablet and the large screen tv.

6   Discussion

The first goal of this experiment was to determine if using virtual characters with life-like animations would have an effect on how often users looked at the virtual characters (**Section 1**). Even though there wasn't a significant difference in this, participants preferred working with virtual characters containing animations. We hypothesized that the amount of time spent looking at the virtual patients would be higher in the tablet condition and even though we did not observe a significant result, we did observe that the tablet condition gives us the ability to distinguish when participants are looking at either the virtual mother or the virtual child, which isn't as clear in the other two conditions where the virtual environment is smaller. Also, we hypothesized that participants would spend most of their time looking at the virtual patients, which wasn't the case. Participants spent most of their time looking at the bank of questions, which may be because the participants were freshman nursing students with no experience interviewing patients. Participants spent the least amount of time looking at Sidnie (the nursing assistant), which may be because of how much time the nursing students spent focused on the task and not the interaction. Overall, our system resulted in high scores on the System Usability Scale in all conditions. In the debriefing interview, the participants were very positive towards the system and reported that they would love to use it again.

7 Future Work

The results of this experiment yielded valuable suggestions on improvements. The gaze plot data provided us with examples of how users interact with our visual interface. We plan to use the results to modify and improve the layout of our interface to give us finer detail on how users look at the individual characters. We would also like to obtain eye tracking data for mobile tablet use.

Acknowledgements. This research was supported, in part, by the NSF Graduate Research Fellowship Program (fellow numbers 2009080400 and 2011095211), and Interdisciplinary Research Innovations Grant from the College of Health Education and Human Development at Clemson University and a grant from the Agency for Healthcare, Research and Quality (RO3#HS020233-01).

References

1. Pence, T.B., Dukes, L.C., Hodges, L.F., Meehan, N.K., Johnson, A.: The effects of interaction and visual fidelity on learning outcomes for a virtual pediatric patient system. In: 2013 IEEE International Conference on Healthcare Informatics (ICHI), pp. 209–218. IEEE (2013)
2. Stevens, A., Hernandez, J., Johnsen, K., Dickerson, R., Raij, A., Harrison, C., DiPietro, M., Allen, B., Ferdig, R., Foti, S.: The use of virtual patients to teach medical students history taking and communication skills. American Journal of Surgery 191(6), 806–811 (2006)
3. Hubal, R.C., Frank, G.A., Guinn, C.I.: Lessons learned in modeling schizophrenic and depressed responsive virtual humans for training. In: Proceedings of the 8th International Conference on Intelligent User Interfaces, pp. 85–92. ACM (2003)
4. Hockenberry, M.J., Wilson, D.: Wong's nursing care of infants and children. Mosby/Elsevier (2007)
5. Planas, L.G., Er, N.L.: A systems approach to scaffold communication skills development. American Journal of Pharmaceutical Education 72(2) (April 15, 2008)

6. Durham, C.F., Alden, K.R.: Enhancing patient safety in nursing education through patient simulation. Patient Safety and Quality: An Evidence-Based Handbook for Nurses 6(3), 221–250 (2008)

7. Ball, J.W., Bindler, R.C., Cowen, K.: Child health nursing. Prentice Hall (2013)

8. Chant, S., Jenkinson, T., Randle, J., Russell, G.: Communication skills: some problems in nursing education and practice. Journal of Clinical Nursing 11(1), 12–21 (2002)

9. Johnsen, K., Dickerson, R., Raij, A., Lok, B., Jackson, J., Shin, M., Hernandez, J., Stevens, A., Lind, D.S.: Experiences in using immersive virtual characters to educate medical communication skills. In: Proceedings of Virtual Reality, pp. 179–186. IEEE (2005)

10. Péruch, P., Vercher, J.L., Gauthier, G.M.: Acquisition of spatial knowledge through visual exploration of simulated environments. Ecological Psychology 7(1) (1995)

11. DeVault, D., Artstein, R., Benn, G., Dey, T., Fast, E., Gainer, A., Georgila, K., Gratch, J., Hartholt, A., Lhommet, M.: Simsensei kiosk: a virtual human interviewer for healthcare decision support. In: Proceedings of the 2014 International Conference on Autonomous Agents and Multi-Agent systems, pp. 1061–1068. International Foundation for Autonomous Agents and Multiagent Systems (2014)

12. Gulz, A., Haake, M.: Design of animated pedagogical agents – a look at their look. International Journal of Human-Computer Studies 64(4), 322–339 (2006)

13. Jacob, R.J., Karn, K.S.: Eye tracking in human-computer interaction and usability research: Ready to deliver the promises. Mind 2(3), 4 (2003)

14. Poole, A., Ball, L.J.: Eye tracking in hci and usability research. In: Ghaoui, C. (ed.) Encyclopedia of Human-Computer Interaction (2006)

15. Riley, W., Davis, S., Miller, K., Hansen, H., Sainfort, F., Sweet, R.: Didactic and simulation nontechnical skills team training to improve perinatal patient outcomes in a community hospital. Joint Commission Journal on Quality and Patient Safety 37(8), 357–364 (2011)

16. Law, B., Atkins, M.S., Kirkpatrick, A.E., Lomax, A.J.: Eye gaze patterns differentiate novice and experts in a virtual laparoscopic surgery training environment. In: Proceedings of the 2004 Symposium on Eye Tracking Research & Applications, pp. 41–48. ACM (2004)

17. Mello-Thoms, C., Nodine, C.F., Kundel, H.L.: What attracts the eye to the location of missed and reported breast cancers? In: Proceedings of the 2002 Symposium on Eye Tracking Research & Applications, pp. 111–117. ACM (2002)

18. (Gazepoint), http://gazept.com/

19. Dukes, L.C., Pence, T.B., Hodges, L.F., Meehan, N., Johnson, A.: Sidnie: scaffolded interviews developed by nurses in education. In: Proceedings of the 2013 International Conference on Intelligent User Interfaces, pp. 395–406. ACM (2013)

20. Nielsen, J.: The nielsen norman group (2002)

21. Brooke, J.: Sus-a quick and dirty usability scale. Usability Evaluation in Industry 189, 194 (1996)

22. Mortensen, J., Vinayagamoorthy, V., Slater, M., Steed, A., Lok, B., Whitton, M.: Collaboration in tele-immersive environments. In: Proceedings of the Workshop on Virtual Environments, pp. 93–101. Eurographics Association (2002)

23. Salvucci, D.D., Goldberg, J.H.: Identifying fixations and saccades in eye-tracking protocols. In: Proceedings of the 2000 Symposium on Eye Tracking Research & Applications, pp. 71–78. ACM (2000)

Personalization and Personification:
A Constructive Approach
Based on Parametric Agents

Fabrice Popineau, Georges Dubus, and Yolaine Bourda

SUPELEC Systems Sciences (E3S),
Computer Science Department,
Gif-sur-Yvette, France
{fabrice.popineau,georges.dubus,yolaine.bourda}@supelec.fr

Abstract. In this paper, we illustrate PAGE – for Parametric AGEnts, a constructive way to design personalized or personified virtual agents starting from a plain rational agent. We chose a scenario about the personification of a virtual agent in a serious game for training communication skills. We start from an agent program that does not take into account any kind of agent profile. We show how our PAGE approach allows us to derive different agent programs tailored to different agent profiles while retaining complete control on the resulting agent behavior.

1 Scenario

We address a scenario inspired from [1] and [7]. In a serious game for training communication skills, a player plays the role of a real estate agent to convince a non-player character, played by a virtual agent, to visit a property. During the discussion, the player can ask questions to discover the wishes of the IVA and can communicate information, interpretations and opinions in order to convince the IVA that the property meets its expectations, by highlighting the qualities of the property that echoes the wishes of the buyer. The IVA may also ask questions to get the information he wants, give opinions, and make the decision to visit the property or terminate the conversation.

The PAGE framework is an enhanced and refined version of the work presented in [4]. Two traits of the IVA personality are modeled: the *extraversion* and the *agreeableness* of the Five Factor model [6]. These features are modeled at a coarse grain, without considering for example the facets and schemes of the NEO PI-R model [3].

In [7], the IVA is driven by a BDI agent whose beliefs are the knowledge the IVA has on the property, whose goals are to obtain information and to make a decision, and whose plans are conversation strategies to achieve the goals. The pseudocode in listing 1 illustrates how the personality of the IVA is implemented: the behaviors are given in the form of conditional expressions depending on the psychological profile of the agent. This approach suffers from the multicriterion bloat: the complexity grows exponentially with the number of traits.

T. Bickmore et al. (Eds.): IVA 2014, LNAI 8637, pp. 339–344, 2014.

Listing 1. Pseudocode for selecting the type of information

```
if (agreeable) then                  /* Boolean                    */
   if (extrovert) then               /* Boolean                    */
      if (probability > .5) then     /* With  equal  chance:       */
         return: tell(wish)          /* Tell  a  wish              */
      else
         return: tell(opinion)       /* Tell  an  opinion          */
   else                              /* Act  introvert:            */
      return: tell(fact)             /* Tell  fact  about  the  house */
else                                 /* Act  non—agreeable:        */
   return: tell(fact)                /* Tell  fact  about  itself  */
```

The evaluations published in [1] and [7] about this scenario show the usefulness of the personification of the agent. An agent expressed with BDI can be
translated into an agent expressed in Golog while keeping the same architecture
as shown in [8], but the multicriterion bloat complexity will be inherited. Our
PAGE approach solves this problem by giving an appropriate transformation of
the program for a given profile.

2   PAGE Process

The PAGE process has been enhanced on several points since [4]. This process
is based on a set of transformations that are recursively applied to the original
Golog program. The transformation process is driven by the profile we consider.
The application designer provides a connection table which relies the traits in
the profile to actions that are related to these traits. The first goal of these
transformations is to allow to prefer actions which are more geared towards the
profile. The notion of *families of actions* and *families of procedure* have been
refined to open up the set of available ways to achieve a given result. In addition
to preferences (denoted by *pref+* and *pref-* later on), we also have introduced
the ability to block or force the use of certain ways to achieve results: some
behaviors may be required (*req*) or banned (*ban*). Last, actively sensing user
actions is essential for an agent interacting with humans and requires online
planning ability. Our transformation process can transform programs as a whole,
hence is not subject to the sensing barrier contrarily to other approaches like
DT-Golog [2] [9] [5].

This gives us a rich set of operations that enables us to transform a profile
independent Golog program into one which is either personalized or personified.
We detail an example of the latter below.

proc *shareInformation*   (1)   **proc** *evaluate(message)*   (2)
  shareWish $\pi f; message = tell(f)?;$
  | *shareOpinion*   **if** $f = Fact(\_)$
  | *shareFactAboutHouse*   **then** *assert(f); ackApprove(f)*
  | *shareFactAboutItself*   **else** $\neg incompatible(f)?;$ *assert(f); ackApprove(f)*
endProc | *ackReject(f)*
                                         endIf
                                       endProc

3   Agent Modification

The buyer agent can be personified in many ways. We show two of them, and show that they interact seamlessly. Transformations will be applied on procedures 1 and 2.

Selecting the type of information to share. The agent can choose to share information with the player (eq:shareInformation). The standard agent will choose randomly between *shareWish*, *shareOpinion*, *shareFactAboutHouse* and *shareFactAboutItself*. An *extrovert* character will tend to express his wishes and opinions, while an introvert will express facts and ask questions. An *agreeable* character will tend to ask about the house or the environment, while a disagreeable character will tend to talk about himself. In the implementation of [1], this personalization is done by enumeration of the possibilities (listing 1).

We express *introvert* as the negation of *extrovert* (*neg(extrovert)*). That way, the introvert agent will avoid actions associated with extrovert, and vice versa. Given the description of the traits *agreeable* and *extrovert*, we define the function *attributes*:

$$attributes(shareWish) = attributes(shareOpinion) = \{agreeable, extrovert\}$$
$$attributes(shareFactAboutHouse) = \{agreeable, neg(extrovert)\}$$
$$attributes(shareFactAboutItself) = \{neg(agreeable), neg(extrovert)\}$$

The definition of *attributes* enables the automatic transformation by the PAGE process of the *shareInformation* procedure according to a profile. The results for various profiles are given in table 1 where the names have been shortened (the prefix *share* has been removed). This approach gives us variations in programs, and thus let us define complex behaviors without having to state the result of each trait combination.

Table 1. Transformation of the *shareInformation* procedure under different profiles

agreeable	extrovert	Transformed procedure
pref-	pref-	shareFactAboutItself 〉 shareFactAboutHouse 〉 (shareWish | shareOpinion)
pref-	neutral	shareFactAboutItself 〉 (shareWish | shareOpinion | shareFactAboutHouse)
pref-	pref+	(shareWish | shareOpinion | shareFactAboutItself) 〉 shareFactAboutHouse
neutral	pref-	(shareFactAboutHouse | shareFactAboutItself) 〉 (shareWish | shareOpinion)
neutral	neutral	shareWish | shareOpinion | shareFactAboutHouse | shareFactAboutItself
neutral	pref+	(shareWish | shareOpinion) 〉 (shareFactAboutHouse | shareFactAboutItself)
pref+	pref-	shareFactAboutHouse 〉 (shareWish | shareOpinion | shareFactAboutItself)
pref+	neutral	(shareWish | shareOpinion | shareFactAboutHouse) 〉 shareFactAboutItself
pref+	pref+	(shareWish | shareOpinion) 〉 shareFactAboutHouse 〉 shareFactAboutItself

Accepting interpretations. When the player gives the agent information, the agent can accept or reject it. Facts are always accepted, because the agent consider the player doesn't lie. Opinions and interpretations may be rejected if they contradict the knowledge base. This behaviour is defined in the procedure *evaluate* (2).

To personify the agent, we extend the basic behavior of *ackApprove()* and *ackReject()* (acknowledge approval or rejection in a neutral manner) by defining two families of procedures. First, the procedure *ackApproveWithOpinion* (3) lets the agent acknowledge approval while giving his opinion. It is only available if the agent has an opinion on the subject. It is associated with an *extrovert* behaviour. The second procedure *ackApproveSilently* (8), lets the agent say nothing after accepting an information. A third procedure *ackRejectSilently* (9) lets the agent reject an information without saying anything. Both procedures are different because they are part of different families: the first one can be used when accepting a piece of information, the other one when rejecting. Both are associated with a *disagreeable* behaviour. Two families (10 and11) state what procedures can be used instead of others. Finaly, we state (7) that adding a message to the knowledge base is associated to the trait *agreeable*. The PAGE process uses these families to replace *ackApprov* and *ackReject* by other procedures that are more suitable for the profile.

For an extrovert agent ({*extrovert* : *pref+*, *agreeable* : *neutral*}), the result of the transformation is procedure 12. The differences with (2) are underlined. For each family of procedures, (*ackApprove* and *ackReject*), each member of the family is ranked with regard to the profile. Thus *ackApproveWithOpinion* is of class *pref+*, since its unique attribute is *extrovert* with value *pref+* in the profile. Similarly, *ackRejectSilently* and *ackApproveSilently* are of class *pref-* and *ackApprove* and *ackReject* have no class. Procedures of negative classes are dismissed, and the others are replaced by a choice between the remaining procedures in families with a preference for procedures of the highest rank: *ackApprove(f)* is replaced by (*ackApproveWithOpinion(f)*⟩*ackApprove(f)*. This is the only change that has an effect in this example. For a disagreeable agent({*extrovert* : *neutral*, *agreeable* : *pref-*}), the result is procedure 13.

Combining transformations. Both transformations apply to different parts of the program, hence it is possible to apply them simultaneously to get an agent having both alterations of his behavior. Problems only arise in cases where alterations deal with the same parts of the program, in which case the transformation process may give several results. For this reason, we believe that the process has to stay semi-automatic: the designer of the application may want to validate the result of the transformation.

proc *ackApproveWithOpinion(f)*

$$(3)$$

$\pi predicate, opinion$
$f = \_(predicate, \_)$
$\quad \wedge KB(Opinion(predicate, opinion))?$
if *opinion* > 0.5 **then**
$\quad acknowledge(accept\_ happy)$
else
$\quad acknowledge(accept\_ unhappy)$
endIf
endProc

attributes(ackApproveWithOpinion)

$$(4)$$

$= \{extrovert\}$
attributes(ackApproveSilently) $\quad (5)$
$\quad = \{neg(agreeable)\}$
attributes(ackRejectSilently) $\quad (6)$
$\quad = \{neg(agreeable)\}$
attributes(assert(f)) $= \{agreeable\}$

$$(7)$$

proc $ackApproveSilently(f)$ (8) $family(\{ackApprove,$ (10)
    nil $ackApproveWithOpinion,$
endProc $ackApproveSilently\})$
proc $ackRejectSilently(f)$ (9) $family(\{ackReject,$ (11)
    nil $ackRejectSilently\})$
endProc

proc $evaluate(message)$ (12)   **proc** $evaluate(message)$ (13)
    $\pi f; message = tell(f)?;$ $\pi f; message = tell(f)?;$
    if $f = Fact(\_)$ **then**   **if** $f = Fact(\_)$ **then**
       $assert(f);$ $assert(f);$
       $\overline{(ackApproveWithOpinion(f)}$ $\overline{(ackApproveSilently(f)}$
       $\overline{\rangle ackApprove(f))}$ $\overline{\rangle ackApprove(f))}$
    else   **else**
       $\neg incompatible(f)?; assert(f);$ $\overline{ackRejectSilently(f)\rangle ackReject(f)}$
       $\overline{(ackApproveWithOpinion(f)}$ $\overline{\rangle \neg incompatible(f)?; assert(f);}$
       $\overline{\rangle ackApprove(f))}$ $\overline{(ackApproveSilently(f)\rangle ackApprove(f))}$
       $| ackReject(f)$ **endIf**
    endIf   **endProc**
endProc

4 Conclusion

We have illustrated how to use our PAGE approach on a real-case scenario which has been previously assessed. We have shown that our approach allows for a simpler and clearer expression of the behavioral change than a classical approach. Our next step is to provide an interactive tool so that the agent designer can chose what transformations to apply at each point in the program. Families of actions have also to be investigated from an ontological point of view. Last, we have considered personalization and personification as exclusive transformations, but we will find extremely interesting to address the problem of giving both behaviors to an agent program.

References

1. Van den Bosch, K., Brandenburgh, A., Muller, T.J., Heuvelink, A.: Characters with personality! In: Nakano, Y., Neff, M., Paiva, A., Walker, M. (eds.) IVA 2012. LNCS, vol. 7502, pp. 426–439. Springer, Heidelberg (2012)
2. Boutilier, C., Reiter, R., Soutchanski, M., Thrun, S., et al.: Decision-theoretic, high-level agent programming in the situation calculus. In: AAAI/IAAI, pp. 355–362 (2000)
3. Costa, P.T., McCrae, R.R.: The NEO PI-R professional manual. Psychological Assessment Resources, Odessa (1992)
4. Dubus, G., Popineau, F., Bourda, Y., Sansonnet, J.P.: Parametric reasoning agents extend the control over standard behaviors. In: 2013 IEEE/WIC/ACM International Joint Conferences on Web Intelligence (WI) and Intelligent Agent Technologies (IAT) (2013)

5. Ferrein, A., Fritz, C., Lakemeyer, G.: Using golog for deliberation and team coordination in robotic soccer. KI 19(1), 24 (2005)
6. Goldberg, L.R.: An alternative description of personality: The Big-Five factor structure. Journal of Personality and Social Psychology 59, 1216–1229 (1990)
7. Muller, T.J., Heuvelink, A., van den Bosch, K., Swartjes, I., et al.: Glengarry glen ross: Using bdi for sales game dialogues. In: AIIDE (2012)
8. Sardina, S., Lespérance, Y.: Golog speaks the BDI language. In: Braubach, L., Briot, J.-P., Thangarajah, J. (eds.) ProMAS 2009. LNCS, vol. 5919, pp. 82–99. Springer, Heidelberg (2010)
9. Soutchanski, M.: An on-line decision-theoretic golog interpreter. In: IJCAI, pp. 19–26. Citeseer (2001)

Interpersonal Attitude of a Speaking Agent in Simulated Group Conversations

Brian Ravenet[1], Angelo Cafaro[2], Magalie Ochs[2], and Catherine Pelachaud[2]

[1] Institut Mines-Télécom; Télécom Paristech; CNRS LTCI
[2] CNRS LTCI ; Télécom Paristech, 37/39 rue Dareau, 75014 Paris, France
{ravenet,cafaro,ochs,pelachaud}@telecom-paristech.fr

Abstract. Embodied Conversational Agents have been widely used to simulate dyadic interactions with users. We want to explore the context of expression of interpersonal attitudes in simulated group conversations. We are presenting a model that allows agents to exhibit a variety of nonverbal behaviors (e.g gestures, facial expressions, proxemics) depending on the interpersonal attitudes that they want to express within a group while talking. The model combines corpus-based and theoretical-based approaches and we present a preliminary implementation of this model.

1 Introduction

While embodied conversational agents (ECAs) have been mainly studied in dyadic interaction settings, there is also a growing interest for small group situations. A dyadic interaction is a 2-interactant configuration, whereas a small group situation implies generally three to twenty interactants [1]. We propose an agent's model that allows them to adapt and exhibit different nonverbal behaviors when talking, depending on the interpersonal attitudes that they want to express. Interpersonal attitude is an "affective style that can be naturally or strategically employed in an interaction with a person or a group of persons"[2]. We are using the representation from Argyle to manipulate agent's interpersonal attitudes [3]. In order to model the influence of such interpersonal attitudes on an ECA's nonverbal behavior, our approach is based on a combination of behavior models coupling a data-based model of conversational gestures and a rule-based model of group formation that simultaneously influence the ECAs' nonverbal behavior from the literature of Human and Social Sciences. Previous work with similar setting was either missing the influence of interpersonal attitudes on agent's exhibited behavior [4–6] or was not considering group formation behavior (i.e. simulated group conversation) [16, 7, 8].

2 Our Augmented *Behavior Planner*

Our model works as a *Behavior Planner* but instead of considering only a set of possible nonverbal behaviors for an intention, we propose an augmented model that takes into account the interpersonal attitudes the agent wants to express

T. Bickmore et al. (Eds.): IVA 2014, LNAI 8637, pp. 345–349, 2014.

in order to select the most appropriate behavior. Interpersonal attitudes can be expressed with nonverbal behavior in both dyadic [9, 10] and small group interactions [11]. A more dominant person tends to do more gestures [9] and mutual gaze is a sign of dominance or friendliness [10]. In [11], Mehrabian describes eye gaze, posture and distance as important behaviors that impact the evaluation of attitude in small group interactions.

2.1   Two-Stage Influence

Central to our model is the Behavior Planner component. On one hand we are influencing the nonverbal behavior related to conversational and performative intents (e.g. facial expression, gestures, head orientation). On the other hand, we are influencing the behavior related to group formations and cohesion (e.g. gaze behavior, interpersonal distance and body orientation). We limited the generated conversational nonverbal behavior only for the ECA that is speaking but we plan to consider other conversation roles in the future. As we are integrating two models that both influence the nonverbal behavior of an agent, we define the following mechanism to combine them: on each modality, the two stages are given a weight (which sum equals to 1) to indicate the degree of influence each model has on the modality. We are now presenting the first stage. The nonverbal conversational behavior that we are considering in our model is the following: presence of gestures and head movements, type of facial expressions, head orientation, presence of gaze avoidance, spatial extent and power of the gestures. Depending on the speech act and the desired expressed attitude, the nonverbal behavior generated should vary. In order to do this we integrated the model developed in [12] with the current model. We are manipulating the probabilities to select particular values for our parameters following this network. A possible outcome for a dominant attitude would be for instance wide and powerful gestures and an upward head, no gaze avoidance and a neutral facial expression. For a friendly attitude, the agent might perform the speech act using a smiling face, tilting his head on the side with wide and smooth gestures. The second stage of our Behavior Planner is the influence of the attitude on the ECA behavior that manages the group formation and cohesion, in particular the interpersonal distance, the gaze behavior and the body orientation. Based on Hall's proxemics [13] and Kendon F-Formation [14] theories, our model adds on top of these a set of rules to configure this spatial organization depending on the social attitude. When performing a speech act, the model chooses for the speaking agent which other member (human or agent) is its preferred target for a glance, the importance of maintaining an body orientation related to the group or to the adressee and how close it wants to stand to each other member within its social space. For instance, the agent should have a higher probability to glance at the group member towards which it expresses submissiveness or friendliness, stand closer with group members towards which it expresses friendliness or a neutral status level and it should orient its body more directly towards group members with which it expresses submissiveness [11].

2.2 Combining the Models

This Behavior Planner takes as input the interpersonal attitudes of the agent towards all the other agents. The first stage computes the upper body nonverbal behavior (facial expression, presence of gestures and head movement, head orientation, spatial extent and power of gestures) for this speech act and the interpersonal attitude towards the adressee. The other stage, computes the body orientation, the interpersonal distance and the group member which is looked at within an F-Formation. On top of this, the combined model computes the preferred target, the weights for the body orientation modality (more weight from the group formation model resulting in an orientation more consistent with the group and less towards the adressee) and the desired interpersonal distances between all characters in their social spaces.

3   Implementation

This paper describes a preliminary implementation of our model extended to small group of ECAs in a simulated conversation. The implementation relies on two separate technologies, the VIB platform and the Impulsion AI engine. VIB is a SAIBA compliant platform for the generation and realization of multimodal behavior for ECAs. In [12], we extended the *Behavior Planner* of this platform with our bayesian network to generate the agents' nonverbal behavior to express different social attitudes in dyadic interactions. The Impulsion AI engine is a software platform developed to improve ECAs nonverbal behavior in social simulations with particular emphasis on F-formation systems (i.e. group conversations) and gatherings (e.g. multiple groups sharing the same environment). The engine is grounded on Scheflen's human territories and Kendon's F-Formation [14] theories and it provides ECAs with autonomous generation and realization of gaze, proxemics and body orientation behavior supporting a simulated group conversation. Both VIB and Impulsion have been deployed within the Unity3D game engine. In this preliminary implementation of our model we geared up a set of ECAs with an integrated version of VIB and Impulsion. On a software engineering perspective, we have coordinated this integration by allowing VIB to control the upper body part of our characters (gestures and facial expressions, the head orientation is not handled by VIB in this implementation), while Impulsion is controlling the character's interpersonal distance, body orientation and gaze behavior. This integration is still work in progress and presents two challenging issues that we need to address. First the whole orchestration of nonverbal behavior needs to be consistent with the intended social attitudes that we aim to express. Secondly, at a lower level, we are working on blending the resulting animations corresponding to the behaviors exhibited.

4   Conclusion

In this paper, we have presented a model for conversational groups of humans and agents and a preliminary implementation of the Behavior Planner of this model. We have used an approach combining two models of social interaction, one dedicated to conversational nonverbal behavior and the other for small group formation and territorial cohesion. This is a novel approach, however it introduces some challenging issues that we need to address: on a theoretical level, we need to assess if two separate models of social behavior are compatible when combined together to generate believable and consistent behavior. We are aware that the model for attitudes in dyadic interactions cannot simply be migrated to small group interactions. This new social context has different requirements due to the different spatial arrangements of the ECAs involved and the need to clearly define the addressee for each separate nonverbal modality (e.g. body oriented towards a participant while gazing at another).

Acknowledgment. This research has been supported by the Media Seventh Framework Program FP7 under grant agreement 287723 (REVERIE).

References

1. Beebe, S.A., Masterson, J.T.: Communication in small groups: principles and practices. Pearson Education, Inc., Boston (2009)
2. Scherer, K.: What are emotions? and how can they be measured? Social Science Information (2005)
3. Argyle, M.: Bodily Communication. University paperbacks. Methuen (1988)
4. Prada, R., Paiva, A.: Believable groups of synthetic characters. In: Proceedings of the Fourth International Joint Conference on Autonomous Agents and Multiagent Systems, pp. 37–43. ACM (2005)
5. Traum, D., Rickel, J.: Embodied agents for multi-party dialogue in immersive virtual worlds. In: Proceedings of the First International Joint Conference on Autonomous Agents and Multiagent Systems: Part 2, pp. 766–773. ACM (2002)
6. Pedica, C., Hogni Vilhjálmsson, H.: Spontaneous avatar behavior for human territoriality. Applied Artificial Intelligence 24(6), 575–593 (2010)
7. Lee, J., Marsella, S.: Modeling side participants and bystanders: The importance of being a laugh track. In: Hogni Vilhjálmsson, H., Kopp, S., Marsella, S., Thórisson, K.R. (eds.) IVA 2011. LNCS, vol. 6895, pp. 240–247. Springer, Heidelberg (2011)
8. Damian, I., Endrass, B., Huber, P., Bee, N., André, E.: Individualized agent interactions. In: Allbeck, J.M., Faloutsos, P. (eds.) MIG 2011. LNCS, vol. 7060, pp. 15–26. Springer, Heidelberg (2011)
9. Carney, D.R., Hall, J.A., LeBeau, L.: Beliefs about the nonverbal expression of social power. Journal of Nonverbal Behavior 29, 105–123 (2005)
10. Burgoon, J.K., Buller, D.B., Hale, J.L., de Turck, M.A.: Relational Messages Associated with Nonverbal Behaviors. Human Communication Research 10(3), 351–378 (1984)
11. Mehrabian, A.: Significance of posture and position in the communication of attitude and status relationships. Psychological Bulletin 71(5), 359 (1969)

12. Ravenet, B., Ochs, M., Pelachaud, C.: From a user-created corpus of virtual agent's non-verbal behavior to a computational model of interpersonal attitudes. In: Aylett, R., Krenn, B., Pelachaud, C., Shimodaira, H. (eds.) IVA 2013. LNCS, vol. 8108, pp. 263–274. Springer, Heidelberg (2013)
13. Hall, E.T.: The hidden dimension, vol. 1990. Anchor Books, New York (1969)
14. Kendon, A.: Conducting interaction: Patterns of behavior in focused encounters, vol. 7. CUP Archive (1990)
15. Niewiadomski, R., Bevacqua, E., Mancini, M., Pelachaud, C.: Greta: an interactive expressive eca system. In: Proceedings of the 8th International Conference on Autonomous Agents and Multiagent Systems, AAMAS 2009, vol. 2, pp. 1399–1400. International Foundation for Autonomous Agents and Multiagent Systems, Richland (2009)
16. Gillies, M., Crabtree, I.B., Ballin, D.: Customisation and context for expressive behaviour in the broadband world. BT Technology Journal 22(2), 7–17 (2004)

Birth Control, Drug Abuse, or Domestic Violence? What Health Risk Topics Are Women Willing to Discuss with a Virtual Agent?

Jingjing Ren[1], Timothy Bickmore[1], Megan Hempstead[2], and Brian Jack[2]

[1] College of Computer and Information Science, Northeastern University, Boston, MA, USA
{renjj,bickmore}@ccs.neu.edu
[2] Boston University School of Medicine, Boston Medical Center, Boston, MA, USA
{megan.hempstead,brian.jack}@bmc.org

Abstract. The results of a study investigating which health issues women are willing to discuss with a virtual agent are presented, focusing on 108 risks related to maternal and child health. We find that women's perceived importance of a health issue, along with general self-efficacy and comfort discussing the topic are significant predictors of whether they will address it.

Keywords: Relational agent, embodied conversational agent, preconception care, medical informatics, health informatics, social desirability.

1 Introduction

There are an increasing number of virtual agents used in the role of health counselors, for a wide range of applications, including interventions for exercise, diet, and hospital discharge. Virtual agents have also been used to screen and/or counsel individuals on potentially sensitive and stigmatizing health-related behaviors, such as drug and alcohol abuse [1] and mental illness [2]. However, it is unclear what range of health-related topics users would choose to discuss with a virtual agent, given the choice. It is also unclear what factors might drive these decisions, ranging from perceived importance of a health risk, comfort discussing a particular topic, or demographic or personality traits of the user. Such knowledge is important in designing new agent-based health interventions for particular user groups, since it would help determine whether a virtual agent should be used at all for a particular health risk and user demographic and, if a virtual agent is used, which health topics and decision factors need to be the foci of effort in intervention design.

The context of this research is an automated system we are developing to provide "preconception care" (PCC) to young African American women. These women are twice as likely to deliver a low birth weight baby and have twice the infant mortality rate compared to White women in the US. In a recent survey, 108 risks in 12 domains were identified as possible factors in determining infant health in this demographic [3] (Table 1). The domains range from substance abuse to nutrition and exercise, and

T. Bickmore et al. (Eds.): IVA 2014, LNAI 8637, pp. 350–359, 2014.

individual risks span flu vaccinations to alcoholism. The majority of these risks must be addressed well before pregnancy and traditional prenatal care, thus this area of preventive medicine is referred to as "preconception care" [4]. As just one example, folic acid should be taken at least four weeks *before* pregnancy to prevent neural tube defects.

Table 1. Domains of Health Risks Addressed in the Preconception Care System

Domain	Example Risk
Health care and programs	having health insurance
Relationships	physical or sexual abuse
Reproductive health	not using birth control
Health conditions and medicines	asthma
Genetic health history	ethnicity-based health risk
Emotional and mental health	depression
Immunizations and vaccines	need HPV vaccine
Infectious diseases	at risk for sexually-transmitted infection
Substance use	tobacco use
Nutrition and activity	overweight
Environmental issues	toxoplasmosis
Men and health care	partner does not have a physician

Users are enrolled into the PCC system by first completing a survey questionnaire that attempts to determine which of the 108 risk factors they may need to address. In our pilot work, we have discovered that the average woman in our target demographic has 23 (range 13-37) preconception risks [5]. Thus, preconception care represents an application domain in which many health behaviors need to be changed, with the set of behaviors potentially different for each user, and many of which require longitudinal counseling support. In order to help women address their preconception risks, we have developed a virtual agent (Figure 1) that counsels women over the course of a year on how to incrementally address their risks. During each session with the agent, the agent recommends that the user discuss the risk that has the highest clinical importance for preconception care, as rated by a team of family physicians. However, users are free to select any of the topics on their list of risks to discuss with the agent, and are also free to state that they feel any particular risk factor is not relevant to them.

We have recently completed a randomized clinical trial of the preconception care system, and present the results of an analysis of the topics women chose to discuss with the virtual agent. Our primary research questions are:

RQ1. What health risks do women choose to discuss with a virtual agent?
RQ2. What factors predict the risks women choose to discuss?
RQ3. What factors predict uptake on the agent's suggested risk to discuss?

2   Related Work

Many of the PCC health risk topics are very personal and may be uncomfortable for some women to talk about with others, even health professionals. Such stigma is related to social desirability bias, which is the tendency for someone to put themselves in a favorable light with respect to social norms. Kang et al. [6, 7]investigated users' socially desirable responses given different amount of self-disclosure and behavioral realism of virtual agent interviewers, finding that users disclose more with agents who have high behavioral realism and high self-disclosure. Vardoulakis explored social desirability effects in a virtual agent that queried college students about their alcohol consumption, finding that participants self-reported more frequently to a text-based interface than a virtual agent, but with interaction time accounting for the difference (the agent interface took longer to use)[8].

Discussion of personal topics, such as birth control and domestic violence, also constitutes a form of intimate self-disclosure, which generally requires some level of trust between interlocutors, according to social penetration theory [9]. Bickmore and Cassell [2] found that relational conversational strategies, such as small chat, can be used by a virtual agent, to build such a trusting relationship.

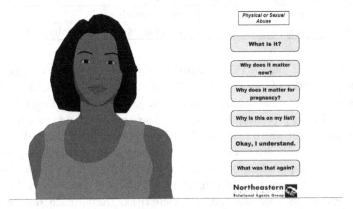

Fig. 1. Virtual Agent Interface used in Preconception Care System

3   Context of the Study: The Preconception Care Virtual Agent

The Preconception Care (PCC) System is a web-based intervention that begins when a user completes a survey questionnaire to identify her PCC risks. Following this, she can conduct sessions as often as she likes to help her address her risks. The intervention is designed for a recommended weekly session over a one year period of time. Users are guided through each session by a virtual agent (Figure 1). Following the survey, the agent introduces the "My Health To-Do List" (Figure 2, Right) and lets users select the identified risks they want to discuss. The agent then describes each risk and why it is important, and offers users the opportunity to take action on it.

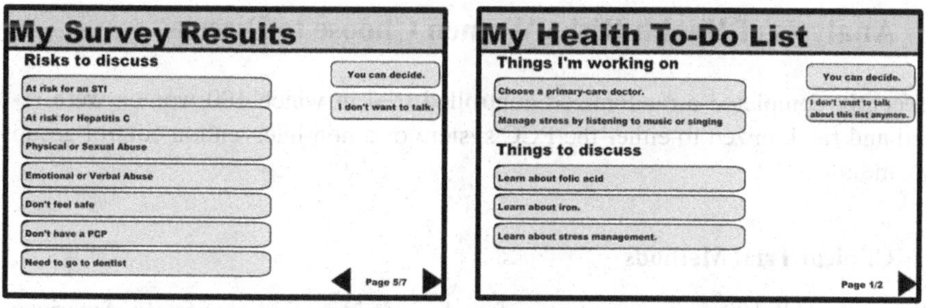

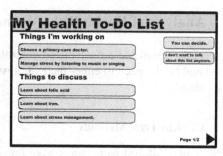

Fig. 2. Sample Survey Results (Left) and "My Health To Do List" (Right)

The agent is rendered in a web-based (Adobe) Flash plugin, using the LiteBody framework [10], with speech output produced on the server with a commercial speech synthesizer. Dialogues are scripted using a custom hierarchical transition network-based scripting language. Agent nonverbal conversational behavior is generated using BEAT [11], and includes beat (baton) hand gestures and eyebrow raises for emphasis, gaze away behavior for signaling turn-taking, and posture shifts to mark topic boundaries, synchronized with speech. User input is obtained via multiple choice selection of utterances.

After a user completes her risk questionnaire her lists of risks is displayed in order of clinical importance (Figure 2, left). At this point she can either pick a risk off the list herself, or ask the agent to choose ("You can decide."), in which case the risk with the highest clinical importance is selected for discussion.

A sample introductory dialogue about a specific risk is shown in Figure 3.

```
Agent: You mentioned that you have been a victim of physical
       or sexual abuse.
User:  What is it?
Agent: Abuse is any physical or sexual harm done to you. It
       can come from any person, including family, someone you
       are dating, someone you live with, or even strangers.
User:  Why does it matter for pregnancy?
Agent: Since you are not pregnant now and are not planning on
       being pregnant soon, this is a great chance for you to
       focus on yourself and being as healthy as you can, both
       physically and emotionally. If you were abused in the
       past or are being abused now, it could make it harder to
       have a healthy baby later on. … …
User:  OK, I understand.
Agent: What best describes your attitude about getting out of a
       physically or sexually abusive situation.
User:  I plan to do this in next 6 months.
```

Fig. 3. Sample Initial Dialogue for Domestic Violence Risk

4   Analysis of Health Risks Women Choose to Discuss

We recently completed a randomized controlled trial in which 100 women were re-cruited and randomized to either the PCC system or a non-intervention control group for six months.

4.1   Clinical Trial Methods

Participants. All 100 participants were female, self-identified as African American or Black, aged 18-34, had regular access to telephone and internet, spoke English, and were self-reported not pregnant at the time of enrollment. Participants were recruited from across the US.

Measures. Participant demographics (age, race, education), generalized self-efficacy (the confidence to overcome obstacles [12]), and health literacy (the ability to read and act on written medical information [13]), were assessed at intake. All participant actions in the PCC system were logged to a database for subsequent analysis. At the conclusion of the six-month intervention, all participants were contacted by phone and asked about each of risks identified by the Risk Assessment to determine their current status with each risk.

Protocol. Following consent, baseline assessment, and randomization, intervention participants were emailed a link to the web-based PCC survey, a Tips Sheet with in-structions for using the PCC system and the study contact information. Intervention participants were emailed periodically to remind them to use the system.

4.2   Auxiliary Data

In order to determine the factors underlying decisions about whether women would discuss a particular health risk or not, we conducted an additional survey of women who were not in the clinical trial. In this survey, we asked women to assess the sensi-tivity and perceived importance of each of the 108 PCC health risks. We reasoned that many women may be uncomfortable discussing certain health risks, even with a vir-tual agent, given social desirability biases (the tendency for someone to put them-selves in a favorable light with respect to social norms).

Sensitivity was assessed by asking "How comfortable would you be discussing this topic with a health professional you don't know?" on a 7-point scale (from 1="Extremely Uncomfortable" to 7="Extremely Comfortable").

Perceived Importance was assessed by asking "How important do you think this risk is for your personal health?" on a 7-point scale (from 1="Extremely unimportant" to 7="Extremely important").
The survey was distributed to 17 women (aged 22 to 29), and 15 complete data sets were obtained.

Each PCC risk was also rank-ordered in importance by a team of family physi-cians, based on the CDC's Select Panel on Preconception Care's publication on the clinical content of preconception care[3]. The Panel considered not only clinical importance, but also the strength of existing evidence and efficacy of available interventions. The development of the Gabby screening questionnaire has been previously published[5]. The perceived importance of risks was significantly correlated with the clinical importance ranking, Spearman's rho=0.259, p<0.05. However, there were many surprising differences between clinicians' importance ranking and perceived importance by lay women. For example, use of the "withdrawal method" of birth control was ranked #5 in importance by clinicians, while lay women ranked it #93 (Table 2).

Table 2. Comparison of Clinician Importance and Perceived Importance by Lay Women of Preconception Care Risk Factors (those with most significant differences)

Risk Topic	Clinician Importance	Perceived Importance
Withdrawal Method	5	93
Multivitamin with folic acid	6	86
'Over the Counter' medicines	24	99
Household chemicals	27	101
Physical or Sexual Abuse	79	9

4.3   Results

Here we focus exclusively on the 42 women (aged 26.02+/-3.4) randomized to the PCC intervention who completed the screening questionnaire, and for whom the screening questionnaire found at least one health risk. These women completed an average of 4.19 (range 1 to 13) interactions with the virtual agent over the six months of the study. The screening questionnaire identified 23.19 (sd 6.12) risks per user and, of these, women chose to discuss an average of 6.33 (sd 7.16) risks with the virtual agent over the duration of the intervention.

RQ1. What health risks do women choose to discuss with the virtual agent?
Table 4 shows those risks women were most and least likely to discuss with the agent, once they had screened positive for the risk and agreed that it was a potential problem for them. Most women who needed HPV vaccine, were sexually active without birth control, or at risk for Hepatitis B discussed these risks with the agent, whereas none of the women who needed more Vitamin D, did not have a primary care physician, or needed more Omega-3 Fatty Acids in their diet chose to discuss these risks with the agent.

RQ2. What factors predict the risks women choose to discuss?
As we hypothesized, there are significant correlations between the perceived importance of a risk and women's likelihood of discussing it (Kendall's tau = -0.168, p<0.05).

Table 3. Risks Most and Least Frequently Discussed For risks that at least 10% of women had and for likelihood of being discussed over 50% or under 5%. Columns as in Table 5

Most Discussed Risks	% total	% dis /acpt	Least Discussed Risks	% total	% dis /acpt
Need HPV vaccine	22%	65%	Need more Vitamin D	20%	0%
No Birth Control	19%	64%	Don't have a PCP	14%	0%
At risk for Hepatitis B	10%	56%	Need more Omega-3 Fatty Acids	10%	0%
'Over the Counter' medicines	13%	56%	Workplace chemicals and dangers	10%	0%
Multivitamin with folic acid	26%	52%	Stress	8%	0%
Born low birth-weight or preterm	16%	50%	Personal History of Health Condition	6%	0%
Alcohol	22%	50%	Don't feel safe	6%	0%
Toxoplasmosis	19%	50%	Depression	4%	0%

Table 4. Logistic Regression to Predict Decision to Discuss Risk

Predictor	Coefficient	p
(Intercept)	-1.941	0.087
S_i	-0.165	0.088
PI_i	0.307	**0.039**
$Total_j$	-0.032	**0.015**
Age_j	-0.044	**0.046**
GSE_j	0.056	**0.001**
$REALM_j$	-0.004	0.311

However, we did not find a significant correlation between the rated sensitivity (comfort discussing a risk) and women's likelihood of discussing it (Kendall's tau = -0.0148, n.s.).

In order to determine the range of factors and their relative contributions to the decision process, we performed a logistic regression on the decision to discuss each risk a woman screened positive for and agreed was potentially relevant to her. Predictors included(also see Table 5):

S_i - Sensitivity of risk i

PI_i - Perceived Importance score of risk i

$Total_j$ - Total number of risks woman j has

Age_j - Age of woman j

GSE_j - General Self-Efficacy of woman j

$REALM_j$ – Health Literacy of woman j has

Table 5. Attributes of the Most Common Risks Reported in the Clinical Trial **# total** is number of women who have the risk; **# reject** is number of women who said that the screening result was incorrect; **# discussed** is number of women who chose to discuss the risk with the agent; **% discussed** = # discussed/ # total; **%dis/acpt** = #discussed/(#total-#reject); **CI** is the clinician importance rank (1=most important); **PI** is the perceived importance rank (from survey); **S** is the risk sensitivity (1-7, from survey).

Risk Topic	# total	# reject	% reject	# dis-cussed	% dis-cussed	% dis/acpt	CI	PI	S
Ethnicity-Based Health Risk	41	5	12.2%	12	29.3%	33.3%	51	75	3.56
Caffeine	41	10	24.4%	6	14.6%	19.4%	105	102	2.19
Listeriosis	39	15	38.5%	9	23.1%	37.5%	83	42	2.31
At risk for an STI	38	8	21.1%	7	18.4%	23.3%	75	69	4
Bad diet or food choices	35	0	0.00%	7	20.0%	20.0%	104	49	2.69
Plastic Water Bottles	33	6	18.2%	10	30.3%	37.0%	57	109	1.94
Partner needs Re-productive Life Plan	30	8	26.7%	7	23.3%	31.8%	65	105	3.06
Need more Iron	29	1	3.5%	9	31.0%	32.1%	26	85	1.59
Not been tested for an STI	27	2	7.4%	4	14.8%	16.0%	77	57	3.75
Multivitamin with folic acid	23	0	0.00%	12	52.2%	52.2%	6	86	1.59
Exercise	23	0	0.00%	2	8.7%	8.7%	68	34	2.13
At risk for Hepatitis C	23	6	26.1%	5	21.7%	29.4%	76	61	3.38
Need more Calcium	22	3	13.6%	7	31.8%	36.8%	25	81	1.59
At risk for Malaria	21	8	38.1%	6	28.6%	46.2%	71	62	2.5
Exposure to Lead	21	9	42.9%	4	19.0%	33.3%	78	83	2.13
...									

Results (using the "glm" function in the R statistical analysis program) are shown in Table 4. Women's decision to discuss a risk is driven primarily by their perceived importance of the risk, but also by their general self-efficacy. The likelihood of discussing any given risk decreases with the total number of risks a woman has, indicating there may be a fixed amount of time women are willing to spend working on their health risks. The probability of discussing risks also decreases with a woman's age. The sensitivity of a risk approached significance as a predictive factor (p=.088), but its influence was in the predicted direction: more sensitive risks were less likely to be discussed.

RQ3. What factors predict uptake on the agent's suggested risk to discuss?
Finally, we investigated what factors predicted when users would choose what risk they wanted to discuss vs. simply letting the agent select the risk with the highest clinical importance. The number of risks already discussed was the primary predictor of this decision. There is a general trend for women to let the agent decide more frequently the more risks they have already discussed (Figure 4). The reason for this could be that once they have already discussed the few risks that are most important to them (by choosing to discuss them), they are satisfied to let the agent choose the order of the remaining ones.

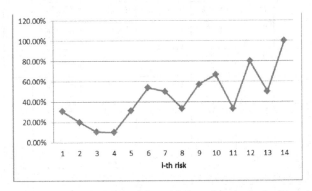

Fig. 4. Percentage of Risk Decisions Abdicated to Agent, by Decision

5   Discussion, Conclusions, and Future Work

We found that women were comfortable and willing to discuss a wide range of health risks with a virtual agent, including many topics that may have significant stigma associated with them, such as domestic violence. The women in our study only discussed 6.3 of the 23.2 health risks they screened positive for with a virtual health counseling agent. However, there was a large variation in their likelihood of discussing different risks with the agent, ranging from 65% (needing HPV vaccine) to 0% (needing more Vitamin D). We found that some of the factors that contribute to this difference include the perceived importance of the risk, a woman's generalized self-efficacy, and her comfort discussing the risk.

There are several limitations to our study and analysis. The participants in the clinical trial did not complete the surveys of importance and sensitivity themselves, thus the data obtained may not match their own assessments of these factors. We also did not compare our results to decisions to discuss these risk factors with a human health counselor, which would have told us much more about women's attitudes towards virtual agents as health counselors.

We have just started another clinical trial of the PCC system in which 530 women will be randomized to the system or a non-intervention control group for a year-long period of time. Future work includes expanding the system's functionality in various ways, such as the ability for the agent to counsel women on developing a reproductive life plan. Our intent is that this effort will ultimately address the significant disparities in infant health in the US.

Acknowledgments. This work has been supported by the Agency for Healthcare Research and Quality (AHRQ), the Health Resources and Services Administration (HRSA), and the National Institute on Minority Health and Health Disparities (NIMHD). We thank the rest of the PCC team, including Daniel Schulman, Juan Fernandez, Leanne Yinusa-Nyahkoon, and Ekaterina Sadikova, Suzanne Mitchell, Paula Gardiner, Fatima Adigun, Divya Mehta and Karla Damus.

References

1. McNair, S., Checchi, K., Rubin, A., Marcello, T., Bickmore, T., Simon, S.: A Pilot Study of a Computer-Based Relational Agent to Screen for Substance-Use Problems in Primary Care. In: Society of Behavioral Medicine 2013 Annual Meeting (2013)
2. Bickmore, T., Puskar, K., Schlenk, E., Pfeifer, L., Sereika, S.: Maintaining Reality: Relational Agents for Antipsychotic Medication Adherence. Interacting with Computers 22, 276–288 (2010)
3. Atrash, H., Jack, B., Johnson, K.: Where is the "w"oman in MCH? American Journal of Obstetrics and Gynecology 199(suppl.), S259–S265 (2008)
4. Centers for Disease Control and Prevention: Recommendations for improving preconception health and health care. Morbidity and Mortality Weekly Report 55(RR-6), 1–23 (2006)
5. Gardiner, P., Hempstead, M.B., Ring, L., Bickmore, T., Yinusa-Nyahkoon, L., Tran, H., Paasche-Orlow, M., Damus, K., Jack, B.: Reaching Women Through Health Information Technology: The Gabby Preconception Care System. Am. J. Health Promotion 27, 11–20 (2013)
6. Kang, S.-H., Fort Morie, J.: Users' socially desirable responding with computer interviewers. In: Conference Users' Socially Desirable Responding with Computer Interviewers, pp. 229–234. ACM
7. Kang, S.-H., Gratch, J.: Exploring Users' Social Responses to Computer Counseling Interviewers' Behavior
8. Vardoulakis, L.M.: Social desirability bias and engagement in systems designed for long-term health tracking. Northeastern University Boston (2013)
9. Altman, I., Taylor, D.: *Social penetration: The development of interpersonal relationships. Holt, Rinhart & Winston, New York (1973)
10. Bickmore, T., Schulman, D., Shaw, G.: DTask and LiteBody: Open Source, Standards-Based Tools for Building Web-Deployed Embodied Conversational Agents. In: Ruttkay, Z., Kipp, M., Nijholt, A., Vilhjálmsson, H.H. (eds.) IVA 2009. LNCS, vol. 5773, pp. 425–431. Springer, Heidelberg (2009)
11. Cassell, J., Vilhjálmsson, H., Bickmore, T.: BEAT: The Behavior Expression Animation Toolkit. In: Conference BEAT: The Behavior Expression Animation Toolkit, pp. 477–486
12. Schwarzer, R., Jerusalem, M.: Generalized Self-Efficacy scale. In: Weinman, J., Wright, S., Johnston, M. (eds.) Measures in Health Psychology: A User's Portfolio, pp. 35–37 (1995)
13. Davis, T., Long, S., Jackson, R., et al.: Rapid estimate of adult literacy in medicine: a shortened screening instrument. Fam. Med. 25, 391–395 (1993)

Evaluating the Impact of Anticipation on the Efficiency and Believability of Virtual Agents

Quentin Reynaud[1,2,3], Jean-Yves Donnart[3], and Vincent Corruble[1,2]

[1] Université Pierre et Marie Curie – Paris 6, LIP6, Paris, France
[2] CNRS, LIP6, Paris, France
{quentin.reynaud,vincent.corruble}@lip6.fr
[3] THALES Training & Simulation, Osny, France
jean-yves.donnart@thalesgroup.com

Abstract. We propose a model of cognitive process allowing virtual agents to exhibit anticipatory abilities. With user experiments, we show that this mechanism brings about an improvement in the efficiency of the behavior generated, and check that external observers are able to perceive it. We also confirm that this improvement in efficiency leads, up to a point, to an improvement in believability as judged by human observers. Beyond this level of efficiency, believability reaches a plateau.

Keywords: virtual agents, hybrid architectures, anticipation, believability, user evaluation, agent-based simulation.

1   Introduction

The field of virtual agents is particularly rich, and finds applications in various domains. In this paper we address primarily applications to urban simulation, though our results are relevant to other domains. In urban simulation, one has to be able to deal with a large number of agents, in real-time, and in a rich environment. These constraints often lead toward using reactive agents which are known to have limitations in terms of believability [1] and are not adequate when the behaviors to simulate become complex. For that reason, the idea of combining reactive and cognitive abilities in hybrid agent architectures is useful [4]. In this paper we tackle the issue of enriching the decision process of virtual agents with anticipatory abilities, one of the most important skills recognized as cognitive. Our claim is that these abilities increase the behaviors efficiency of the virtual agents, and consequently the believability (as perceived by human observers) of these behaviors. We study this claim by integrating the corresponding module in a agent architecture [2] and by evaluating it with a user experiment focusing on the perceived efficiency and believability of the agent's behaviors.

We consider classically that believability is the capacity of an agent to "suspend the disbelief" of observers [3]. Over the last years, the role of anticipation has appeared as an important feature in agent's decision processes and in virtual agent's

T. Bickmore et al. (Eds.): IVA 2014, LNAI 8637, pp. 360–363, 2014.
© Springer International Publishing Switzerland 2014

believability, to such an extent that [1] claimed: "only cognitive systems with anticipation mechanisms can be credible, adaptive, and successful in interaction with both the environment and other autonomous systems and humans".

2   Anticipatory Module

The anticipatory module proposed here takes some inspiration from [5]. Its goal is to provide agents with an ability to make predictions about themselves and their environment, using predictive models. This module is based on an evaluation of future individual satisfaction levels rather than future states as often done in state anticipation. This leads to a better generality, because it is possible to provide the agents with their own model of satisfaction, largely independent from the environment used.

Our anticipatory module uses predictive models. These include a model able to calculate a level of *satisfaction* based on the internal states of the agent. It also includes predictive models about the *environment*, the *actions*, and the *internal states*, which are traditionally used in anticipatory mechanisms. Additionally, a decision model is required to produce predictions on the future *decisions* of the agent. These models can come from several sources: they can be handcrafted by the agent designer, but they can also be learned. A third possibility is to assume that the anticipatory module is fully introspective: it can directly use the various models at work in the agent architecture to run them for predicting their future outputs. We made this simplifying assumption in the experiments reported further below.

We give below a synthetic algorithm of the anticipatory process proposed:

```
Data:
A is an agent;
tc is the current time;
Initialization:
t = tc;
while (StoppingCondition is
false), repeat:
PredictNextAction(A,t);
PredictEndOfAction(A,t);
PredictFutureState(A,t);
EvaluateFutureSatisfaction(A,t);
SearchAnticipatoryPlan();
end
```

StoppingCondition(A,t): is the stopping condition of the algorithm.
PredictNextAction(A,t): predicts the action of A at time t.
PredictEndOfAction(A,t): uses the action model to estimate the time remaining until the completion of the predicted action.
PredictFutureState(A,t): uses the environment model to predict the changes occurring in the environment.
EvaluateFutureSatisfaction(A,t): uses the satisfaction model and the predicted situation to predict the satisfaction (S) at time t .

SearchAnticipatoryPlan: attempts to find a plan that leads to a satisfaction (SP) higher than S. Each plan found by this method is called an *anticipatory plan*: a plan using prediction abilities to attempt to be more efficient. These plans have a grade attached Q, depending on both G the predicted gain in satisfaction, and C a confidence level. In this paper, we consider that the goal of the anticipatory module is only to propose these plans.

3   Empirical Evaluation

In order to validate our model, the anticipatory module is integrated in an agent hybrid architecture, described in [2,6]. Agents are driven by a set of behavior sources (*high-level modules*) that propose behaviors. These proposals are fed into a *decision module*, in charge of the integration of all behavior proposals. By default two simple high-level modules were used: a module based on motivations [7], and a schedule module. The anticipation module is therefore introduced as a third high-level module.

In the following experiments, we assume a fully introspective anticipatory module. Satisfaction is based on the number and priority levels of all behavior proposals received by the agent's decision module, and the stopping condition for anticipation is defined as a maximum number of anticipated actions, set to 3.

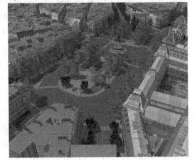

Experiments were carried out with the simulator described in [7], and all simulations take place in the virtual environment of Place de la République area in Paris, which covers 1.6 km², 5000 buildings, and 100 points of interest, with about 20 actions available to the agents.

The goal of these experiments is to evaluate the following hypotheses: (H_1) the anticipatory module improves the behaviors efficiency; (H_2) the anticipatory module improves the behaviors believability; (H_3) an improvement in the behaviors efficiency brings an improvement in the behaviors believability. The user experiments were conducted through an online survey and involved 144 participants.

Table 1. The participants were presented with two short videos showing the proceedings of an agent's morning. The agent starts at home and then goes to work and stays there until noon. Only in the second video, the agent has an anticipatory module activated. Participants were first asked to grade the *efficiency* of the behaviors shown in both videos on a Likert scale, from 1 to 7 (results in Table 1), then the *believability* of the same behaviors (results in Table 2).

Table 1. Efficiency of behaviors with and without anticipation, on a Likert scale from 1 to 7

	Average score	st. dev.	Mode
Without anticipation	3.69	1.60	4
With anticipation	4.64	1.74	6

Table 2. Believability of behaviors with and without anticipation, on a Likert scale from 1 to 7

	Average score	st. dev.	Mode
Without anticipation	4.44	1.53	5
With anticipation	4.96	1.65	6

We can see that both efficiency and believability are improved by anticipation, the first more markedly. Both improvements are significant as confirmed by two student's t-tests (with a confidence level below 0.01). Hence both H_1 and H_2 are validated.

We consider now the evolution of behavior believability as a function of behavior efficiency, in order to check H_3, and based on the graph shown in Figure 1.

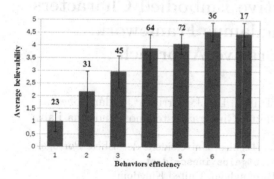

Graph obtained by gathering results from two previous questions: two sets of 144 couples of efficiency and believability scores. From these 288 couples, we obtain the average believability score associated with each efficiency grade. Standard deviations appear as vertical segments, and number of observations on top of bars.

Fig. 1. Average Behavior Believability, Function of Behavior Efficiency

At first, each gain in efficiency brings a significant gain in believability. Above an efficiency score of 4, believability reaches a plateau, and one could even hypothesize the beginning of a decrease in believability. One could say that H_3 is confirmed only when the perceived efficiency is low or medium.

4   Conclusion

In this paper we presented a model of anticipatory module based on the maximization of an agent satisfaction level, that was integrated within a virtual agent architecture. We confirmed that anticipation brings an improvement in the perceived efficiency and believability. Furthermore, we showed a link between the efficiency and the believability of a behavior, though gains in believability are only obvious when efficiency is low or medium. In conclusion, we can argue that adding anticipatory abilities is a crucial step toward increasing agents believability even though we highlighted some limitations to this result, which would require further research.

References

1. Pezzulo, G., Butz, M.V., Castelfranchi, C., Falcone, R. (eds.): The Challenge of Anticipation. LNCS (LNAI), vol. 5225. Springer, Heidelberg (2008)
2. de Sevin, E., Reynaud, Q., Corruble, V.: FlexMex: Flexible Multi-Expert Meta-Architecture for Virtual Agents. In: 1st Conf. on Advances in Cognitive Systems (2012)
3. Bates, J.: The role of emotion in believable agents. Communications of the ACM 37(7), 122–125 (1994)
4. Wooldridge, M., Jennings, N.: Agent theories, architectures, and languages: a survey. Intelligent agents (1995)
5. Davidsson, P., Astor, E., Ekdahl, B.: A framework for autonomous agents based on the concept of anticipatory systems. In: Cybernetics and Systems (1994)
6. Reynaud, Q., Corruble, V.: Un mécanisme de composition de comportements pour agents virtuels. In: 21èmes Journées Francophones sur les Systèmes Multi-Agents, Lille (2013)
7. de Sevin, E., Thalmann, D.: A motivational model of action selection for virtual humans. In: Computer Graphics International, pp. 213–220 (2005)

Developing Interactive Embodied Characters Using the Thalamus Framework: A Collaborative Approach

Tiago Ribeiro[1], Eugenio di Tullio[1], Lee J. Corrigan[2], Aidan Jones[2],
Fotios Papadopoulos[2], Ruth Aylett[3], Ginevra Castellano[2], and Ana Paiva[1]

[1] INESC-ID & Instituto Superior Técnico, Universidade de Lisboa, Portugal
`tiago.ribeiro@gaips.inesc-id.pt`
[2] University of Birmingham, United Kingdom
[3] School of Mathematical and Computer Sciences, Heriot-Watt University,
Edinburgh, UK

Abstract. We address the situation of developing interactive scenarios featuring embodied characters that interact with users through various types of media easily presents as a challenge. Some of the problems that developers face are on collaborating while developing remotely, integrating all the independently developed components, and incrementally developing a system in such way that the developed components can be used since their incorporation, throughout the intermediate phases of development, and on to the final system. We describe how the Thalamus framework addresses these issues, and how it is being used on a large project that targets developing this type of scenarios. A case study is presented, illustrating actual development of such scenario which was then used for a Wizard-of-Oz study.

Keywords: Embodied characters, component integration framework, social robotics, BML.

1 Introduction

As scientists, we envision the creation of autonomous artificial characters that are able to interact with humans in a natural way. It seems that interactive technologies are evolving enough to provide this; however we still strive to figure out how to integrate artificial characters, virtual environments, and our physical world in a seamless interaction. Current applications that feature interactive embodied agents tend to integrate several technologies together, into larger holistic systems.

One particularly interesting field of application that features these kind of holistic systems are the ones involving socially interactive robots [3]. Our work is part of the EU FP7 EMOTE Project[1]. The project aims at developing empathic robotic tutors that can interact with school children through multimedia applications in order to improve learning.

---

[1] `http://www.emote-project.eu/`

T. Bickmore et al. (Eds.): IVA 2014, LNAI 8637, pp. 364–373, 2014.

In this field of human-robot interaction, users interact with an agent, embodied as a robot. This robot is normally regarded by the user as the actual artificially intelligent being. However, it frequently turns out that technically, the robot acts solely as an embodiment and does not actually contain what is regarded as the artificial intelligence. This intelligence will most likely be running on separate computers which communicate with and control the robot [4]. It is also becoming common to have external third-party components extending the interaction environment, such as capture devices (e.g. Microsoft© Kinect©[2]) or touch-tables. Current mobile devices can also be used to extend the interaction, providing the physical robot with a ubiquitous virtual form, in a process called migration [9].

The requirements for this type of tutor and interaction environment thus aims us at exploring component-based embodied agents in which components can be reused in different scenarios.

This paper describes Thalamus, our component integration framework, developed in order to support the development of interactive agents that can seamlessly integrate the agent's logic with components for both various embodiments (virtual or robotic) and mixed environments (virtual and physical). We describe how it is being used in EMOTE for collaboratively developing the overall system that includes a robotic character (tutor), a touch-based video-game, perceptual components, and high-level behaviour control. We present a case study in which the tutor is controlled in a Wizard-of-Oz setting, and how the same components can still be used when we replace the wizard with an autonomous agent.

2   Related Work

Several authors have faced the kind of problems we refer to, and as such, have proposed other architectures before. Schröeder developed the SEMAINE API, which was used in the EU FP7 Semaine Project[3]. This is a component integration framework, based on the principles of asynchronous messaging middleware. Its architecture, however, has a pipeline message flow, meaning that it follows in the traditional sense-think-act loop of interactive agents. The author points out two key requirements for a framework of this kind: Infrastructure, meaning that components must be able to run on different programming languages and operating systems; and Communication, meaning that components must follow suitable representation formats, which should be standards where possible[8].

CMION was developed in the context of the EU FP7 LIREC[4]. It is a mind-body framework for integrating sensors and actuators through various degrees of abstraction. It was designed especially for allowing agent migration (transferring the agent's identify to a different embodiment). As such, it abstractly encapsulates functionalities of an embodiment into what they call competencies. These competencies share information through a blackboard component. By defining

---

[2] http://www.microsoft.com/en-us/kinectforwindows/
[3] http://www.semaine-project.eu/
[4] http://lirec.eu/

an embodiment as a set of competencies, agents can then migrate to other embodiments, as long as those implement the same type of competencies[2].

Thalamus was first also developed for the same LIREC project[6]. I was initially developed as an embodiment-independent BML scheduler which was used to run BML on robots. It also provided interaction between high-level perception structures (PML) and the BML plans, so that an agent's behaviour could be planned to interact with asynchronous events from the environment.

More recently, the same authors have presented the Censys Model[7]. Censys serves as a theoretical-to-technical foundation on how developers can design and structure agents following some concepts taken from philosophy and neuroscience, in order to break the sense-think-act loop of traditional agents. What Censys proposes is that there is no need to explicitly define a Mind or a Body in an agent. The Mind process can be built out of several interacting processes, which exchange information. The Body processes would be all the processes that are capable of turning the higher-level behaviour instructions onto low-level body actions, and the low level perceptual data into higher-level representations that can be understood by other components. The behaviour realization components do not event have to be the same as the perception components. This allows to more easily reuse components in different applications, by replacing only specific parts of the system. In a Censys architecture, the flow of communication is asynchronous and does not follow a predefined path (pipeline). This allows several modules to perform lower-level autonomous behaviour, while other modules simultaneously process and provide higher-level information.

ROS - Robot Operating System is a popular middleware for robotics that provides a common communication layer to enable different types of sensors, motors and other components to exchange data[5]. ROS is module-based, meaning that a ROS-based robot actually runs several different modules, being each one of them responsible for controlling one or more components of the robot. They communicate based on a message oriented middleware (MOM). This is accomplished through a publish-subscribe pattern, in which each module specifies the type of messages it wants to receive (subscription), so that each time another module produces that message (publication), the subscribed modules receive it.

3   Thalamus as a Modular Framework for Interactive Embodied Agents

Thalamus was initially developed as a cross-media body interface for artificial embodied characters[6]. It was based on the SAIBA framework [1], and developed mostly as a BML scheduler, with the additional capability of supporting abstract perceptions which could interact with BML actions, in order to allow for continuous interaction with a character. By providing only the scheduling and not the realization functionality of BML, it can be used with different embodiments, both virtual and robotic.

3.1 Motivation

We have now adapted Thalamus to follow on the Censys model[7], thus turning it into a more general component-integration framework. Traditionally, the body of an embodied agent framework contains all the physical interfaces of the character, both in terms of actuation and perception. However, we consider that the interface with the environment can be composed of several components.

An example of this would be an interactive scenario featuring an expressive robot and a Kinect© camera for perceiving the user. An interactive system should be modular enough to allow replacing the robot by another one for the expressive function, while keeping the Kinect© for the perceptual function.

By building on Censys, we do not designate any specific component as being either the *body* or the *mind*. This also makes it easier to have a character that interacts both with the physical environment and with a virtual one.

Taking as example an interactive setting with the robot, the Kinect©, and a touch surface/screen, these three components all provide an interface with the user and the physical environment. However, the touch screen will most likely be running another application which provides a virtual environment. On such a setting, we do not consider it appropriate to strictly define the body as a specific component of our system.

The main new feature we have introduced into Thalamus is the MOM mechanism, which is designed to integrate with the scheduler. This integration between scheduler and MOM allows to have the asynchronous and abstract sides of communication given by the MOM, while still supporting synchronously distributed behaviours that run in a BML-like manner. However, the Thalamus scheduler is more abstract than BML, which allows it to synchronize actions and events that do not only originate from BML-based behaviour.

3.2 Architecture

Figure 1 shows an overview of how Thalamus is currently structured. The Thalamus Master (Master) is the main node which centralizes all communication that runs between different Thalamus Modules. Both the Master and each of the Modules can run either in the same or in different computers, as the communication is established over some type of network protocol. As described on the Censys model, each Module can subscribe and publish both Actions and Perceptions.

In Thalamus, both of these are treated as Events. We distinguished them mostly for easier design, development and comprehension of the agents. The figure also shows the MOM-based manager as the central part of the framework, and how it is tightly linked with the scheduler.

The Master maintains a proxy to each of the Modules that are connected, in order to manage the communication between these two parts. Each Module actually communicates with it's specific Module Proxy, both to subscribe, announce, publish and receive events. Every time the configuration of the connected modules changes (i.e, some module connects or disconnects from the system), all the

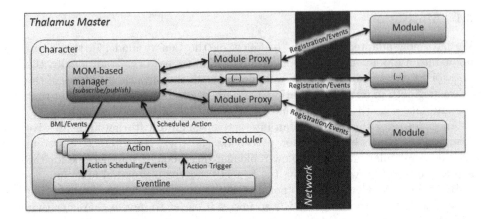

Fig. 1. The current Thalamus Framework architecture

available Event definitions are broadcast to all Modules. This allows Modules to know what is currently available in the system, and if necessary, adapt the way they behave.

Models that exchange the same type of Events must all follow a pre-defined Event structure in order to consider the same parameters for the transmitted Event. These are specified outside of any Module, in shared libraries. Each library can contain several groups of Events, which we called Interfaces. These Interfaces are defined externally by the agent developers, and should include all the Events that are necessary for implementing a specific kind of functionality.

Figure 2 shows an example in which several Modules subscribe and publish to Events which are defined by Interfaces in separate libraries. By subscribing to a specific Interface, the Module subscribes to all Events defined in it. Each Module can subscribe or publish to as many Interfaces as the agent developers consider the Module to be responsible for.

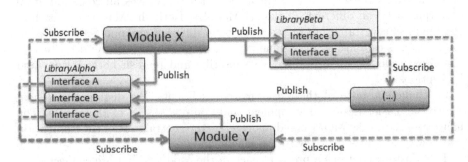

Fig. 2. Example scheme of how different modules publish and subscribe to events

3.3   Implementation and Development Workflow

Thalamus is currently implemented in C#/dotnet. It can run either as a library, or as a standalone application, with its own GUI. The Master node generally runs in the standalone form. All the other Modules run as separate applications by implementing the ThalamusClient class. In order to publish events, each Module also contains an instance of a ThalamusPublisher class. We are currently using the XML-RPC.Net[5] library for remote message invocation between the Modules and the Master.

The framework is open-source, and is currently available through a Mercurial repository in Sourceforge[6]. There is a README.txt file which includes the basic workflow with Thalamus, and a Documentation folder with instructions on how to start writing modules.

Thalamus also includes a simple GUI which provides features like:

- Creating a Character, which will automatically receive connections from any Modules;
- Viewing the Modules that are connected to such Character;
- Manually triggering Actions and Perceptions, for debugging and testing purposes;
- Event viewer with filters.

4   Case Study: The Modular Wizard-of-Oz

Thalamus is currently being use as the backbone integration platform in the European FP7 EMOTE project. Several partners are using it collaboratively to develop different Modules that communicate with each other in order to achieve the project's goals. The project aims at developing empathic robotic tutors that can interact with school children through multimedia applications in order to improve learning.

4.1   Collaborative Platform for Large-Scale Agent Development

Several things in Thalamus were developed with collaborative development in mind. We highlight the method of defining Event Interfaces as separate libraries that can be shared by different Modules. The Thalamus Master has no knowledge of these Interfaces and Events. They are all abstracted when sent to the Master, so that the Master relies only on the type of Event that is being transmitted, and the rules that it has for who to broadcast it to. This has allowed developers to work independently on different Modules that communicate with each other by simply sharing a library which contains the necessary Events.

By having anticipated that a large scale interactive scenario would include several logical, virtual and physical components, we have made the integration

---

[5] http://xml-rpc.net/

[6] http://sourceforge.net/projects/thalamus/

process as easy and flexible as possible. Besides the shared Interfaces, all Modules and the Master have a network communication layer that allows them to find each other and connect automatically across a local network, and maintain such connection even when one Module, or even the Master fails for some reason (normally during development and debugging of new features). It would be extremely tedious to require setting up connections manually, and having to restart all the modules every time something failed.

4.2   Interactive Scenarios

In EMOTE, the tutor is being developed for two different interactive scenarios, both using a robotic embodiment, and a large touch-table. The touch-table runs a multimedia interactive application (like a video-game). The user interacts with the system by using the game application. The system also interacts back through the robotic embodiment, which provides a character with expressive behaviour.

In a large-scale project, it is common to run tests with initial versions of the system in order to collect data about how users interact with all the components that are being developed. In our case, before implementing the final autonomous robotic tutor, we are going through several mock-up and wizard-of-oz (WoZ) experiments. This section briefly describes how Thalamus was used to integrate the components used in a recent WoZ experiment.

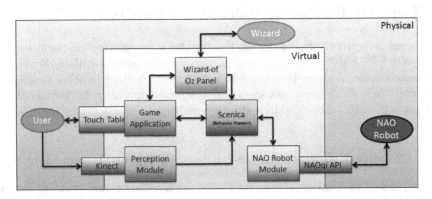

Fig. 3. Structure of the Wizard-of-Oz setting. The physical and virtual components are distinguished.

Figure 3 shows how the current system is structured for the WoZ experiment. Our physical components are a NAO robot[7], a multi-touch table (MTT), and a Microsoft© Kinect©.

The MTT provides both a virtual environment (Game Application) that is shared by the agent and the user, and is also used for input from the user. The Kinect captures the user. Currently it is used only for head-tracking.

[7] http://www.aldebaran.com/en

The NAO Robot provides an embodiment that exhibits expressive behaviour towards the user. Such expressive behavior is generated and managed by a behavior planner module which we call Scenica. This module is constantly updated with information from the Perception module (which interfaces with the Kinect). It also receives coordinate information from the Game Application, in order to be able to instruct the robot to gaze, point or wave towards specific points on the screen. Scenica also provides some semi-autonomous behaviour. It manages gazing behaviour so that the Wizard does not have to deal with all that.

The Wizard uses the WoZ panel to control the flow of the game, to parametrize some of Scenica's semi-autonomous behaviour, and to manually select high-level FML utterances. These utterances are dialogue acts which were previously written and tagged both with non-verbal and game instructions. The FML is broken down in Scenica into BML actions and game-actions. The actions are then sent through Thalamus to be scheduled and/or routed to other modules (NAO Robot Module and Game Application).

As stated earlier, all the modules communicate over a network. That allows for easy deployment of different Modules across different machines. The NAO Robot Module runs on the actual robot, using Mono[8]. The Game Application runs on the MTT, while the remaining modules (Scenica, Perception and WoZ) run on another computer. As we are implementing more intensive algorithms for the Perception module, in the future we may decide to deploy this to a dedicated machine with specific hardware.

4.3 Feedback from the Developers

EMOTE's technical team has been collaboratively developing the described system. All of them have experience and degrees related with Computer Science, and are either pursuing a PhD degree, or working as post-doc in the project. They were questioned regarding the strengths and weaknesses of Thalamus. Their qualitative feedback is reported in the following paragraphs.

A. Strengths
   Development
   - Modules can easily be added, removed and reused;
   - Easy to debug with the event viewer;
   - Simple concept of events and actions;
   - Underlying mechanics are abstracted. The modules' internal logic are separated from the communication level;
   - Easy to specify what information a Module publishes and easy to discover what you can subscribe to;
   - Made it easy to work with NAO robot by using BML;
   - Distributed computing allows distributing resources;
   - Concentration on developing primary code without actually knowing which other modules the interface would need to communicate with;
   - Run on different OS and easy to interop with different languages.

---

[8] http://www.mono-project.com/Main_Page

- Each Module synchronizes its internal clock with the Master, in order to provide logging with near-matching time-stamps;

Collaboration

- Collaboration with other developers enhanced thanks to the independence of each Module;
- Each developer is abstracted away from the concerns of others;
- Development is easily separated, implementation within modules can be changed simply and easily without affecting other modules;
- Each developer needed only to agree on the specification of their requirements for the Events' format (name and parameters);
- Development was not drastically affected by partners changing requirements on a near daily basis;
- After specifying the interfaces, each developer works on its own module, and once ready, things fit easily.

Networking

- A module can crash and then reconnect to Thalamus without causing any issues to other modules;
- No need for set-ups e.g. ip-addresses or names;

B. Weaknesses

Development

- Some limitations on the type of data that can be sent or received from the clients;
- Complex classes or enumerators are not well managed (even though they can be used);
- Sometimes Thalamus Standalone crashes;
- All modules should be running the same version of Thalamus (from sourceforge) otherwise they can't communicate;

Networking

- The discovery of the Thalamus Master can be improved.
- Impossible to select which network adapter to use;
- On some versions of Windows©, requires removing UAC[9] and firewall protection to work;
- Network failure sometimes caused some repeated messages;

5   Conclusions and Future Work

We have described how the Thalamus framework is being used in a large project in which different developers working remotely are able to collaborate on building an interactive scenario featuring a robotic character. The developers have pointed out some of the main benefits and handicaps collected during their experience of working together. We believe that on projects integrating so many technologies, there should be focus on how the backbone tools and frameworks are adequate for the needs of the developers. International projects often require development across different countries, habits, and time zones. We also address the re-usability

---

[9] User Access Control.

of components in different scenarios as a benefit of planning ahead with an easily extensible and modular framework. The kind of abstraction and high-level integration we provide with Thalamus is also directed towards more recent applications, which often integrate virtual and physical environments, with virtual and physical characters.

There are, of course, points we still consider to be missing. One of them is a mechanism for managing conflicts, in the case of several Modules publishing or subscribing to the same type of Messages. This will highly depend on what is the purpose of the agent, which Modules are being used, and how each of them works. As such, we intend to provide Thalamus only with mechanisms for establishing rules, while the actual rules should be established by the developers.

There are still some network issues to be solved. In the future we may want to replace the XML-RPC-based communications layer with a more stable and efficient implementation.

Acknowledgments. This work was partially supported by the European Commission (EC) and was funded by the EU FP7 ICT-317923 project EMOTE and partially supported by national funds through FCT - Fundação para a Ciência e a Tecnologia, under the project PEst-OE/EEI/LA0021/2013.

References

1. Kopp, S., Krenn, B., Marsella, S.C., Marshall, A.N., Pelachaud, C., Pirker, H., Thórisson, K.R., Vilhjálmsson, H.H.: Towards a common framework for multimodal generation: The behavior markup language. In: Gratch, J., Young, M., Aylett, R.S., Ballin, D., Olivier, P. (eds.) IVA 2006. LNCS (LNAI), vol. 4133, pp. 205–217. Springer, Heidelberg (2006)
2. Kriegel, M., Aylett, R., Cuba, P., Vala, M., Paiva, A.: Robots Meet IVAs: A Mind-Body Interface for Migrating Artificial Intelligent Agents. In: Vilhjálmsson, H.H., Kopp, S., Marsella, S., Thórisson, K.R. (eds.) IVA 2011. LNCS, vol. 6895, pp. 282–295. Springer, Heidelberg (2011)
3. Leite, I., Martinho, C., Paiva, A.: Social Robots for Long-Term Interaction: A Survey. International Journal of Social Robotics 5(2), 291–308 (2013)
4. Pereira, A., Prada, R., Paiva, A.: Socially present board game opponents. In: Nijholt, A., Romão, T., Reidsma, D. (eds.) ACE 2012. LNCS, vol. 7624, pp. 101–116. Springer, Heidelberg (2012)
5. Quigley, M., Gerkey, B.: ROS: an open-source Robot Operating System. In: ICRA Workshop on Open Source Software, vol. 3(3.2) (2009)
6. Ribeiro, T., Vala, M., Paiva, A.: Thalamus: Closing the mind-body loop in interactive embodied characters. In: Nakano, Y., Neff, M., Paiva, A., Walker, M. (eds.) IVA 2012. LNCS, vol. 7502, pp. 189–195. Springer, Heidelberg (2012)
7. Ribeiro, T., Vala, M., Paiva, A.: Censys: A Model for Distributed Embodied Cognition. In: Aylett, R., Krenn, B., Pelachaud, C., Shimodaira, H. (eds.) IVA 2013. LNCS, vol. 8108, pp. 58–67. Springer, Heidelberg (2013)
8. Schröder, M.: The SEMAINE API: A component integration framework for a naturally interacting and emotionally competent Embodied Conversational Agent. Ph.D. thesis (2012)
9. Segura, E.M., Cramer, H., Gomes, P.F., Paiva, A.: Revive! Reactions to Migration Between Different Embodiments When Playing With Robotic Pets Categories and Subject Descriptors, pp. 88–97 (2012)

The Right Agent for the Job?
The Effects of Agent Visual Appearance on Task Domain

Lazlo Ring, Dina Utami, and Timothy Bickmore

College of Computer and Information Science, Northeastern University,
Boston, MA, USA
{lring,dinau,bickmore}@ccs.neu.edu

Abstract. The visual design of virtual agents presents developers with a very large number of choices. We conducted a series of studies using Amazon's Mechanical Turk that demonstrate that there are no design universals for characters, optimal design of character proportion and rendering style depends on the task domain and user characteristics. Specifically, we found these adjustments to an agent's appearance directly effected how users rated it based on whether it was discussing social or medical content. The results of this research aim to help create visual guidelines for the development of domain specific virtual agents.

Keywords: Virtual Agents, Rendering Styles, Character Proportions.

1 Introduction

There are many design decisions that must be made when creating a virtual agent for a new application and user demographic. These decisions range from the species of the agent (humanoid, animal, robot, etc.), genre of the character (anime, cartoon proportioned, realistic), the apparent role of the character, demographic parameters (gender, race, age), selection of clothing and accessories, hairstyle, and rendering style. Although several studies have attempted to systematically explore parts of this design space [17,4] they have all constrained their investigations to single application domains, such as entertainment. However, the most appropriate character design for one domain is not necessarily the most appropriate for another. For example, a toon-shaded anime style character may be ideal in a social networking application but possibly inappropriate as the interface to a retirement planning system.

In this paper, we further investigate the visual design space for intelligent virtual agents, but include in our research the systematic manipulation of task type. This work is motivated by our experience building health counseling agents [21] in which it is usually not obvious whether more playful, cartoony agents would be preferred, because they may increase engagement, or more realistic agents are better, because of the seriousness of the health topics being discussed (e.g., chemotherapy protocols for cancer patients). We have made many design decisions based on small sample user studies or anecdotal feedback, and wanted

T. Bickmore et al. (Eds.): IVA 2014, LNAI 8637, pp. 374–384, 2014.

a more systematic answer to the question of which character design is the most appropriate in any given situation.

Given our application domains of interest, we have limited our exploration to humanoid characters (no monkeys or parrots), hold behavioral realism (animation) and character environment constant, and systematically explore rendering style and character proportions in correlation with genre of the character's design across task domains. Based on our experience and previous studies (Section 2) our primary hypotheses relate character realism and the levity/seriousness of a task domain as follows.

H1: Realism will be judged more appropriate for task domains high in seriousness.

H2: Frivolity (non-realism) will be judged more appropriate for domains low in seriousness.

In the remainder of this paper we briefly review related studies on character design and describe our experimental methodology, before presenting two design studies and conclusions.

2 Related Work

Several researchers have investigated the effects of visual design choices on user perceptions of a virtual agent. In this section we review the concept of the how realism, rendering style and character proportion have been shown to change people's attitudes towards virtual agents, and why these may be influenced by the task domain.

2.1 Effects of Rendering Styles

Using the concept of the Uncanny Valley [18], McDonnell et al. investigated how different rendering styles affect how users perceive a 3D character [17]. Using ten points along the realism spectrum, ten shaders were created and applied to a 3D model of a human. Using these variants, two studies were conducted to investigate how users evaluated the different rendered models on social aspects such as friendliness, trustworthiness and appeal of the character. The results of this study showed that toon shaded and highly realistic models were best received by participants across the various social aspects, with the toon shaded version slightly outperforming the high quality version in the majority of comparisons.

2.2 Effects of Character Proportions

The proportions of animated characters have also been explored as ways to understand and work around the uncanny valley. Kenn McDonald, a Sony Pictures Imageworks animator said that "A good way to avoid the uncanny valley is to move a character's proportions and structure outside the range of human.'" and attributed the success of Gollum from the Lord of The Rings and Grendel in Beowulf to their disproportion. His reasoning is that when viewers see the characters, they will think that they are not human and will not judge them by the same rule as if they were [11].

2.3   Effects of Realism

Several researchers have studied the effects of realism on user perceptions. There are two kinds of realism studied: appearance realism and behavior realism. For appearance realism, Kang et al. [15] found that social co-presence is higher when dynamic high iconic avatars are used in mobile video telephones. For behavioral realism, Garau et al. [10] and Bailenson et al. [3] found that a large mismatch between behavioral realism and appearance realism of avatars lowered social realism. Bailenson and Yee [4] also found that the more realistic the behavior of the agent, the more persuasive the agent is. Finally, Guadagno et al. [12] and Bailenson [2] found that social influence within immersive virtual environments is higher with virtual humans with high behavioral realism. Furthermore, in their study, the researchers found that this effect was moderated by the gender similarity between human and the avatar. In 2007, Yee et al. conducted a meta-analysis of 25 experimental studies of anthropomorphism, embodied agents, or agent realism and found that human-like representations with higher realism generated more positive subjective user ratings than representations with lower realism [24].

Researchers have also compared the effects of watching cartoons vs. videos of humans. Han et al. [14] showed using fMRI studies that different parts of the human brain are used when presented with cartoons compared to videos of real people. Chen, et al. demonstrated that exposure to cartoon video clip shifts preferences of human faces towards larger eyes [9].

2.4   Effects of Agent Appearance on Tasks

Many studies have also investigated task-specific effects of different character designs. Several researchers have shown that the gender [5,6,12,16] and race [5,13,19] of pedagogical agents have significant effects on a student's self efficacy and motivation. However these generalizations have been shown to be context dependent. For example, female agents are more effective in trying to convince students of the merits of engineering as a career regardless of user gender [1].

An agent's attractiveness, coolness and age have also been shown to be influential in pedagogical agents. While undergraduate female students are more likely to identify themselves with young, attractive, and cool female agents, they tend to choose to learn more about engineering from male agents that were attractive but uncool [7,20,1].

3   The Renderlab System

In order to conduct systematic investigations into the effects of agent appearance on user perceptions, we developed an online system integrated into Amazon's Mechanical Turk with real-time support to dynamically alter a 3D agent's graphical appearance. The platform uses a Unity-based 3D environment to render animated virtual agents over the web. The agents interact with users in brief dialogue sessions using a hierarchical state-machine-based dialogue engine, template-based text generation, conversational nonverbal behavior generation using BEAT [8], and synthesized speech. User contributions to the dialogue are made via a multiple-choice menu. Since task domain is a focus of our studies, we felt it was important that users engage in interactive dialogue rather than just passively listen to the agents. The Unity-based animation engine run in users' web browsers included support for the dynamic loading of Cg/HLSL shaders for the agent (3D rigged models) at runtime. A single set of animation files were also incorporated into the agent via Unity's Mecanim system to ensure that there were no variations between the animations the agents performed between study conditions. All virtual agents used the same range of nonverbal behavior including: visemes and eyebrow raises synchronized to speech, head nods, facial displays of emotion, posture shifts, gazing at and away from the user, and idle behavior (blinking, etc.).

In each of the following studies, we created and used dialogue scripts for social interaction and medical counseling. Each dialogue was 6 to 10 turns long. The social interaction scripts discussed the user's favorite books and movies, while the medical scripts discussed two about cancer related topics (Table 1).

Table 1. Sample Dialogue Excerpts

Medical Dialogue
Agent: Hi, today I would like to talk to you about the importance of having regular colorectal screening for cancer.
User: Go on.
Agent: Screening is the process of looking for cancer in people who have no symptoms of the disease.
User: Sure.
Agent: Colorectal cancer is the third most common cancer diagnosed and is the third leading cause of cancer-related deaths in the United States... It also allows more colorectal cancers to be found earlier, when the disease is easier to cure.
Social Dialogue
Agent: Hi, do you like watching movies?
User: Yes.
Agent: Great! Me too!
User: Sure.
Agent: So, what kind of movie do you like?

Common Measures: In both of the following studies, we assessed user attitudes towards the agent using ten 7-point Likert-scale self-report questions following each interaction with an agent. The items assessed were: *realism, appeal, familiarity, eeriness, friendliness, trustworthiness, easiness to interact with, desire to continue working with, likability, caring, appropriateness, and the quality of motion.* Two open-ended questions were also given, one asking the user how they would describe the character appearance and one for general comments about the agent.

4 Experiment 1: Shading Styles

In our first experiment, we sought to replicate part of McDonnell's Render Me Real? study by investigating the impact of rendering style on user perceptions, but in two different task domains.

4.1 Methods

We selected commercial shaders to match two of the conditions used in the Render Me Real? study (Human High Quality 1 we refer to as Realistic, and (Toon Shaded) as closely as possible for a human-proportioned character (Figure 1). To create the Toon Shaded version of the model, the MatCaps shader library from the Unity assest store was integrated into the client for real time render support.

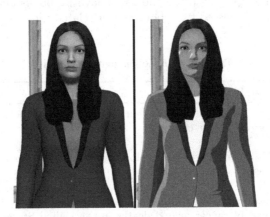

Fig. 1. Screenshot of Realistic (left) and Toon Shaded (right) agent

4.2 Participants

Participants were recruited on Amazon's Mechanical Turk for a counterbalanced, within-subjects experiment in which they interacted with four variants of the agent, Shaded-Social, Realistic-Social, Shaded-Medical and Realistic-Medical.

4.3 Results

Sixty-seven participants (36 Males, 31 Females) successfully completed the study, resulting in a total of 268 agent interactions (4 interactions per user). A 2x2 (rendering style vs. task) repeated measures ANOVA was performed using the ex package in R. Table 2 and 3 show the main results and interaction effects of the study.

Table 2. Main Effects in Study 1

| | Medical | | Social | | p-value | |
	Shaded	Realistic	Shaded	Realistic	Rendering	Dialogue
Realistic	4.24(1.59)	4.76(1.44)	4.03(1.68)	4.39(1.47)	<0.01	<0.01
Friendly	4.96(1.34)	4.88(1.31)	5.48(1.19)	5.07(1.48)	0.04	0.02
Familiar	4.6(1.82)	4.99(1.68)	4.2(1.92)	4.31(1.84)	0.18	<0.01
Trustworthy	5(1.4)	4.93(1.51)	4.58(1.35)	4.46(1.47)	0.43	<0.01
Appropriate	5.37(1.48)	5.49(1.39)	4.87(1.57)	5.15(1.53)	0.15	<0.01
Desire to Cont.	4.45(1.73)	4.36(1.77)	4.48(1.8)	4.24(1.87)	0.24	0.76
Likeable	4.42(1.6)	4.49(1.73)	4.72(1.6)	4.25(1.78)	0.19	0.82
Caring	4.13(1.83)	4.25(1.84)	4(1.83)	3.76(1.73)	0.66	0.06

4.4   Manipulation Check

The *realism* question was used as a manipulation check. This test was found to be significant in the expected direction, with users rating the Realistic agent significantly higher on the *realism* question compared to the Shaded version of the agent $F(1,66) = 11.10$, p <.01.

Table 3. Interaction effect beween dialogue condition vs rendering style in Study 1

	Interaction p-value
Friendly	0.16
Familiar	0.44
Appropriate	0.56
Desire to Continue	0.46
Likeable	0.03
Caring	0.08

4.5   Outcome Analysis

We found main effects of task on appropriateness, $F(1,66) = 7.83$, trustworthiness, $F(1,66) = 13.77$, and familiarity, $F(1,66) = 14.97$, p <.01, with these factors being rated higher for medical task compared to the social task. Two main effects were also found on friendliness, with the agent being rated as more friendly in the social task $F(1,66) = 6.97$, p <.05, and the shaded version, $F(1,66) = 4.33$, p <.05.

A significant interaction of task and rendering style was found on likeability, $F(1,66) = 5.22$, p <.05, with the shaded agent being rated as more likeable than the the realistic agent, but only for the social task. The interaction of task and rendering style on caring was found to be trending towards significance, $F(1,66)$ = 3.18, p = 0.08, with the realistic agent being rated as more caring for the medical task, and the shaded agent being rated as more caring for the social task.

4.6 Discussion

This experiment demonstrated that there are significant effects of agent rendering on a user's impressions of it, particularly in social tasks. We found that for social dialogue the Toon Shaded agent was rated as being more likeable and caring. This finding replicates the results of McDonnell's study, in which the more cartoon like character was rated higher than the realistic ones on these measures. However, in the medical task we only found this result for friendliness. One possible explanation for this is that the medical scripts were more task oriented than the social dialogue, in which there was a clear primary purpose to the dialogue (education in this case).

5 Experiment 2: Character Proportions

In our second study we explored the effects of character proportions (cartoony vs. realistic, Figure 2) on user attitudes across tasks.

5.1 Methods

We used a modified version of the Toon-Shaded agent from Experiment 1, and compared it to a cartoon-proportioned character that was otherwise equivalent in dress, hairstyle and skin tone (Figure 2).

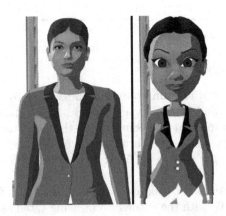

Fig. 2. Screenshot of Human (left) and Cartoon (right) proportioned agents

5.2 Results

Forty-seven participants (31 Males, 16 Females) participated in this study, resulting in a total of 188 agent interactions. A 2x2 (rendering style vs. task) repeated measures ANOVA was performed using the ex package in R. Table 4 shows the main results of the study.

Table 4. Main Effects for Study 2

	Medical		Social		p-value	
	Shaded	Realistic	Shaded	Realistic	Rendering	Dialogue
Realistic	4.82(1.48)	4.23(1.73)	4.71(1.69)	4.15(1.98)	<0.01	0.49
Friendly	4.58(1.23)	5.06(1.2)	4.86(1.77)	5.36(1.31)	0.02	0.06
Familiar	4.71(1.56)	4.85(1.62)	4.54(1.73)	4.4(1.73)	0.91	0.05
Trustworthy	5.04(1.28)	5.21(1.17)	4.67(1.53)	4.91(1.27)	0.22	0.02
Appropriate	5.36(1.37)	5.08(1.57)	4.67(1.64)	5.21(1.57)	0.59	0.08
Desire to Cont.	4.42(1.73)	4.96(1.65)	4.54(1.75)	4.70(1.59)	0.29	0.55
Likeable	4.47(1.63)	4.77(1.61)	4.54(1.75)	4.70(1.59)	0.40	0.94
Caring	4.40(1.71)	4.67(1.74)	4.06(1.74)	4.23(1.80)	0.31	<0.01

5.3 Manipulation Check

Significance was found for how realistic the agent was in the predicted direction, with the human proportioned character being rated as more realistic than the cartoon proportion character $F(1,47) = 7.23$, p <.01.

5.4 Outcome Analysis

Similar main effect results were found for familiarity, trustworthiness, appropriateness and caring for the social and medical tasks as compared to Experiment 1. The minor discrepancy in significance between the two experiments may be due to having fewer subjects in Experiment 2 compared to Experiment 1. For friendliness however, an additional main effects of cartoon proportioned was found, $F(1,46) = 6.94$, p <.05, in which the cartoon proportioned character were rated as being significantly friendlier than the human proportioned character.

A significant interaction of task and character proportion was also found on approriateness $F(1,46) = 7.12$, p <.05, with participants rating the realistic agent as being significantly more appropriate for the medical task, while rating the cartoon proportioned character as being significantly more appropriate for the social task (Figure 3).

5.5 Discussion

This experiment suggests that the design rules for the visual appearance of an agent may not be universal, but depend on the application domain. Although

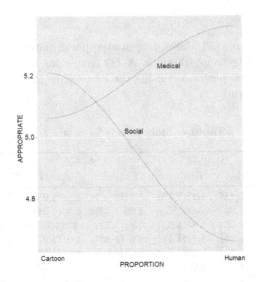

Fig. 3. Interaction effect of agent proportion and appropriateness

participants found the cartoon-proportioned character to be friendlier regardless of dialogue content, they found it more appropriate for the human proportioned character to talk to them about medical content. The effect of character proportions on friendliness is supported by character design heuristics that specify that larger-eyed characters can more easily express emotion [22]. The interaction of proportion and task on appropriateness, however, may be caused by participants' mental model of what they think of as a medical professional, which is most likely not a cartoon character.

6   Conclusion

In this paper we explored the effects of an agent's appearance and application domain on user perceptions of the agent. We found partial support for our hypotheses relating agent realism and task seriousness on user perceptions of the agent. Specifically, we found that changes in an agent's appearance effected how users rated its friendliness, likability, caring, and appeal depending on the content of its dialogue.

For our first experiment we investigated the effects of manipulating an agent's rendering styles, comparing toon shaded and realistic looking agents. This experiment found that toon shaded characters were rated as being more likable, and caring when compared to realistic characters in social task contexts.

In our second experiment we looked at changing an agent's proportions, comparing a human and cartoon proportioned character. Through this investigation we found that cartoon proportioned characters were rated as being more friendly regardless of task domain, but found that more realistic characters were rated as being more appropriate for medical tasks.

The findings from these studies suggest designing an agent may not be as simple as make the most realistic or cartoony agent possible. Our results suggest that a purely medical system a highly realistic agent may be a better design, whereas for a social system a cartoon like agent may work better.

Our studies have many limitations, including the relatively small convenience samples recruited on Mechanical Turk that may not generalize to any particular user demographic for a target application. We have also only explored a tiny corner of the very large space of design parameters for virtual agents. In future studies we aim to further explore this space by looking at various other graphic manipulations such as lightning and color, and also investigate how these effects change over time in longitudinal tasks.

References

1. Ashby Plant, E., Baylor, A.L., Doerr, C.E., Rosenberg-Kima, R.B.: Changing middle-school students' attitudes and performance regarding engineering with computer-based social models. Computers & Education 53(2), 209–215 (2009)
2. Bailenson, J.N., Blascovich, J., Beall, A.C., Loomis, J.M.: Interpersonal distance in immersive virtual environments. Personality and Social Psychology Bulletin 29(7), 819–833 (2003)
3. Bailenson, J.N., Swinth, K., Hoyt, C., Persky, S., Dimov, A., Blascovich, J.: The independent and interactive effects of embodied-agent appearance and behavior on self-report, cognitive, and behavioral markers of copresence in immersive virtual environments. Presence: Teleoperators and Virtual Environments 14(4), 379–393 (2005)
4. Bailenson, J.N., Yee, N.: Digital chameleons automatic assimilation of nonverbal gestures in immersive virtual environments. Psychological Science 16(10), 814–819 (2005)
5. Baylor, A.L., Kim, Y.: Pedagogical agent design: The impact of agent realism, gender, ethnicity, and instructional role. In: Lester, J.C., Vicari, R.M., Paraguaçu, F. (eds.) ITS 2004. LNCS, vol. 3220, pp. 592–603. Springer, Heidelberg (2004)
6. Baylor, A.L., Kim, Y.: Simulating instructional roles through pedagogical agents. International Journal of Artificial Intelligence in Education 15(2), 95–115 (2005)
7. Baylor, A.L., Rosenberg-Kima, R.B., Plant, E.A.: Interface agents as social models: the impact of appearance on females' attitude toward engineering. In: CHI 2006 Extended Abstracts on Human Factors in Computing Systems, pp. 526–531. ACM (2006)
8. Cassell, J., Vilhjálmsson, H.H., Bickmore, T.: Beat: the behavior expression animation toolkit. In: Life-Like Characters, pp. 163–185. Springer (2004)
9. Chen, H., Russell, R., Nakayama, K., Livingstone, M.: Crossing the "uncanny valley": adaptation to cartoon faces can influence perception of human faces. Perception 39(3), 378 (2010)
10. Garau, M., Slater, M., Vinayagamoorthy, V., Brogni, A., Steed, A., Sasse, M.A.: The impact of avatar realism and eye gaze control on perceived quality of communication in a shared immersive virtual environment. In: Proceedings of the SIGCHI Conference on Human Factors in Computing Systems, pp. 529–536. ACM (2003)
11. Geller, T.: Overcoming the uncanny valley. IEEE Computer Graphics and Applications 28(4), 11–17 (2008)

12. Guadagno, R.E., Blascovich, J., Bailenson, J.N., Mccall, C.: Virtual humans and persuasion: The effects of agency and behavioral realism. Media Psychology 10(1), 1–22 (2007)

13. Gulz, A., Haake, M., Tärning, B.: Visual gender and its motivational and cognitive effects–a user study. Lund University Cognitive Studies 137 (2007)

14. Han, S., Jiang, Y., Humphreys, G.W., Zhou, T., Cai, P.: Distinct neural substrates for the perception of real and virtual visual worlds. NeuroImage 24(3), 928–935 (2005)

15. Kang, S.H., Watt, J.H., Ala, S.K.: Social copresence in anonymous social interactions using a mobile video telephone. In: Proceedings of the SIGCHI Conference on Human Factors in Computing Systems, CHI 2008, pp. 1535–1544. ACM, New York (2008), http://doi.acm.org/10.1145/1357054.1357295

16. Kim, Y., Baylor, A.L., Shen, E.: Pedagogical agents as learning companions: The impact of agent emotion and gender. Journal of Computer Assisted Learning 23(3), 220–234 (2007)

17. McDonnell, R., Breidt, M., Bülthoff, H.H.: Render me real?: investigating the effect of render style on the perception of animated virtual humans. ACM Transactions on Graphics (TOG) 31(4), 91 (2012)

18. Mori, M.: The uncanny valley. Energy 7(4), 33–35 (1970)

19. Pratt, J.A., Hauser, K., Ugray, Z., Patterson, O.: Looking at human–computer interface design: Effects of ethnicity in computer agents. Interacting with Computers 19(4), 512–523 (2007)

20. Rosenberg-Kima, R.B., Baylor, A.L., Plant, E.A., Doerr, C.E.: The importance of interface agent visual presence: Voice alone is less effective in impacting young women's attitudes toward engineering. In: de Kort, Y.A.W., IJsselsteijn, W.A., Midden, C., Eggen, B., Fogg, B.J. (eds.) PERSUASIVE 2007. LNCS, vol. 4744, pp. 214–222. Springer, Heidelberg (2007)

21. Schulman, D., Bickmore, T.W., Sidner, C.L.: An intelligent conversational agent for promoting long-term health behavior change using motivational interviewing. In: AAAI Spring Symposium: AI and Health Communication (2011)

22. Thomas, F., Johnston, O., Thomas, F.: The illusion of life: Disney animation. Hyperion, New York (1995)

23. van Vugt, H.C., Konijn, E.A., Hoorn, J.F., Veldhuis, J.: Why fat interface characters are better e-health advisors. In: Gratch, J., Young, M., Aylett, R.S., Ballin, D., Olivier, P. (eds.) IVA 2006. LNCS (LNAI), vol. 4133, pp. 1–13. Springer, Heidelberg (2006)

24. Yee, N., Bailenson, J.N., Rickertsen, K.: A meta-analysis of the impact of the inclusion and realism of human-like faces on user experiences in interfaces. In: Proceedings of the SIGCHI Conference on Human Factors in Computing Systems, pp. 1–10. ACM (2007)

Exploring Gender Biases with Virtual Patients for High Stakes Interpersonal Skills Training

Diego J. Rivera-Gutierrez[1], Regis Kopper[2], Andrea Kleinsmith[1],
Juan Cendan[3], Glen Finney[1], and Benjamin Lok[1]

[1] University of Florida, Gainesville, FL 32611, USA
[2] Duke University, Durham, NC 27708, USA
[3] University of Central Florida, Orlando, FL 32816, USA
djrg@cise.ufl.edu

Abstract. The use of virtual characters in a variety of research areas
is widespread. One such area is healthcare. The study presented in this
paper leveraged virtual patients to examine whether virtual patients are
more likely to be correctly diagnosed due to gender and skin tone. Medical students at the University of Florida College of Medicine interacted
with six virtual patients across two sessions. The six virtual patients
comprised various combinations of gender and skin tone. Each virtual
patient presented with a different cranial nerve injury. The results indicate a significant difference in correct diagnosis according to patient
gender for one of the cases. In that case, female patients were correctly
diagnosed more frequently than their male counterpart. The description
of that case required that the virtual patient present with a visible bruise
on the forehead. We hypothesize the results obtained could be due to a
transfer of a real world gender bias.

Keywords: virtual patients, healthcare, virtual humans, intelligent
agents, autonomous agents, gender bias, user studies, cranial nerve palsies.

1 Introduction

Virtual characters have been used in a number of different research areas. For
instance, virtual characters have been implemented to examine cultural differences [1], social phobias such as fear of public speaking [2] and social anxiety [3],
emotion expression and perception [4], etc. Virtual characters have also become
widely used in medical situations, such as training medical students' interpersonal and interviewing skills. Because of this widespread use of virtual characters,
it is important to understand how the presentation of the character may affect
decisions made by the humans in the interactions [5]. Indeed, Zanbaka et al [6]
found that a virtual human's ability to persuade users is affected by its gender
and visual realism.

Psychological research suggests that unconscious bias and stereotyping are normal aspects of human cognition [7]. Recent data suggest that provider bias, defined as negative attitudes, beliefs and behaviors towards one group by another,

T. Bickmore et al. (Eds.): IVA 2014, LNAI 8637, pp. 385–396, 2014.
© Springer International Publishing Switzerland 2014

may contribute to healthcare disparities [8]. Implicit bias, or the unintentional use of stereotypes, appears to be more common in interpersonal interactions [9]. Social psychologists have shown that when complex decision making is required, the use of stereotypes is more likely [10]. Medical research suggests that physicians demonstrate implicit biases that affect their beliefs, interpersonal interactions with patients and their clinical decision-making [11]. For instance, it has been shown that some diseases are diagnosed more often in men than in women (e.g., COPD (chronic obstructive pulmonary disease)) partially due to social factors [12].

The study presented in this paper leveraged virtual patients to examine whether virtual patient gender and skin tone has an effect on the primary diagnosis determined by third year medical students. The initial results indicate that there may indeed be a transfer of a real world bias, with the gender of the virtual patient affecting the likelihood that the medical students correctly diagnose the virtual patient. Female virtual patients were correctly diagnosed significantly more often than their male counterpart. Both the male and female virtual patients were modeled with a bruise on the forehead. We hypothesize that the visual representation of a bruise on the female virtual patient's head may have led the medical students to treat her pain as more serious than the male virtual patient's pain. While there is work on realism with virtual characters, the authors are unaware of existing research showing that physical manifestation of an injury on a female virtual patient may lead to higher rates of correct diagnosis.

2   Related Work

The ability of virtual humans to elicit realistic reactions from humans during interpersonal simulation tasks and training is well documented. For instance, several studies have shown that people with a fear of public speaking react with anxiety to an audience of virtual humans (e.g., [2]). Studies also indicate that the same virtual audiences can be used to treat a fear of public speaking; reducing avoidance of public speaking [13] and anxiety levels [2]. Similarly, a study by Pan et al [3] found that stress levels of men with social anxiety in relationships decreased over prolonged interaction with a female virtual human.

Virtual humans have also been used in cultural training to teach social conversational verbal and nonverbal protocols in the setting of south Indian culture [14]. Participants who learned and practiced social behaviors with a virtual human performed significantly better in a testing session than those who learned from an illustrated instructions booklet. Virtual humans and environments have also been employed by the US military to aid personnel in familiarization with cross-cultural interactions using VECTOR (Virtual Environment Cultural Training for Operational Readiness) [1].

In the last 10 to 15 years, there has been a considerable amount of research on the use virtual humans in medical training. For instance, virtual patients have been used to train medical students in interpersonal communication skills [15]. Research by Johnsen et al [16] examined doctors' performance in interview skills of a real person compared to a virtual human. Results indicated that there is a significant correlation between the performance of medical students interviewing a real person (standardized patient actor) and a virtual patient.

Other investigators have successfully used virtual patients to study skin tone bias among healthcare providers and students. Kenny et al [17] employed virtual patients of different ethnicities to demonstrate bias among novice mental health clinicians. Haider and colleagues [18] reported that medical students demonstrated an unconscious preference for white people and those in the upper social class. Results from a study by Rossen et al [19] found that medical students demonstrated racial bias to a level comparable with real world bias when interacting with virtual patients.

Gender bias between patient and provider is another area in which research has been conducted using virtual patients. However, the focus has been on investigating differences in pain assessment and management [20], [21], [22] [23]. In these studies, facial expressions of virtual patients were manipulated to show expressions of pain. In general, overall results demonstrated that healthcare provider participants exhibited biases in pain assessment due to patient gender differences. The participants were more likely to recommend female virtual patients to get medical help more often than male virtual patients, to treat female virtual patients' pain with opioid medications vs. non-opioid medications, and to rate female virtual patients as having higher pain intensity and pain unpleasantness.

3 System Description

The Neurological Examination Rehearsal Virtual Environment (NERVE) is a virtual human simulation environment in which medical students can interview virtual patients presenting cranial nerve palsies (see Figure 1). Cranial nerve palsies present asymmetric eye movement or facial responses and often are an indication of underlying potentially life threatening conditions.

NERVE allows medical students to perform an interview and physical examination of the virtual patient.

The interview is performed using text input. The text input is matched to a database of possible questions and the virtual patient responds with an appropriate response. The virtual human responds using pre-recorded speeches and animations.

The physical examination is performed using a set of virtual tools available to the student. These virtual tools allow students to perform simplified versions of the physical examinations performed on real patients suffering from cranial nerve palsies. Three virtual tools are available: a virtual hand, a virtual ophthalmoscope, and a virtual eye chart.

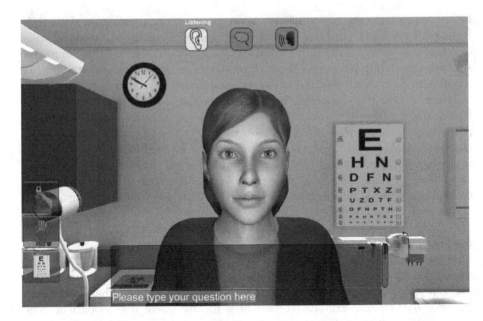

Fig. 1. Sample interaction with a virtual patient in NERVE

- Using the virtual hand tool, students can ask the virtual patients to: a) follow a finger with their eyes to check extraocular movements, b) count the number of fingers the patient saw to test for diplopia, and c) ask if they could see the finger shaking to perform a visual field examination.
- Using the virtual ophthalmoscope, students can: a) check the patients' pupillary response to light, and b) perform a funduscopic exam.
- Using the virtual eye chart students can ask the virtual patient to read different lines to check for visual acuity.

For the complete study, six different cases were used, as summarized in Table 1. Although the CN3 cases are mentioned for completeness of the study, they are not included in the analysis as they were included to investigate another research question which is outside the scope of this paper. For cases CN4, MG, CN6 and CN7 four versions were created. The differences between these four versions were only skin-tone and gender of the virtual patient and correspond to: 1) African-American female, 2) Caucasian female, 3) African-American male and 4) Caucasian male. Figure 2 displays all four visual appearances. Notice that for the CN4 case it was necessary to add a bruise on the forehead of the patient. This bruise is relevant only to the CN4 case and was caused by the patient falling from a bicycle. For CN7, which commonly presents with facial paralysis, the right side of the patient's face did not move when the virtual human was speaking or being examined. Finally, for CN6 the patient was overweight as weight is a significant factor to the patient's condition.

Table 1. Case details and descriptions. "Questions" refers to the number of questions that the particular virtual human is able to answer. "Responses" refers to the number of answers the particular virtual human is able to give.

Case	Questions & Responses	Description
Cranial nerve 4 (CN4)	1290 & 224	The patient presents with a lesion of the left cranial nerve 4. The patient suffered a bicycle accident 3 days previous to the encounter and lost consciousness after the accident. The accident produced a bruise on the head, headaches and double vision.
Myasthenia gravis (MG)	1253 & 223	The patient presents with blurry vision during the evening and when tired. The blurry vision worsens when trying to focus in activities like reading and watching TV. The patient does not present with headaches or head trauma.
Cranial nerve 6 (CN6)	1077 & 215	The patient presents with a lesion of the left cranial nerve 6. The patient has been suffering from double vision for 2 weeks. The patient suffers from diabetes and is overweight by 80lbs.
Cranial nerve 7 (CN7)	1081 & 215	The patient presents with a lesion of the right cranial nerve 7. The patient has lost movement on the right side of the face and reports the right eye feels dry. The problem started the morning of the patient encounter.
Cranial nerve 3 - Reassuring (CN3R)	1242 & 224	The patient presents with a left ischemic cranial nerve 3 palsy. The patient has double vision and pupils are reactive. The patient is a 55 year old diabetic and should make a full recovery with rest.
Cranial nerve 3 - Worrisome (CN3W)	1142 & 222	The patient presents with a left compressive cranial nerve 3 palsy. The patient has double vision starting with a bad headache and the left pupil is not reactive. The patient is not a diabetic and likely requires surgery.

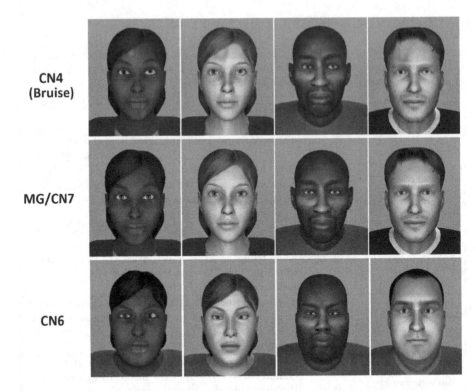

Fig. 2. Comparison between the virtual humans for all four cases considered. For CN4, the virtual humans display both a bump on the head and a deviation of the left eye inward and upward. For MG and CN7, the same visual appearance was used with the difference that the CN7 characters showed facial paralysis on the right side of their face. For CN6, the virtual humans are overweight and display a deviation of the left eye inward.

4   User Study

The primary goal of the user study was to evaluate the effects of gender and skin-tone in correct diagnosis of cranial nerve related illnesses.

Figure 3 summarizes the study procedure. The procedure consisted of two sessions. Each session lasted approximately one hour. During the first session, students 1) completed a demographics survey, 2) went through a tutorial of the system and 2) interviewed three virtual patients. The cases for the virtual patients in the first week were CN4, either CN3R or CN3W, and finally MG. During the second session, students interviewed another three virtual patients. The cases for the virtual patients in the second week were CN6, the other CN3 case(e.g., if the student interacted with CN3W on the first week, they would interact with CN3R), and finally CN7. Cases CN4, MG, CN6 and CN7 (highlighted in green in Figure 3) were randomized so that each participant saw all four combinations of skin-tone (Caucasian or African-American) and gender (male or female).

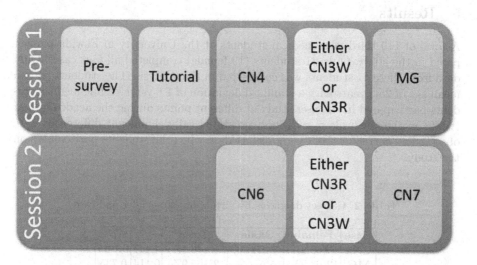

Fig. 3. Procedure of the user study. Yellow squares correspond to introductory steps, green squares correspond to the cases used for the presented study, light blue squares correspond to unrelated study.

The order of the cases was not randomized because the focus of the user study was on gender and skin-tone.

For each virtual patient, the students filled out a Clinical Skills Evaluation Patient Note that included their findings and their diagnosis of the patient. In this patient note, students gave up to 3 possible diagnoses for each patient. Students were asked to list the diagnoses in order of likelihood. The diagnoses given were coded by the authors as either correct or incorrect based on expert knowledge. A student was considered to have reached a correct diagnosis of a patient if they listed the right cranial nerve palsy or related disease as any of the three possible diagnoses for the patient.

The user study took place over a full academic year. The population for the study consisted of third-year medical students from the University of Florida during their neurology rotation. Each rotation had between 5 and 10 students and lasted three weeks. The first session of the user study took place during the first week of the rotation and the second session during the second week. Each session was held in a conference room and supervised by one of the researchers. Students worked individually in all sessions and used headphones to avoid interfering with each other. In some cases, students were not able to make the sessions due to scheduling problems. In those cases, the students were encouraged to finish the exercise at home on their own computers.

Hypothesis 1: Gender of the virtual patient will affect correctness of diagnosis of the virtual patient's condition.

Hypothesis 2: Skin-tone of the virtual patient will affect correctness of diagnosis of the virtual patient's condition.

5 Results

A total of 119 third-year medical students at the University of Florida participated in the study. Only 41 students (19 female) completed all four cases. Only
data from these 41 students was considered in the analysis. The students had an
mean age of 25.2 years with a standard deviation of 1.6 years. While medical students participated in the user study at different points during the academic year
(while on their neurology rotation), no statistically significant differences were
observed on correctness of diagnosis based on when the students participated on
the study.

Table 2. Correct diagnosis by virtual human gender and case

Case	Female	Male	Total	χ^2	p
CN4	14(60.9%)	5(27.8%)	19(46.3%)	4.447	**0.035**
MG	12(63.2%)	15(68.2%)	27(65.9%)	0.114	0.735
CN6	16(72.7%)	15(78.9%)	31(75.6%)	0.214	0.644
CN7	18(85.7%)	19(95.0%)	37(90.2%)	1.003	0.317
Total	60(73.2%)	54(65.9%)	114(69.5%)	1.03	0.308

Table 2 contains the breakdown of correct diagnosis by virtual patient gender
for each of the four cases analyzed in this study. Chi-square tests of independence were conducted to examine the relation between correctness of the diagnosis reported by the students and the gender of the virtual patient. As shown
in Table 2, the relationship was statistically significant for the CN4 case only,
$\chi^2(1, N = 41) = 4.447, p = 0.035$. Male virtual patients suffering from a CN4
lesion were less likely to be diagnosed correctly than female virtual patients with
the same condition. This result was only observed for this particular case. We
used log-linear analysis to test that this difference in correctness of diagnosis
was not correlated to the virtual human's skin tone, the participant's ethnicity
or the participant's gender.

Analysis also showed that 1) the participant's ethnicity, 2) participant's gender, and 3) virtual human skin-tone did not significantly correlate with correctness of diagnosis for any of the cases ($p > 0.05$).

The average interaction with the virtual humans lasted 7 minutes 34 seconds
with a standard deviation of 57 seconds. On average students asked 26.17 questions to each virtual human with a standard deviation of 10.34 questions. Table 3
includes the average number of questions asked by case. Paired samples t-tests
were conducted between all case combinations and no significant differences in
terms of amount of questions asked were found.

Table 3. Number of questions asked per case

Case	Mean	Standard Deviation
CN4	24.48	8.37
MG	27.71	13.17
CN6	26.17	9.29
CN7	26.34	10.13
Total	26.17	10.34

6 Discussion

The fact that gender was a significant factor for the students correctly diagnosing only the virtual patient with the CN4 was an unexpected finding. When comparing the CN4 case to the other three cases considered (MG,CN6, and CN7), the main difference between them is the visual representation of the bruise on the patient's forehead. Based on an assessment by the students' instructor, all four cases are similar in difficulty. MG is considered to be the easier case and CN6 the hardest case to diagnose. Moreover, the instructor also confirmed that gender does not play a role in a CN4 injury. We postulate that possible gender biases due to prosocial factors may have contributed to the students' ability to correctly diagnose the female virtual patient. Because of the visible bruise, the female virtual patient may have been perceived as being in more pain than the male counterpart, thus students may have unconsciously made a stronger effort to diagnose the female. As discussed in Section 2, results from Hirsh et al [21] found that participants recommended female virtual patients to get medical help more often than male virtual patients. They also found that participants rated female virtual patients as having higher pain intensity and pain unpleasantness than male virtual patients.

There is a considerable amount of research regarding gender biases in patient diagnosis and treatment as reported in [24] [20]. Research has shown that female patients have longer doctor visits than male patients, and that more explanations are provided for female patients than for male patients [25]. We examined this possibility in the CN4 case by analyzing possible differences due to gender according to length of interaction and number of questions asked. Our thought was perhaps the participants were able to accurately diagnose the female virtual patient due to significantly longer interaction duration and therefore significantly more questions asked of the female virtual patient. However, an independent samples t-test revealed no significant differences in number of questions participants asked female virtual patients (M=22.54, SD=7.99) and male virtual patients (M=19.07, SD=6.91), $t(39) = 1.4$, $p = .085$. This finding is in line with the lack of significant differences in overall length of interaction as described in Section 5.

7   Limitations

The primary limitation of the study is that the order of cases according to cranial nerve injury was not randomized; CN4 was always the first case to be examined by the students. This could confound the results based on lack of familiarity with the system. However, it is important to notice that students completed an interactive tutorial of the system before interacting with the first patient. The tutorial included a short test interaction with the tutorial character and all the relevant information on how to interact with the virtual patient and how to perform a cranial nerve examination using the NERVE system.

8   Conclusions

In the presented user study, a group of third-year medical students at the University of Florida College of Medicine interviewed six virtual patients that included various combinations of gender and skin-tone. The results of the user study show that the students were more likely to reach a correct diagnosis of one of the cases with a female virtual patient than with a male virtual patient. The particular case included a visual representation of a bruise on the forehead of the virtual patient resulting from a bicycle accident that produced the condition. This bruise is the main difference between the case with statistically significant differences for gender and the other cases that did not show such differences. We have postulated that the observed differences might be related to possible gender biases due to prosocial factors may have contributed to the students ability to correctly diagnose the female virtual patient. Such biases could have produced the students to perceive of the female virtual human to be in more pain than the male virtual human. While we speculate that the findings may be due to the transfer of real world biases onto virtual patients, additional studies are needed to support this claim more definitively.

Acknowledgments. Research reported in this paper was supported by the National Institutes of Health (NIH) under award number 1R01LM010813-01. The content is solely the responsibility of the authors and does not necessarily represent the official views of the National Institutes of Health.

References

1. Deaton, J.E., Barba, C., Santarelli, T., Rosenzweig, L., Souders, V., McCollum, C., Seip, J., Knerr, B.W., Singer, M.J.: Virtual environment cultural training for operational readiness (vector). Virtual Reality 8(3), 156–167 (2005)
2. Slater, M., Pertaub, D.P., Barker, C., Clark, D.M.: An experimental study on fear of public speaking using a virtual environment. CyberPsychology & Behavior 9(5), 627–633 (2006)
3. Pan, X., Gillies, M., Barker, C., Clark, D.M., Slater, M.: Socially anxious and confident men interact with a forward virtual woman: an experimental study. PloS One 7(4), e32931 (2012)

4. McRorie, M., Sneddon, I., de Sevin, E., Bevacqua, E., Pelachaud, C.: A model of personality and emotional traits. In: Ruttkay, Z., Kipp, M., Nijholt, A., Vilhjálmsson, H.H. (eds.) IVA 2009. LNCS, vol. 5773, pp. 27–33. Springer, Heidelberg (2009)
5. MacDorman, K.F., Coram, J.A., Ho, C.C., Patel, H.: Gender Differences in the Impact of Presentational Factors in Human Character Animation on Decisions in Ethical Dilemmas. Presence 19(3), 213–229 (2010)
6. Zanbaka, C., Goolkasian, P., Hodges, L.: Can a virtual cat persuade you?: the role of gender and realism in speaker persuasiveness. In: Proceedings of the SIGCHI Conference on Human Factors in Computing Systems (2006)
7. Fiske, S.T.: Stereotyping, prejudice, and discrimination at the seam between the centuries: Evolution, culture, mind, and brain. European Journal of Social Psychology 30(3), 299–322 (2000)
8. Van Ryn, M.: Research on the provider contribution to race/ethnicity disparities in medical care. Medical Care 40(1), I-140 (2002)
9. Cooper, L.A., Roter, D.L., Carson, K.A., Beach, M.C., Sabin, J.A., Greenwald, A.G., Inui, T.S.: The associations of clinicians' implicit attitudes about race with medical visit communication and patient ratings of interpersonal care. American Journal of Public Health 102(5), 979–987 (2012)
10. Bodenhausen, G.V., Lichtenstein, M.: Social stereotypes and information-processing strategies: The impact of task complexity. Journal of Personality and Social Psychology 52(5), 871 (1987)
11. Sabin, J.A., Rivara, F.P., Greenwald, A.G.: Physician implicit attitudes and stereotypes about race and quality of medical care. Medical Care 46(7), 678–685 (2008)
12. Chapman, K.R., Tashkin, D.P., Pye, D.J.: Gender bias in the diagnosis of copd. CHEST Journal 119(6), 1691–1695 (2001)
13. Harris, S.R., Kemmerling, R.L., North, M.M.: Brief virtual reality therapy for public speaking anxiety. Cyberpsychology & Behavior 5(6), 543–550 (2002)
14. Babu, S., Suma, E., Barnes, T., Hodges, L.F.: Can Immersive Virtual Humans Teach Social Conversational Protocols? In: IEEE Virtual Reality Conference, pp. 215–218 (2007)
15. Deladisma, A.M., Gupta, M., Kotranza, A., Bittner IV, J.G., Imam, T., Swinson, D., Gucwa, A., Nesbit, R., Lok, B., Pugh, C., et al.: A pilot study to integrate an immersive virtual patient with a breast complaint and breast examination simulator into a surgery clerkship. The American Journal of Surgery 197(1), 102–106 (2009)
16. Johnsen, K., Raij, A., Stevens, A., Lind, D., Lok, B.: The validity of a virtual human experience for interpersonal skills education. In: Proceedings of the SIGCHI Conference on Human Factors in Computing Systems, pp. 1049–1058. ACM (2007)
17. Kenny, P., Parsons, T.D., Gratch, J., Leuski, A., Rizzo, A.A.: Virtual patients for clinical therapist skills training. In: Pelachaud, C., Martin, J.-C., André, E., Chollet, G., Karpouzis, K., Pelé, D. (eds.) IVA 2007. LNCS (LNAI), vol. 4722, pp. 197–210. Springer, Heidelberg (2007)
18. Haider, A.H., Sexton, J., Sriram, N., Cooper, L.A., Efron, D.T., Swoboda, S., Villegas, C.V., Haut, E.R., Bonds, M., Pronovost, P.J., et al.: Association of unconscious race and social class bias with vignette-based clinical assessments by medical students. JAMA 306(9), 942–951 (2011)
19. Rossen, B., Johnsen, K., Deladisma, A., Lind, S., Lok, B.: Virtual humans elicit skin-tone bias consistent with real-world skin-tone biases. In: Prendinger, H., Lester, J.C., Ishizuka, M. (eds.) IVA 2008. LNCS (LNAI), vol. 5208, pp. 237–244. Springer, Heidelberg (2008)

20. Hirsh, A.T., Hollingshead, N.A., Matthias, M.S., Bair, M.J., Kroenke, K.: The influence of patient sex, provider sex, and sexist attitudes on pain treatment decisions. The Journal of Pain (2014)
21. Hirsh, A.T., Alqudah, A.F., Stutts, L.A., Robinson, M.E.: Virtual human technology: Capturing sex, race, and age influences in individual pain decision policies. Pain 140(1), 231–238 (2008)
22. Wandner, L.D., Stutts, L.A., Alqudah, A.F., Craggs, J.G., Scipio, C.D., Hirsh, A.T., Robinson, M.E.: Virtual human technology: patient demographics and healthcare training factors in pain observation and treatment recommendations. Journal of Pain Research 3, 241–247 (2009)
23. Hirsh, A.T., George, S.Z., Robinson, M.E.: Pain assessment and treatment disparities: a virtual human technology investigation. Pain 143(1), 106–113 (2009)
24. Elderkin-Thompson, V., Waitzkin, H.: Differences in clinical communication by gender. Journal of General Internal Medicine 14(2), 112–121 (1999)
25. Waitzkin, H.: Information giving in medical care. Journal of Health and Social Behavior, 81–101 (1985)

A Qualitative Evaluation of Behavior during Conflict with an Authoritative Virtual Human

Andrew Robb[1], Casey White[2], Andrew Cordar[1], Adam Wendling[1], Samsun Lampotang[1], and Benjamin Lok[1]

[1] University of Florida, Gainesville, FL 32611, USA
[2] University of Virginia, Charlottesville, VA, USA

Abstract. This research explores the extent to which humans behave realistically during conflict with a virtual human occupying a position of authority. To this end, we created a virtual team to train nurses how to manage conflict in the operating room; the team's virtual surgeon engages in reckless behavior that could endanger the safety of the team's patient, requiring nurses to intervene and correct the virtual surgeon's behavior. Results from post-hoc behavioral analysis and semi-structured interviews indicate that participants behaved realistically during conflict, as compared against existing behavioral frameworks. However, some participants reported perceiving their virtual teammates as strangers, which they felt may have caused them to behave differently than they would with their normal teammates.

Keywords: virtual humans, human behavior, user study, medicine, conflict.

1 Introduction

There is a growing interest in using virtual humans for interpersonal skills training. Training systems have been developed that use virtual humans to teach people to conduct medical interviews [11], perform physical exams [16], practice negotiation skills [5], and cope with bullying [9]. Studies using these systems have shown that interacting with virtual humans can help people build important interpersonal skills.

Authority hierarchies often play an important role in interpersonal interactions. Up till now, most virtual human research has focused on scenarios where humans possess more authority than the virtual humans they work with (e.g. medical students interviewing a virtual patient [11]). Other research has explored scenarios where there are no clear authority figures (e.g. an American soldier negotiating with a virtual Afghani physician [5]). Comparatively little research has investigated scenarios where humans are subordinate to a virtual human.

The study described here examines how humans behave while working with a virtual human occupying a position of authority; specifically, we studied how nurses attempted to resolve conflict with a virtual surgeon. Our goals for this research were to explore how nurses behave during conflict with the virtual

T. Bickmore et al. (Eds.): IVA 2014, LNAI 8637, pp. 397–409, 2014.
© Springer International Publishing Switzerland 2014

surgeon and to compare their behavior against existing research describing how conflict is managed among human beings.

While behavior can be examined quantitatively, a deeper understanding of behavior requires exploring people's motivations and thought processes, which are best assessed qualitatively [8]. Qualitative methods can help identify motivational differences that quantitative methods might miss. For instance, if a nurse fails to speak up when a surgeon makes a dangerous decision, it is important to understand whether the nurse agreed with the surgeon's decision or whether she did not agree with it, but was unwilling to confront the surgeon. We employed qualitative methods to explore how participants behaved during conflict with the virtual surgeon, and also to assess what motivated them to use these methods. We describe our qualitative methods further in Section 3.

In this paper, we describe our implementation of a virtual operating room team, led by a virtual surgeon whose behavior clearly disregards official safety protocols and could potentially endanger a patient's safety. We classify participants' behavior according to two existing behavioral frameworks, and report on one factor that participants believed may have influenced their behavior during conflict with the virtual surgeon. Finally, we report on participants' perspectives on the use of virtual humans to prepare people for conflict with authority figures.

2   Related Work

In this section, we review research that explored how people behave with virtual humans, compared to real-world standards. We also review several important qualitative studies exploring interactions with virtual humans, and discuss two theories describing how people behave during conflict, in terms of influence tactics used during conflict and outcomes reached after conflict.

Realistic Behavior with Virtual Humans. Numerous studies have suggested that people's interactions with virtual humans are governed by the same rules that govern interactions among human beings. Bailenson et al. found that participants maintained typical interpersonal distances when interacting with a virtual human, and that participants disliked virtual humans who violated their personal space [1]. Rossen et al. found that users with real-world racial biases exhibited these biases during interactions with a dark-skinned virtual patient [17]. Pertaub et al. observed that negative virtual audiences evoked anxiety in participants practicing public speaking [15]. Kotranza et al. found that students expressed empathy towards a mixed-reality human (MRH) when practicing breast exams [13]. Kotranza also compared students' interactions with the MRH to their interactions with a human standardized patient (an actor who trains medical students), and found that students used comforting and reassuring touches with similar frequencies for both the MRH and the standardized patient.

Qualitative Research and Virtual Humans. While qualitative methods are not frequently used in virtual human research, there have been several studies that used them to explore how users behaved with virtual humans. Bickmore conducted a qualitative evaluation of two agents: REA (a real estate agent) and Laura (an exercise coach) [2]. His qualitative evaluations helped develop a nuanced understanding of how users perceived REA's small talk capabilities and the importance of Laura's relational capabilities, as they related to improving exercise performance. Vardoulakis et al. explored how older adults talked with a companion agent over multiple sessions [20]. Their qualitative evaluation helped reveal what topics older adults wanted to talk about with companion agents, including personal storytelling, family, and attitudes toward aging. Hall et al. conducted a qualitative evaluation of the virtual characters in FearNot, a virtual learning environment designed to help children develop coping strategies for bullying [9]. Their qualitative evaluation revealed that while children were accepting of lower quality, cartoonish graphics, they were more critical of lower quality animations and facial gestures. These studies highlight how qualitative methods can improve our understanding of how humans interact with virtual humans.

Behavior During Conflict in the Real World. Kipnis et al. describe eight different influence tactics people employ in the workforce when trying to gain compliance: Rationality, Assertiveness, Upward Appeal, Coalitions, Ingratiation, Sanctions, Blocking, and Exchanges [12]. People use different influence tactics based on the relative status of the person they seek to influence. Rationality is used most frequently when seeking to influence a superior. Ingratiation, exchange, and upward appeal are used most frequently with co-workers and subordinates. Assertiveness and sanctions are used most frequently with subordinates. Blocking is used without regard to status.

Van Dyne et al. proposed a conceptual framework that describes outcomes to conflict in the work place using two factors: behavior (remain silent or speak out) and motive (acquiescence, self-protection, and other-orientation) [6]. Motive modifies behavior – for example, people can engage in either self-protective silence (withholding damaging information) or self-protective voice (speaking out to redirect conflict away from oneself). Acquiescence offers no objection to the conflict, either out of resignation or feelings of low self-efficacy. Self-protection actively seeks to direct the conflict away from oneself, either by actively proposing ideas that shift attention away from oneself or by withholding information to protect oneself. Other-orientation seeks to resolve conflict through proposing solutions or withholding confidential information.

3   Methodological Approach

Participants' behavior during this study was video recorded; these videos were transcribed for use during our qualitative analysis. Borrowing from Gordens Coding Interview Responses [7], two of the authors analyzed each participant's transcript and coded the outcome of his or her conflict with the virtual surgeon. After finishing the initial coding, the two authors discussed their observations and agreed that each participants' behavior could be described using one of the five outcomes shown in Table 1. They then re-coded the transcripts using the five outcomes as a guide. After the second round of coding, the coders were in complete agreement on all but two participants. The differences with these two participants were discussed and quickly reconciled, resulting in 100% agreement and perfect inter-rater reliability.

After finalizing the coding of the conflict outcomes, the same two authors then analyzed and coded the language participants used during conflict, using Kipnis' influence tactics [12] as a guide. After finishing the initial coding, the two authors discussed their observations and more precisely defined how each influence tactic applied to this population, using specific examples they had found in the transcripts. They then analyzed and re-coded the transcripts using these updated definitions. After the second round of coding, the coders were in complete agreement on all but four participants. The differences with these four participants were discussed and quickly reconciled, resulting in 100% agreement and perfect inter-rater reliability.

4   The Speaking Up Exercise

This research was conducted in conjunction with the nursing management team at a major academic medical center. Working with the nursing management team responsible for the hospital's operating rooms, we developed a training exercise that placed nurses in conflict with a virtual surgeon, whose reckless behavior endangered the safety of a simulated patient. During the exercise, the virtual surgeon attempts to start the surgery even though replacement blood is not available – the team forgot to send blood samples to the blood bank while preparing the patient for surgery. Rather than following hospital policy and waiting for results from the blood bank, the virtual surgeon pushes to start the surgery immediately, saying that if they send the samples now, the blood bank will be able to process them before replacement blood will be needed.

The nursing management team believed that all nurses should recognize that this practice could endanger the patient. If this were to occur in real life, the nursing management team would want nurses to speak up about the patient-safety issue and ask the surgeon to wait until the blood results were back. If the surgeon was to ignore the nurse or refuse to stop, the nurse should "stop the line" and call for assistance from a charge nurse or nursing management.

We developed two virtual humans (see Figure 1) for the exercise: a virtual surgeon and a virtual anesthesiologist. To reduce the possibility of gender and racial confounds, both the virtual surgeon and the virtual anesthesiologist were modeled to look like average Caucasian men. This combination of race and gender is representative of the majority of surgeons and anesthesiologists practicing in the U.S [3]. The patient in this exercise was developmentally-delayed and non-verbal, which prevented him from interacting with the team. The patient was in surgery for a scoliosis repair, a high-risk surgery associated with considerable blood loss.

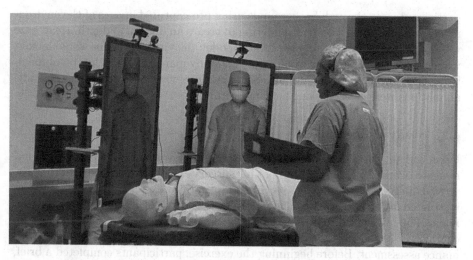

Fig. 1. A participant working with the virtual anesthesiologist and the virtual surgeon, who are standing behind the mannequin patient simulator

4.1 The Virtual Human Technology

The virtual humans used in this exercise were life-size and interacted with participants using speech and gesture. The virtual humans' speeches were prerecorded by voice actors, and gestures were created using motion capture. The virtual humans were controlled by a Wizard-of-Oz; human-factors researchers frequently use Wizard-of-Ozs to reduce confounding effects that can be introduced by speech recognition errors or speech understanding errors [2,4,16,20]. The wizard controlled both the surgeon and the anesthesiologist simultaneously, using an interface which allowed him to trigger the virtual humans' speeches using pre-specified lists. This interface was organized by character and topic, to allow for rapid selection. The interface also intelligently suggested responses based on the last action performed. The wizard followed a specific script for each stage of the interaction, but made adjustments when participants behaved unexpectedly. The virtual humans were capable of making nine generic statements, such as "Yes", "No", "OK", and "I'm not sure", which allowed the wizard to respond to unexpected questions or statements. In order to create a consistent experience for each participant, the same wizard was used during the entire study. To reduce suspicion that the virtual humans were controlled by a human, participants were told that the virtual humans were fully autonomous and were required to complete a speech recognition training session and wear a microphone during the exercise. The exercise took place in a former operating room which had been converted to a simulation lab.

The virtual humans were embedded in the simulation lab using high-physicality ANDI units (shown in Figure 1), as described by Chuah [4], which include the following features: rendered life-size on 42" televisions, head tracking with a Microsoft Kinect, which allows the virtual humans to make eye contact with participants, see-through backgrounds using pre-captured images of the environment, and perspective-correct rendering to create an illusion of depth. Head gaze was controlled through a simple Markov model; the virtual humans would look at whoever was speaking, but would also randomly glance at the other team members. They also blinked and mimicked idle motions when not speaking – these idle animations were created using motion capture.

4.2   Study Procedure

Upon arrival, participants were told they would be working with two virtual humans to prepare a simulated patient for surgery. They were not warned that the virtual surgeon would behave recklessly during the exercise. Participants were instructed to treat the virtual humans exactly like they would treat real humans. They were also told that their behavior during the exercise would remain completely confidential, and that the exercise was not being used as a performance assessment. Before beginning the exercise, participants completed a brief, interactive tutorial involving a virtual nurse, who explained how to interact with virtual humans.

The exercise was split into two stages: the briefing stage and the timeout stage. In *the briefing* stage, participants worked with a virtual surgeon and a virtual anesthesiologist to ensure that the patient was ready for the start of anesthesia. The virtual surgeon guided this stage, working through a checklist used in the hospital operating rooms. The virtual surgeon addressed questions to the participant and the virtual anesthesiologist as needed. The virtual anesthesiologist occasionally interrupted the virtual surgeon to ask a question. Participants could also interrupt with questions or comments. At the end of the briefing, the virtual surgeon learned that blood samples had not been drawn and instructed the virtual anesthesiologist to draw the blood after anesthetizing the patient.

After the virtual surgeon completed the checklist, participants moved on to *the timeout* stage. In this stage, participants worked with the virtual surgeon and the virtual anesthesiologist to confirm that the patient was ready for the incision. The virtual surgeon guided this stage, working through a second, shorter checklist. After asking the participant several basic questions, the virtual surgeon asked the virtual anesthesiologist if the blood was now available. The virtual anesthesiologist reported that he had forgotten to send the blood to the lab. This angered the virtual surgeon, who berated the virtual anesthesiologist and then announced that, because they were running late, the team needed to send the blood samples immediately and start the surgery without waiting for the results. This is a reckless course of action and is against hospital policy, because the patient might need blood sooner than expected, and because the patient's blood could have antibodies, which would slow the blood preparation processes.

If participants spoke up to the virtual surgeon and asked him to wait, he would repeatedly object to their concerns. His objections were: that the patient was unlikely to have antibodies because he had never been transfused before, that there was sufficient time to get blood before it would be needed, and that waiting could harm the patient because of the additional time he would be under anesthesia (these objections were developed in collaboration with nursing management and an anesthesiologist). After a participant spoke up three times, the virtual surgeon announced that he was not going to listen to the participant anymore and that he was going to begin the surgery. At this point participants were forced to either back down or "stop the line" and call a supervisor.

A semi-structured interview was conducted with each participant after they had completed the timeout. This semi-structured interview focused on exploring what motivated participants' behavior. Participants were specifically asked to explain why they had handled the incident with the missing blood the way they did, and to compare the experience to how they might behave in the real world, with real teams.

4.3   Participants

A total of 26 participants (20 female) took part in the exercise. All participants were nurses who were currently working in the hospital operating rooms. The average participant age was 43 years old; ages ranged from 25 to 67. Participants had been working as a nurse for an average of 24.5 years, and as a nurse in the OR for an average of 19 years. Of the 26 participants, 16 reported their race as White, 5 as Asian, and 4 as Black. One participant did not report her race.

5   Results and Discussion

In this section, we compare participants' behavior to existing conflict-management research, look at what motivated participants' actions, and discuss one factor which participants felt may have caused them to behave differently with a virtual team, compared to the teams they usually work with. Participants' behavior, on the whole, was consistent with existing research about how people behave during conflict. When discussing what motivated their behavior, participants generally spoke in terms of their real-world experience. Participants mentioned one factor that may have caused them to behave differently than they would with real teams: their unfamiliarity with the virtual humans; in the real world, our participants are almost always familiar with their teammates. They felt that being unfamiliar with the specific virtual humans may have caused them to behave differently. We discuss these results in more detail below.

5.1   Participant Behavior during the Speaking Up Moment

Outcomes Reached by Participants. Post-hoc analysis of the exercise revealed that participants reached five different outcomes (Table 1), which are consistent with Van Dyne's framework that describes outcomes to conflict [6].

Stopping the line is *other-oriented voice*, where the participant voiced concern for the patient's safety. Filing an incident report and shifting responsibility are *self-protective voice*. These participants attempted to protect themselves from patient-safety repercussions by establishing that he or she had objected to the

Table 1. The resolution methods are ordered based on the degree of resistance participants offered to the surgeon, in descending order. The number of people who exhibited each behavior is shown in the # column.

Outcome	#	Description
Stopped the line	5	Refused to let the surgeon begin the operation
Incident report	2	Agreed to proceed, but filed a report on the incident
Shifted responsibility	5	Voiced concern, but left the decision up to the surgeon
Gave in	3	Voiced concern, but backed down to the surgeon
No Objections	11	Raised no objections to the surgeon's decision

surgeon's proposed course of action, but had been unable to stop him from proceeding. Giving in and offering no objections are either *acquiescent voice*, *acquiescent silence*, or *self-protective silence*; the specific categorization depends on why participants offered no objection. *Other-oriented silence*, which was not observed, was not applicable to this exercise. Observing each of the relevant conflict-management outcomes described by Van Dyne suggests that humans view conflict with virtual humans in the same terms as conflict with real humans. Observing self-protective behavior is particularly interesting, given that participants knew that failure to protect the simulated patient would not result in any real-world consequences. Participants' experience with conflict in the real world may have led them to resort to self-protective behavior once they were unable to convince the virtual surgeon to delay the surgery, in spite of the simulated nature of the exercise.

That only five participants stopped the line was not surprising, given that the traditional hierarchy between surgeons and nurses often makes speaking up difficult [18]. Nurses sometimes also feel that a surgeon's extensive medical training makes him or her more qualified to make decisions about patient care [14]. Participants mentioned both of these difficulties during the exercise. Six participants deferred to the virtual surgeon for hierarchical reasons, using phrases like "You're the surgeon, it's up to you". Three participants stated that the virtual surgeon's experience and position made him more qualified to make the decision. From a training perspective, participants' difficulty speaking up to the virtual surgeon is encouraging, as it suggests that virtual humans can be used to help people overcome reluctance about speaking up during conflict.

Persuasion Strategies Employed By Participants. We used Kipnis' eight influence tactics [12] to classify participants' behavior during the conflict with the virtual surgeon (Table 2). Fifteen participants used one or more influence tactics; the remaining 11 participants offered no objections to the surgeon's behavior.

Rationality was the most frequently used influence tactic. All but one participant who engaged in conflict with the surgeon employed rationality when seeking to convince the surgeon to wait. The one participant who did not employ rationality attempted to use assertiveness and ingratiation, but gave in when these tactics failed to stop the surgeon. The high number of participants

Table 2. The number of participants who used an influence tactic are shown in the # column. Participants frequently used more than one influence tactic when attempting to get the surgeon to delay the surgery.

Influence Tactic	#	Example
Rationality	14	"You know it takes 45 minutes for a type-and-screen to be done, and then if the patient has antibodies it's extra time."
Assertiveness	11	"We have to send two ABO samples, and we haven't even sent the first one yet."
Upward Appeal	5	"I think that we should wait. I'm going to call the charge nurse and talk to her about it."
Coalitions	3	"I'll call the blood bank and see how long they think it will take to process the blood sample"
Ingratiation	3	"I understand you're on a tight time schedule, but we need to proceed with caution, as we would with any other patient."
Sanctions	1	"That's fine, if that's your choice, but I'll have to make sure that it's noted in his chart."
Blocking	1	"I'm waiting on the blood."
Exchange	0	*Examples of exchange would include calling on past services or offering future services/favors in return for compliance*

who used rationality is consistent with Kipnis' finding that rationality is the most commonly used tactic during conflict with superiors. However, it is somewhat surprising that eleven participants used assertiveness, given that Kipnis found that assertiveness is most commonly used during attempts to influence subordinates. The high number of participants who employed assertiveness may be explained by the virtual surgeon's unwillingness to be convinced by reason; of the eleven participants who used assertiveness, seven used it only after first failing to convince the virtual surgeon using rationality. The remaining six tactics were used infrequently, which is consistent with Kipnis' findings that they were used most frequently with co-workers and subordinates.

Participants typically used more than one influence tactic when attempting to convince the surgeon to wait. Five participants used two tactics, four used three tactics, two used four tactics, and one used five tactics. Only three participants used a single tactic. Two of the three participants who used a single tactic gave in to the surgeon. The other participant who used a single tactic shifted responsibility to the surgeon.

5.2 Real World Motivations for Participant Behavior

During post-exercise interviews, participants generally explained their behavior in terms of real-world experience, for instance, referencing their knowledge of the procedure, their assessment of how long it would take to get blood, and their beliefs about a nurse's role in the operating room.

Participants who stopped the line explained their behavior in three ways. Two cited how scoliosis surgeries incur a large amount of blood loss, which would need to be replaced with blood from the blood bank. Two cited past experience with needing blood during a surgery. Four cited their role as a patient advocate, which means they must protect the patient's safety, even if it leads to conflict with an authority figure.

Participants who did not stop the line explained their behavior in many ways. Eight believed that there was enough time to get replacement blood before the patient would need it. Four did not believe the surgery would incur significant blood loss. Six deferred to the surgeon, believing that he knew best. Three felt the virtual anesthesiologist gave implicit consent to continue when he did not object to the surgeon's proposal to move forward. Others also justified moving forward based on past experiences in the operating room, the availability of emergency blood, and the ability to pause the surgery before losing blood.

5.3   Impressions about Training with Virtual Humans

Participants reported that the exercise provided a good opportunity to practice speaking up to a surgeon. Multiple participants reported feeling like they had been speaking up to a real surgeon, commenting on his tone of voice, his anger and impatience, and the arguments he raised. Participants were also positive about the interaction with the entire virtual team, saying that the way the virtual humans looked at participants, interacted with each other, and responded verbally to participants made them feel like they were working with a real team.

Several participants reported feeling more confident and more motivated to speak up after practicing with the virtual humans. Other participants reported that they did not find it personally useful because they already felt comfortable speaking up; however, they did feel that it would be useful for less experienced nurses who did not already know how to speak up. Intriguingly, three of these nurses did not stop the line, indicating that they either were not completely comfortable speaking up, or failed to identify the patient safety issue. This inconsistency between participants' self-assessment and their behavior underscores the importance of this type of training.

Despite being pleased with the exercise, seven participants said one aspect of the simulation may have caused them to behave differently than they would in the real world: the virtual humans felt like human strangers, not familiar co-workers. Participants explained that, in the real world, they work with the same team members almost every day. Being familiar with their co-workers produces a sense of rapport, which participants said helps them to feel comfortable with their teammates, even during conflict. This sense of rapport was missing with the virtual humans, because the virtual humans were unfamiliar; this made speaking up more difficult for some participants.

In addition to generating a sense of rapport, participants said that familiarity with their team members allows them to anticipate how their teammates may react during conflict, which makes speaking up easier. Some participants felt that speaking up to the virtual surgeon was difficult because they were not familiar enough with him to predict how he would respond to being challenged. Coming from a different perspective, two participants expressed that it was actually easier to speak up to the virtual surgeon, because they knew they would not be working with him on a regular basis. These participants were more comfortable with the possibility of antagonizing the virtual surgeon because there would not be any long-term consequences if he got upset.

This is a key point – when people are familiar with their co-workers, being unfamiliar with a virtual human may lead them to alter their behavior; this is especially true during high-stakes interactions, like conflict with an authority figure. Depending on a person's perspective, conflict may become easier or harder. If people focus on the lack of long-term consequences, they may manage conflict more aggressively than they would in real life. Others may respond more timidly, because they lack rapport with their virtual team members and can not predict how an unfamiliar virtual authority figure will respond to being challenged.

This observation is consistent with research showing that existing relationships can increase people's willingness to share information and make concessions, reduce the use of competitive or coercive tactics, and improve task performance by reducing social uncertainty and concerns about acceptance [10,19]. Given that familiarity with team members can influence people's behavior, cultivating a sense of familiarity with virtual team members may be important when training people who work with familiar teams. It may be possible to cultivate familiarity by priming people using storytelling techniques, demonstrating key aspects of a virtual human's personality during a tutorial (e.g. the virtual human gets very upset, or exhibits patience and forgiveness), or by modeling the virtual human's appearance and behavior after an individual known to the participant.

6   Conclusions and Future Work

This study explored how nurses behaved during conflict with an authoritative virtual human. We created a virtual operating room team, led by a virtual surgeon whose reckless behavior could endanger the team's patient. This behavior required nurses to speak up and stop him from beginning the surgery. We examined participants' behavior during conflict with the virtual surgeon and found that it was consistent with two real-world behavioral frameworks proposed by Van Dyne and Kipnis. Participants reached each of the five relevant outcomes described by Van Dyne, and employed seven of the eight influence tactics described by Kipnis. In short, participants approached conflict with the virtual surgeon using the same techniques employed during real conflict with humans. While it is possible that a specific individual may behave differently during conflict with real and virtual humans, it appears that, in aggregate, people approach conflict with virtual humans and real humans using the same methods. This conclusion is also supported by participants' tendency to explain their behavior using real-world motivations.

Another contribution of this study is the observation that some nurses felt that working with virtual humans was like working with human strangers.

This finding is important as humans sometimes behave differently when working with strangers, compared to familiar individuals. While this is likely acceptable in settings where participants regularly work with strangers (e.g. interviewing a virtual patient or working in ad hoc teams), it may be undesirable when simulating interactions where participants are familiar with the people they work with (e.g. established teams). In these situations, it may be important to allow participants to build rapport with their virtual teammates, and to help participants anticipate how their virtual teammates will react during the simulation.

An important limitation of this study is the gender imbalance among participants. Given that nurses are predominately women, our findings about conflict and the importance of familiarity may not generalize to other, more heterogeneous, populations. This limitation is especially important given that gender effects are not uncommon when examining social behavior. Future work is required to explore whether these results can be generalized to other populations.

We are currently working with nursing management at the hospital to integrate the Speaking Up exercise into nurses' annual continuing education training. We are also expanding the Speaking Up scenario to support training surgical technicians (who are also subordinate to surgeons). Future research will explore how working with a second human teammate affects how people behave during conflict with virtual authority figures.

Acknowledgments. The authors would like to thank Theresa Hughes, Terry Sullivan, and David Lizdas for their help in developing the Speaking Up exercise and recruiting participants, as well as the nurses who agreed to participate in this study. This work was supported in part by NSF Grant 1161491.

References

1. Bailenson, J.N., Beall, A.C., Loomis, J.M.: Interpersonal Distance in Immersive Virtual Environments. Personality and Social Psychology Bulletin 29(7) (2003)
2. Bickmore, T.W.: Relational Agents: Effecting Change through Human-Computer Relationships. PhD thesis (2003)
3. Castillo-Page, L.: Diversity in the Physician Workforce: Facts & Figures 2010. Association of American Medical Colleges (2010)
4. Chuah, J., Robb, A., White, C., Wendling, A., Lampotang, S., Kooper, R., Lok, B.: Exploring agent physicality and social presence for medical team training. Presence: Teleoperators & Virtual Environments 22(2), 141–170 (2013)
5. Core, M., Traum, D., Lane, H.C., Swartout, W., Gratch, J., van Lent, M., Marsella, S.: Teaching Negotiation Skills through Practice and Reflection with Virtual Humans. Simulation 82(11), 685–701 (2006)
6. Dyne, L., Ang, S., Botero, I.: Conceptualizing Employee Silence and Employee Voice as Multidimensional Constructs*. Journal of Management Studies (September 2003)
7. Gordon, R.: Basic Interviewing Skills. F. E. Peacock, Itasca (1992)
8. Guest, G., Namey, E., Mitchell, M.: Collecting Qualitative Data: A field manual for applied research (2012)

9. Hall, L., Vala, M., Hall, M., Webster, M., Woods, S., Gordon, A., Aylett, R.S.: FearNot's Appearance: Reflecting children's expectations and perspectives. In: Gratch, J., Young, M., Aylett, R.S., Ballin, D., Olivier, P. (eds.) IVA 2006. LNCS (LNAI), vol. 4133, pp. 407–419. Springer, Heidelberg (2006)
10. Jehn, K., Mannix, E.: The dynamic nature of conflict: A longitudinal study of intragroup conflict and group performance. Academy of Management Journal 44(2), 238–251 (2001)
11. Johnsen, K., Raij, A., Stevens, A., Lind, D., Lok, B.: The validity of a virtual human experience for interpersonal skills education. In: Proceedings of the SIGCHI Conference on Human Factors in Computing Systems, pp. 1049–1058. ACM (2007)
12. Kipnis, D., Schmidt, S.M., Wilkinson, I.: Intraorganizational influence tactics: Explorations in getting one's way. Journal of Applied Psychology 65(4) (1980)
13. Kotranza, A., Lok, B., Deladisma, A., Pugh, C., Lind, D.: Mixed reality humans: Evaluating behavior, usability, and acceptability. IEEE Transactions on Visualization and Computer Graphics 15(3), 369–382 (2009)
14. Makary, M.A., Sexton, J.B., Freischlag, J.A., Holzmueller, C.G., Millman, E.A., Rowen, L., Pronovost, P.J.: Operating room teamwork among physicians and nurses: teamwork in the eye of the beholder. Journal of the American College of Surgeons 202(5), 746–752 (2006)
15. Pertaub, D., Slater, M., Street, G., Wce, L., Barker, C.: An Experiment on Public Speaking Anxiety in Response to Three Different Types. Presence: Teleoperators & Virtual Environments 11(1), 68–78 (2002)
16. Robb, A., Kopper, R., Ambani, R., Qayyum, F., Lind, D., Su, L.-M., Lok, B.: Leveraging Virtual Humans to Effectively Prepare Learners for Stressful Interpersonal Experiences. In: 2013 IEEE Virtual Reality, VR (2013)
17. Rossen, B., Johnsen, K., Deladisma, A., Lind, S., Lok, B.: Virtual humans elicit skin-tone bias consistent with real-world skin-tone biases. In: Prendinger, H., Lester, J.C., Ishizuka, M. (eds.) IVA 2008. LNCS (LNAI), vol. 5208, pp. 237–244. Springer, Heidelberg (2008)
18. Thomas, E.J., Sexton, J.B., Helmreich, R.L.: Discrepant attitudes about teamwork among critical care nurses and physicians. Critical Care Medicine 31(3), 956–959 (2003)
19. Valley, K., Neale, M., Mannix, E.: Friends, lovers, colleagues, strangers: The effects of relationships on the process and outcome of dyadic negotiations. Research on Negotiation in Organizations (1995)
20. Vardoulakis, L.P., Ring, L., Barry, B., Sidner, C.L., Bickmore, T.: Designing relational agents as long term social companions for older adults. In: Nakano, Y., Neff, M., Paiva, A., Walker, M. (eds.) IVA 2012. LNCS, vol. 7502, pp. 289–302. Springer, Heidelberg (2012)

Steps towards a Challenging Teachable Agent

Annika Silvervarg[1], Camilla Kirkegaard[1], Jens Nirme[2], Magnus Haake[2],
and Agneta Gulz[1]

[1] Dept. Computer and Information Science, Linköping University, Linköping, Sweden
{annika.silvervarg,camilla.kirkegaard,agneta.gulz}@liu.se
[2] Cognitive Science, Lund University, Kungshuset, Lundagård, Lund, Sweden
{jens.nirme,magnus.haake}@lucs.lu.se

Abstract. This paper presents the first steps towards a new type of pedagogical agent – a Challenger Teachable Agent, CTA. The overall aim of introducing a CTA is to increase engagement and motivation and challenge students into deeper learning and metacognitive reasoning. The paper discusses desired design features of such an agent on the basis of related work and results from a study where 11-year old students interacted with a first version of a CTA in the framework of an educational software for history. The focus is on how students respond when the CTA disagrees and questions their suggestions, and how groups of students, differing in response behavior and in self-efficacy, experience the CTA.

Keywords: Teachable agent, challenge, interaction, learning, experience.

1 Introduction and Background

This paper explores students' interaction with and responses to a new type of pedagogical agent – a challenger teachable agent (CTA). In brief, a teachable agent (TA) is an embodied computer agent which is taught or trained by a student where AI techniques guide the agent's behaviour based on what the agent is taught [1]. Importantly, a TA has no knowledge to begin with, but the knowledge that it gains reflects, more or less, what it is being taught by the student.

Overall, teachable agents have proven pedagogically powerful as an implementation of the *learning by teaching* pedagogy [2, 3]. Our goal is to boost this pedagogical power even further by introducing a teachable agent with a more explicit agency or "will of its own". To our knowledge, the TAs developed so far do not show much of a "will". They do not, for example, argue with a student on whether a piece of information is adequate for a task or not, or indicate that they find a particular topic uninteresting.

Regarding pedagogical agents in general, Frasson and Aïmeur [4] proposed *troublemaker agents* as a subset of learning companions that would question and challenge a student. Such an agent suggests a solution and then asks the student if she agrees or not. If the student does not agree, the troublemaker will argue for her or his own solution – whether it is correct or not – until the student either agrees or the troublemaker runs out of arguments. The students are thereby encouraged to question

T. Bickmore et al. (Eds.): IVA 2014, LNAI 8637, pp. 410–419, 2014.

their own knowledge and be more motivated as teachers. Several studies show learning gains from troublemaker agents, particularly for high-achieving students, e.g. [4, 5].

Even one of the seminal papers on teachable agents by Brophy et al. [1] proposed a teachable agent that "may be impetuous, not listen or collaborate well". The implementation and study presented in this article is, however, the first practical attempt in this direction. In an educational software for learning history, we introduce a CTA that, during learning activities where the CTA and student work together and take turns, questions and challenges the student in various ways.

The main motive for introducing a CTA is to stimulate deep learning (c.f. [5]). By being questioned and challenged at times by his or her TA we hope the student becomes encouraged to think once more and perhaps reorganize or rephrase the material he/she is teaching [6]. We also wish to stimulate metacognitive abilities, i.e. reflection on problem solving and learning, abilities that have a transitive value for students when faced with future challenges [7]. In addition, our previous studies have shown that students frequently ask for a TA "with more of an attitude". It can be boring to interact with an agent that is always positive, compliant and cheerful – and such agents are weak in believability [8].

In the longer run, we are implementing the following set of challenging behaviours in our CTA.

1. The CTA inducing confusion or cognitive disequilibrium by contradicting the student with the aim to provoke the student to reflect on what is true, thereby processing the material at a deeper level [9].
2. The CTA requesting clarification of a solution in a learning activity, thus creating opportunities for debating the study material before accepting it, potentially prompting a desire in the student to share meaning and be understood [10]. This kind of teachable agent behaviour is represented in *SimStudent* [11] where the TA interacts with the student in natural language while solving equations. The TA tries to solve a problem step-by-step and the user verifies the correctness of each step. The TA can ask follow-up questions during this process, which forces the student to reflect on the concepts in the current problem and to show how well he/she understands the material.
3. The CTA occasionally introducing erroneous facts during the learning activities. This will hopefully provoke the student to justify his/her answers [4]. Training to distinguish between right and wrong solutions is also a means to achieve higher confidence in a domain.
4. The CTA prompting the student to choose a task at a more challenging level.

For the study presented in this paper we focus on this first aspect, i.e. the CTAs questioning of the students' proposals – both in cases where the students' proposal is correct and when it is not. To question someone you are collaborating with means to introduce a conflict. Several authors discuss the educational potential of conflict or dissonance in other areas than that of teachable agents. For instance, one of the five modes that Weinberger and Fischer [12] lift forth in their analysis of different "social modes of co-construction" in students' collaborative activities is that of

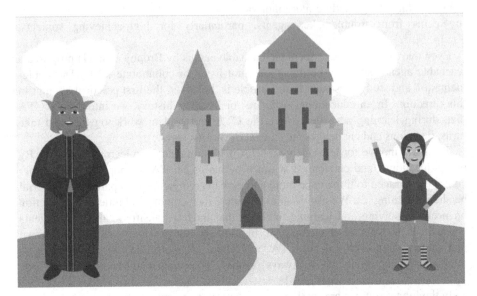

Fig. 1. The Castle of Time with the Guardian of History to the left and the Time elf (the teachable agent) to the right

"conflict-oriented consensus building". In this mode, a conflict is the starting point wherefrom critical reasoning at some point leads to a further step taken together, i.e. in consensus.

Therefore, as a first step in the design of a CTA, this paper presents a study of students' responses when their TA questions their proposals in a collaborative learning activity. Our two main research questions were:

1. "What do students do when the CTA questions their proposals?"
2. "How do students perceive collaboration with a CTA with respect to the agent's questioning and/or challenging behaviour?"

We predicted that the answers to both research questions would vary for students with high and low self-efficacy respectively, i.e. with a strong vs. weak belief in their own competence.

2   The Guardian of History – TA-Based Learning Environment

"The Guardian of History" is an educational software for history for age 10-12 year. The narrative centres on securing a successor to the Guardian of History, who is in charge of the Castle of Time but about to retire, see Fig. 1. The student takes on a teacher role and his/her task is to teach a time elf, i.e. a teachable agent, about history so that the time elf can qualify as successor to the Guardian of History. To do this, the student must first learn for him-/herself. Thereafter the student teaches the time elf

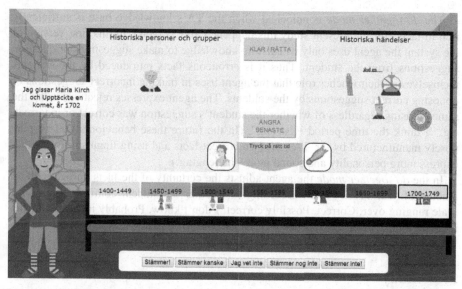

Fig. 2. The timeline learning activity. The time elf has suggested that Maria Kirch discovered a comet in 1702 and the student can choose to confirm or reject this proposal.

during various game-like learning activities. The learning activity used in this study focuses on basic facts where a person is linked to an event and a time period, and placed on a timeline, see Fig. 2.

The time elf (TA) can be taught in two different modes:

1. By watching the student perform the learning activity on his/her own
2. Through performing the learning activity together with the student.

In the latter case, the student and TA take turns suggesting a fact and giving feedback to one another's suggestions via a multiple choice dialogue. When the TA suggests a fact the student can confirm or reject it, and similarly, when the student makes a proposal the TA can say that it believes it to be correct or incorrect. If the TA rejects the student's proposal, the student can chose to nevertheless affirm it – or the student can ask the TA to suggest an alternative instead, for example:

Student [*suggests*]: "Galileo Galilei invented the telescope between 1650 and 1700."
TA [*rejects*]: "I think the time period is wrong. Are you sure?"
Student [*affirms*]: "I am sure." [*or withdraws*]: "Do you have another suggestion?"

The TAs knowledge base consists of facts, i.e. <Person, Event, Time period>, that have a certainty between 1 and 10. The TA starts out with an empty knowledge base and learns by adding new facts with certainty 1 when it observes the student working on the timeline activity. If a fact is repeated the agent increases the certainty with 1. If the student adds facts that are incorrect or contradicting, e.g. <Galileo Galilei, Invented telescope, 1600-1649>, which is correct, and <Galileo Galilei, Invented telescope, 1650-1699>, which is incorrect, they are both added to the TA's knowledge base.

The *do together mode* is unlocked when the TA's knowledge base is sufficiently rich in facts (for the present study this happened after 5 facts). In this first version of the system the agent uses only its existing knowledge to make suggestions or question suggestions from the student. Thus it is erroneous facts introduced by the students themselves in their teacher role that the agent uses in making incorrect suggestions or opposing correct suggestions by the students. The agent expresses rejections using the same phrasing regardless of whether the student's suggestion was correct or incorrect, e.g. "I think the time period is wrong". (In the future these behaviours will be purposely manufactured by the TA based on correct facts and using linguistic forms that express more personality and sound more challenging.)

In the *do together mode* the agent adjusts the certainty of the facts known with an amount of: +2, +1, 0, -1, -2, according to whether the student confirms them on a scale ranging over: Correct, Possibly correct, I don't know, Probably incorrect, Incorrect (see Fig. 2.) If a fact reaches a certainty of zero or below it is removed from the TA's knowledge base.

3   Study

20 female and 15 male 11-year olds from two classes in a Swedish school participated in the study. The students used the educational software and interacted with their TAs during two subsequent lessons, each with a duration of 25-35 minutes. The students' actions and choices were logged by the software. After the last session the students filled out a questionnaire regarding their experience of using the software and their view on the role of the teachable agent, the TA's willingness to cooperate, and different aspects of performing learning activities together with the TA. They were also asked about what they thought about their own ability to teach the TA (i.e. their self-efficacy). The questionnaire used a 5 point Likert scale ranging from "Strongly disagree" to "Strongly agree".

The logs of the students' behaviour showed that the students proposed a total of 161 correct propositions, of which the TA rejected 40 (25%), and 615 incorrect propositions, of which the TA rejected 137 (22%), see Fig. 3. Thus, the TA rejected approximately one fourth (23%) of all propositions suggested by the students.

3.1   Research Question 1 – Students Responses to CTA Behaviour

Turning to our first research question: "What do students do when the CTA questions their proposals?" the log data showed that (see Fig. 3):

— *Case 1:* the students incorrectly withdrew 21 of 40 (53%) of their originally correct proposals when the proposal was rejected by the CTA.
— *Case 2:* the students correctly withdrew 117 of 137 (85%) of their originally incorrect proposals after having the proposal rejected by the CTA.

Thus, the students correctly withdrew significantly more of their proposals when they were correctly rejected by the CTA (Case 2) as evaluated by a Mann-Whitney's U test (Case 1: median = 0.5, mean rank = 19.1; Case 2: median = 1.0, mean rank = 28.8; $U = 172.5; Z = -2.484; p < .05; r = .35$).

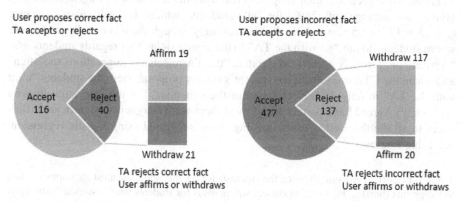

Fig. 3. The pie charts show how the TA reacts to users' correct or incorrect suggestions, and the stacked bar charts show how the user in turn reacts to the agents incorrect or correct rejection of their suggestions.

For the students that answered "Strongly disagreed" or "Disagreed" versus "Agreed" or "Strongly agreed" on the questionnaire item "The TA rejects my suggestions too often", no overall pattern could be secured due to few data points. Students who experienced that their TA rejected their suggestions "too often" withdrew 42% of their originally correct proposals compared to 74% for the students who didn't experience that the TA rejected their suggestions "too often" (see Fig. 4). Regarding the situation of an originally incorrect proposal by a student that was questioned by the TA, the students who experienced that the TA rejected their suggestions "too often" withdrew their proposals in 81% of the cases, compared to 95% for students who didn't experience that the TA rejected their suggestions "too often".

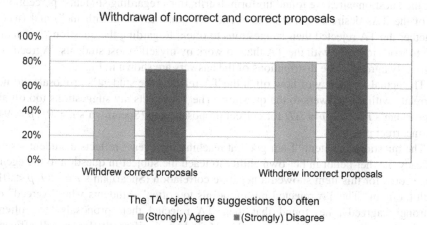

Fig. 4. The figure shows how often students withdrew correct/incorrect proposals for the two groups "(Strongly) Agree" and "(Strongly) Disagree" to "TA rejects my suggestions too often".

One striking result is how strongly inclined the students were to "go with the TA" when the TA objected to their proposal (138 withdrawals out of 177 agent rejections) giving an average of 78% for all students which is well above chance $(\chi^2(1, N = 177) = 55.4, p < .001)$. But interestingly enough there is one diverging case where students do not "go with the TA" to the same extent. This regards students who "Agreed" or "Strongly agreed" to the item "the TA rejects my suggestions too often" and where the CTA questioned the student's correct proposal. Here the students "went with the TA" in only 42% (see above) of the situations. For the case students who "(Strongly) Agreed" and correct withdrawal there was (marginally) significant differences to all the three other cases (see Fig. 4) as suggested using logistic regression, see Table 1 below.

Table 1. Logistic regression showing the contrasts for a:i, d:c, and d:i against a:c corresponding to the groups (bars) in Fig. 4: (a:c) correct withdrawals for students who answered "(Strongly) Agree"; (a:i) incorrect withdrawals for students who answered "(Strongly) Agree"; (d:c) correct withdrawals for students who answered "(Strongly) Disagree"; (d:i) incorrect withdrawals for students who answered "(Strongly) Disagree".

Contrasts	Z	p
a:c vs. a:i	2.439	0.015 *
a:c vs. d:c	1.743	0.081 .
a:c vs. d:i	2.729	0.007 **

. $p < 0.1$ * $p < 0.05$ ** $p < 0.01$ *** $p < 0.001$

3.2 Research Question 2 – Perception of Collaboration with the CTA

Our second research question was: "How do students perceive collaboration with a CTA with respect to the agent's questioning and/or challenging behaviour?" Analysing the questionnaires we found uniform distributions regarding students' perceptions: (i) of the TAs desire to collaborate ("The TA wants to work with me") and (ii) on whether the TA rejected their suggestions to often. Regarding the question "It is more fun to work together with the TA than to work by myself" most students "Agreed" or "Strongly agreed". The distributions of the answers are shown in Fig. 5.

The actual frequency of how often the TA rejected the student's proposals did not correlate with the answers to the question "The TA rejects my suggestions too often" (Spearman's $r = -.17, p = .37$) for correct proposals, and (Spearman's $r = .01, p = .94$) for incorrect proposals.

The questionnaire item "I am good at teaching the agent" reflects a student's self-efficacy, i.e. her belief in her own ability to teach the subject in question to the agent. The scores for this item showed a negative correlation (Spearman's $r = -.59, p < .01$) with the item "The TA rejected my proposals too often". Students who "Agreed" or "Strongly agreed", i.e. found that their TA rejected their proposals "too often" (Self-efficacy: median = 4, mean rank = 16.7) had significantly lower self-efficacy (Mann-Whitney's U test: $U = 104.5, Z = 2.51, p < .05$) than those who

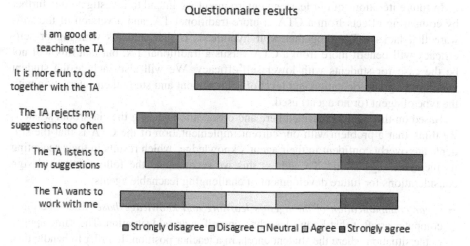

Fig. 5. The distribution of answers on a 5 point Likert scale from "Strongly disagree" to "Strongly agree" for questionnaire questions regarding the cooperation with the CTA.

"Strongly disagreed" or "Disagreed", i.e. did not find that their TA rejected their proposals "too often" (Self-efficacy: median = 2, mean rank = 9.0)[1].

4   Conclusions and Future Work

With respect to the first research question on students' responses to a CTA, the overall result was that students generally went along with their CTA's objections rather than holding on to their own initial proposal. Since they did so even when they were initially correct we did not achieve the desired result of improving the students' learning. However, most students experienced it was more fun to do the learning activity together with the CTA than to do the same activity by themselves. This is a positive result in view of our continued development of a CTA-based software, but how and when the CTA challenges the student needs to be improved. Some suggestions are discussed below as design recommendations for future development.

Regarding the students' attitudes towards their CTA, the most salient result was that students with higher self-efficacy (i.e. who saw themselves as good teachers for their CTA) did not experience that their CTA questioned them too often, whereas students with lower self-efficacy did experience this. In contrast, the *actual frequency* of challenging/questioning by the CTA did not affect the extent to which the students *experienced* that the TA was challenging/questioning them "too often". In other words, the experience of being challenged seems more strongly connected to students' personal preferences than actual occurrence of challenge by the CTA.

---

[1] The self-reported self-efficacy displayed a medium effect size correlation (Spearman's $r = .38, p < .04$) with the number of proposed correct propositions by the students, i.e. with a measurement of actual ability/performance.

In future iterations of our learning environment we intend to investigate this further by comparing effects from a CTA, a more traditional TA, and a version of the software that lacks a TA altogether. Our hypothesis is that students with higher self-efficacy will benefit more from a CTA versus a traditional TA, but that this will not be the case for students with lower self-efficacy. We will also include the student variables of goal-orientation and level of achievement and study their interaction with the type of agent (or no agent) used.

Based on the results presented here and observations during the classroom sessions we think that a problem with our current implementation of the CTA is that the students are overly confident in their agent's knowledge, which results in their accepting its incorrect suggestions. To address this we recommend the following two design considerations for future development of challenging teachable agents:

— *Clear communication of the agent's learning and knowledge base.* Encountering a computer artefact that knows less than oneself is an odd situation. The same applies to the situation where the student enrols in a teacher position. In order to handle this, we will develop a stronger narrative for the software that emphasizes that the CTA has *no initial knowledge* and that its knowledge state basically is a reflection of what the student has taught it. We will also let this be reflected in how the CTA voices its rejections to student proposals so that it does not seem too confident and knowledgeable but more as a tutee. The more the CTA is exposed to a certain fact the more certain it should become, but initially it should be quite uncertain.

— *Adjust magnitude, frequency and timing of challenging behaviour.* A student must stand on a solid ground to meet challenges in the form of rejection or errors from the CTA. Students need to have mastered the learning material to a certain degree before they are challenged, and/or the magnitude of the errors must be adjusted to the students' knowledge level so that they can be detected. We will address this by letting the student initially engage in each learning activity *without* the CTA in order to build a threshold knowledge level before starting to teach and work together with the CTA.

References

1. Brophy, S., Biswas, G., Katzlberger, T., Bransford, J., Schwartz, D.: Teachable Agents: Combining Insights from Learning Theory and Computer Science. In: Lajoie, S.P., Vivet, M. (eds.) Artificial Intelligence in Education, pp. 21–28. IOS Press, Amsterdam (1999)
2. Chase, C., Chin, D., Oppezzo, M., Schwartz, D.: Teachable Agents and the Protégé Effect: Increasing the Effort Towards Learning. J. Sci. Educ. Technol. 18(4), 334–352 (2009)
3. Blair, K., Schwartz, D., Biswas, G., Leelawong, K.: Pedagogical Agents for Learning by Teaching: Teachable Agents. Educational Technology: Special Issue on Pedagogical Agents 47(1), 56–61 (2007)
4. Frasson, C., Aïmeur, E.: A Comparison of Three Learning Strategies in Intelligent Tutoring Systems. J. Educ. Comput. Res. 14(4), 371–383 (1996)
5. Aïmeur, E., Dufort, H., Leibu, D., Frasson, C.: Some Justifications About the Learning By Disturbing Strategy. In: du Boulay, W., Mizoguchi, R. (eds.) Artificial Intelligence in Education, pp. 1–14. IOS Press, Amsterdam (1997)

6. Schwartz, D., Chase, C., Chin, D., Oppezzo, M., Kwong, H.: Interactive Metacognition: Monitoring and Regulating a Teachable Agent. In: Hacker, D.J., Dunlosky, J., Graesser, A.C. (eds.) Handbook of Metacognition in Education, pp. 340–358. Routledge (2009)

7. Chin, D.B., Dohmen, I.M., Cheng, B.H., Oppezzo, M.A., Chase, C.C., Schwartz, D.L.: Preparing Students for Future Learning with Teachable Agents. Educ. Technol. Res. Dev. 58(6), 649–669 (2010)

8. Cassell, J., Thórisson, K.R.: The Power of a Nod and a Glance: Envelope vs. Emotional Feedback in Animated Conversational Agents. Appl. Artif. Intell. 13, 519–538 (1999)

9. D'Mello, S., Lehman, B., Pekrun, R., Graesser, A.: Confusion can be Beneficial for Learning. Learning and Instruction 29, 153–170 (2014)

10. Schwartz, D.: The Productive Agency that Drives Collaborative Learning. In: Dillenbourg, P. (ed.) Collaborative Learning: Cognitive and Computational Approaches, pp. 197–218. Permagon, Amsterdam (1999)

11. Carlson, R., Keiser, V., Matsuda, N., Koedinger, K.R., Penstein Rosé, C.: Building a Conversational SimStudent. In: Cerri, S.A., Clancey, W.J., Papadourakis, G., Panourgia, K. (eds.) ITS 2012. LNCS, vol. 7315, pp. 563–569. Springer, Heidelberg (2012)

12. Weinberger, A., Fischer, F.: A Framework to Analyze Argumentative Knowledge Construction in Computer-Supported Collaborative Learning. Computers & Education 46(1), 71–95 (2006)

Large-scale Collection and Analysis of Personal Question-Answer Pairs for Conversational Agents

Hiroaki Sugiyama[1], Toyomi Meguro[1],
Ryuichiro Higashinaka[2], and Yasuhiro Minami[1]

[1] NTT Communication Science Labs., Kyoto, Japan
{sugiyama.hiroaki,meguro.toyomi,minami.yasuhiro}@lab.ntt.co.jp
[2] NTT Media Intelligence Labs., Kanagawa, Japan
higashinaka.ryuichiro@lab.ntt.co.jp

Abstract. In conversation, a speaker sometimes asks questions that relate to another speaker's detailed personality, such as his/her favorite foods and sports. This behavior also appears in conversations with conversational agents; therefore, agents should be developed that can respond to such questions. In previous agents, this was achieved by creating question-answer pairs defined by hand. However, when a small number of persons create the pairs, we cannot know what types of questions are frequently asked. This makes it difficult to know whether the created questions cover frequently asked questions; therefore, such essential question-answer pairs for conversational agents are possibly overlooked. This study analyzes a large number of question-answer pairs for six personae created by many question-generators, with one answer-generator for each persona. The proposed approach allows many questioners to create questions for various personae, enabling us to investigate the types of questions that are frequently asked. A comparison with questions appearing in conversations between humans shows that 50.2% of the questions were contained in our question-answer pairs and the coverage rate was almost saturated with the 20 recruited question-generators.

Keywords: system personality, conversational system, crowdsourcing.

1 Introduction

Recent research on dialogue agents has actively investigated on casual dialogue [13,10,17,8,4], because conversational agents are useful not only for entertainment or counseling purposes but also for the improvement of performance in task-oriented dialogues [2]. In conversation, people often ask questions related to the personality of the person with whom they are speaking, such as the person's favorite foods and already experienced sports [16]. Nishimura et al. showed that such personal questions were also appearing in conversations with conversational agents [9], so the capability to answer personal questions is an essential factor for development of conversational agents.

T. Bickmore et al. (Eds.): IVA 2014, LNAI 8637, pp. 420–433, 2014.
© Springer International Publishing Switzerland 2014

Most previous research on the personality of dialogue agents has investigated the agent's personality using roughly-grained categories, such as Big-Five in PERSONAGE [3,5,6]. They focused on parameterizing the personalities, but did not deal with specific subjects of the personalities, which are required to answer personal questions. To answer a user's personal questions, Batacharia et al. developed the Person DataBase (PDB), which consists of question-answer pairs (*QA pairs*) evoked by a pre-defined persona *Catherine*, who is a 26 year-old female living in New York [1]. Their approach searches the PDB for questions similar to the user's question utterances and generates answers relevant to the questions. Even though this approach seems reasonable, when the PDB is developed by a few persons, it is difficult to know whether the developed PDB covers frequently asked questions; therefore, essential QA pairs for conversational agents may be overlooked.

To investigate the types of questions that are frequently asked, we adopt an approach that lets many participants create personal questions evoked by pre-defined personae. Since many questions are intensively created for each persona and will be overlapped, we can identify frequently asked questions and investigate the types of such questions. This approach is a kind of crowdsourcing [14]. Rossen et al. shows that the idea of crowdsourcing is effective to develop a domain-specific conversational agent which works with many stimuli-response pairs [11]. Their work limited domains of the stimuli, consists of many stimuli-response pairs. However, our work does not specify the domains of the questions. Since domains are not limited, the number of possible questions of our work will be much larger than that of domain-specific stimuli as in [11]. To examine the effectiveness of our approach, it is important to investigate the property of the collected questions, such as the coverage of created questions in real conversations. We report a detailed analysis of the developed PDB, by the classification of the answers and a comparison with questions appearing in conversations between humans.

2 Development of a PDB

To create a number of question-answer pairs (*QA pairs*) related to an agent's personality, one approach lets people create such QA pairs for a pre-defined persona. However, when just a few people create them, it is difficult to know what kind of questions are frequently asked; thus, they might overlook essential questions for conversational agents. To deal with this problem, we adopt an approach that allows many participants create question sentences for pre-defined personae. Figure 1 illustrates the collection procedure of QA pairs.

First, we recruited 42 Japanese-speaking participants (*questioners*) balanced for gender and age to create the question sentences. Each questioner created 100 or more question sentences for each of the following six personae listed in Table 1. The robot personae are expected to evoke different types of questions from the human personae. Each questioner created the sentences with following five rules: (A) create sentences about he/she want to ask naturally, (B) create sentences

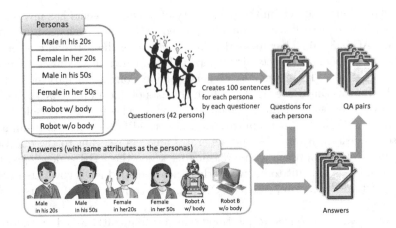

Fig. 1. Overview of collection of QA pairs

without omissions, (C) create one sentence for each question (no partition), (D) do not create duplicated questions for a persona (e.g., *"where do you live?"* and *"where is your current address?"*), and (E) do not copy questions from other sources like the web. Table 1 shows that we collected 26595 question sentences.

Next, a participant called *an answerer* (not the questioner) who had the same attributes as one of the personae created answers for the questions associated to the persona based on the following instructions: (a) create answers based on your own experiences or favorites, (b) create the same answers for the questions that represent identical subjects, (c) create as many *Yes/No* answers as possible (called *Yes/No* restrictions). Instruction (a) suppresses inconsistency between answers, such as *"Yes"* for *"Do you have a dog?"* and *"No"* for *"Do you have a pet?"* However, for robot personae, the answerers create answers based on a robot character they imagined themselves. If the various answers are created for identical-subject questions, it is difficult to classify and analyze the answers. To suppress the variation of the answers, we designed instructions (b) and (c). Instruction (b) directly suppresses variations. Instruction (c) is effective for question sentences that are answerable with *"Yes/No"* but are expected to be answered with specific subjects, such as *"Do you have a pet?"*.

After the collection, the question-answer sentence pairs (*QA-pairs*) are classified to question categories that represent each identical subject by another participant (not the author, not the questioner, and not the answerer) called *an information annotator*. This approach enables us to identify frequently-asked question subjects based on the number of question sentences in each question category. Table 1 shows that the question sentences are classified to 10082 question categories.

Finally, the information annotator annotated the following information described in Table 2 to the collected QA pairs. We call QA pairs with such information a *Person DataBase (PDB)*. Table 3 illustrates examples of the collected PDB.

Table 1. Persona attributes and statistics of the collected PDB

Persona attributes	# of question sentences	# of question categories
(1) Human (male in his 20s)	4431	2537
(2) Human (female in her 20s)	4475	2263
(3) Human (male in his 50s)	4438	2732
(4) Human (female in her 50s)	4458	2279
(5) Robot (with body)	4426	2232
(6) Robot (without body)	4367	2665
Summation	26595	10082

Table 2. Information annotated to PDB (Examples are translated by the authors)

Information	Description	Examples
Question sentences	Created question sentences	*Who are you?*
Question categories	Categories that consist of question sentences which denote the same subjects	Names
Answer sentences	Created answer sentences	*I'm Taichi.*
Topic labels	Labels that consist of question categories which denote the similar subjects	Names
Answer types	Labels that represent types of answers	Name: person names
Extended named entities	Labels that represent ENE of answers	Name: person
Persona types	Attributes of persona	male in 20s

3 Analysis of the PDB

We analyzed the statistics of our obtained PDB such as frequently asked questions based on the annotated information and investigated the differences between the questions in PDB and real conversations.

3.1 Question Categories

Statistics. At first, we analyzed the number of question sentences in each question category to examine the deviation of the sentences. Figure 2 shows their distribution, which is long-tailed (half of the question sentences belong to the top 11% (1110) categories), and 65.1% (6568) of the question categories have only one sentence.

To reveal the frequently asked question categories and investigate the differences depending on the frequency, we sort the question categories by their

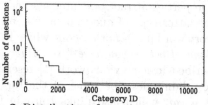

Fig. 2. Distribution of question sentences contained by each question category

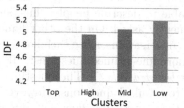

Fig. 3. Averaged IDF values of questions of the clusters

Table 3. Examples of PDB (All columns except Extended Named Entities (ENEs) are translated by authors)

Question sentences	Question categories	Answer sentences	Topic labels	Answer types	ENEs	Persona
How accurately can you understand what people say?	How accurately you can understand what people says	98%	How accurately you understand Japanese	Quantity: Other	Percent	Robot B
Do you want to hold a wedding ceremony at overseas?	Whether you want to hold a wedding ceremony at overseas	Yes	Whether you want to be married/Ideal marriage or family	Yes/No	No ENE	20s Male
When is your birthday?	Birthday	Sep., 10th, 1986.	Birthday	Quantity: Date	Date	20s Male
Do you usually eat pancakes?	Whether you usually eat pancakes	No	Favorite sweets/Whether you like sweets	Yes/No	No ENE	20s Male
Do you buy groceries by yourself?	Whether you buy groceries by yourself	No	Preparation of dishes/grocery shopping	Yes/No	No ENE	50s Female
Do you have persimmon trees in your garden?	Whether you have persimmon trees in your garden	No	Arrangement of houses or rooms	Yes/No	No ENE	50s Female
Do you have any pets?	Whether you have some pets	No	What you have some pets	Yes/No	No ENE	20s Female
Can you edit videos?	Whether you can edit videos	No	Whether you can edit videos	Yes/No	No ENE	20s Male

frequencies and divide them into four almost equal-sized clusters. Figure 3 illustrates the Inverse Document Frequencies (IDFs) calculated using sentences in the conversation corpus that we describe later (see Sec. 3.1.2). All of the differences were significant (Independent Student's t-test; $p < .01$). The difference between the top- and the high-ranked clusters is the largest. This indicates that the top-ranked cluster contains questions with less subject-specific words (e.g., proper nouns) and the question sentences of the high-ranked cluster consist of many subject-specific words.

Table 4 shows the examples and the statistics of the top, high, medium, and low frequency ranked clusters. The top-ranked question categories consist of two types of questions: properties that all persons have, such as *Name* or *Living place*, and conversation triggers with which we can easily expand a conversation, such as *Whether you like to cook* or *Whether you have a pet*. Such properties (the former type of questions) are unchanging for each person during at least several years and have large variances among persons. These characteristics are suitable to describe people; thus, such properties attract our interests and are frequently asked. On the other hand, the latter type of questions are useful to fuel conversations, since each has a category word like *pet* or *cooking*, which leads to more fine-grained questions: "*What kind of pet do you have?*" or "*Have you ever baked a cake?*". The questions described in a previous work [1] resemble our top-ranked questions. However, they didn't describe some of the top 10 questions (e.g., *Whether you can drive a car*, which also ranks third in the ranking by females in their 20s). This indicates that some essential questions may be overlooked in those created by just a few people.

Table 4. Examples of question categories

(a) Top-ranked categories (15 or more sentences, 1st-258th, 7403 sentences)

Question categories	#
Name	155
Birth place	111
Living place	98
Whether you can drive a car	97
Whether you have a pet	84
Whether you smoke	77
Whether you like to cook	75
Favorite color	75
Work	73
Whether you are married	73

(b) High-ranked categories (5 to 14 sentences, 259th-1110th, 6511 sentences)

Question categories	#
The number of siblings	14
Frequency of drinking alcohol	14
Time to make yourself up	14
Whether you play fishing	10
Favorite school meals	10
Whether you like museums of art	10
Color of your hair	5
Favorite rice ball ingredients	5
Favorite TV stations	5
Biggest regret	5

(c) Mid-ranked categories (2 to 4 sentences, 1111th-3514th, 6113 sentences)

Question categories	#
The most memorable dramas recently	4
How many dramas you watch in a week	4
Whether you have disguised as a woman	4
Anxiety about the future	3
Desirable travel companions	3
Whether you have corrected your teeth	3
Weak points (for robots)	3
Where you look at strangers	2
Whether you eat till you recover the cost in a buffet stype restaurant	2
Whether you go to public baths	2

(d) Low-ranked categories (1 sentences, 3515th-10082th, 6568 sentences)

Question categories	#
Whether something is in fashion in your generation	1
Whether you request life-prolonging treatments	1
Whether you make accessories	1
Favorite tastes of snow cones	1
Whether you have sports heroes in childhood	1
Frequencies of shaving in a day	1
Preferences of ties	1
Whether you become sensitive to earthquake after the 3.11 earthquake	1
Whether you like a ball game	1
The way you search for new information	1

The high- and mid-ranked question categories shown in Table 4(b) and 4(c) contain question categories that are related to the top-ranked question categories, such as *Favorite colors* and *Color of your hair*. While the high- and mid-ranked clusters are similar, mid-ranked questions have more specific subjects than high-ranked ones and adjuncts like *recently* in *The most memorable dramas recently*.

Some of the low-ranked question categories shown in Table 4(d) contain question categories subdivided from more frequent ones for the following reasons: overly narrow subjects, limited conditions, grammatical tenses, and the *Yes/No* restriction. For example, *Whether you request life-prolonging treatment* asks about life-prolonging treatment that is subdivided from medical treatment. The question *Whether you have sports heroes in childhood* is subdivided from a more frequent question category *Whether you have sports heroes* because of the limitations of the term *childhood*. The question *Whether you go to public baths* is subdivided from *Whether you have been to public baths* based on different grammatical tenses. The question *Whether you go to a hot spring* is subdivided from *Your favorite hot springs* since the former should be answered with *Yes/No* but the latter should not because of the *Yes/No* restriction.

Figure 4 illustrates the variation of the number of cumulative question categories while the number of questioners increases. The top-, high- and mid-

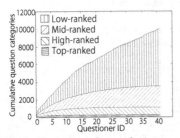

Fig. 4. Variation of cumulative question categories of each cluster while increasing the number of questioners

Table 5. Ranking correlations of the orders of top- and high-ranked question categories among personae. While correlations of human-human personae show high scores, that of human-robot personae shows negative correlations.

	20s M	20s F	50s M	50s F	Robot A	Robot B
20s M	1.00	0.53	0.37	0.37	-0.23	-0.06
20s F	0.53	1.00	0.25	0.47	-0.26	-0.05
50s M	0.37	0.25	1.00	0.41	-0.19	-0.09
50s F	0.37	0.47	0.41	1.00	-0.22	-0.10
Robot A	-0.23	-0.26	-0.19	-0.22	1.00	0.38
Robot B	-0.06	-0.05	-0.09	-0.10	0.38	1.00

ranked clusters were saturated with only 5, 15 and 35 questioners respectively. In contrast, even though we expected that the increase of the low-ranked cluster became slow with 40 questioners, the low-ranked cluster did not saturate and increased almost linearly. This indicates that the number of conceivable personal questions is huge.

Table 5 shows the ranking correlations of the orders of top- and high-ranked question categories among the personae. This shows that the orders between human personae are not so different (0.25 − 0.53 of rank correlations). Male in his 50s shows lower correlations than the other human personae, especially the correlation with female in her 20s is the lowest (0.25). One characteristic difference between human personae is that questions of similar subjects are described differently depending on the life stages, such as, *Whether you have a boyfriend/girlfriend?* and *Whether you are married*. In contrast, the rank correlations between the human and robot personae are negative. Table 6 illustrates the most frequently asked questions whose associated personae include Robot A or Robot B and their ranks in a ranking, which is prepared with question sentences for human personae. This shows that some of the questions do not appear for the human personae. For example, *Whether you can run* and *Whether you have emotion* are related to robot abilities or properties that are obvious for humans. Therefore, to develop a PDB that can be used for conversational agents, it is necessary to collect questions for such robot personae.

Comparison with the Conversation Corpus. To compare the personality questions in PDB with those in real conversations, we extracted personality questions from the conversation corpus gathered by Higashinaka et al. [4] that contains 3680 text chat based conversations (with 134 K sentences). From 183 sampled conversations, we harvested 490 personality questions (7.8% of all the sentences and 72.0% of all the questions) with corresponding question categories labeled by two annotators (not the authors). The agreement rate of the labeled question categories between the annotators was 0.816.

The followings are the number of questions classified in each cluster (Fig. 5): 85 (17.3%) top-ranked, 52 (10.6%) high-ranked, 29 (5.9%) middle-ranked, and 36

Table 6. Examples of question categories of robot personae. *Rank* means a rank in a ranking, which is created with question sentences for human personae (N/A means that the category does not appear for human personae).

(a) Robot A (embodied)

Question categories	Rank
Name	1
Weights	42
Place of production	N/A
Whether you can cook	13
Height	29
Whether you can write a character	N/A
Whether you can run	N/A
Birthday	33
Whether you can sing a song	59
Whether you can drive a car	6

(b) Robot B (no body)

Question categories	Rank
Name	1
Whether you can sing a song	59
Whether you are male or female types	42
Birth place	2
Manufactured purpose	N/A
Birthday	33
Whether you can change your voice	N/A
Whether you have emotion	N/A
Age	17
Manufacturer's name	N/A

(7.3%) low-ranked. The other 288 questions (58.7%) were not contained in our PDB. Since the clusters have similar number of question sentences, we expected that these numbers were almost the same each other; however, the top-ranked cluster was associated with many questions in the conversation corpus. This is because of the short length of our corpus, which averaged 36.5 sentences for each conversation.

Figure 6 shows the cumulative number of the question sentences in the conversation corpus that were contained in our PDB while the number of the questioners is increased. This demonstrates that only one questioner could create most of the top-ranked questions; however, some of the top-ranked questions were overlooked and few questions assigned to the other clusters were created. The coverage rate improved linearly till about 20 questioners, and over 20 questioners, the improvement of each cluster except low-ranked saturated. Consequently, we consider 20 questioners are reasonable to collect personal questions sufficiently. Even though a larger size of a PDB possibly contains more questions in the corpus since the low-ranked cluster improved steadily, it seems insufficient when considering the slowdown of improvement at 20 questioners.

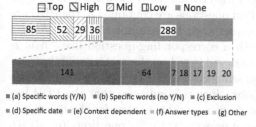

Fig. 5. Cluster assignment of the questions in the conversation corpus

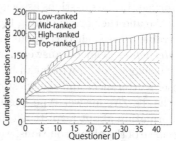

Fig. 6. Cluster assignment of the questions in the conversation corpus

To answer the rest of the questions (*None* in Fig. 5), it is important to analyze the reason why they are not contained in our PDB. Table 7 shows the classification of

Table 7. Reasons why questions were not contained in PDB

Reason	Examples	#
(a) Limited by specific words (answer type: Yes/No)	Do you know Gero-onsen spa?	141 (48.9%)
(b) Limited by specific words (answer type: not Yes/No)	What is your recommendation for Italy?	64 (22.2%)
(c) Includes words that exclude a specific word (e.g., except for)	What did you play any other instrument except the clarinet?	7 (2.4%)
(d) Limited to a specific date or time (e.g., to-day's lunch)	What did you eat for lunch today?	18 (6.2%)
(e) Assumes a conversation context	What was up that you couldn't sleep till morning?	17 (5.9%)
(f) Different answer types (Yes/No or factoid questions)	How long have you lived at your current address?	19 (6.5%)
(g) Other	What do you have delicious dishes that you have cooked?	20(6.9%)

the reasons and their examples, and Fig. 5 illustrates the proportion of each reason. In Fig. 5, 71.1% (205) of the reasons were (a) and (b). They contain specific words, such as *Gero-onsen spa* or *for Italy*, which limit the question subjects. For questions whose answer type is *Yes/No*, specific questions can be easily created with typical phrases and such specific words as "*Do you know Gero-onsen spa?*" or "*Do you like Gero-onsen spa?*". Even though (a) seems to be answerable since the answer type is *Yes/No*, it is difficult to maintain the consistency with the other answers. The answer "*No*" will help to avoid the inconsistency, but such agents that always say "*No*" would irritate users. The questions for reason (b) can also be answered using stochastic response generation methods [15], which generate sentences related to user utterances by leveraging word dependencies in a corpus; however, it is also difficult to avoid inconsistency. The questions of reason (e) are more difficult to answer, since such questions require understanding of deep contexts of conversation to generate answers.

On the other hand, (c) and (d) can be easily answered by substituting the other question categories without such limitations or exclusions as *today* or *except the clarinet*. In the questions associated with reason (f), those whose answer type is *Yes/No* and the corresponding factual questions are contained in the PDB are answerable with such corresponding questions. For example, "*Do you have a favorite actor?*" can be answered with a corresponding question like "*Who is your favorite actor?*", which can be retrieved based on the sentence similarity of the user's utterances and the question sentences in the PDB. When the PDB has only the *Yes/No* answer type questions, since this indicates that the PDB has no information about favorite actors, *No* is a suitable answer for the questions.

Because of the above solutions, we can recover 44 (15.2%) questions [(c),(d),(f)] with the PDB itself; this improvement increases the coverage rate to 50.2% (246/490), which seems almost the upper bound of this approach. Even though the other 141 (48.9%) questions of (a) are answerable with a large text corpus and 64 (22.2%) questions of (b) are potentially answerable with stochastic response generation methods, they potentially conflict with other answers.

3.2   Answer Types and Extended Named Entities

The classification of the answers gives us another view of the analysis that reveals the subjects of frequently-asked questions. Table 8 shows the distribution of the answer types with associated Extended Named Entities (ENEs) [12] that consists of about 200 Named Entity types. The answer types were originally defined in Nagata et al. [7]. We added a small modification that integrates *Explanation: cause* and *Explanation: principle* to *Explanation: reason* and obtained 21 answer types.

The most frequent answer type was *Yes/No* with 60% of the PDB. PDB contains so many noun-driven questions such as *"Do you like sushi?"* or *"Do you know Woodstock from Snoopy?"* because they can be created to match the number of nouns. The *Yes/No* restriction also accelerates the appearance of such answer types. In the conversation corpus, the most frequent answer type is *Yes/No* (143/202, 70.7%), and the second is *Name: named entity* (41/202, 20.2%); the other answer types scarcely appeared in the corpus.

Table 8. Answer types and Extended Named Entities (ENEs)

Major type	Sub type	ENE examples
Yes/No (16255)	Yes/No (16255)	No ENE (16225)
Explanation (2528)	Association (70)	Person (18)Dish (18)No ENE (16)
	Reputation (447)	No ENE (447)
	Reason (56)	No ENE (56)
	True identity (2)	No ENE (2)
	Method (243)	No ENE (242),Dish (1)
	Meaning (64)	No ENE (59),Product_Other (5)
	Other (1646)	No ENE (1632),Incident_Other (7)
Quantity (2337)	Money (235)	Money (235)
	Period (354)	Period_Time (251),Period_Year (84)
	Hour (31)	Time_Top_Other (19),Era (8)
	Time (134)	Time (134)
	Date (135)	Date (135)
	Other (1448)	Frequency (276),N_Product (239),Age (218)
Name (4339)	Organization name (320)	Company (192),Show_Organization (48)
	Location name (836)	Province (260),Country (144)
	Named entity (2571)	Dish (415),Product_Other (337)
	Person name (444)	Person (444)
	Web site (11)	Product_Other(11)
	Other (157)	No ENE (151),Name_Other (6)
Other (1136)	Selection (1012)	No ENE (275),Dish (169)
	Description (2)	No ENE (2)
	Phrase (122)	No ENE (121),Public_Institution (1)

Except for *No ENE*, most ENEs are annotated to the questions whose answer types are *Name* or *Quantity*, since the ENEs are defined to categorize such entities. Table 9 shows the frequently appearing ENEs and example sentences for each of the answer types. Over half of the questions associated with the *Name* answer type were labeled with the most frequently 10 ENEs. In the conversation corpus, except for *No ENE*, the most frequent ones were *Dish* (10), *Movie* (9) and *Music* (5). Since the speakers in our conversational corpus used pseudonyms to speak to another speaker, the questions with ENE *Person* did not appear in the conversation corpus.

In the answer types *Explanation* and *Quantity*, the most frequent subtype was *Other*, which indicates that our answer types were inadequate to classify them. Even though the ENEs complemented the classification of *Quantity*, they could not complement the classification of the questions whose answer type was *Explanation*, since the answers associated with these questions are described with sentences, not with the words for which the ENEs are designed.

Table 9. Frequent ENEs

(a) Name (# is 4339)

ENE name	# of sentences
Person	444 (10%)
Dish	415 (9%)
Product_Other	348 (8%)
Province	260 (5%)
Company	192 (4%)
Position_Vocation	192 (4%)
Music	161 (3%)
Country	144 (3%)
Sport	125 (2%)
Food_Other	115 (2%)

(b) Quantity (# is 2337)

ENE name	# of sentences
Frequency	276 (11%)
Period_Time	251 (10%)
N_Product	239 (10%)
Money	235 (10%)
Age	218 (9%)
N_Person	173 (7%)
Date	135 (5%)
Time	134 (5%)
Physical_Extent	114 (4%)
Period_Year	84 (3%)

3.3 Topic Labels

We annotated *Topic labels* to aggregate question categories. These labels are designed to integrate the question categories that have similar subjects but are divided because of the difference of limitations, answer types, and grammatical tenses. We expect that these labels enable us to investigate the subjects of the questions more clearly. The information annotator aggregated question categories into topic labels based on the following aggregation types.

(a) **Specific words.** This aggregates question categories with specific words into one with more abstract words: e.g., *Whether you tend to be angry* and *Whether you are romantic* into *Your Character*.

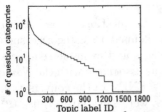

Fig. 7. Distribution of question categories by topic labels

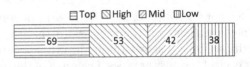

Fig. 8. Questions in conversation corpus assigned to each topic label cluster

Table 10. Examples of topic labels

(a) Top-ranked labels (20 or more categories, 1st-77th, 2576 categories, 5779 sentences, average number in each category is 2.24)

Topic labels	# of category
Favorite foods or dishes	137
Character	121
Opinions to politics	78
Available movements	64
Your appearances	62
Meal style/custom	62
Policy of child cares/education	55
Ideal sort of marriage partner	54
School lives	54
Relationship with your family	51

(b) High-ranked labels (19 to 11 categories, 78st-171th, 2384 categories, 6682 sentences, average number in each category is 2.80)

Topic labels	# of category
Something with which you played in childhood	19
Whether you play sports/Exercise habits	19
Whether you have a child/Personality of the child	19
Whether you have a favorite place	19
Using SNS	18
Person who chooses your clothes	11
Whether you like/dislike bugs	11
Whether you enjoy works	11
Weak point/Inferiority complex	11
Whether you like yourself	11

(c) Mid-ranked labels (10 to 6 categories, 172st-337th, 2561 categories, 6995 sentences, average number in each category is 2.73)

Topic labels	# of category
Favorite books/Whether you like reading books	10
Whether you like trips	10
Favorite downtown	10
Whether you like art/art museums	10
The way you take a bath	7
Your favorite rice	7
Whether you like sea or mountain	6
Amusement parks where you have been	6
Frequency of going beauty shop	6
Favorite sushi	6

(d) Low-ranked labels (5 to 1 categories, 338th-1178th, 2561 categories, 7139 sentences, average number in each category is 2.78)

Topic labels	# of category
Whether you agree to invite the Tokyo Olympic	5
Whether you have a debt/Sum of a debt	5
Whether you have a credit card	5
Political affiliates	5
Whether you are a morning or nocturnal person	5
Mental age	1
Whether you want to cosplay	1
Whether you take sunglasses	1
Whether you have hit someone	1
Whether you came the first love	1

(b) **Resemble questions.** This integrates similar question categories with nuanced differences: e.g., *Whether you like cooking, Whether you are good at cooking* and *Whether you can cook.*

(c) **Negative questions.** This integrates negative and question categories with the opposite meaning: e.g., *Whether you don't have some disliked foods* with *Whether you have some disliked foods.*

(b) **Answer types.** This integrates question categories, of which only the answer types are different: e.g., *Whether you like favorite sports* and *Your favorite sports.*

First, we counted the question categories in each topic label to examine how the topic labels aggregate the question categories. Figure 7 illustrates the distribution of the numbers of question categories in each topic. The total was 1763, the average number of question categories by each topic was 5.71, and the average number of answer types by each topic was 1.95. While only 40% of the question categories are associated with two or more question sentences, 70% of the topics consist of two or more question categories.

Next, we sorted and classified the topic labels into four clusters in the same manner as the question categories. Table 10 shows the clusters of the topic labels. Figure 8 illustrates the number of questions assigned to each cluster. Table 10(a) shows that the top-ranked topic labels contained over 50 question categories. Since the subjects of question categories contained with these topic labels had subject-specific words such as *Ethnic* in "*Do you like Ethnic dishes?*", these topic labels were composed of a large number of question categories. On the other hand, in the low-ranked topic labels, the subject of categories was too specific such as *cosplay*; this is the reason why such categories were not integrated with the other categories.

4   Conclusion

We proposed an approach that collects many questions about personality to develop a large scale Person Database (PDB). We analyzed the statistics of our PDB and the differences with questions from real conversations. Our analysis shows that a PDB, composed of over 26 K questions, contains 50.2% of the questions from the conversations. This coverage rate was almost saturated with about 20 question-generators.

Future work will apply the created PDB to conversational agents. To answer personal questions, recognizing question categories is a promising approach. Filtering with other information, such as answer types, will also improve the performance of generating reasonable answers. Generating questions in the PDB is another interesting way to improve such agents. The collected questions are suitable to be asked to any person and to trigger new conversation subjects; these are essential abilities for conversational agents.

Acknowledgement. We would like to thank the members of Advanced Speech and Language Technology Group, Audio, Speech, and Language Media Project, NTT Media Intelligence Laboratories for jointly creating the PDB.

References

1. Batacharia, B., Levy, D., Catizone, R., Krotov, A., Wilks, Y.: CONVERSE: a conversational companion. Machine Conversations, pp. 205–215 (1999)
2. Bickmore, T., Cassell, J.: Relational Agents: A Model and Implementation of Building User Trust. In: Proceedings of the SIGCHI Conference on Human Factors in Computing Systems, pp. 396–403 (2001)
3. Caspi, A., Roberts, B.W., Shiner, R.L.: Personality development: stability and change. Annual Review of Psychology 56, 453–484 (2005)

4. Higashinaka, R., Imamura, K., Meguro, T., Miyazaki, C., Kobayashi, N., Sugiyama, H., Hirano, T., Makino, T., Matsuo, Y.: Towards an open domain conversational system fully based on natural language processing. In: Proceedings of the 25th International Conference on Computational Linguistics (2014)
5. John, O.P., Srivastava, S.: The Big Five trait taxonomy: History, measurement, and theoretical perspectives. No. 510 (1999)
6. Mairesse, F., Walker, M.: PERSONAGE: Personality generation for dialogue. In: Proceedings of the Annual Meeting of the Association For Computational Linguistics, pp. 496–503 (2007)
7. Nagata, M., Saito, K., Matsuo, Y.: Japanese natural language retrieval system: Web Answers. In: Proceedings of the Annual Meeting of the Association of Natural Language Processing, p. B2–2 (2006) (in Japanese)
8. Meguro, T., Higashinaka, R., Minami, Y., Dohsaka, K.: Controlling Listening-oriented Dialogue using Partially Observable Markov Decision Processes. In: Proceedings of the 23rd International Conference on Computational Linguistics, pp. 761–769 (2010)
9. Nisimura, R., Nishihara, Y., Tsurumi, R., Lee, A., Saruwatari, H., Shikano, K.: Takemaru-kun: Speech-oriented Information System for Real World Research Platform. In: Proceedings of the First International Workshop on Language Understanding and Agents for Real World Interaction, pp. 70–78 (2003)
10. Ritter, A., Cherry, C., Dolan, W.: Data-Driven Response Generation in Social Media. In: Proceedings of the 2011 Conference on Empirical Methods in Natural Language Processing, pp. 583–593 (2011)
11. Rossen, B., Lok, B.: A crowdsourcing method to develop virtual human conversational agents. International Journal of Human-Computer Studies 70(4), 301–319 (2012)
12. Sekine, S., Sudo, K., Nobata, C.: Extended Named Entity Hierarchy. In: LREC (2002)
13. Shibata, M., Nishiguchi, T., Tomiura, Y.: Dialog System for Open-Ended Conversation Using Web Documents. Informatica 33, 277–284 (2009)
14. Singh, P., Lin, T., Mueller, E.T., Lim, G., Perkins, T., Zhu, W.L.: Open Mind Common Sense: Knowledge Acquisition from the General Public. In: Meersman, R., Tari, Z. (eds.) CoopIS/DOA/ODBASE 2002. LNCS, vol. 2519, pp. 1223–1237. Springer, Heidelberg (2002)
15. Sugiyama, H., Meguro, T., Higashinaka, R., Minami, Y.: Open-domain Utterance Generation for Conversational Dialogue Systems using Web-scale Dependency Structures. In: Proceedings of the 14th Annual SIGdial Meeting on Discourse and Dialogue, pp. 334–338 (2013)
16. Tidwell, L.C., Walther, J.B.: Computer-Mediated Communication Effects on Disclosure, Impressions, and Interpersonal Evaluations. Human Communication Research 28(3), 317–348 (2002)
17. Wong, W., Cavedon, L., Thangarajah, J., Padgham, L.: Strategies for Mixed-Initiative Conversation Management using Question-Answer Pairs. In: Proceedings of the 24th International Conference on Computational Linguistics, pp. 2821–2834 (2012)

Design Guidelines for a Virtual Coach
for Post-Traumatic Stress Disorder Patients

Myrthe Tielman[1], Willem-Paul Brinkman[1], and Mark A. Neerincx[1,2]

[1] Delft University of Technology, Delft, The Netherlands
[2] TNO Human Factors, Soesterberg, The Netherlands

Abstract. Patients with Post Traumatic Stress Disorder (PTSD) often
need to specify and relive their traumatic memories in therapy to relieve
their disorder, which can be a very painful process. One new development
is an internet-based guided self-therapy system (IBGST), where people
work at home and a therapist is remotely involved. We propose to enrich
an IBGST with a virtual coach to motivate and assist the patient during
the therapy. We have created scenarios and requirements for an IBGST
coach and discussed these with 10 experts in structured interviews. From
these interviews, we have identified 10 important guidelines to assist with
the design of a virtual coach assisting with PTSD treatment.

Keywords: Virtual coach, PTSS, Guidelines, Structured interviews.

1 Introduction

An important upcoming role for virtual agents is coaching, the task of motivating
and assisting people to achieve their goals. Blanson-Henkemans et al. [1] show
that a virtual coach can motivate and support people successfully. Rizzo et al.
[2] present a virtual coach which can be used to assist Post-Traumatic Stress
Disorder (PTSD) patients by guiding them towards information.

PTSD is a mental disorder following one or more traumatic experiences with
symptoms such as intrusive memories of the traumatic event, dissociative reactions and irritable behavior [3]. One of the most practiced treatments for PTSD
is Cognitive Behavioral Therapy (CBT) with exposure, which is the process of
exposing the patient to stimuli which are related to the traumatic memory and
will elicit a fear response.

A new development within the treatment of PTSD is an internet-based guided
self-therapy (IBGST) system, where people work at home and a therapist is only
remotely involved. In this paper we will focus on the Multi-Model Memory Restructuring (3MR) system [4], which allows patients to structure memories and
follow exposure-therapy on their own PC through creating memories on a visual
timeline and adding media such as photos, music and text. An additional functionality is the possibility to recreate personal memories in a 3D environment.
One difficulty is that exposure treatments can be very painful and possibly de-
motivating at times. For this reason, we believe that a virtual coach would be
a very useful addition to the system. Such a coach could be capable of offering

T. Bickmore et al. (Eds.): IVA 2014, LNAI 8637, pp. 434–437, 2014.
© Springer International Publishing Switzerland 2014

Table 1. Guidelines for a virtual coach for PTSD

Guideline & Suggestions for use by virtual coach
Motivate: Compliment patients, when they have a hard time, explain that this is normal, remind them of personal goals.
Take patient seriously: Let the patients decide if they are ready to end therapy, do not explain what they already know.
Protect patient: Build in relaxation exercises for when exposure becomes too much, give relapse-prevention.
Be down to earth: Be very factual, never act shocked, do not show many emotions, use simple, unaffected language.
Personalize: When motivating, mention specific things about this person and progress, adapt gender and age to fit patient.
Transparency: Be clear on what is going to happen and the coach's capabilities, explain why the patient needs to do things.
Avoid negative reinforcement: Do not reflect too much on negative things, never give negative feedback, never act disappointed.
Protect patients from themselves: Too much choice can lead to dissatisfaction, discourage avoidance behavior.
Psychoeducation: Put the progress and therapy into a theoretical frame, explain why things need to be done and why they work.
Acknowledge: Acknowledge the tension and emotional state of the patient, let them know the coach has heard them.

Table 2. A decomposition of the guideline of Motivation for a virtual coach for PTSD

Motivational theme	Explanation for use by virtual coach
Compliment	Give concrete, but many compliments
Empathy	Show empathy, but never include strong feelings
Evaluate	Set concrete goals to evaluate progress and outcome
Doing badly is not possible	There is no 'wrong' way to do things
Personalize	Motivate in a personalized way, be as concrete as possible
Be positive	Give positive feedback and reflect most on positive things

personalized and motivational assistance during the therapy process, increasing trust in the therapy and hope in a positive outcome.

In this paper, we present the first steps towards developing such a virtual coach for patients with PTSD working with the IBGST 3MR system. Because of differences between PTSD patients we have chosen to focus on two specific patient groups, namely victims of childhood sexual abuse (CSA) and military veterans.

2 Structured Interviews

To determine the specific user requirements for PTSD patients, we have designed scenarios with discussed these in structured interviews with 10 experts.

We adopted a scenario-based approach to inform the experts on the context in which our coach would be operating. The scenarios represented the types of sessions a patient would follow during treatment including a possible way in which the virtual coach could assist and also described aspects of behavior of the virtual coach which were based on literature on motivation [5] and medical communication guidelines [6]. From the scenarios we identified requirements for the coach, dealing with topics such as facial expressions, giving explanations on the therapy and motivation. From these requirements we formulated strong claims such as 'It would pose a problem if the virtual coach had the same characteristics with each patient' to stimulate a discussion. In structured interviews, we presented the scenarios and claims to 10 experts specialized in trauma treatment. The interviews were conducted in 6 sessions, each with 1 to 3 experts present. Each session discussed between 6 and 24 claims.

All interviews were recorded and the statements of the experts were written down. After this, we determined the underlying guideline and grouped the statements. From this analysis, we derived the guidelines as shown in Table 1. From the contexts, we can also present some suggestions for the use of each guideline. Motivating a patient was mentioned often, so we also considered what the experts said on motivation in more detail and identified six ways of motivating, as shown in Table 2.

3   Discussion and Conclusion

A first observation we can make of our guidelines is that they agree with the principles identified by Miller and Rollnick and Wouda at al. [5,6]. Another thing to consider is the role of our virtual coach. Based on the guidelines identified we can say that the coach can be a safe-guard, an educator and a motivator. These three roles correspond to roles a human therapist would also have, but a virtual coach does have its own limitations and possibilities which set it apart. Opportunities for a virtual coach may lie with being down to earth and personalization. A virtual coach will never have strong emotional reactions to traumatic memories which would need to be kept in check and a virtual coach has the unique quality that appearance, age and gender can be adapted specifically for a patient. Another difference which is connected to personalization is the support of memory retrieval. Therapists typically ask questions to assist patients with remembering, and it is important that these questions are well tailored to the patient. For humans natural language is the key ingredient, which is challenging for a virtual coach. However, because the coach is embedded into a system it has more modalities available. A coach could react to items which are placed in the application, for instance ask who is present in a photograph or a video. Another example is that a coach could notice how many items are added when specific questions are asked to keep track of which questions work well for which patient.

To conclude this paper, we would like to give examples of some of the ways in which our guidelines could be applied to specific functions and behavior of a virtual coach. These are presented in Table 3.

Table 3. Examples of behavior for a virtual coach for PTSD, based on the guidelines

Potential behavior of a virtual coach coach	Guideline
When patients fill in how they feel, mention that you have heard them, i.e. 'I notice you are feeling distressed now.'	Acknowledge
In the beginning of a session, explain what is going to happen.	Transparency
If the patient indicates wishing to quit, remind them of their goals.	Motivate
Let the patient choose the gender of their coach.	Personalization
Be factual in complementing, so do not say 'Great job, amazing, you are wonderful', but 'You completed this task, well done'.	Be down to earth
Never express a negative emotion. Whenever the patient fails to do something, do not punish but ask them why they did not do it.	do not reinforce the negative
If distress is very high, explain that this is normal and will decrease.	Psychoeducation
Monitor symptoms, if these keep increasing, notify a therapist.	Protect patient
Whenever explaining something for the second time, state this explicitly. 'I know you have heard this before, but...'	Take patient seriously
Do not let patients decide when to start with exposure by themselves, assist them in setting a date.	Protect patient from themselves

Acknowledgements. This work is part of the research programme VESP, which is supported by the Netherlands Organization for Scientific Research (NWO), program Creative Industry (project number 314-99-104).

References

1. Blanson-Henkemans, O.A., van der Mast, C.A., van der Boog, P.J., Neerincx, M.A., Lindenberg, J., Zwetsloot-Schonk, B.J.: An online lifestyle diary with a persuasive computer assistant providing feedback on self-management. Technology and Health Care 17, 253–267 (2009)
2. Rizzo, A., Lange, B., Buckwalter, J.G., Forbell, E., Kim, J., Sagae, K., Williams, J., Difede, J., Rothbaum, B.O., Reger, G., Parsons, T., Kenny, P.: Simcoach: an intelligent virtual human system for providing healthcare information and support. In: Proc. 8th Intl Conf. Disability, Virtual Reality & Associated Technologies (2010)
3. American Psychiatric Association: Diagnostic and Statistical Manual of Nental Disorders, 5th edn. American Psychiatric Association (2013)
4. Brinkman, W.P., Vermetten, E., van den Steen, M., Neerincx, M.: Cognitive engineering of a military multi-modal memory restructuring system. Journal of CyberTherapy and Rehabilitation 4(1), 83–99 (2011)
5. Miller, W.R., Rollnick, S.: Motivational interviewing: Preparing people to change addictive behavior. Guilford Press, New York (1991)
6. Wouda, J., van de Wiel, H., van Vliet, K.: Medische communicatie, Gespreksvaardigheden voor de arts. De Tijdstroom (2000)

A Virtual Therapist for Speech and Language Therapy

Sarel van Vuuren[1,2] and Leora R. Cherney[3,4]

[1] University of Colorado Boulder, Institute of Cognitive Science, Boulder, CO, USA
[2] University of Colorado Anschutz Medical Campus, School of Medicine,
Department of Physical Medicine and Rehabilitation, Denver, CO, USA
sarel@colorado.edu
[3] Rehabilitation Institute of Chicago,
Center for Aphasia Research and Treatment, Chicago, IL, USA
[4] Northwestern University, Feinberg School of Medicine,
Department of Physical Medicine and Rehabilitation, Chicago, IL, USA
lcherney@ric.org

Abstract. A virtual therapist (VT) capable of modeling visible speech and directing speech and language therapy is presented. Three perspectives of practical and clinical use are described. The first is a description of treatment and typical roles that the VT performs in directing participation, practice and performance. The second is a description of techniques for modeling visible speech and implementing tele-rehabilitation. The third is an analysis of performance of a system (*AphasiaRx*™) for delivering speech and language therapy to people with aphasia, with results presented from a randomized controlled cross-over study in which the VT provided two levels of cuing. Compared to low cue treatment, high cue treatment resulted in 2.3 times faster learning. The paper concludes with a discussion of the benefits of speech and language therapy delivered by the VT.

Keywords: Virtual agents, virtual therapists, speech and language therapy, aphasia treatment, tele-rehabilitation, tele-care, speech animation.

1   Introduction

For persons with aphasia (PWA), virtualization of treatment is critical given the prevalence of the disorder, effect it has on their ability to communicate, and general lack of access to long-term treatment options. This paper describes the role, implementation and performance of a virtual therapist (VT) for delivering speech and language therapy.

Aphasia is an acquired multi-modality disturbance of language, resulting from focal damage to the portions of the brain responsible for language. It impairs, to varying degrees, understanding and expression of oral language, reading and writing. It occurs with a wide range of neurologic disorders including stroke, brain tumor, cerebral trauma, intracranial surgical procedures, and degenerative neurological disorders [1]. An estimated 80,000 new cases of aphasia per year in the United States result from stroke alone, while the prevalence in the country overall has been estimated to exceed

T. Bickmore et al. (Eds.): IVA 2014, LNAI 8637, pp. 438–448, 2014.
© Springer International Publishing Switzerland 2014

one million people [2]. Effects are chronic and potentially long-term, with reduced language skills limiting participation in social, vocational, and recreational activities.

Services for persons with aphasia (PWAs) have been drastically shortened. Legislation has seriously curtailed the amount of treatment a PWA may receive after hospitalization. Often they may be eligible for only a limited number of treatment sessions for a limited period of time. In some cases, they may not receive any treatment for their communication disorder following their acute hospitalization [3]. Reduced resources (e.g. transportation difficulties, therapist shortages in rural areas) further limit available services. Given this state of affairs, it is imperative that clinicians provide treatment that results in the greatest improvement in the shortest amount of time— motiving a shift within the field to tele-rehabilitation for anywhere-access, and as described in this paper, reliance on a VT to maintain guidance, encouragement and fidelity.

1.1   Treatment with a Virtual Speech Therapist

Script treatment, whether delivered by human [4, 5], or computer [6, 7, 8], has been shown to be highly effective for treating PWAs. In script treatment, therapy is based on the oral production of scripts, which are short functional dialogs structured around communication of everyday activities. A computer program called *AphasiaScripts™* that we developed in 2004 is available from www.ric.org/aphasia, but its use of a proprietary VT with visible speech based on motion capture variable length concatenative synthesis [9], with resulting large footprint and restriction to computer only use, meant it was not suited for tele-rehabilitation across devices. Recently, we developed a new system called *AphasiaRx™*, designed to be more portable and functional, with a new VT that works across devices, and built-in web monitoring, scheduling and communication technologies. Fig. 1 shows a screen image.

The new system is designed to be easy to use by people with developmental and acquired disabilities, who might have fine motor skills difficulties. Navigation is done with a space bar, and in the case of a tablet, with the whole screen as a button. Activities are sequenced, leveled, and adaptive where possible, with guidance and feedback provided interactively by the VT. Because the treatment is repetitive, VT responses are limited to short cues to maximize practice time and treatment intensity.

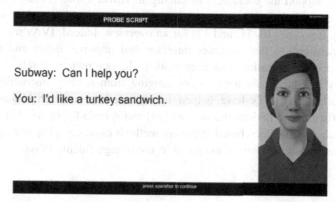

Fig. 1. Screen image from *AphasiaRx™* system with sentence for VT and PWA turn displayed

Treatment is structured around three phases of script practice:

1. The PWA listens to a script while it appears on the screen. The VT is visible and using a high quality recorded female voice, reads aloud, articulating carefully. Each word is read and highlighted on the screen.
2. Each sentence or conversation turn is read aloud twice in unison with the VT. Problem words can then be practiced repeatedly by clicking on them. Finally, the PWA independently reads aloud the whole sentence while it is recorded by the system, and is given the option to listen to the recording or practice the sentence again.
3. The conversation is practiced with assistance provided by the VT. Maximum support includes seeing written words, hearing the VT's voice during choral speaking, and watching her oral-motor movements. As the PWA masters the script, he or she can remove cues one by one, so that eventually practice simulates real conversation.

For the speech-language pathologist (SLP), built-in tools make authoring new scripts and treatment plans, assigning them to their clients, and monitoring their performance easy. Scripts can be typed into the program and recorded. Each spoken word is aligned automatically with each written word. Pause time between sentences and the amount of time allotted for each utterance can be adjusted to provide individualized optimal speaking time for each. Different scripts, treatment plans, and schedules can be assigned to individual clients with a built-in calendar. Data are automatically captured, summarized and available for analyses. During practice, key strokes, item responses and response times are recorded and summarized to provide daily and weekly logs showing how time was spent in each part of the program. Recordings of the speech attempts made by the PWA provide the SLP with additional means of assessing change over time.

1.2   Related Approaches in Other Areas

Many studies support the usefulness of intelligent virtual agents (IVAs) that are conversational, embodied, and/or animated for activities such as interaction, motivation and tutoring. E.g., see [10, 11, and 12] for an overview. Indeed, IVAs seem to add a "human dimension" to the computer interface that improve, direct and encourage participation, communication and accessibility. In our own research, IVAs have helped users in educational applications ranging from reading instruction [13] to science tutoring, and VTs have helped users remediate and rehabilitate speech-language difficulties in Parkinson's disease [14] and aphasia [7, 15, 16, 17]. For aphasia in particular, while video based treatment methods exist, e.g. [18], our approach to script treatment described here is unique in its use of high-fidelity IVAs.

2   Modeling and Implementation

There are many existing approaches for animating agents and speech to varying degrees of accuracy, with tradeoffs in computing, cost, flexibility and availability. Our goal is to implement therapy across a range of devices, yet maintain reasonable accuracy, simplicity, consistency, and control. This section explains briefly how this is done.

2.1   Visual Animation

For local or remote control of the VT's visible speech on computer, web and mobile devices, an approach that decouples modeling and animation is needed. To do this, we use a code book to capture visual variation. We assume that the visual realization of individual sounds vary depending on the phonetic context and manner of speaking, and that the temporal evolution depends predominantly on physiological and acoustic constraints governing movement of the oral-motor articulators during acoustic realization— though at different time scales and rates [19]. Using a code-book ensures that the link between speech and animation is in the choice of timing and indices.

Animation starts with a phoneme sequence and corresponding time-aligned audio, generated using a TTS engine or pre-recorded speech aligned with a speech recognizer [13]. The phoneme sequence is then mapped using a code-book to 3D morphs (or 2D images, depending on the application), so that individual phonemes correspond to a sequence of code-book indices in a one-to-many mapping, where the mapping depends on the dynamic realization of the phoneme as well as co-articulation effects.

Code-book entries represent the extremes of visual realizations of parts of phonemes with indices spanning a low 5-dimensional 'visual articulation' space, shown conceptually in Fig. 2. When rendered, the entries look somewhat like the images in Fig. 3.

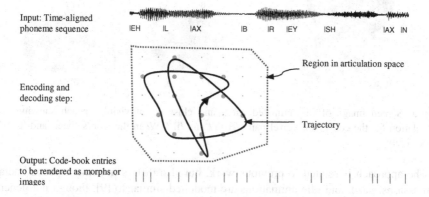

Fig. 2. Conceptual depiction of speech trajectory evolving in visual articulation space and quantization to code-book spanning the space. Actual space is 5 dimensional. The code-book maps a time-aligned phoneme sequence to a corresponding sequence of morphs or images to be rendered.

The space was designed manually using phonological, linguistic and morphological considerations to cover the range of speech locomotion observed in prototypical image sequences and videos that we collected across selected permutations of normally spoken phonemes, syllables and words. For this purpose, we assumed that the dynamic evolution of visible speech is relatively continuous and low-dimensional, so that it can be modeled as a process that traces a continuous trajectory within the space.

Rather than trying to model the articulation space parametrically, the code-book quantizes a convex region of the space on a non-linear sparse grid, allowing the trajectory contained within to be approximated as a sequence of code-book indices. Convexity, monotonicity and smoothness of the space are part of the design so that interpolation and extrapolation can be used. Because indices correspond to grid points, co-articulation, speech rate, and speech effort are modelled by applying transformations directly to the sequences. The transformations are applied at run time and are relatively simple smoothing, blending, scaling and translational functions.

Finally, the resultant sequence of indices are used to recover from the code-book a sequence of high-dimensional morphs (or static images, depending on the application) of the mouth, lips, teeth and tongue, to be interpolated and rendered at the device supported frame rate (Fig. 3). For computer or mobile devices, OpenGL is used to render 3D models, whereas for web applications, HTML5 and WebGL or pure images are used to render 3D models or 2.5D approximations, respectively. We chose this implementation over existing methods (e.g., www.facefx.com), because we wanted full control of the implementation across devices in order to optimize it for tele-rehabilitation.

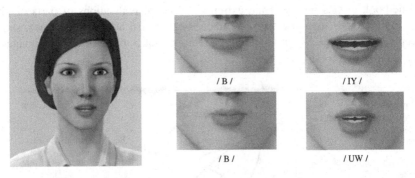

Fig. 3. Screen image of the animated agent and close up of visible speech showing co-articulation for the consonant-vowel pairs /B IY/ and /B UW/ in the words 'beet' and 'boot', respectively.

The approach is related to previous work, but also differs in some aspects. Facial expressions, gaze, and idle animations are modelled similar to [9], though not generated from speech as in [20]. The articulation space is a composite blend of various articulation parameters, making it somewhat different from other parametric approaches [21, 22], but similar in that it allows explicit manipulation of the visible speech. The code-book is designed to allow physiological and articulatory phonetic manipulation of the visible speech, making it different from other data-driven approaches such as video/image stitching [12] and unit-concatenation [9], but similar in that it attempts to model variation using code-book entries, though its entries differ from visemes. The coding scheme, while suitable for transmission, captures visual information at a more linguistic level than the facial animation parameters in the M-PEG 4 standard.

The visible speech produced by the agent has been qualitatively reviewed by speech language pathologists, linguists and audiologists, and we have controlled experiments underway to test the accuracy clinically. Thus, we cannot currently provide specific results regarding visible accuracy or speech intelligibility. Instead, in Section 3 we demonstrate ecological validity with a randomized controlled cross-over study for a speech and language therapy treatment that compared two conditions, one in which the VT modeled speech production, and one with little modeling of speech production.

2.2   Tele-rehabilitation

Implementation follows similar considerations for fidelity and access as [13, 15, 16], but is more flexible and sophisticated in that the system described here can work across a number of different devices. It can operate either as a standalone native application on a computer, tablet, or mobile device, or as a web application in a cloud-based client-server configuration suitable for tele-rehabilitation (Table 1). For the latter, communication, synchronization and access control between the clients (applications) and server are done entirely with the HTTP/S protocol and asynchronous calls.

While this paper focuses on an application for aphasia treatment, the VT and system is suitable for applications that extend beyond virtual speech and language therapy. For example, the architecture's underlying capabilities for web and mobile rehabilitation have been used between Boulder, Denver, and Toronto in a near real-time non-linear context aware prompting system (NCAPS) for people with cognitive disabilities, helping them to navigate and overcome procedural challenges in the workplace [23].

Table 1. The system client-server architecture suitable for tele-rehabilitation

Client-side User Interface (Apps)	Asynchronous HTTP/S Communication	Server-side Control and Data (Cloud)
Computer Web Tablet/Mobile	User and sensor inputs → ← System outputs: Animation control, audio, video, HTML	Task/state management, monitoring, configuration, application and access control, application and user data

3   Clinical Application

A randomized controlled cross-over study using the VT was conducted to investigate the effect of high or low cuing on treatment outcomes over time. It was approved by the IRB of Northwestern University and done at the Rehabilitation Institute of Chicago.

3.1   Methodology

Eight participants were recruited and randomized to receive intensive computer-based script training differing in the amount of high or low cuing provided during treatment. Participants had chronic aphasia resulting from a single left hemisphere stroke (age range 25-66 years, m=52.0, sd = 14.0; time post-onset range 8-59 months, m=26.4, sd=19.2), with severities mild-moderate to severe as measured by the Aphasia Quotient of the Western Aphasia Battery-Revised [24] (range 28.1-80.1, m=58.0, sd=18.5).

In the high cue treatment condition, participants could hear the VT during listening, choral reading and reading aloud, with auditory cues (therapist speaking) and visual cues (therapist's mouth movements) available at the start, during and after practice. In the low cue condition, they received visual and auditory cues when listening to the script being read aloud *initially*, and *after* practice; but did not receive auditory and visual support *during* sentence practice, working instead from the written cues only.

Confounds were controlled for with a cross-over design with three weeks of treatment in one condition, followed by a three week washout period and three weeks of treatment in the second condition; random assignment, and stratification of participants to treatment conditions; control for treatment time; and design and use of similar though different scripts in each condition with scripts matched for length, morphological, phonological and grammatical complexity. Scripts consisted of 10 sentences each.

Scripts were practiced 6 days per week, for up to 90 minutes per day in 3 sessions. Practice and testing were done at home on a loaned laptop with sessions scheduled automatically using the system calendar. Participant responses were measured over time: in 3 sessions before treatment started to establish a baseline, then in separate sessions twice per week during each of the three treatment weeks to assess learning, and finally, once in the week after treatment finished to assess treatment effectiveness.

Performance was measured by averaging the sentence level word accuracy of participants' production of 10 sentences during each assessment session. Sentences were 10 words in length. Accuracy of words were rated using a previously validated 6 point scale and the overall session score expressed on a scale from 0 to 100%. For the time period and measures reported here, a total of 16,000 words (8 participants x 2 conditions x 10 sessions x 10 sentences x 10 words) were collected, recorded and scored. Inter-rater reliability on a 10% subset of sentences was 0.94 (Pearson's r).

In previous work we discussed the implications of this study for speech-language pathology and reported pre- and post-treatment results conditioned on aphasia severity [17]. There, we used Cohen's d to compute effect sizes on gains, with d>0.8 considered a large effect. When combining the high cue and low cue conditions (16 samples, i.e. including all participants for N=8 and two treatment conditions), the effect size for computer treatment was large and statistically significant (d=1.5, p<0.0125).

In the following, we report new results showing the differential effects of high cue and low cue treatment *over time* when delivered by the VT described in Section 2.

3.2   Effect of Cuing on Treatment over Time

Figs. 4a and 4b show the effect of treatment over time. Gain in scores (% accuracy) over baseline are shown before, during and after treatment. Gains in both high and low cue treatment conditions increased rapidly once treatment started.

Fig. 4a shows the effect of treatment and cumulative practice hours for one participant. Practice time in both conditions were matched, and congruent with gains. At the end of treatment gains leveled off. For a perfect score, the participant's maximum attainable gains were limited to 36.6% in the high cue condition and 38.3% in the low cue condition, suggesting possible ceiling effects during the latter half of the treatment period. Limited participant pre-training before the treatment period can also be seen.

Fig. 4b shows average gain scores (% accuracy) over baseline for all 8 participants, with the effects of high cue and low cue treatment shown separately over time. Values were computed by averaging samples for participants in each condition over both the time and value axes. The maximum gain that could be attained depended on the participant's starting level and ranged from 14.8% to 38.3% in the low cue treatment condition, and 15.2% to 37.3% in the high cue treatment condition.

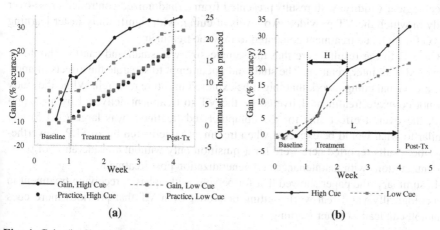

Fig. 4. Gain (in % accuracy) over baseline for high and low cue treatment conditions. Gains increased rapidly once treatment started, with gains for high cue increasing faster than low cue treatment. **(a)** Gains and cumulative hours practiced for one participant. **(b)** Average gains for N=8 participants. Participants receiving high cue compared to low cue treatment reached the same level of gain faster, in about half the time.

Of the eight participants, six learned faster in the high cue condition. Indeed, gains supported findings from a post-treatment survey reported in [17] where 6 of 8 participants said they liked high cue treatment better.

High cue treatment on average led to faster learning and higher gains, with an estimated overall speedup of L/H=2.3 using the averages from Fig. 4b. This meant that when participants received high cue treatment, they on average learned more than twice as fast as when they received low cue treatment, reaching the same level of proficiency in less than half the time (1.3 weeks compared to 2.9 weeks from start of treatment).

Preliminary analyses with mixed effects models – often used in pharmacological studies of treatment and dosage response over time [25], showed the effect is statistically significant. A logistic mixed effects model fitted to the gains for all 8 PWAs and conditions, showed that cue level differentially and significantly affected gain over the treatment period $(\chi^2(1) = 10.98, p < 0.0009)$ [paper in preparation]. From the model, the predicted speedup for the difference in time to reach the same level of gain between the two conditions was L/H=2.34, similar to the non-parametric estimate from Fig. 4b.

4   Discussion and Conclusions

The paper described a virtual therapist (VT) for delivering speech and language therapy to persons with aphasia (PWA). Three different perspectives focusing on role, implementation and performance were provided, namely: how the VT directed participation, practice and performance in much the same way an SLP does; modeling and implementation considerations for visible speech and tele-rehabilitation; and evidence of ecological validity, with results presented from a randomized controlled cross-over study in which the VT provided two levels of cuing, with significantly faster learning (2.3x) for high cue treatment compared to low cue treatment.

Caveats to the results were that the sample size was small and caution should be exercised with interpretation. The study did not attempt to separate the effects of auditory and visual cuing– work that might be explored in future research. While the study did not compare treatment delivered by the VT to treatment delivered by an expert SLP, the overall effect size for the computerized treatment was large (d=1.5) and similar to what would be expected when treatment is delivered by an SLP. Nevertheless, the results reported here were for acquisition only without consideration of possible interactions with maintenance and generalization post-treatment.

In summary, the paper showed that for persons with aphasia, receiving treatment in an ecologically valid real-world setting delivered by a VT that provides more cues than not, can lead to faster learning.

Acknowledgements. Supported by the National Institute on Deafness and Other Communication Disorders, National Institutes of Health, Award 1R01DC011754 (to S.V.V. and L.R.C.). Animation research supported by University of Colorado Boulder, and platform research supported in part by the National Institute on Disability and

Rehabilitation Research, U.S. Department of Education, Award H133E090003 (to C. Bodine, www.rerc-act.org). The content is solely the responsibility of the authors and does not necessarily represent the official views of the funding organizations. Endorsement by the Federal Government should not be assumed. The authors do not have a financial interest in the product. Thanks are extended to Julia Carpenter, Rachel Hitch, Rosalind Hurwitz, Rosalind Kaye, Jaime Lee, Anita Halper, Audrey Holland, Michael C. Mozer, Nattawut Ngampatipatpong, Robert Bowen and Taylor Struemph.

References

1. Albert, M.L., Goodglass, H., Helm, N.A., Rubens, A.B., Alexander, M.P.: Clinical Aspects of Dysphagia. Springer, New York (1981)
2. NIH Pub No. 97-4257: National Institute on Deafness and Other Communication Disorders, Facts Sheet: Aphasia. Bethesda, MD: Author (2008)
3. Elman, R.J., Simmins-Mackie, N., Kagan, A.: Clinical services for aphasia: Feast or famine? Paper presented at the Annual Meeting of the American Speech-Language-Hearing Association, Chicago, Illinois (2003)
4. Holland, A., Milman, L., Munoz, M., Bays, G.: Scripts in the management of aphasia. Paper presented at the World Federation of Neurology, Aphasia and Cognitive Disorders Section Meeting, Villefranche, France (2002)
5. Youmans, G.L., Holland, A.L., Munoz, M., Bourgeois, M.: Script training and automaticity in two individuals with aphasia. Aphasiology 19, 435–450 (2005)
6. Cherney, L.R., Halper, A.S.: Novel Technology for Treating Individuals with Aphasia and Concomitant Cognitive Deficits. Topics in Stroke Rehabilitation 15(6), 542–554 (2008)
7. Lee, J.B., Kaye, R.C., Cherney, L.R.: Conversational script performance in adults with non-fluent aphasia: Treatment intensity and aphasia severity. Aphasiology 23(7), 885–897 (2009)
8. Manheim, L.M., Halper, A.S., Cherney, L.: Patient-Reported Changes in Communication after Computer-Based Script Training for Aphasia. Archives of Physical Medicine and Rehabilitation 90(4), 623–627 (2009), doi:10.1016/j.apmr.2008.10.022
9. Ma, J., Cole, R., Pellom, B., Ward, W., Wise, B.: Accurate visible speech synthesis based on concatenating variable length motion capture data. IEEE Transactions on Visualization and Computer Graphics 12(2), 266–276 (2006)
10. Moreno, R., Mayer, R., Spires, H., Lester, J.: The Case for Social Agency in Computer-Based Teaching: Do Students Learn More Deeply When They Interact with Animated Pedagogical Agents? Cognition and Instruction 192(2), 177–213 (2001)
11. Gratch, J., Rickel, J., André, E., Badler, N., Cassell, J., Petajan, E.: Creating interactive virtual humans: Some assembly required. IEEE Intelligent Systems 17(4), 54–63 (2002)
12. Cosatto, E., Ostermann, J., Graf, H.P., Schroeter, J.: Lifelike talking faces for interactive services. Proceedings of the IEEE: Special Issue on Human-Computer Multimodal Interface 91(9), 1406–1429 (2003)
13. Van Vuuren, S.: Technologies that power pedagogical agents. Educational Technology 24(1), 4–10 (2007)
14. Cole, R., Halpern, A., Ramig, L., Van Vuuren, S., Ngampatipatpong, N., Yan, J.: A Virtual Speech Therapist for Individuals with Parkinson Disease. Educational Technology 24(1), 51–55 (2007)

15. Cherney, L., Babbit, E., Kwang-Youn, K., Van Vuuren, S., Ngampatipatpong, N.: Aphasia Treatment over the Internet: A Randomized Placebo-Controlled Clinical Trial. In: Clinical Aphasiology Conference, Ft. Lauderdale, FL, May 31-June 4 (2011)
16. Cherney, L., Van Vuuren, S.: Telerehabilitation, Virtual Therapists and Acquired Neurologic Speech and Language Disorders. Seminars in Speech and Language 33(3), 243–257 (2012) PubMed PMID: 22851346
17. Cherney, L., Kaye, R., Van Vuuren, S.: Acquisition and Maintenance of Scripts in Aphasia: A Comparison of Two Cuing Conditions. American Journal of Speech-Language Pathology 23, S343–S360 (2014)
18. VAST speech aid. SpeakinMotion (2014), http://www.speakinmotion.com
19. Yang, H.H., Van Vuuren, S., Sharma, S., Hermansky, H.: Relevance of time-frequency features for phonetic and speaker-channel classification. Speech Communication 31(1), 35–50 (2000)
20. Marsella, S., Xu, Y., Lhommet, M., Feng, A., Scherer, S., Shapiro, A.: Virtual character performance from speech. In: Proceedings of the 12th ACM SIGGRAPH/Eurographics Symposium on Computer Animation, pp. 25–35. ACM (2013)
21. Cohen, M., Massaro, D.: Modeling coarticulation in synthetic visual speech. In: Thalmann, N.M., Thalmann, D. (eds.) Models and Techniques in Computer Animation, pp. 141–155. Springer (1994)
22. Pelachaud, C.: Visual Text-to-Speech. In: Pandzic, I.S., Forchheimer, R. (eds.) MPEG4 Facial Animation - The Standard, Implementations and Applications. John Wiley & Sons (2002)
23. Melonis, M., Mihailidis, A., Keyfitz, R., Grzes, M., Hoey, J., Bodine, C.: Empowering Adults With a Cognitive Disability Through Inclusion of Non-Linear Context Aware Prompting Technology (N-CAPS). In: RESNA Conference Proceedings, June 30 (2012)
24. Kertesz, A.: Western Aphasia Battery-Revised. PsychCorp., San Antonio (2007)
25. Pinheiro, J.C., Bates, D.M.: Mixed-Effects Models in S and S-PLUS. Springer (2000)

AsapRealizer 2.0: The Next Steps in Fluent Behavior Realization for ECAs

Herwin van Welbergen, Ramin Yaghoubzadeh, and Stefan Kopp*

Sociable Agents Group, CITEC, Fac. of Technology,
Bielefeld University, Germany

Abstract. Natural human interaction is highly dynamic and responsive: interlocutors produce utterances incrementally, smoothly switch speaking turns with virtually no delay, make use of on-the-fly adaptation and (self) interruptions, execute movement in tight synchrony, etc. We present the conglomeration of our research efforts in enabling the realization of such fluent interactions for Embodied Conversational Agents in the behavior realizer 'AsapRealizer 2.0' and show how it provides fluent realization capabilities that go beyond the state-of-the-art.

Keywords: AsapRealizer, Fluent Behavior Realization, BML 1.0, BMLA.

1 Introduction

Human conversations are highly dynamic, responsive interactions. In such interactions, utterances are produced incrementally [1,2], subject to on-the-fly adaptation (e.g. speaking louder to keep a challenged turn) and (self) interruptions. While listening, plans for next speaking contributions are constructed, allowing very rapid turn transitions [3]. Furthermore, conversations are characterized by interpersonal synchrony [4], including the alignment of movement rhythm (e.g. alignment of walking rhythm, exercise motion, postural sway or even breathing patterns) and smooth meshing/intertwining of behavior between the interlocutors (e.g., smooth turn-taking and backchannel feedback).

To enable such fluent interaction in Embodied Conversational Agents (ECAs) we must steer away from the traditional turn-based non-incremental interaction paradigm in which the ECA first fully analyzes user contributions and subsequently fully plans its contribution, which is then executed entirely ballistically (providing no adaptation in nor interruption of ongoing behavior). Although fluent interaction has recently become a hot research topic (see [5] for an overview), others have focused their research efforts mainly at incremental dialogue understanding and behavior planning (for example: [6]). Truly fluent interaction in ECAs *additionally* requires highly flexible behavior realization. This is a topic we have given a great deal of attention in the development of ECAs and dialogue systems within our two research groups (the Sociable Agents

---

* This research and development project is funded by the German Federal Ministry of Education and Research (BMBF) within the Leading-Edge Cluster Competition and managed by the Project Management Agency Karlsruhe (PTKA). The authors are responsible for the contents of this publication. The development of AsapRealizer 1.0 was conducted in collaboration with the Human Media Interaction group at the University of Twente.

T. Bickmore et al. (Eds.): IVA 2014, LNAI 8637, pp. 449–462, 2014.
© Springer International Publishing Switzerland 2014

Group at Bielefeld University and the Human Media Interaction Group at the University of Twente) in the last 10 years.

We present the conglomeration of our research in AsapRealizer, a BML 1.0 behavior realizer that unifies the fluent behavior realization capabilities that were required in several projects tackled within our research groups. AsapRealizer builds on two existing realizers from both our groups, that have focused on either incremental multimodal utterance construction [7] or interactional coordination [8] as isolated problems. In earlier work [9] we show that by combining the realization capabilities for incremental multimodal behavior construction and interactional coordination in a single realizer, we can enable interaction scenarios that go beyond the capabilities of these individual realizers.

While the preliminary version of AsapRealizer (1.0) [9] provided the specification of and an architecture framework for fluent behavior realization, it provided its implementation mainly for gesture. AsapRealizer 2.0 –discussed in this paper– generalizes AsapRealizer 1.0's capabilities by additionally implementing fluent realization capabilities for speech, gaze and facial expression. This required us to implement a novel adaptive gaze model and to embed a recently developed incremental and adaptive Text-To-Speech system [10].

In this paper we summarize and motivate AsapRealizer fluent realization capabilities and provide a more detailed description of the implementation of its novel capabilities. Additionally, we contribute a thorough comparison of AsapRealizer with the state-of-the-art in behavior realization in terms of incremental realization plan construction and on the fly adaptation of behavior.

2   Motivation

Over the course of more than 10 years, our research groups have developed several research applications in which fluent behavior realization played a key role (see Fig. 1 for some examples).

One of our first applications requiring fluent interaction was the virtual construction instructor Max [11]. Max cooperated with users in a construction task in Virtual Reality. While the interaction with Max was mostly turn-based, he still required incremental behavior realization from a fluent stream of multiple utterances, in which gestures were to be fluently connected. This required its realizer to adjust the timing and shape of ongoing behavior.

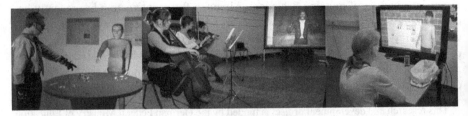

Fig. 1. Fluent behavior realization applications. Left: the virtual construction instructor Max, middle: the virtual conductor (photo: Henk Postma, Stenden Hogeschool), right: the daily assistant Billie

At the University of Twente, we have been interested in investigating and implementing ECA behavior for interactions in which there is simultaneous expressive behavior by a human interlocutor and an ECA. Prototypical applications for such behavior are a virtual dancer that aligns her movement both to movement of a human dance partner and to live music, a virtual orchestra conductor that conducts a real orchestra, and a virtual trainer that exercises together with a human trainee (see [12] for an overview). In all these applications the ECA exhibits tight coordination of movement timing with the interlocutor, which required both synchronization based on *predictions* from the ECA's own performance and that of the interlocutor and very flexible behavior realization in which the timing and shape (e.g. amplitude of movement) of behavior can be adapted on the fly. In Bielefeld, similar adaptivity in behavior realization was required in robotic speech-gesture synchronization [13]: the unreliable timing of robotic movement required an adaptable execution process in which the timing of speech is modified on-the-fly.

In more traditional dialog-based interfaces, both of our research groups have looked at going beyond turn-based interaction paradigms and providing attentive speakers that adapt their ongoing behavior based on interlocutor feedback and active listeners that continuously signal their understanding to a human speaker [14,15,16]. The implementation of behavior realization for attentive speakers is especially challenging. It requires graceful interruption of utterances (in speech, gesture, gaze, facial expression), the modification of ongoing behavior (e.g. speaking louder to keep the turn), partial rephrasing of ongoing behavior realizations (while keeping the rest of the realization plan intact) and the employment of several strategies to provide (the illusion of) very reactive behavior. The latter include the use of fillers (e.g. uhm) to keep the turn and gain some time for behavior planning, and the preplanning of (multiple alternative) utterances for instant later execution.

Beyond application in laboratory settings, we are currently employing AsapRealizer in a cooperation project (VASA/Verstanden) with a health care provider. The project aims to ascertain the feasibility (and acceptability) of spoken-language controlled daily assistants for people with cognitive impairments. Starting from the first Wizard-of-Oz prestudies, interruptible generation was employed, which in combination with the low latency led to easy recovery in situations with disputed floor. Quick and seamless generation and incremental processing are of paramount importance for the system, since participants understand small sequential chunks of information best [17].

In summary, incremental behavior plan construction, graceful interruption and adaptation of ongoing behavior have been essential capabilities for fluent behavior realization with AsapRealizer (see also Table 1). Adaptations of behavior may be steered: 1) by the behavior planner (top-down adaptations), for example when requesting the ECA to speak louder, 2) by the AsapRealizer itself (bottom-up adaptations), for example to achieve co-articulation between gestures on the fly and 3) by external constraints from the environment, for example to align the ECAs exercise movement to that of a user.

3   Fluent Behavior Realization Capabilities

We have developed the BML extension BMLA [5] to allow the specification of Asap-Realizer's fluent behavior realization capabilities. Within AsapRealizer, these capabili-

Table 1. Motivation for AsapRealizer's fluent behavior realization capabilities

Capability	Motivating Project(s)
Incremental plan construction	[11,12,13,14,15,16,17]
Graceful interruption	[14,15,16,17]
Top-down adaptation of ongoing behavior	[14,15,16]
Bottom up adaptation of ongoing behavior	[11,13]
Adaptations of ongoing behavior to the changing environment	[12]

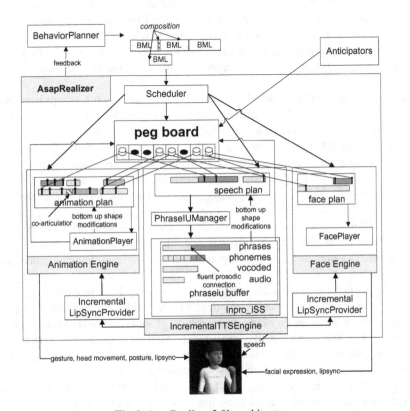

Fig. 2. AsapRealizer 2.0's architecture

ties are implemented both with a flexible architecture (see Fig. 2) to manage the behavior plan and with the implementation of modality specific flexibility for the behaviors themselves.

3.1 Incremental Plan Construction

Constructing a plan out of small increments allows AsapRealizer to start realizing behavior early and to do part of its plan construction while it is executing previous increments, thus making the ECA more reactive. Such incrementality has a biological basis: psycholinguistics has identified incrementality as an important property of fluent human language production (e.g. [2]). While speech can be seen as a concatenation of increments that are smaller than a sentence [1], the increments connect smoothly, and as a result prosodic properties that are *suprasegmental* (e.g. rhythm, sentence intonation) are observed in speech. A similar incrementality has been proposed in gesture research. According to McNeill's segmentation hypothesis [18], speech and gesture are produced in successive increments that each contain one prosodic phrase in speech and one co-expressive gesture phrase. Gesture movement between the strokes of two successive gestures (in two successive increments) depends on their relative timing, and may range from retracting the arm to an in-between rest position, to a smooth direct transition movement to the next gesture.

Incremental plan construction in AsapRealizer therefore not only requires specifying sequential relations between the increments, but also the implementation of smooth connections between the increments. AsapRealizer supports incremental plan construction from increments specified in BML blocks. Since the occurrence of smooth connection between increments (or the lack thereof) can well have a communicative function (e.g. marking information boundaries [19]) we allow the behavior planner to have control over whether or not it should occur. To this end, we provide specification mechanisms in BMLA, that allow a detailed specification of how BML blocks are to be composed (see [5] for examples and syntax). AsapRealizer's automatic gesture co-articulation is implemented using functionality first developed for ACE [7], which was generalized to BML (see [9] for implementation details). Fluent prosodic connection is achieved by embedding the Inpro_iSS [10] incremental Text-To-Speech (TTS) system. Unlike current mainstream TTS systems that requires a the full utterance in advance to generate its intonation, Inpro_iSS can incrementally construct utterances with appropriate intonation from small increments. Fluent speech realization is achieved by the implementation of an IncrementalSpeechEngine that embeds Inpro_iSS. The IncrementalSpeechEngine executes a speech plan containing IncrementalSpeechUnits, which are constructed on the basis of the BML specification of the desired speech. In Inpro_iSS, the current utterance plan is represented by a buffer of PhraseIUs. PhraseIUs are Incremental Units that typically represent part of a sentence. This PhraseIU buffer forms a stretch of continuous speech to be uttered. When devising a phrase's prosody, the whole buffer is used as context. For each IncrementalSpeechUnit, a corresponding PhraseIU is created in Inpro_iSS. AsapRealizer's PhraseIUManager fills (and empties) the buffer based on the (predicted) timing of the IncrementalSpeechUnits in the plan. Its goal is to keep the buffer as full as possible, allowing the maximum quality of prosody, given the currently known speech plan. The timing of the ongoing utterance is subject to change (e.g. subject to timing changes caused by prosody enhancements or parameter changes). These timing changes are automatically communicated to behavior in aligned other modalities (e.g. lipsync, gesture) using AsapRealizer's PegBoard (see also Section 3.3).

In addition to incremental production, humans employ fillers (e.g. uhm) to keep or take a turn without having a plan at hand [3]. Bauman and Schlangen show that a dialog system that uses such fillers is preferred by users over one that waits with speaking until all information is available [20]. However, in certain situations the usage of those fillers may communicate unintended communicative functions and should be avoided.

We therefore allow the behavior planner to specify both the occurrence of fillers and whether or not they are to be automatically skipped if a new increment concatenated after the filler is scheduled on time. The latter bears resemblance to the skipping of the retraction phase of gestures and is implemented in a similar fashion. Automatic

---

BML Example 1 Incremental speech construction.

```
<bml id="bml1">
  <speech bmlis:generatefiller="true" id="s1">
    <text>The car goes around the corner and</text>
  </speech>
</bml>
<bml id="bml2" bmla:chunkAfter="bml1">
  <speech id="s1"><text>turns right.</text></speech>
</bml>
```

---

filler insertion is illustrated in BML Example. 1: first the bmlis:generatefiller attribute specifies that a filler may be generated in the first speech behavior; secondly, the bmla:chunkAfter attribute specifies that bml2 is chunked directly after bml1, allowing filler-skipping. If bml2 is not scheduled in time, the sentence "The car goes around the corner and uhm.. turns right." is produced, otherwise the filler is omitted and and a fluent prosodic connection between bml1 and bml2 is established. We have implemented automatic filler insertion using Inpro_iSS's HesitationIUs. HesitationIUs are realized as "uhm" if they are last in the buffer, and skipped otherwise. The PhraseIUManager adds both a PhraseIU and a HesitationIU to the buffer for each IncrementalSpeechUnit that is constructed from a speech behavior with the generatefiller attribute. For these IncrementalSpeechUnits the relax phase occurs during the filler. New BML blocks can be chunked after them, skipping their relax phase (and thus the filler).

To achieve even higher reactivity, AsapRealizer provides the capability to preplan BML blocks that can be instantly activated at later time (see [5] for examples and syntax). This allows very reactive behavior realization, e.g. in contexts where only few ECA responses are valid; each response can then be pre-planned while a user is speaking and then the 'appropiate' one can be activated without scheduling delay once user input is analyzed and the ECA has the floor.

3.2 Graceful Interruption

A behavior planner may interrupt ongoing behavior using BMLA interrupt behaviors (see [5] for the syntax). Interrupting behavior in a natural manner entails more than simple halting e.g. speech or gesture. AsapRealizer makes use of the BML 1.0 notion of *ground state* for postures and gaze targets and generally implements an interruption by gracefully restoring the ECA's ground state. Gestures are interrupted by automatic insertion of a transition motion that guides the ECA's arms to the posture ground state; gaze is interrupted by the insertion of a new gaze motion to the gaze target ground state;

facial expressions are interrupted by inserting a transition motion to a neutral facial expression. Speech may be interrupted instantly, or at phoneme or word boundaries. The ground states themselves are changed using postureShift and gazeShift behaviors respectively.

3.3   Adaptation of Ongoing Behavior

AsapRealizer realizes a stream of BML blocks, each of which specifies the timing (e.g. sync points X of behavior A and Y of behavior B should occur at the same time) and shape (e.g. behavior A should be performed with the left hand) of the desired behaviors. Generally, BML blocks are under-specified and leave realizers freedom in their actual realization. Realizers can make use of this to achieve natural looking motor behavior, e.g. by setting a biologically plausible duration of a gesture preparation. AsapRealizer employs a flexible behavior plan representation –the PegBoard. The PegBoard maintains a set of TimePegs that symbolically link to the synchronization points of behaviors that are constrained to be at the same time. The timing of these TimePegs may be updated, which moves the timing of the associated synchronization points, but maintains the time constraints specified upon them. The PegBoard thus allows one to do timing modifications of the behavior plan as it is being executed, but in such a way that BML constraints remain satisfied and no expensive re-scheduling is needed (see [21] for implementation details).

Additionally, adaptation of ongoing behavior requires e.g. animation and speech realizations in which certain parameters of ongoing behavior can be changed on the fly. AsapRealizer provides a facial animation system in which the intensity of ongoing morph based, MPEG-4 based, Action Unit based or emotional animation can be changed [22]. We provide a procedural animation system which allows arbitrary mathematical formulas and parameter sets to be used for motion specification and allows the parameters of ongoing animation to be changed (see [8] for implementation details). This design is more flexible than traditional procedural animation models that define motion in terms of splines or other predefined motion formulas and that use fixed parameter sets (e.g. [23,24]). To demonstrate that our procedural motion captures such models as a subset, we have semi-automatically converted several motion units from Greta [23] as procedural animations in our system and provide on-the-fly adaptation of their spatial extent, fluidity and power parameters. Ongoing speech is adjusted through Inpro_iSS, which currently supports on-the-fly adaptations of speech pitch, loudness and speaking rate.

Top-down Adaptation of Ongoing Behavior. Our BMLA parametervaluechange behavior allows the behavior planner to adapt ongoing behavior elements (see [5] for syntax). Such adaptations allow the behavior planner to, for example, raise the loudness of ongoing speech to keep a challenged turn (see BML Example 2).

Bottom-up Adaptation of Ongoing Behavior. Bottom up adaptation of gesture is required since the preparation and retraction phases need to be constructed on the fly because the start position of the preparation, the hand position at the start/end of the

BML Example 2 Change the volume of the bml1:speech1 from its current value to 90, over a linear trajectory.

```
<bmla:parametervaluechange target="bml1:speech1" paramId="volume"
    start="bml1:speech1:s1" end="bml1:speech1:s1+1">
  <bmla:trajectory type="linear" targetValue="90"/>
</bmla:parametervaluechange>
```

stroke and the posture ground state at the end of the gesture are all subject to change during gesture execution. The initial hand position may vary by previously executed motion and/or posture changes, the hand position at the start/end of the stroke may vary by top-down parameter adjustments in the gesture, and the rest posture state may change as a result of posture shifts. We have implemented an adaptive timing process for the preparation and retraction of gestures, which is described in detail in [9]. Similarly, the timing of preparation and retraction of gaze is subject to changes in the position of the gaze target, the position of e.g. the head and eyes at the start of the gaze, and the gaze ground state. To realize adaptive, full body gaze in which the timing of the preparation and retraction of gaze is automatically determined, AsapRealizer provides a novel biologically motivated gaze model and the implementation of the gaze 'ground state', which keeps track of the current gaze target and automatically creates motions to it whenever the selected body parts (e.g. eyes, neck, spine) for the ground state are not occupied with other movement that has higher priority. The BML 1.0 gazeShift behavior has been implemented to change the desired gaze ground state. AsapRealizer's gaze model is based on [25], and introduces some improvements to it: the eyes reach the target first and then lock on to it, that is, they overshoot their end rotation and then move back while remaining locked on the target (implementing [26]), the maximum speed of the eye and its velocity profile are biologically motivated (implementing [27]) and the eyes adhere to their biological rotation limits (obtained from [28]).

Adaptation to a Changing World. AsapRealizer's flexible plan representation is also used to allow tight synchronization with interlocutor behavior. On the specification side this is achieved by allowing the synchronization of behaviors to time events provided by *anticipators* (see BML Example. 3 for an example). An anticipator manages TimePegs

BML Example 3 Aligning the start of a speech behavior to occur slightly before the predicted end of interlocutor speech.

```
<speech start="anticipators:turnStopAnticipator:turnStop-0.1">..</speech>
```

within AsapRealizer's PegBoard that may be used to make adjustments to the timing of behavior that is synchronized to them. Anticipators use perceptions of the real world to continually update the timing of these TimePegs, by extrapolating these perceptions into predictions of the timing of future events (e.g. the end of an interlocutor turn, the next beat in music) that correspond to the managed TimePegs. We have implemented an anticipator to predict tempo events in real-time music for a virtual dancer or conductor [29], an anticipator that predicts the timing of fitness exercises of a user that exercises together with a virtual trainer [30], and several anticipators for wizard of Oz experiments that provide time events on button presses.

4   Comparison with Other Realizers

Table 2 provides a summary of AsapRealizer 2.0's fluent behavior realization capabilities in comparison with other Realizers. The listed capabilities are a selection of the capabilities offered by the different realizers for 1) incrementally constructing a plan out of multiple BML blocks and 2) adapting ongoing behavior (in e.g. timing and shape), as gathered from the papers describing them, their manuals and personal communication with their authors.

The first version of AsapRealizer [9] combined the incremental behavior realization capabilities of ACE [7] with Elckerlyc's capabilities for interactional coordination [8]. AsapRealizer 2.0 enhances AsapRealizer 1.0's capabilities by implementing the capabilities that were only available for gesture in AsapRealizer 1.0 also for speech, gaze and facial expression. It also provides incremental plan construction capabilities for prepending (rather than just appending), which is useful for the insertion of short delays and rephrases, while keeping the original behavior plan mostly intact.

The capabilities for the incremental construction of the behavior out of multiple BML blocks in the state-of-the-art Realizers SmartBody [31], EMBOT realizer [32], and the BML realizer of the Greta ECA [23] is limited to the specification and realization of sequential relations between BML blocks (but not fluently connecting them) and instantly merging BML blocks with ongoing behavior.

Unlike AsapRealizer, ACE, and Elckerlyc, each of these realizer has a rigid underlying behavior plan representation. The SmartBody scheduling algorithm resolves a BML block to a fixed plan in which all behaviors are assigned absolute timestamps ([31], p154) and animation is represented by specialized controllers. EMBOT Realizer represents its ongoing behavior in EMBRScript, an animation layer in which all elements have absolute time stamps and only absolute space descriptions may be used ([24], p513). In Greta, increments (with one gesture as their smallest granularity) of ongoing behavior are sent to a dedicated MPEG-4 player, which does not allow the adaptation of its ongoing movement ([23], p5). Because of their rigid plan representations, these realizers lack the ability to adapt their ongoing behavior and do not provide interruption capabilities beyond cutting of their speech. This is true to a lesser extent in SmartBody, which allows changes in shape, but not timing of ongoing behavior. SmartBody employs this flexibility mostly in allowing a rich behavior repertoire for interaction with the environment. Most realizers provide some autonomous behavior (e.g. blinking, breathing) and allow top-down control over some of its parameters (e.g. frequency), which can, for example, be used by the behavior planner to express some emotion of the ECA.

Beyond the capabilities offered by AsapRealizer, SmartBody offers a wider set of behaviors to interact with the world, including 'events' to communicate information to the outside world in tight synchrony to ongoing behavior. This functionality is typically used

Table 2. Fluent behavior realization capabilities of different Realizers

	EMBOT realizer	Greta	SmartBody	ACE	Elckerlyc	AsapRealizer 1.0	AsapRealizer 2.0
Incremental plan construction							
Merging increments	✓	✓	✓	✓	✓	✓	✓
Immediate/high priority increments	✓	✗	✗	✗	✗	✗	✗
Appending increments	?	?	✓	✓	✓	✓	✓
Prepending increments	✗	✗	✗	✗	✗	✗	✓
Preplanning and activation	✗	✗	✗	✗	✓	✓	✓
Chunking increments	✗	✗	✗	✓	✗	✓	✓
On-the-fly gesture co-articulation	✗	✗	✗	✓	✗	✓	✓
On-the-fly incremental intonation	✗	✗	✗	✗	✗	✗	✓
Automatic speech fillers	✗	✗	✗	✗	✗	✗	✓
Graceful interruption							
Speech	?	?	✓	✗	✓	✓	✓
Gesture	✗	✗	✗	✗	✗	✓	✓
Gaze	✗	✗	✗	✗	✗	✗	✓
Facial expression	✗	✗	✗	✗	✗	✗	✓
Top-down adaptation							
Speech	✗	✗	✗	✗	✗	✗	✓
Gesture	✗	✗	✗	✗	✓	✓	✓
Facial expression	✗	✗	✗	✗	✓	✓	✓
Breathing	✓	?	✓	✓	✓	✓	✓
Blinking	✓	?	✓	✓	✓	✓	✓
Bottom-up adaptation							
Speech	✗	✗	✗	✓	✗	✗	✓
Gesture	✗	✗	✗	✓	✗	✓	✓
Facial expression	✗	✗	✗	✗	✗	✗	✗
Interacting with a changing world							
Gaze at moving targets	?	✗	✓	✓	✓	✓	✓
Manipulate moving targets	✗	✗	✓	✗	✗	✗	✗
Point at moving targets	✗	✗	✓	✓	✓	✓	✓
Follow/walk to moving targets	✗	✗	✓	✗	✗	✗	✗
Maintain endeffector constraints	✗	✗	✓	✗	✗	✗	✗
Emit (synchronized) events to indicate world changes	✗	✗	✓	✗	✗	✗	✗
On-the-fly synchronization to predicted (external) time events	✗	✗	✗	✗	✓	✓	✓

for inter-ECA communication, but has applications beyond that (for example, communicating that an ECA pressed the light switch to the environment it is in). EMBOT realizer offers the unique capability to specify that an increment requires immediate, high priority execution. These increments are performed as soon as possible, overriding existing elements.

5 The Bigger Picture: The Articulated Social Agents Platform

AsapRealizer is the behavior realization component of the Articulated Social Agents Platform(Asap)[5], a platform specifically designed for the development of ECAs that allow fluent interaction with their human interlocutors. Asap provides a collection of software for social robots and virtual humans jointly developed by our two research groups. In addition to a collection of tools, we also provide the means (through middleware and architecture concepts (see Fig. 3)) to compose virtual human or robot applications in which the tools are embedded. Asap embeds the SAIBA architecture for behavior realization ([33], left side of Fig. 3) and enhances it with two essential features for fast and fluent virtual human behavior: a close bi-directional coordination between input processing and output generation, and incremental processing of both input and output. In this paper we have show how these two features play a part in the behavior realization within AsapRealizer. In [5] and on the Asap website [1] we illustrate in several scenarios how AsapRealizer's realization capabilities play out in concert with fluent intent and behavior planning and input processing.

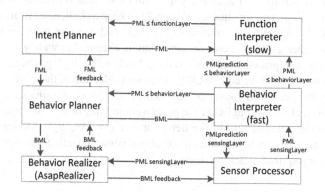

Fig. 3. The Asap Architecture

6 Discussion

We have presented AsapRealizer 2.0, a BML behavior realizer that has several fluent behavior realization capabilities that, in most aspects, go beyond the state of the art. AsapRealizer is eminently suitable for behavior realization in very dynamic contexts.

---

[1] http://www.asap-project.org

Fluent behavior realization is however not the only important aspect of a realizer, and other realizers may have an edge over AsapRealizer in e.g. the realism of their behavior repertoire, which might make them more suitable in contexts where less flexible behavior suffices.

While we model how ECA behavior is changed through changes in the environment, we currently provide no means to model how an ECA steered by AsapRealizer changes the environment. We are planning to implement a mechanism inspired by SmartBody's event system to achieve this. In our applications, we plan to use such events e.g. to adapt a traditional user interface in reaction to the behavior of an embedded ECA or to make changes in the calendar used by the daily assistant Billie.

Our flexible plan representation using the PegBoard has recently been adapted in the Thalamus robotic framework [34], where it provides flexible (input) event based control of interactive robots. Achieving speech-gesture synchronization is challenging in current robotic systems that do not allow changes in ongoing behavior, since the exact timing of robotic gesture can typically not be predicted very precisely beforehand by standard robot software [35]. We propose that AsapRealizer's capability to adjust the timing of ongoing behavior can potentially be used to achieve speech-gesture synchrony for robots on the fly (see [35] for details).

AsapRealizer's fluent behavior realization capabilities open up many exciting possibilities for behavior and intent planning. In particular, we are currently interested in fluent turn-taking. Using AsapRealizer, we can model turn-taking that goes beyond the state of the art in 1) allowing the ECA to interrupt the user (e.g when something urgent comes up, to instantly correct a mistake made by the user or to indicate that the ECA no longer understands the user at an early moment rather than providing such feedback after the user is completely finished speaking), 2) to keep a challenged turn (e.g. to provide a last bit of important information to the user) and 3) to let itself be interrupted in a graceful manner. Each of these use cases can be executed in widely varying ways. For example, one can grab the turn by speaking loud, with a high pitch, fast and/or by gazing at the interlocutor (see e.g. [36,37]). The exact selection of these surface features modulates e.g. the perceived conversational skill, friendliness, dominance and naturalness (perceived realism) of the ECA, the perceived urgency of the message she/he has to deliver, and the effectiveness of the behavior (see e.g. [38,39]). In future work we aim to model the relations between such social and communicative parameters and the surface behavior required to achieve them.

References

1. Howes, C., Purver, M., Healey, P.G.T., Mills, G., Gregoromichelaki, E.: On incrementality in dialogue: Evidence from compound contributions. Dialogue & Discourse 2(1), 297–311 (2011)
2. Levelt, W.J.M.: Speaking: From Intention to Articulation. The MIT Press (1989)
3. Clark, H.H.: Using language. Cambridge University Press (1996)
4. Bernieri, F.J., Rosenthal, R.: Interpersonal coordination: Behavior matching and interactional synchrony. In: Feldman, R.S., Rimé, B. (eds.) Fundamentals of Nonverbal Behavior. Studies in Emotional and Social Interaction. Cambridge University Press (1991)

5. Kopp, S., van Welbergen, H., Yaghoubzadeh, R., Buschmeier, H.: An architecture for fluid real-time conversational agents: integrating incremental output generation and input processing. Journal on Multimodal User Interfaces (2013) (online first article)
6. Traum, D., DeVault, D., Lee, J., Wang, Z., Marsella, S.: Incremental dialogue understanding and feedback for multiparty, multimodal conversation. In: Nakano, Y., Neff, M., Paiva, A., Walker, M. (eds.) IVA 2012. LNCS, vol. 7502, pp. 275–288. Springer, Heidelberg (2012)
7. Kopp, S., Wachsmuth, I.: Synthesizing multimodal utterances for conversational agents. Computer Animation and Virtual Worlds 15(1), 39–52 (2004)
8. van Welbergen, H., Reidsma, D., Ruttkay, Z.M., Zwiers, J.: Elckerlyc: A BML realizer for continuous, multimodal interaction with a virtual human. Journal on Multimodal User Interfaces 3(4), 271–284 (2010)
9. van Welbergen, H., Reidsma, D., Kopp, S.: An incremental multimodal realizer for behavior co-articulation and coordination. In: Nakano, Y., Neff, M., Paiva, A., Walker, M. (eds.) IVA 2012. LNCS, vol. 7502, pp. 175–188. Springer, Heidelberg (2012)
10. Baumann, T., Schlangen, D.: Inpro iSS: A component for just-in-time incremental speech synthesis. In: ACL System Demonstrations, pp. 103–108. ACL (2012)
11. Kopp, S., Jung, B., Leßmann, N., Wachsmuth, I.: Max - a multimodal assistant in virtual reality construction. Künstliche Intelligenz 17(4), 11–17 (2003)
12. Nijholt, A., Reidsma, D., van Welbergen, H., op den Akker, R., Ruttkay, Z.: Mutually co-ordinated anticipatory multimodal interaction. In: Esposito, A., Bourbakis, N.G., Avouris, N., Hatzilygeroudis, I. (eds.) HH and HM Interaction. LNCS (LNAI), vol. 5042, pp. 70–89. Springer, Heidelberg (2008)
13. Salem, M., Kopp, S., Joublin, F.: Generating finely synchronized gesture and speech for humanoid robots: a closed-loop approach. In: HRI, pp. 219–220 (2013)
14. Reidsma, D., de Kok, I., Neiberg, D., Pammi, S., van Straalen, B., Truong, K.P., van Welbergen, H.: Continuous interaction with a virtual human. Journal on Multimodal User Interfaces 4(2), 97–118 (2011)
15. Buschmeier, H., Kopp, S.: Towards conversational agents that attend to and adapt to communicative user feedback. In: Vilhjálmsson, H.H., Kopp, S., Marsella, S., Thórisson, K.R. (eds.) IVA 2011. LNCS, vol. 6895, pp. 169–182. Springer, Heidelberg (2011)
16. Buschmeier, H., Baumann, T., Dosch, B., Schlangen, D., Kopp, S.: Combining incremental language generation and incremental speech synthesis for adaptive information presentation. In: SIGdial, pp. 295–303 (2012)
17. Yaghoubzadeh, R., Kramer, M., Pitsch, K., Kopp, S.: Virtual agents as daily assistants for elderly or cognitively impaired people. In: Aylett, R., Krenn, B., Pelachaud, C., Shimodaira, H. (eds.) IVA 2013. LNCS, vol. 8108, pp. 79–91. Springer, Heidelberg (2013)
18. McNeill, D.: Hand and Mind: What Gestures Reveal about Thought. University of Chicago Press (1995)
19. Kendon, A.: Gesticulation and speech: Two aspects of the process of utterance. In: Key, M.R. (ed.) The Relation of Verbal and Nonverbal Communication, pp. 207–227. Mouton (1980)
20. Baumann, T., Schlangen, D.: Interactional adequacy as a factor in the perception of synthesized speech. In: ISCA Speech Synthesis Workshop (2013)
21. van Welbergen, H., Reidsma, D., Zwiers, J.: Multimodal plan representation for adaptable BML scheduling. AAMAS 27(2), 305–327 (2013)
22. Paul, R.: Realization and high level specification of facial expressions for embodied agents. Master's thesis, University of Twente (2010)
23. Anh, L.Q., Huang, J., Pelachaud, C.: A common gesture and speech production framework for virtual and physical agents. In: ICMI Workshop on Speech and Gesture Production (2012)

24. Heloir, A., Kipp, M.: Real-time animation of interactive agents: Specification and realization. Applied Artificial Intelligence 24(6), 510–529 (2010)
25. Grillon, H., Thalmann, D.: Simulating gaze attention behaviors for crowds. Computer Animation and Virtual Worlds 20(2-3), 111–119 (2009)
26. Radua, P., Tweed, D., Vilis, T.: Three-dimensional eye, head, and chest orientations after large gaze shifts and the underlying neural strategies. Journal of Neurophysiology 72(6), 2840–2852 (1994)
27. Carpenter, R.H.S.: Movements of the Eyes, 2nd edn. Pion Ltd. (1988)
28. Tweed, D.: Three-dimensional model of the human eye-head saccadic system. Journal of Neurophysiology 77(2), 654–666 (1997)
29. Reidsma, D., Nijholt, A., Bos, P.: Temporal interaction between an artificial orchestra conductor and human musicians. Computers in Entertainment 6(4), 1–22 (2008)
30. Reidsma, D., Dehling, E., van Welbergen, H., Zwiers, J., Nijholt, A.: Leading and following with a virtual trainer. In: International Workshop on Whole Body Interaction, University of Liverpool (2011)
31. Thiebaux, M., Marshall, A.N., Marsella, S., Kallmann, M.: Smartbody: Behavior realization for embodied conversational agents. In: Proceedings of AAMAS, pp. 151–158 (2008)
32. Kipp, M., Heloir, A., Schröder, M., Gebhard, P.: Realizing multimodal behavior. In: Safonova, A. (ed.) IVA 2010. LNCS, vol. 6356, pp. 57–63. Springer, Heidelberg (2010)
33. Kopp, S., Krenn, B., Marsella, S.C., Marshall, A.N., Pelachaud, C., Pirker, H., Thórisson, K.R., Vilhjálmsson, H.H.: Towards a common framework for multimodal generation: The behavior markup language. In: Gratch, J., Young, M., Aylett, R.S., Ballin, D., Olivier, P. (eds.) IVA 2006. LNCS (LNAI), vol. 4133, pp. 205–217. Springer, Heidelberg (2006)
34. Ribeiro, T., Vala, M., Paiva, A.: Thalamus: Closing the mind-body loop in interactive embodied characters. In: Nakano, Y., Neff, M., Paiva, A., Walker, M. (eds.) IVA 2012. LNCS, vol. 7502, pp. 189–195. Springer, Heidelberg (2012)
35. Lohse, M., van Welbergen, H.: Designing appropriate feedback for virtual agents and robots. Position paper at RO-MAN 2012 Workshop "Robot Feedback in Human-Robot Interaction: How to Make a Robot "Readable" for a Human Interaction Partner" (2012)
36. Kendon, A.: Some functions of gaze direction in social interaction. Acta Psychologica 26, 22–63 (1967)
37. Esposito, R., Yang, L.: Acoustic correlates of interruptions in spoken dialogue. In: ESCA Workshop on Interactive Dialogue in Multi-Modal Systems (1999)
38. Goldberg, J.A.: Interrupting the discourse on interruptions: An analysis in terms of relationally neutral, power- and rapport-oriented acts. Journal of Pragmatics 14(6), 883–903 (1990)
39. ter Maat, M., Truong, K.P., Heylen, D.: How turn-taking strategies influence users' impressions of an agent. In: Safonova, A. (ed.) IVA 2010. LNCS, vol. 6356, pp. 441–453. Springer, Heidelberg (2010)

A Data-Driven Method for Real-Time Character Animation in Human-Agent Interaction

David Vogt[1], Steve Grehl[1], Erik Berger[1],
Heni Ben Amor[2], and Bernhard Jung[1]

[1] Institut für Informatik,
Technische Universität Bergakademie Freiberg,
Bernhard-von-Cotta Str. 2, 09599 Freiberg, Germany
erik.berger@informatik.tu-freiberg.de
http://www.informatik.tu-freiberg.de
[2] Institute for Robotics and Intelligent Machines,
Georgia Institute of Technology,
801 Atlantic Drive, Atlanta, GA 30332-0280, USA
hba7@mail.gatech.edu
http://robotics.gatech.edu/

Abstract. We address the problem of creating believable animations for virtual humans that need to react to the body movements of a human interaction partner in real-time. Our data-driven approach uses prerecorded motion capture data of two interacting persons and performs motion adaptation during the live human-agent interaction. Extending the interaction mesh approach, our main contribution is a new scheme for efficient identification of motions in the prerecorded animation data that are similar to the live interaction. A global low-dimensional posture space serves to select the most similar interaction example, while local, more detail-rich posture spaces are used to identify poses closely matching the human motion. Using the interaction mesh of the selected motion example, an animation can then be synthesized that takes into account both spatial and temporal similarities between the prerecorded and live interactions.

Keywords: character animation, interaction mesh, virtual agent, interactive characters.

1 Introduction

Intelligent virtual agents have found widespread applications ranging from computer games [1,2], to educational software [3,4], or even shopping assistants [5]. Advances in sensing and graphics technology have significantly affected the development of avatars and their acceptance by users. An important example for this development is the introduction of affordable, low-cost motion tracking cameras. Instead of relying on artificial interfaces between humans and virtual agents, e.g. graphical user interfaces or joysticks, we can now directly analyze the user's body movement and thereby allow for a much more natural interaction.

T. Bickmore et al. (Eds.): IVA 2014, LNAI 8637, pp. 463–476, 2014.

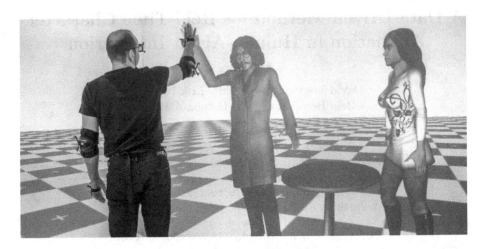

Fig. 1. A virtual agent's animation is calculated based on live human motion data. For that we first analyze the user's current and previous postures to select the interaction he's currently in. After matching temporal as well as spatial aspects we further optimize the character's response with interaction meshes. In this way, a virtual agent can react to ongoing human motions for different interactions in real-time.

However, the ability to track human motion also introduces two key challenges to the design of intelligent avatars: (1) recorded motion needs to be classified and (2) adequate responses by the avatar need to be triggered. A prevalent approach to solving this task is to use machine learning algorithms in order to identify the semantics of a recorded movement and then trigger a recorded movement or behavior as a response [6,7]. Such classification-based approaches typically require the human movement to be seen entirely before a response can be triggered. In addition, they often do not generalize to different variations of the movement.

In this paper, we investigate a method for human-agent interaction which allows a virtual agent to react to ongoing human motions interactively and in real-time. Towards this end, we propose a data-driven approach to reactive motion generation based on motion capture data and multivariate time series analysis. First, human-human interactions are recorded in order to create a library of appropriate responses. Then, during human-agent interactions, the user's live motion is analyzed in segmented low-dimensional spaces. In doing so, we identify suitable responses by aligning the observed motion to the templates in our library. The resulting response is then optimized utilizing *Interaction Meshes* [8] to allow for fine grade adaptation to the observed human motion. We extend the Interaction Mesh approach by adding a context-aware decision layer that allows multiple two-person interactions to be triggered. Temporal contexts are embedded implicitly in the low-dimensional space which enable temporal drifts and varying motion speeds.

The remainder of the paper is organized as follows. In section 2, we review existing techniques and outline key advantages of our approach. In section 3, we introduce the concept of global and local posture spaces and describe the motion matching algorithm. Consequently, we present an algorithm for interactive generation of responses for virtual characters. In section 4, we present different experiments that were performed using an human-sized virtual character in an immersive CAVE environment.

2 Related Work

Enabling a virtual human to engage in interactions with users that involve complex motions has long been a goal of researchers. Towards that end different example-based approaches have been proposed. In [9] for example the authors propose a framework for online action recognition using histograms. In doing so, they map live motions to existing motion capture datasets with a dynamic timewarp implementation. The temporal context of postures is preserved by using dynamic programming.

Camporesi et al. describe a data-driven method for virtual agent animation based on demonstrated user motions [10]. For that several examples are recorded using a motion capture system with a reduced set of markers. During runtime character movements are computed by blending example motions to new situations. The underlying minimization problem is solved efficiently which allows for real-time motion generation.

Naour et al. [11] propose a method based on Laplacian mesh editing [12], which has proven to be well suited for animating close interactions. Here interaction meshes [13] are defined with respect to their temporal correlations in the original animation. Motion optimization is achieved by solving two minimization problems. The first penalizes deformations that results from Laplacian coordinate manipulation and the second preserves the length of motion segments over time.

The approaches presented so far allow interactive motion manipulation of a virtual character, however, live human motions are usually not incorporated and, thus human-agent interactions are not supported.

In contrast to that, Taubert et al. [14] presented an approach based on a hierarchical probabilistic model (GP-LVMs with a GPDM on top) to capture recorded motions for live human-agent interactions. During runtime different emotional styles of movements can then be synthesized. However, due to the computational expensive nature of the underlying probabilistic algorithm, model learning is a time consuming process.

Ho et al. [8] propose a method based on two-person motion capture data with a two stage process. First, the postures of the afterwards active interaction partner, i.e the human, and the virtual agent are organized in a kd-tree. This leads to a tree where each leaf stores pairs of poses that have been obtained in the initial recording. Then, for live human-agent interactions the tree is queried for postures that are similar to the current user pose. Here, Euclidean distances among 15-dimensional feature sets, in particular positions of both hands, feet and the pelvis are used as similarity measure. The most similar pose leads then, to the corresponding frame of the initial recording. After that, the characters pose is morphed to match spatial constraints by solving a space-time optimization problem with interaction meshes [13]. In doing so a virtual character can react to an ongoing human interaction in real-time.

However, in their approach Ho et al. synthesize a character's motion solely based on a single user posture and the last neighbor search result. This limits the temporal context of the response generation to two poses since long-range temporal dependencies are not considered. In order to distinguish between interactions that share similar segments, larger memories have to be taken into account to animate the character in a believable/contextual manner. E.g., towards the end of many interactions, one agent returns to the rest pose while the other agent is following-through an interaction-specific finishing motion. To that end, we propose the usage of an interaction memory as well as motion segments rather then single postures to allow wider temporal coherences.

Also, during runtime Ho et al. use 15 dimensions corresponding to 5 Cartesian positions, i.e. both hands, feet and the pelvis to match the current user posture in their kd-tree. However, for complex motions like dancing elbows, knees and the head are often a crucial part of the dance style. In our approach, we propose low-dimensional posture spaces [15] which capture intrinsic information that constitutes the essence of each interaction.

3   Methodology

The goal of this work is to provide a motion synthesis framework that allows virtual characters to engage in two-person interactions with a human counterpart. Our data-driven approach is based on the observation and generalization of a recorded library of human-human interactions. We first record two-person interactions with a motion capture system[1]. The recorded interactions encapsulate information on how the movements of each person affect behavioral responses from his partner. Leveraging this information, we propose an algorithm that automatically identifies the appropriate reaction to be performed by a virtual agent during human-agent interaction.

Our approach is based on the concept of low-dimensional posture spaces [15]. Low-dimensional posture spaces capture the intrinsic correlation among joint positions during motor skill generation. As a result, they can be used to generalize recorded movements to new, unobserved situations while at the same time reducing model complexity. In this paper we show, that movements during two-person interactions can also be captured by a low-dimensional posture space, e.g. the joint movement lies on a low-dimensional manifold.

The proposed method uses dimensionality reduction to extract important correlations during joint behavior. Figure 2 shows an overview of the approach.

---

[1] In our experiments we use a A.R.T DTrack 2 motion capture system.

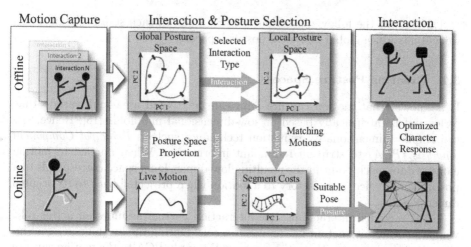

Fig. 2. Overview of the proposed method. First, we record two-person interactions with a motion capture system. Then the data is reduced in dimensionality leading to a global posture space as well as a set of local posture spaces specific to each interaction. To calculate a suitable character response during the online interaction, a reference frame of the original motion has to be identified by first using the global posture space to select an interaction and second by searching for similar motions in the corresponding local posture space. This leads to a pair of poses, i.e. postures of both interactants during the initial recording, which is then used to calculate an optimized posture for the virtual character.

The following description provides a brief overview of the steps involved in our method:

Posture Space Projection The user's live motion is captured and projected into the low-dimensional global posture space.

Selecting an Interaction Type Given the movements in the low-dimensional global interaction space, we identify the interaction type that fits the observation best.

Identifying Matching Motions User postures are projected into the local posture space of the active interaction type. Similarities between the projected trajectory and recorded movements from the library of training data are calculated. The segment with the highest similarity, i.e., a motion with similar postural changes is selected.

Extracting a Suitable Pose A cost matrix which captures distances to the best fitting motion segment is calculated to identify a point, i.e., a pair of poses of the initial recording, which satisfies postural as well as temporal requirements.

Optimizing a Character's Response Since the user's motion will vary as compared to the initial recording, we optimize selected character poses to the new situation by using interaction meshes [13].

Throughout the following sections we will focus on each step in detail. First, we will introduce global and local posture spaces.

3.1 Creating Posture Spaces

It is known, that motion capture data can be treated as a multivariate time series and is intrinsically based on low-dimensional manifolds [15]. Hence, one can employ dimensionality reduction techniques such as *Principal Component Analysis (PCA)* to strip off redundant information. When applied to motion capture data, each point in the resulting low-dimensional space corresponds to a posture and, hence, a trajectory to a motion when projected back to its original dimension.

In the recorded interactions, one interaction partner assumes an *active* role, while the other interactant has an *reactive* role. During the live human-agent interaction, the human is the active partner. We apply PCA to the motion capture data of the active interactant in the demonstrated interactions in several ways. First, we concatenate all motion capture recordings of the active interactant and project them into a single low-dimensional space, called *Global Posture Space* $\mathcal{I}$. Here all poses $x_{i,n}^{\mathcal{I}}$ are reduced to k dimensions. Second, for each demonstrated interaction i a l-dimensional *Local Posture Space* $\mathcal{P}_i$ is calculated to capture small details in the user's motion. To select a suitable amount of principal components k and l respectively we only select Eigenvectors that encode an entropy above 1 percent [15]. Hence, each posture space has a different dimensionality ensuring that enough dimensions are used to preserve small details of motions while at the same time reducing computational costs.

However, if we would consider the motion as a whole, alternations in the relationship of latent variables would not be taken into account [16]. Therefore, we split each interaction type in j segments, using Hotelling's T^2 statistics, which tries to capture changes of the underlying correlation structure. It does so, by minimizing the variance over a segment $\mathcal{S}_{i,j}$ and, consequently, concatenating temporal consecutive postures to motion segments in low-dimensional space. The cost function can be formalized as follows.

$$\mathcal{S}_{i,j} := \left\{ x_{i,n=a}, x_{i,n=a+1}, \ldots, x_{i,n=b} \right\} \tag{1a}$$

$$cost_{T^2}(\mathcal{S}_{i,j}) = \frac{1}{b-a+1} \sum_{j=a_i}^{b_i} T_{i,j}^2 \qquad T_{i,j}^2 = x_{i,n}^T x_{i,n} \tag{1b}$$

The segmented global posture space is now used to select an interaction template in a ongoing human-agent interaction.

3.2 Selecting an Interaction Template

To classify an ongoing human agent interaction the user's posture $y^{\mathcal{H}}$ is projected into the global posture space $\mathcal{I}$ leading to a new point $y^{\mathcal{I}}$. The Euclidean distances d_i between this point and the closest segment centroid of each inter-action i are calculated and added to a so called *interaction memory* D. This is done for the current time step t and the previous q time steps.

$$D = (d_1 \, d_2 \ldots d_i \ldots d_m) \, , \; d_i = \left(d_i^t \, d_i^{t-1} \ldots d_i^{t-q} \right)^T \tag{2a}$$

$$d_i = min(\|y^{\mathcal{I}} - centroid(\mathcal{S}_{i,j}^{\mathcal{I}})\|) \, , i \in \mathbb{N} : [1, m] \tag{2b}$$

Every column i captures the distances to the closest centroid of interaction i. Each row stores the distances of a single time step for all interactions. The interaction with the smallest mean value over all q rows identifies an interaction template.

3.3 Identifying Matching Motions

For believable human agent interactions a character's response highly depends on temporal features of the interaction. In a dance motion for example, it is crucial to be in strict time whereas for a high five movement the interactants' hands have to meet at the right time. In order to allow a virtual character to engage in such interactions past user poses have to be utilized. For that, a set of previous poses is projected into the local posture space of the active interaction, leading to a new motion trajectory $y_o^{\mathcal{P}_i}$.

Then, a similarity value s_{PCA} is calculated for each neighboring posture space segment. By only including the neighborhood, we restrict possible character responses to motions that contain postures similar to the ones obtained in the initial recording. The comparative measurement is defined as the sum of angles between each pair of sub principal components which can be formalized as [17]:

$$s_{PCA} = \frac{1}{l} \sum_{k=1}^{l} \sum_{c=1}^{l} cos^2 \Theta_{kc} = \frac{1}{l} trace(U_{k,l}^T U_{c,l} U_{c,l}^T U_{k,l}) \tag{3}$$

Here, l is the number of principal components for local comparison. Θ_{kc} de-notes the angle between k^{th} principal component (PC) of a segment and the cth sub PC of the user motion. In order to calculate the similarity value efficiently, the equation is reformulated in matrix form where $U_{k,l}$ is the subspace defined by the eigenvectors of the covariance matrix for segment k with dimension l.

In essence, the algorithm assigns high similarity values for segments with PC axes pointing in the same direction. In other words, segments with similar postural changes over time are assigned large similarity values. The segment j that fits the last user motion best is now used for further optimization.

3.4 Extracting a Suitable Pose

Since segment lengths vary for different motion parts of an interaction the follow-ing accumulated cost matrix is employed to identify a temporal matching pose of

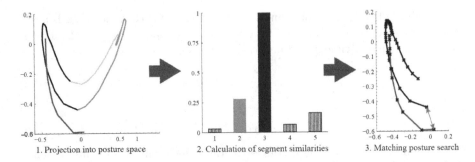

1. Projection into posture space   2. Calculation of segment similarities   3. Matching posture search

Fig. 3. The figure shows all required steps to identify a frame of the initial motion recording for an ongoing human-agent interaction. First the live user movement is projected into low-dimensional space leading to a new trajectory. After that, most similar segments are labeled utilizing Hotelling's T^2 statistics. Finally, the most similar posture is extracted by evaluating a cost matrix.

the original recording [18]. In doing so, we evaluate distances in low-dimensional space of live user poses $y_o^{\mathcal{P}_i}$ and template postures $x_{i,n}^{\mathcal{P}_i}$.

$$
S_{n,o} := \begin{cases}
\sum_{n=a}^{b} \|y_1^{\mathcal{P}_i} - x_{i,n}^{\mathcal{P}_i}\| & \forall n \in \mathbb{N} :]a, b], \ o = 1 \\[2mm]
\|y_o^{\mathcal{P}_i} - x_{i,a}^{\mathcal{P}_i}\| & \forall o \in \mathbb{N} :]1, O], \ n = a \\[2mm]
\begin{aligned} min\{S_{n-1,o-1}, S_{n,o-1}, S_{n-1,o}\} \\ + \|y_o^{\mathcal{P}_i} - x_{i,n}^{\mathcal{P}_i}\| \end{aligned} & \forall n \in \mathbb{N} :]a, b], \ o \in \mathbb{N} :]1, O]
\end{cases} \tag{4}
$$

To summarize, figure 3.3 shows required steps to select a frame of the initial recording that fits the motion context of the selected interaction template while at the same time satisfying postural similarities. The resulting pose is now subject to spatial optimization using interaction meshes.

3.5   Optimizing a Characters Response

In the previous step a frame of the initial recording has been identified that represents the most similar user posture. However, the user's movement will differ from the original motion in form and size and, thus, further optimization is required. To retain the characteristics of the prerecorded interaction, we optimize the selected posture by using interaction meshes [13]. In doing so, we minimize the Laplacian deformation energy [12] of a newly created mesh with regard to the one created during the initial recording. Here, the Laplacian deformation energy is defined as follows:

$$
E_L(V) := \sum_j \frac{1}{2} \|L(x_j) - L(y_j)\|^2 \tag{5}
$$

L is the operator to compute the Laplacian coordinates from given Cartesian coordinates $V = (p_1, \ldots, p_{2m})^T$. x_j are vertex locations (motion capture markers) from the prerecorded motion capture data in the selected frame, whereas y_j are coordinates of markers from the live human-agent interaction. Laplacian coordinates of a vertex are obtained as follows:

$$L(p_j) = p_j - \sum_{l \in N_j} w_l^j p_l \qquad (6)$$

N_j is the one-ring neighborhood of vertex p_j.

Since we want to react to an ongoing user motion, additional positional constraints have to be defined on the interaction mesh.

We treat the current user posture as a hard constraint in our optimization problem. Additionally, we define soft constraints on the character vertices to retain further desired aspects of the interaction, e.g. supporting foot contact and body position. The resulting optimization problem subject to the soft and hard constraints can be reformulated as system of linear equations (cf. [13]):

$$\begin{bmatrix} \mathcal{M}^T \mathcal{M} + F^T \mathcal{W} F & C^T \\ C & 0 \end{bmatrix} \begin{bmatrix} V \\ \lambda \end{bmatrix} = \begin{bmatrix} \mathcal{M}^T \mathcal{B} + \mathcal{F}^T \mathcal{W} f \\ h \end{bmatrix} \qquad (7)$$

where V and λ denote the vertices of the deformed interaction mesh and the Lagrange modifiers respectively. $\mathcal{M}$ is the Laplacian matrix of the original motion. C is the matrix of all constraints which can be separated into the matrix $\mathcal{F}$ of soft constraints, e.g. the virtual agent's position constraints, and the vector h of hard constraints, e.g. the user's current posture. Each soft constraint f is weighted by the weight matrix $\mathcal{W}$. $\mathcal{M}^T \mathcal{B}$ denotes the transformation of the original vertex positions $\mathcal{B}$ in Cartesian coordinates into Laplacian coordinates.

A solution of the system of linear equations is an interaction mesh V that minimizes the Laplacian deformation energy while satisfying the different constraints. However, vertex locations cannot be transferred to a virtual character without further post-processing, since not all joints correspond to a vertex. In order to calculate rotations for each bone we utilize an inverse kinematics solver.

4   Evaluation

To evaluate our method we recorded two-person interactions, namely high five, a hand clapping game, waving at each other and a jive dance. The corresponding 15 dimensional global posture space is illustrated for the first 3 principal components in figure 4. In a live human-agent interaction a user was tasked to high five the virtual agent. As expected its motion varied from the initial recording, however, its trajectory in low-dimensional space stills followed the same direction. This is due to the fact that similar postures were adopted which in turn lead to neighboring low-dimensional points.

On the right hand side of figure 4 the local posture space of the selected interaction is visualized. Here the closest matching motion segment of the initial

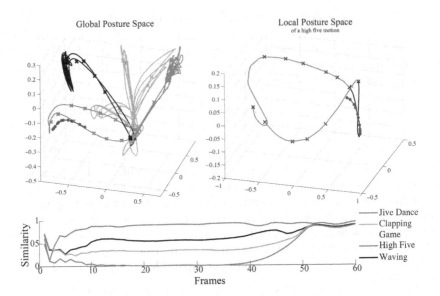

Global Posture Space

Local Posture Space
of a high five motion

Jive Dance
Clapping
Game
High Five
Waving

Similarity

Frames

Fig. 4. In the figure on top the global as well as the selected local posture space is shown. A user was tasked to high five the virtual agent. Below the mean activation in our interaction memory is visualized. As can be seen, a recorded high five motion is most similar to the executed user motion. However, one can also conclude that other motions also exhibit similar poses especially around frame 50 to 60.

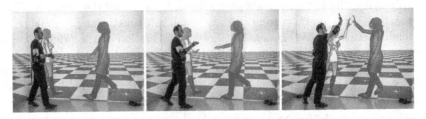

Fig. 5. The virtual agent's postures are optimized for live human agent interactions. In this example a user high fives a virtual character successfully. The agent adopts its motion to meet the users hand at the right time and position.

recording is marked (black trajectory). As can be seen, the user motion (indicated by the red trajectory) also follows the path of the closest segment. After calculating the cost matrix, a matching point is selected and its associated interaction mesh is optimized. The resulting character responses can be seen in figure 5 for 3 frames.

In a second example we utilized the same global posture space to detect a ongoing jive dance motion. The projection of current and recent user postures into the global local low-dimensional spaces are shown in figure 6 top left. As can be seen, its motion matches the shape of the jive template which has been generated from the initial recording. Additionally, the local posture space corresponding to

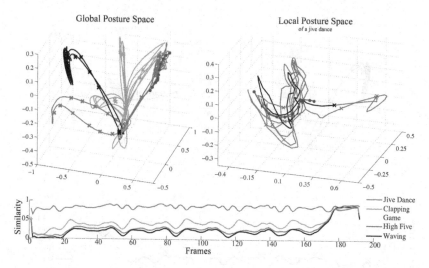

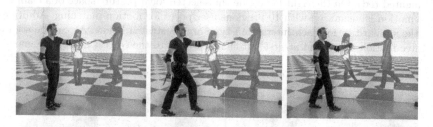

Fig. 6. The global as well as the selected local posture space of a jive dance motion are shown on top. The live user postures are highlighted red. The mean activation for each interaction is outlined below.

Fig. 7. The motion of a virtual character is optimized in real-time using our interaction learning method. As can be seen the agent successfully imitates the behavior shown in the initial recording.

the selected interaction is shown. The most similar segment is highlighted. The final character response can be seen in figure 7.

The similarities of the live user motion to recorded interaction examples are in figure 6 bottom. The reason for the large similarities towards the end of the interactions is that in all our recordings, the active participants returned to a pose with both arms resting aside.

In a third example a hand clapping game is performed with a virtual character. Here the same global posture space that has been created from the initial recordings is used. As shown in figure 8 the projected user postures (highlighted red) match the template created from a clapping game motion. However, as illustrated below the selected interaction type has been a high five at first (see frame 1 to 20) but changed later to the correct interaction. The reason for that

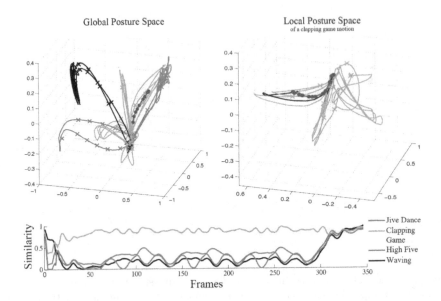

Fig. 8. The figure shows the global posture space and projected live user postures (highlighted red). On the right hand side the selected local posture space of a clapping game motion is visualized with 10 previous user poses for motion matching. Additionally, the similarities for each interaction type are illustrated below. As can be seen a high five motion is selected at first but changed later to the correct clapping game.

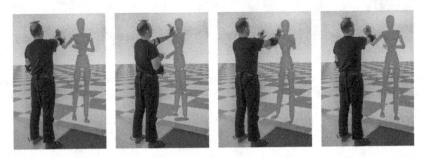

Fig. 9. With our method a virtual character can respond to complex interactions like a clapping game as shown in the figure for 4 key postures. Here the agent's hand has to meet the users palm at the right time and at the right position.

are similar postures that have been obtained in both motion capture recordings. The final character responses are illustrated for 4 key postures in figure 9.

5   Discussion

The presented approach utilizes a so called interaction memory for hysteresis effects and to allow a virtual agent to remain in an interaction. As a result it can potentially lock the agent in one interaction. The sliding window size of the interaction memory obviously affects the overall latency of the system. In our experiments a memory size q of 10 has been proven to be well suited. This leads to memory length of approximately 0.5 seconds at 20 frames per second and to a lag of 300ms on average on a modern Macbook Pro. Selecting a posture in global posture space as well as motion matching in local posture spaces takes on average 0.008s whereas optimizing the interaction meshes itself takes 0.01 seconds. In our current implementation, transforming the resulting vertex coordinates to joint angles utilizing the inverse kinematics solver takes twice as long (0.029 seconds).

Currently, the proposed method does not allow for additional objects to be included in two-person interactions as global as well as local posture spaces are not sensitive to object ownerships. Furthermore, we currently do not track, and thus cannot recreate the interactants' hand shapes during interactions.

6 Conclusion

In this paper, we presented a new, data-driven method for generating real-time responses of an interactive virtual human. Using training data acquired from human-human interactions, we generate low-dimensional representations that allow for the generalization of the observed behavior to different variations thereof. In doing so, crucial characteristics of an interaction as well as small details of motions are preserved and used to animate a virtual agent. We extended the approach presented by Ho et al. [8] to situations where the temporal context of interactions plays an important role.

Experiments performed in an immersive virtual environment show that the approach can be used for synthesizing context-aware responses in real-time. As a result, a more natural interaction between a virtual agent and a human user can be established.

As a possible extension of the approach, we are currently considering the implementation of time-varying interaction meshes as well as a probability based segmentation to allow for overlapping segments. In addition we are also investigating the use of the proposed approach in the generation of robot responses during human-robot interaction.

References

1. Deng, L., Leung, H., Gu, N., Yang, Y.: Real-time mocap dance recognition for an interactive dancing game. Computer Animation and Virtual Worlds 22(2-3), 229–237 (2011)
2. Kim, J., Seol, Y., Lee, J.: Human motion reconstruction from sparse 3d motion sensors using kernel cca-based regression. Computer Animation and Virtual Worlds 24(6), 565–576 (2013)
3. Weimin, X., Wenhong, X.: E-learning assistant system based on virtual human interaction technology. In: Shi, Y., van Albada, G.D., Dongarra, J., Sloot, P.M.A. (eds.) ICCS 2007, Part III. LNCS, vol. 4489, pp. 551–554. Springer, Heidelberg (2007)

4. Osterlund, J., Lawrence, B.: Virtual reality: Avatars in human spaceflight training. Acta Astronautica 71(0), 139–150 (2012)
5. Chattaraman, V., Kwon, W.-S., Gilbert, J.E.: Virtual agents in retail web sites: Benefits of simulated social interaction for older users. Computers in Human Behavior 28(6), 2055–2066 (2012)
6. Jung, B., Amor, H.B., Heumer, G., Vitzthum, A.: Action capture: A vr-based method for character animation. In: Coquillart, S., Brunnett, G., Welch, G. (eds.) Virtual Realities, pp. 97–122. Springer, Heidelberg (2008)
7. Bouchard, D., Badler, N.I.: Semantic segmentation of motion capture using laban movement analysis. In: Pelachaud, C., Martin, J.-C., André, E., Chollet, G., Karpouzis, K., Pelé, D. (eds.) IVA 2007. LNCS (LNAI), vol. 4722, pp. 37–44. Springer, Heidelberg (2007)
8. Ho, E.S.L., Chan, J.C.P., Komura, T., Leung, H.: Interactive partner control in close interactions for real-time applications. ACM Trans. Multimedia Comput. Commun. Appl. 9, 21:1–21:19 (2013)
9. Barnachon, M., Bouakaz, S., Boufama, B., Guillou, E.: Ongoing human action recognition with motion capture. Pattern Recognition 47(1), 238–247 (2014)
10. Camporesi, C., Huang, Y., Kallmann, M.: Interactive motion modeling and parameterization by direct demonstration. In: Allbeck, J., Badler, N., Bickmore, T., Pelachaud, C., Safonova, A. (eds.) IVA 2010. LNCS, vol. 6356, pp. 77–90. Springer, Heidelberg (2010)
11. Le Naour, T., Courty, N., Gibet, S.: Spatiotemporal coupling with the 3d+t motion laplacian. Computer Animation and Virtual Worlds 24(3-4), 419–428 (2013)
12. Sorkine, O., Cohen-Or, D., Lipman, Y., Alexa, M., Rössl, C., Seidel, H.-P.: Laplacian surface editing. In: Proceedings of the 2004 Eurographics/ACM SIGGRAPH Symposium on Geometry Processing, SGP 2004, pp. 175–184. ACM, New York (2004)
13. Ho, E.S.L., Komura, T., Tai, C.-L.: Spatial relationship preserving character motion adaptation. ACM Trans. Graph. 29 (July 2010)
14. Taubert, N., Löffler, M., Ludolph, N., Christensen, A., Endres, D., Giese, M.A.: A virtual reality setup for controllable, stylized real-time interactions between humans and avatars with sparse gaussian process dynamical models. In: Proceedings of the ACM Symposium on Applied Perception, SAP 2013, pp. 41–44. ACM, New York (2013)
15. Ben Amor, H.: Imitation Learning of Motor Skills for Synthetic Humanoids. PhD thesis, Technische Universität Bergakademie Freiberg (2010)
16. Bankó, Z., Abonyi, J.: Correlation based dynamic time warping of multivariate time series. Expert Systems with Applications 39(17), 12814–12823 (2012)
17. Krzanowski, W.J.: Between-groups comparison of principal components 74, 703–707 (September 1979)
18. Vlachos, M., Hadjieleftheriou, M., Keogh, E.J., Gunopulos, D.: Indexing multidimensional trajectories for similarity queries. In: Spatial Databases, pp. 107–128 (2005)

Compound Gesture Generation: A Model Based on Ideational Units

Yuyu Xu[1], Catherine Pelachaud[2], and Stacy Marsella[1]

[1] Northeastern University, Boston, MA 02115, USA
[2] CNRS - LTCI, Telecom ParisTech, France

Abstract. This work presents a hierarchical framework that generates continuous gesture animation performance for virtual characters. As opposed to approaches that focus more on realizing individual gesture, the focus of this work is on the relation between gestures as part of an overall gesture performance. Following Calbris' work [3], our approach is to structure the performance around ideational units and determine gestural features within and across these ideational units. Furthermore, we use Calbris' work on the relation between form and meaning in gesture to help inform how individual gesture's expressivity is manipulated. Our framework takes in high level communicative function descriptions, generates behavior descriptions and realizes them using our character animation engine. We define the specifications for these different levels of descriptions. Finally, we show the general results as well as experiments illustrating the impacts of the key features.

1 Introduction

Gestures play an important role in everyday communications. People use gestures to indicate location, describe an imaginary object, express attitudes, or regulate conversation flow [8]. Effective speakers use gestures as a tool to better convey ideas. For example, a clinician's use of gestures can impact the clinician-patient relation [6].

Our desire is to generate gestural performances for life-like virtual characters. At the level of individual gestures, gestures have a complex feature structure. There are the phases of gestural motion including the rest, preparation, stroke, holding and relax phases [8], as well as the form of the motion, its location and changing handshapes. However, our interest lies beyond realizing these features in individual gestures. We model an approach to integrating individual gestures' features into an overall fluid performance involving gesture sequences (a.k.a. gesture units [7,9]).

Specifically, the goal of this work is to realize gesturing for virtual characters that takes into account that human gesturing has a hierarchical structure that serves important demarcative, referential and expressive purposes [3]. Within a gesture performance, some features such as handshape, movement or location in space, may be coupled across gestures while other features serve at times a key role in distinguishing individual gestures, both physically and at the level of its

T. Bickmore et al. (Eds.): IVA 2014, LNAI 8637, pp. 477–491, 2014.

meaning, from one another. For example, the hands may go into a rest position between gestures to indicate the end of an idea, a change of handshape can serve to indicate the start of a new idea in the discourse or one gesture's location may serve to refer to a preceding gesture.

We layout an approach that uses this higher level of organization to realize gesture performances. This approach a) determines when and which features are common versus which ones must be distinguishable and b) addresses issues concerning the physical coordination or co-articulation between gestures within gesture units, including when gestures go into relax, rest positions or holds. Closely leveraging the work of Calbris [3], we use the concept of ideational unit, which Calbris argues structures the discourse and the kinesic segmentation of gestures. Specifically, ideational units serve to impose requirements on gestural features in an overall performance. Further, we use Calbris' work on the relation of form and meaning in gesture [3] to help inform how a gesture's expressivity is manipulated.

In this paper, we propose a model of this kinesic segmentation. We then describe an implementation that satisfies these requirements by selecting and flexibly modifying the performances of gestures. Finally we present results and suggest areas for further improvements.

2   Background Theory

To ground our model, we leverage research from Calbris [3], a French semiologist, that views shape and movement of communicative gestures as abstraction of physical objects and actions (e.g. putting the hands in the shape of a bowl as a sign of offering; using the back-front line to indicate temporal information). She also studied how gestures are organized one from other.

First, Calbris argues for a structuring of verbal and nonverbal behaviors into larger ideational units, a coupling of related ideas that can span multiple gestures for example. This coupling plays important demarcative functions as well as helping to convey meaning and is therefore critical to gesture specification and realization.

Specifically, consistency of aspects of the form or motion across gestures serve a demarcative function of illustrating a common overriding topic while changes in gestural form and movement can serve a demarcative function of indicating a topic shift. In other words, changes convey information. So going from one gesture to the next in one overriding conversational topic, a gesturer tends to not make changes in motions or handshapes that are not meaningful. To do otherwise risks undesired false implicatures, misinterpretations by an observer. Related to that, one can view a gesture's motion as a form of optimization, avoiding unnecessary exertion.

Additionally, the ideational units can be divided up into tighter rhythmic-semantic units by the type of change from one gesture to the next, change that provides information and performs a referential function. In other words, consecutive motions that have similar features or referential relations construct a rhythmic-semantic unit. For example, in enumeration there are similarities in the motion and form, contrast requires a certain symmetry and elaboration suggests repetition.

Second, Calbris argues that human conversation both verbally and non-verbally, is often grounded in metaphors, especially physical metaphors. So abstract concepts like an idea, an agreement or a relationship can be represented through gesture as physical objects or actions. Further, properties of, and actions on that abstract concept such as the importance of an idea, discarding an agreement or ending of a relationship can be indicated by gesture that suggests size, discarding or cutting of a physical object, respectively. Such metaphoric gestures are common in human speech and in some cultures a quite common form of gesture.

The physical metaphor that underlies a gesture imposes critical constraints on how the gesture is physically realized. So to convey the ending of a relationship, a speaker may gesture with a cutting motion that involves a vertical acceleration of the hand in a flat configuration with the edge of the hand leading the motion, as if it were a knife. Each of these features is critical, with the acceleration representing the knife's chopping motion, the flat palm representing the knife and the edge of the palm representing the knife's edge. So as a consequence, any animation system that realizes this behavior must obey these constraints that arise from the embodiment of virtual agent. In particular, attempts to fit the timing of the gesture to co-occurring speech or gestures that precede or follow must not override these constraints.

Similarly, we argue that the underlying metaphor can inform how we want to realize and manipulate the gesture's expressivity. For example, if the importance of an idea is conveyed by a two-handed gesture that frames an imaginary object, then a very important idea can be conveyed by framing a larger object. Similarly discarding an idea with prejudice might be indicated by a particularly strongly accelerated sweeping motion.

Finally the grounding in physical concepts and space means location matters across gestures. The delineation of a concept as an object in physical space means subsequent references to that object must refer back to that location.

3 Gesture Model Description

Our model for gesture works as a system of constraints, containing three categories based on hierarchical structuring of gesture performances. The first category, the one most central to this paper, is the constraints on gestural features within and across coupled gesture sequences, established by structuring into ideational units. The second category deals with the connection between individual gestures. The last category focuses on the constraints on individual gestures, such as timing of the stroke that are common to gesture work [17].

We first discuss the overall structuring of the model then we go into greater details into the constraints that operate on these structures.

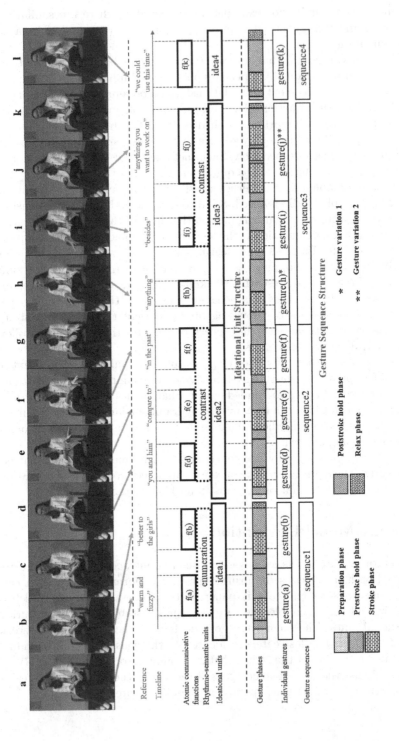

Fig. 1. Compound gesture model example

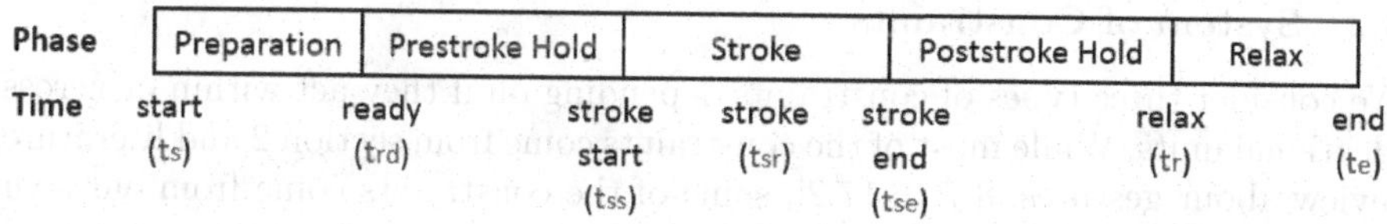

Phase	Preparation	Prestroke Hold	Stroke	Poststroke Hold	Relax
Time	start (t_s)	ready (t_{rd})	stroke start (t_{ss})	stroke (t_{sr}) stroke end (t_{se})	relax (t_r)	end (t_e)

Fig. 2. *Gesture Phases*: $Preparation[t_s, t_{rd}]$ defines the period when gesture leaves body posture and arrives to gesture space. $PrestrokeHold[t_{rd}, t_{ss}]$ is a pause before real stroke motion happens. $Stroke[t_{ss}, t_{se}]$ is where gesture motion conveys its meaning, it's the most essential part of a gesture. $PoststrokeHold[t_{se}, t_r]$ is a hold period after stroke phase is done. $Relax[t_r, t_e]$ is when gesture goes back to body posture from gesture space.

We use an annotated turn within a dialog, shown in Figure 1, to illustrate some of these constraints. The dialog is a part of a role play between a clinician and a person pretending to be a client suffering from depression. The clinician is saying she is willing to talk about anything except what the client's husband is complaining about. First section of the figure (above first horizontal dash separator) lists a sequence of images in correspondence to the phrases the clinician used. The images without an arrow connecting the phrases indicate the rest positions. Second section (between first and second horizontal dash separator) demonstrates the ideational unit structure which represents the utterance in ideation space. Third section (below second horizontal dash separator) presents the example's gesture sequence structure in gesture space. The lines between second section and third section indicates the one to one mapping between ideation space and gesture space.

In what follows, we use standard notions concerning the time markers and phases of gestures [8], as described in Figure 2.

3.1 Hierarchical Unit Structure

We refer to Calbris' first argument and define structures accordingly. As seen in Figure 1, the hierarchical structure of the gesture performance is composed of two major types of units.

- **Ideational Unit/Gesture Sequence.** As we see in Figure 1, an ideational unit can be a compound or coupling of atomic ideas (communicative functions) - the willingness to talk about anything except what the husband wants constitutes one ideational unit, it can also contain what Calbris [3] referred to as rhythmic-semantic units. For example, contrast or enumeration tightly relate atomic communicative functions and their associated gestures to each other. Ideational unit is in correspondence to gesture sequence (gesture unit), which is formed by one or more individual gestures.
- **Atomic Communicative Function/Individual Gesture.** This level is comprised of communicative functions that are associated with corresponding individual gestures [8], such as "anything", $f(h)$ in Figure 1.

3.2   System of Constraints

We consider three types of constraints depending on if they act within or across ideational units. While most of the constraints come from section 2 and literature review about gestures [8,7,16,17,2], some of the constraints come from our own observations of human data.

Within and Across Ideation Units/Gesture Sequences This category of constraints are based on the arguments from section 2. It defines the constraints for gesture performance according to the structure of the ideational units.

- *To serve the purpose of demarcating ideas, hands tend to rest or relax at the end of ideational units (see first section in Figure 1), but do not go to rest between gestures within ideational units.* Whether hands rest between gestures within ideational units depends on whether there is sufficient timing between gestures (for example, notice in Figure 1 between $gesture(f)$ and $gesture(h)$, there's no time left to go back to rest position.)
- *Consecutive gestures should have distinctive features within ideational unit.* In effect, they should be visibly distinguishable one from the other with notable provisos: features that are not relevant to what current gesture is conveying, persist from previous gestures (for example, notice in Figure 1, handshape persists).
- *References between gestures can be through similarities in (i.e., constraints on) the shape, movement or location features.* The reference can be local, e.g. in the case of enumeration, the reference is within ideational unit though potentially it can also be across ideational units. In the case of referencing impacting movement: the movement in the subsequent (referring) case may likely be more abstract (loose repetition of the movement). A gesture that refers to other gestures by physical location should have their stroke-end be at the location of the referred gesture and less critically the referring gesture shape should be the shape of the referred stroke-end gesture. See Figure 1, $gesture(h)$ is a metaphoric gesture that is referred to by $gesture(j)$.

Within An Ideational Unit This category describes the co-articulation constraints between gestures, to be more specific, gesture phase sequence construction between two individual gestures. An example can be found in third section of Figure 1.

- *Co-articulation between gestures eliminates some phases* [8]. Given two gestures, $gesture1$ and $gesture2$, usual co-articulation has the following phase sequence:
  $Stroke(gesture1), PoststrokeHold(gesture1),$
  $Preparation(gesture2), [PrestrokeHold(gesture2)], Stroke(gesture2)$
  Note that the phase specified inside the square bracket usually can be skipped depending on the timing constraints (i.e. if there is not enough time). The gesture can go to a relax phase instead of a hold.
- *The co-articulation from previous gesture to a beat gesture should ensure that the beat gesture should have a preparation phase that allows it to be distinguishable from the previous one.* The dynamic property of the preparation

phase of the beat should come mainly from the beat gesture. This is important when 2 gestures phases (relax phase of previous gesture and preparation phase of following gesture) need to blend with each other; or to co-articulate with one another. Beat gestures often have a quick and accelerated preparation phase: an anticipation of the dynamic quality of the stroke phase of the beat gesture. This constraint comes from our own data analysis.

- When the same gesture is repeated to emphasize a point, it tends to be repeated with a different expressivity quality [2]: the motion between t_{ss} and t_{se} of the repeated gesture have a larger spatial extent; the movement between the t_{ss} and t_{se} is larger (e.g. the hands draw a larger circle); and the velocity of the movement increases.
- Gesture co-articulation fundamentally has to obey the dynamic constraints of the motion (again based on our own observations). Otherwise it will end up in unnatural results that draws the observer's attention and interpretation away from the stroke of the gesture itself. For example, the transition motion speed between gestures can't be very different from the gesture speed before the transition and after, which might cause unexpected acceleration or deacceleration.

Individual Gestures This category of constraints deals with individual gestures, most of them are common to the gesture literature [8,17], but we also incorporate the concept of embodiment into physical gestures [3].

- Gesture with a referential content can be adjusted on the fly according to content's physical properties [3]. For example, representing an abstract concept as a physical object might have its size property, either big or small, be adjusted to reflect the importance of the idea. Gestures that have such variations can be found in Figure 1 marked with *.
- Relax position is different from rest position [16]. At relax position, the hands still stay in the gesture space. The hands may go toward the body a bit and the hand shape takes a more open relax shape.
- Although hold are often described as being necessary for co-articulation, they can also be used for emphasis [8]. Their use is highly dependent on timing constraints between consecutive gesture strokes.
- Strokes have to occur on or slightly before stress words [17].

4   Framework

Our gesture generation system follows the SAIBA ([11]) framework guidelines. The whole process is comprised of two main modules, behavior planning and behavior generation. Behavior planning module takes in high level communicative function descriptions as input using function markup language (FML) and generates behavior descriptions using behavior markup language (BML). Behavior realization module takes in BML descriptions outputs a description of the character's animation in terms of joint rotations.

4.1   Behavior Planning

The behavior planning module contains communicative function derivation and behavior mapping processes that maps ideational units (described by FML) to gesture behaviors (described by BML).

```
<fml>
....
<ideational id="i3">
    <function type="container" id="c3" location="center" action="delineate-set"
        modifier="round" attribute="large" reference="anything"/>
    <rhythmic-semantic id="d3" type="elaboration" nucleus="c3"/>
        <function type="movement" action="discard" source="c3" target="right"
            reference="what he wants"/>
        <function type="reference" action="indicate" location="c3" reference="anything"/>
        <function type="reference" id="r1" action="indicate" location="front" reference="you"/>
        <function type="emphasis" reference="you want to work on"/>
    </ rhythmic-semantic >
</ideational>
...
</fml>
<bml>
...
<gesture-sequence rest="sp1:T117" constraint-rest="true" constraint-handiness="true"
        constraint-handshape="true">
    <gesture move-lexeme="sweep-dome" hand-lexeme="flat" palm-orient="down"
        extent="large" location="center" stroke="sp1:T92"/>
    <gesture move-lexeme= "push" hand-lexeme="flat" palm-orient-right="down"
        palm-orient-left= "right" extent="large" location= "right" stroke="sp1:T98"/>
    <gesture move-lexeme="sweep-dome" hand-lexeme="flat" palm-orient="down"
        extent="large" location="center" stroke="sp1:T104"/>
    <gesture move-lexeme= "forward" hand-lexeme="flat" palm-orient="oblique-forward"
        location="front" stroke="sp1:T108">
        <gesture-overlay move-lexeme="forward-down" hand-lexeme="flat" palm-orient="down"
location="front" stroke="sp1:T110"/>
    <gesture/>
</gesture-sequence>
...
</bml>
```

Fig. 3. Example FML and BML snippet

Our FML descriptions use extended FML specifications to reflect our compound model and particularly to reflect the ideational unit structure. We add three type of tags: <ideational>, <rhythmic-semantic> and <function>. They are in correspondence to ideational unit, rhythmic-semantic unit and atomic communicative function respectively. <function>'s attributes can be found in Table 1. Note that <function> not only defines communicative function, but also specifies actions which usually only appear in BML domain. The reason is the actions in FML are not the real physical actions, but rather a description of the communicative function in terms of an underlying embodied metaphor.

Our BML descriptions extend standard BML specifications and add <gesture-sequence>, <gesture> and <gesture-overlay> to reflect the gesture sequence structure. <gesture-sequence> is the behavior space mapping of an ideational unit, its attributes for this tag represent the features within and across ideational

Table 1. FML <function>'s attributes

Specification	Description	Example
id	identity name for the function	c1, c2
type	type of communication function	reference, emphasis, movement, container
location	location of metaphoric object	center, left, right, up, down, front, back
action	action	listing, delineate, move, discard
modifier	modifier for the action	finger, round
attribute	attribute for metaphoric object	large, further
reference	reference to utterance	warm and fuzzy

unit. Similarly, <gesture> is the behavior space mapping of the atomic utterance content, its attributes reflect features within the same communicative function unit. <gesture-overlay> describes repeated gestures happen inside an unitary gesture which is a result of derivative process from features needed for gesture performance. An example snippet of FML and BML description can be found in Figure 3.

We use a rule based system approach (as in [15,13,4,14]) as our behavior planner and extend its rules to support features in the model. The key role for these rules is to map from FML descriptions to BML descriptions. As part of this mapping, the rules need to resolve the referential content's location accordingly to their ids (see Table 1). Also they must map FML aspects like emphasis to behavioral manifestations like repetitions, such as in the following rule example.[1]

```
emphasis_function
if
    fcn($functionType,$modifier,$start1,$end1,$priority1)
    fcn(emphasis,$modifier1,$start1,$end2,$priority2)
    check $end1 < $end2
then
    fcn($functionType,overlay,$end1,$end2,$priority1)
```

4.2 Behavior Realization

The behavior realization module generates the animation. The animation platform we use, SmartBody [21], supports both procedural and data driven techniques, but in the case of gesture generation, we rely on key-frame or mocap animations to get natural and smooth results. Based on the animation framework, we developed an algorithm that animates the BML output descriptions provided by the previous behavior planning module.

Behavior realization has two steps. <gesture-sequence> defines the selection of individual gesture animations with given all the constraints as requirements

---

[1] Variables in the example rule refer to Table 1.

(these animations will combine to be the final animation sequence). Then the blending techniques are used to adjust individual gesture animation to achieve certain constraints or variations, such as to modify gesture so it can refer to location of previous gesture or depict a metaphoric object's physical size.

We assume a motion database with each gesture motion tagged with labels including communicative function, type of action, handedness, handshape, action modifier such as big and small. We run Algorithm 1 to realize step one as mentioned above.

We use $M = \{m\}$ to define our gesture motion database and each motion has a set of tags $T_m(m) = \{tag\}$, given input BML behavior set $B = \{b\}$ with each behavior with tag $T_b(b) = \{tag\}$, we are trying get a final animation sequence $A_{final} = \{...\}$. $ConstraintFunc$ applies the constraints defined in the section 3, for example, consecutive gestures should have the same handshapes. $ChooseBest$ looks at possible animation sequences $VectorA$ and tries to find the best one. Here, we simplify $ChooseBest$ by just hand picking the best one[2].

```
1.  motion subset for behavior b M'[b] = {φ}
2.  for i ← 1 to behaviorSetSize do
3.     for j ← 1 to motionSetSize do
4.        if T_m(j) is a subset of T_b(i) then
5.           Append(M'[b], M(j))
6.        end if
7.     end for
8.  end for
9.  VectorA = []
10. for i ← 1 to behaviorSetSize do
11.    temporary animation sequence A = {φ}
12.    motionSubSetSize = size(M'(i))
13.    for j ← 1 to motionSubSetSize do
14.       if A is empty then
15.          A ← M'(i)(j)
16.       end if
17.       a =last element of A
18.       meetConstraints = ConstraintFunc(M'(i, j), a)
19.       if meetConstraints is TRUE then
20.          Append(A, M'(i, j))
21.       else
22.          Prune M'(i, j) or a by priority and hands go back to rest position
23.       end if
24.    end for
25.    Append(VectorA, A)
26. end for
27. A_final = ChooseBest(VectorA)
```

Algorithm 1. Animation Sequence Generation Algorithm

---

[2] We visually choose the one that is the smoothest and the most natural in the overall performance.

Then we utilize the SmartBody blending controller, based on a barycentric parametric blending technique [5], so that it can flexibly adjust individual gesture animations. Similar gesture animations are grouped offline to define an animation blend space and adjustment parameters are extracted (automatically by calling SmartBody's API). During run-time execution, control parameters are given as an input from the BML descriptions and used to calculate the weights for each motion inside the blend. Take *sweep-dome* gesture for example, there can be two similar motions, one depicts a small object with modifier label as "small" and one depicts a large object with modifier label as "large". If BML descriptions input a sweep-dome gesture with a modifier "medium", we interpret that in parameter space, infer the distance needed for two hands and use it to compute the weights for motions. Similarly we can do that for adjusting locations of the hand.

5   Related Work

Many techniques have been explored to generate gestures, differing in terms of input data used, underlying model and framework. Many researchers have focused on gesture generation. ACE [10] focuses on deictic and iconic gestures, it takes text input and looks for specific words in order to display associated gestures with timing based on prosody analysis. NVBG [13] is a rule based system that uses the communicative intent embedded in the surface text as well as the agent's cognitive processing such as internal goals and emotion states. Cerebella [15,14] used an improved communication function inference mechanism along with prosodic analysis. Kopp et al. [12] based their system on the *Sketch Model* [20] and can create gestures from arbitrary form specifications and handle co-articulations. Kipp et al. [9] introduced a system that generates gestures in particular styles based on probabilistic reproduction of data captured from a human subject, and an extension that includes dynamics [18].

Among all these works our method resembles [9] the most in terms that we all deal with a sequence of gesture movements that go beyond the structure of individual gestures. The difference is they capture the regularities indirectly through data analysis. In our approach, we are explicitly modeling the constraints and features that are carried on within and in between ideational units.

6   Results

To illustrate the approach, we annotated five videos drawn from a simulated role play corpus, an example of which is depicted in Figure 1. FML descriptions were created for these videos (see Figure 3) to provide input for our framework which then generated gesture performances. In order to examine the impact of *within* and *across ideational units* constraints, we removed individual constraints one by one to check its impact. We created side by side comparison videos, one with all constraints active (on), the other missing one constraint, as can be seen from link

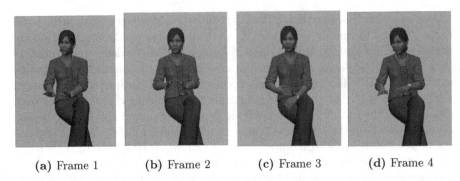

(a) Frame 1   (b) Frame 2   (c) Frame 3   (d) Frame 4

Fig. 4. A sample performance from an animation video: the above sequence shows the key strokes for the performance generated for: "Okay, let's just backup for a second then, what's happening right now? So when we were talking, you find yourself kind of drifting off, what's going on?"

http://youtu.be/A-3Ic-zCqnM.[3] Alternatively, you can also find an example performance depicted Figure 4 and a comparison example from Figure 5.

Studies. We also did studies to specifically test the impact of the "hands going to rest or relax position constraint at the end of ideational units but not going to rest position within ideational units" constraint. We consider two conditions here, one is hands never go to rest or relax position and the other is hands always go to rest position after finishing individual gestures. Leveraging Amazon Mechanical Turk [1], we ask the participants to select which video they think is closer to how humans gesture and give their strength of preference (scaled from 1 to 5 and 5 is strongest) after watching the comparison video. We randomize both the order between video pairs and the overall order of videos being watched by participants. Each comparison video is assigned to 50 workers.

First study is designed to test the first condition, we only use three examples since two of them only contain one ideational unit, which won't be able to show the constraint impact across the ideational unit. Video with all constraints active is preferred with a percentage of 71.1%, strength of preference 3.79, while video with hands never go to rest or relax position is preferred with a percentage of 29.9%, strength of preference 3.11. Binomial test is run on preferences with significant value $p < 0.001$. The result of the study shows strong impact of the constraints.

Second study covers the second condition, all five examples are used. Video with all constraints on and video with hands always go to rest position has a preference rate of 40.6% and 59.4% respectively, although people who pick the

---

[3] The video is organized as follows: it first provides five overall results, then four comparison videos, followed by videos presenting adjustment of metaphoric size of an object and gesture referential location using parametric blending technique, finally we present a video showing the repeated gesture inside individual gesture used for emphasizing a point.

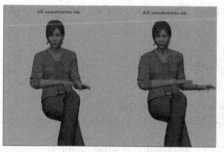 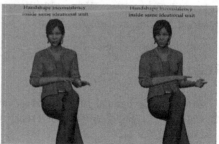

(a) All constraints on   (b) Inconsistent handshapes

Fig. 5. A comparison example: each image shows two frames of the performance. Left image has all constraints active and right image disables one constraint - the handshape consistency within the same ideational unit.

video with all constraints on has a strength of preference value of 3.46 which is higher than 3.25 when they pick the video with hands always go to rest position. Binomial test is run on preferences with significant value $p < 0.001$. The gestures in the video are located closed to the rest position. So visually, there are not much differences between both videos. The rule needs to be further verified on other examples.

We haven't done study yet for other constraints like handshapes and handiness consistency. However, based on our visual inspections, it was fairly obvious to the authors that violating these constraints caused visual awkwardness.

7 Discussion

In this paper we present a novel sequential gesture model that looks at ideational structures to provide guidelines for the gesture performances.

The main contribution in turns of implementation includes creating behavior planning rules to map from FML descriptions to BML descriptions and a behavior realization algorithm. Results and studies show that these constraints play an important role in natural human gesturing that without it the performance would not look right.

The second study also identified a key issue with how we implemented the model. Although our model posits the distinctions between relax and rest pose within the ideational unit, we didn't realize it in our implementation, that might be the reason of the failure for the second study. To be more specific, our implementation uses a hold which is often utilized to emphasize a point, instead of relaxing after t_{se} of a gesture during the transition to the other gesture within the same ideational unit, this causing an unnatural result.

For the future work, we are hoping to test our sequential gesture model on different behavior realizers such as Greta [19].

Acknowledgments. We would like to thank Teresa Dey for all the animations provided for our motion database.

References

1. Amazon: Mechanical turk, https://www.mturk.com/mturk/
2. Calbris, G.: The Semiotics of French Gestures, vol. V. Indiana University Press (1990)
3. Calbris, G.: Elements of Meaning in Gesture. Gesture studies. John Benjamins Publishing Company (2011)
4. Cassell, J., Vilhjálmsson, H.H., Bickmore, T.: Beat: The behavior expression animation toolkit. In: Proceedings of the 28th Annual Conference on Computer Graphics and Interactive Techniques, SIGGRAPH 2001, pp. 477–486. ACM, New York (2001)
5. Feng, A.W., Xu, Y., Shapiro, A.: An example-based motion synthesis technique for locomotion and object manipulation. In: ACM SIGGRAPH Symposium on Interactive 3D Graphics and Games, Costa Mesa, CA (March 2012)
6. Hall, J.A., Harrigan, J.A., Rosenthal, R.: Nonverbal behavior in clinician patient interaction. Applied and Preventive Psychology 4(1), 21–37 (1995)
7. Kendon, A.: Gesture: Visible Action as Utterance. Cambridge University Press (2004)
8. Kendon, A.: Some relationships between body motion and speech. Pergamon Press (1972)
9. Kipp, M., Neff, M., Kipp, K., Albrecht, I.: Towards natural gesture synthesis: Evaluating gesture units in a data-driven approach to gesture synthesis. In: Pelachaud, C., Martin, J.-C., André, E., Chollet, G., Karpouzis, K., Pelé, D. (eds.) IVA 2007. LNCS (LNAI), vol. 4722, pp. 15–28. Springer, Heidelberg (2007)
10. Kopp, S., Jung, B., Leßmann, N., Wachsmuth, I.: Max - a multimodal assistant in virtual reality construction. Künstliche Intelligenz 17(4), 11 (2003)
11. Kopp, S., Krenn, B., Marsella, S.C., Marshall, A.N., Pelachaud, C., Pirker, H., Thórisson, K.R., Vilhjálmsson, H.H.: Towards a Common Framework for Multimodal Generation: The Behavior Markup Language. In: Gratch, J., Young, M., Aylett, R.S., Ballin, D., Olivier, P. (eds.) IVA 2006. LNCS (LNAI), vol. 4133, pp. 205–217. Springer, Heidelberg (2006)
12. Kopp, S., Wachsmuth, I.: Synthesizing multimodal utterances for conversational agents. Computer Animation and Virtual Worlds 15(1), 39–52 (2004)
13. Lee, J., Marsella, S.C.: Nonverbal behavior generator for embodied conversational agents. In: Gratch, J., Young, M., Aylett, R.S., Ballin, D., Olivier, P. (eds.) IVA 2006. LNCS (LNAI), vol. 4133, pp. 243–255. Springer, Heidelberg (2006)
14. Lhommet, M., Marsella, S.C.: Gesture with meaning. In: Aylett, R., Krenn, B., Pelachaud, C., Shimodaira, H. (eds.) IVA 2013. LNCS, vol. 8108, pp. 303–312. Springer, Heidelberg (2013)
15. Marsella, S., Xu, Y., Lhommet, M., Feng, A.W., Scherer, S., Shapiro, A.: Virtual character performance from speech. In: Symposium on Computer Animation, pp. 25–35 (2013)
16. McNeill, D.: Hand and Mind: What Gestures Reveal about Thought. University of Chicago Press (1992)
17. McNeill, D.: Gesture and Thought. University of Chicago Press (2005)

18. Neff, M., Kipp, M., Albrecht, I., Seidel, H.P.: Gesture modeling and animation based on a probabilistic re-creation of speaker style. ACM Transactions on Graphics (2008)
19. Niewiadomski, R., Bevacqua, E., Mancini, M., Pelachaud, C.: Greta: an interactive expressive ECA system. In: International Conference on Autonomous Agents and Multiagent Systems, pp. 1399–1400 (2009)
20. de Ruiter, J.P.: The production of gesture and speech. Cambridge University Press (2000)
21. Thiebaux, M., Marsella, S., Marshall, A.N., Kallmann, M.: Smartbody: Behavior realization for embodied conversational agents. In: Proceedings of the 7th International Joint Conference on Autonomous Agents and Multiagent Systems, AAMAS 2008, vol. 1, pp. 151–158. International Foundation for Autonomous Agents and Multiagent Systems, Richland (2008)

Statistical Dialog Manager Design Tool for Health Screening and Assessments

Ugan Yasavur, Christine Lisetti, and Napthali Rishe

School of Computing and Information Sciences
Florida International University
Miami, FL, 33199, USA
ugan.yasavur@fiu.edu, {lisetti,rishen}@cs.fiu.edu

Abstract. We focus on creating a programming tool which enables to create dialog managers for speech-enabled IVA applications in the standardized health screening and assessment domain. Our approach aims to bridge the gap between the intelligent virtual agents (IVA) and the spoken dialog systems (SDS) research communities for the delivery of standardized health interviews by embodied conversational agents (ECA).

Keywords: spoken dialogue system, partially observable Markov decision processes (POMDP), reinforcement learning, embodied conversational agent (ECA), intelligent virtual agents (IVA), brief intervention, behavior change, alcoholism.

1 Introduction and Related Research

Latest progress in speech recognition technology, together with advances in the field of conversational intelligent virtual agents (IVA), have created new possibilities to develop a variety of useful applications to address contemporary healthcare challenges. Because current automatic speech recognizers (ASR) are still regarded as a noisy input channels, they need to be backed up with a mechanism to operate against noisy recognitions. In the spoken dialog systems (SDS) area, recent research has mostly concentrated on addressing this problem by employing stochastic and data-driven dialog management (DM) methodologies, namely reinforcement learning based approaches [8]. These approaches, however, have not been widely used by IVA researchers so far.

There are a number of IVA applications in health-related domains such as fitness and activity promotion applications [1], virtual support agents for post traumatic stress disorder [4], health interventions for drinking problems [3]. As an interaction modality, some researchers use ECAs with menu-based inputs [1,3], others use speech as input modality with simple dialog management [5] and, Morbini et al. [4] uses free-text as input modality.

We aim to bridge the gap between SDS and IVA research, and to use findings from the SDS community for DM in the applications of IVAs in the health domain. The goal of our approach is to create a tool to design custom dialog managers which employs POMDPs as an underlying mechanism. Using our tool,

T. Bickmore et al. (Eds.): IVA 2014, LNAI 8637, pp. 492–495, 2014.

a dialog designer can just specify the content-related information (e.g. question to be asked, information that needs to be provided) and connections between each question in the interview. To facilitate the process, we created an API to design dialog managers. Our tool can be used to create spoken dialog systems for initial screening of patients, conducting brief health interventions and information-providing applications.

2 Approach

Brief Interventions for Behavior Change. We focussed our current approach on an IVA-delivered behavior change brief intervention for excessive alcohol consumption. For the content of the behavior change dialog, we strictly follow the pocket guide from National Institute on Alcohol Abuse and Alcoholism (NIAAA) for alcohol screening and brief interventions for youth [2], which is publicly available online. The initial screen and brief intervention has 3 steps: **1)** Step 1: Ask the two screening questions; **2)** Step 2: *a)* Guide Patient, *b)* Assess Risk **3)** Advise and Assist.

Dialog Management. The dialog manager has to track a dialog state which usually contains some important dialog state attributes such as: ASR confidence level, grammar type, information about whether the received answer is confirmed or not, number of re-asks. Each state is mapped to a dialog action that is called *Dialog Policy*. To optimize the system, a reward function is designed. We can formalize the defined mechanism with the Markov decision processes (MDP) framework. MDP assumes that the entire state space is fully observable. However, it is partially observable in SDSs because of imperfect ASR outputs.

An SDS with a partially observable Markov decision processes (POMDP) model attempts to address the partially observable nature of SDS state spaces [7]. According to SDS-POMDP model, at each dialog turn, a user has a goal g in mind (e.g. provide an answer as to the number of days in week s/he drinks, or as to whether alcohol consumption causes any health problems). The system takes a dialog action a (e.g. how many days in a week do you drink alcoholic beverage?) and the user replies with action u ("I usually drink on weekends"). The speech recognizer outputs the N-best list of recognitions $\nu = \{\nu_1, \nu_2, ..., \nu_n\}$ with the estimated confidence scores indicating the likelihood of each recognition being correct, $P(u|\nu)$, while processing the audio. A history variable h keeps track of the relevant dialog history (e.g. receipt of each piece of information, confirmation status of each piece of information). Because ASR is a noisy sensor, g, u, h are not fully observable by the system. Instead, the system maintains a distribution b over these values. Given some existing distribution $b(g, h)$, and observations a and ν', an updated distribution $b'(g', h')$ can be computed [7,6]:

$$b'(g', h') = k \sum_{\nu'} P(u'|\nu') \sum_{h} P(u'|g', h, a) P(h'|g', u', h, a) \sum_{g} P(g'|a, g) b(g, h)$$

$$(1)$$

where $P(u'|g', h, a)$ computes how likely are user actions; $P(h'|g', u', h, a)$ computes how the dialog history evolves; $P(g'|a, g)$ computes how the user's goal may change; and k is a normalizing factor.

POMDPs grow exponentially with the number of possible user goals, and it is not possible to calculate this update in real time. This means that POMDP usually suffer from scalability issues [7]. To overcome this problem, a distribution over the set of partitions of user goals $\{p_1, p_2, ..., p_n\}$ is maintained: each partition p_n indicates a collection of user goals, and each user goal can be belong to exactly one partition. The belief in a partition is the sum of the dialog states it contains.

It is assumed that the user's goal is fixed during the interaction, and that error-prone ASR confusions between recognitions that are not on the ASR N-best list are uniform. These two assumptions allow to compute [9]:

$$b'(g', h') = k \sum_{\nu'} P(u'|\nu') \sum_{h \varepsilon p'} P(u'|p', u', h, a) P(p'|p) b(g, h) \qquad (2)$$

where $P(p'|p)$ shows the fraction of belief in p which p' would have if p were split into p' and $p - p'$: $P(p'|p) = b_0(p')/b_0(p)$ and $P(p - p'|p) = b_0(p - p')/b_0(p)$, where $b_0(p)$ is the prior probability of a partition p [9].

The partitioning is performed in the following way: first each recognition in the N-best list is compared to each existing partition; if user action can split the partition, the partition is divided. Then the belief in each partition (and dialog histories) is updated using Equation (2). To avoid exponential growth of the number of partitions, low confidence partitions are combined by summing up their beliefs. This approach usually allows to take into account 2-3 N-best recognitions [9]. This problem is addressed by applying incremental partition recombination for tracking dialog states by using a larger number of N-best recognitions [6]. We use the incremental partition combination approach in dialog state tracking [6].

A Tool for Representing Patterns in Health Brief Interviews as Programatic Objects. The goal of our approach is to create a tool to design custom dialog managers which employs POMDPs as an underlying mechanism. As a result, a dialog designer can just specify the content-related information (e.g. question to be asked, information that needs to be provided) and transitions between each question in the screening. To facilitate the process, we created an API to design dialog managers. Each question represented as an object which encapsulates the dialog policies and the transition information. In other words, each question object consists of a POMDP with transition information to successor step. Since the most of the dialog actions have similar purposes such as asking a question, confirmations, and re-asking a question, it is possible create parameterized patterns that are encapsulated in programmatic objects. Basically, each question object contains all the underlying basic functionality for each piece of information which can be customized. The questions objects can be considered as nodes of a graph, the transitions between questions can be considered as edges that require a key value to transit from one node to another. The key value is a piece of information that the system tries to get from a user in a particular question.

A dialog designer needs to instantiate a question object with at least 4 parameters: 1) the question text, 2) the semantic keys which are used to create edges from current node to successor nodes, 3) the prior node which indicates which is the prior of the current node, and 4) the semantic-key-to-connect indicates which edge of the prior node it should connect. Creating question objects which encapsulates POMDP mechanism is as easy as specifying some content-related parameters.

3 Conclusion and Future Work

We created dialog manager design tool for creating dialog managers for delivery of standardized health interviews, which will increase the accessibility of state of the art dialog management approaches to non-experts. We also adapted methodologies currently used by the SDS community to health dialogs. As future work, we plan to test and evaluate our system with real users.

References

1. Bickmore, T.W., Schulman, D., Sidner, C.: Automated interventions for multiple health behaviors using conversational agents. Patient Education and Counseling 92(2), 142–148 (2013)
2. of Health, U.D., Services, H.: Alcohol screening and brief intervention for youth: A practitioner's guide (2011)
3. Lisetti, C., Amini, R., Yasavur, U., Rishe, N.: I can help you change! an empathic virtual agent delivers behavior change health interventions. ACM Transactions on Management Information Systems (TMIS) 4(4), 19 (2013)
4. Morbini, F., Forbell, E., DeVault, D., Sagae, K., Traum, D.R., Rizzo, A.A.: A mixed-initiative conversational dialogue system for healthcare. In: Proceedings of the 13th Annual Meeting of the Special Interest Group on Discourse and Dialogue, SIGDIAL 2012, pp. 137–139. Association for Computational Linguistics, Stroudsburg (2012), http://dl.acm.org/citation.cfm?id=2392800.2392825
5. Turunen, M., Hakulinen, J., Ståhl, O., Gambäck, B., Hansen, P., Rodríguez Gancedo, M.C., de la Cámara, R.S., Smith, C., Charlton, D., Cavazza, M.: Multimodal and mobile conversational health and fitness companions. Computer Speech & Language 25(2), 192–209 (2011)
6. Williams, J.D.: Incremental partition recombination for efficient tracking of multiple dialog states. In: 2010 IEEE International Conference on Acoustics Speech and Signal Processing (ICASSP), pp. 5382–5385. IEEE (2010)
7. Williams, J.D., Young, S.: Partially observable markov decision processes for spoken dialog systems. Computer Speech & Language 21(2), 393–422 (2007)
8. Young, S., Gašić, M., Thomson, B., Williams, J.: Pomdp-based statistical spoken dialog systems: A review (2013)
9. Young, S., Gašić, M., Keizer, S., Mairesse, F., Schatzmann, J., Thomson, B., Yu, K.: The hidden information state model: A practical framework for pomdp-based spoken dialogue management. Computer Speech & Language 24(2), 150–174 (2010)

Towards Learning Nonverbal Identities from the Web: Automatically Identifying Visually Accentuated Words

AmirAli B. Zadeh, Kenji Sagae, and Louis Philippe Morency

Institute for Creative Technologies,
University of Southern California,
12015 E Waterfront Drive, Playa Vista, CA 90094-2546, USA
{zadeh,sagae,morency}@ict.usc.edu

Abstract. This paper presents a novel long-term idea to learn automatically from online multimedia content, such as videos from YouTube channels, a portfolio of nonverbal identities in the form of computational representation of prototypical gestures of a speaker. As a first step towards this vision, this paper presents proof-of-concept experiments to automatically identify visually accentuated words from a collection of online videos of the same person. The experimental results are promising with many accentuated words automatically identified and specific head motion patterns were associated with these words.

1 Introduction

Much progress has been done in recent years in the field of interactive virtual agents. One particular emphasis has been on automatically generating nonverbal behaviors to accompany spoken words of the virtual human. While earlier versions of these nonverbal behavior generators [1, 2, 3, 5] were mostly based on literature review and general observations, new data-driven approaches [4, 6, 7, 8, 9] have been proposed to learn from a corpus of interaction the nonverbal behaviors that are used by a specific person or that generalizes across all participants. Given the significant cost associated with acquiring and annotating such dataset, an important issue is the scalability of these approaches. How can we create a large-scale portfolio of these nonverbal behavior generators for different interaction styles and personalities?

In this paper, we propose a long-term idea of using online multimedia content to help with the issue of scalability and customization of current nonverbal behavior generators. Video hosting websites such as YouTube contain a large amount of videos and channels where people are expressing their opinions about different topics. Each of these speakers has different communicative styles and their behaviors are idiosyncratic.

As a first step towards this vision, we present a proof of concept experiment focusing on visually accentuated words (i.e., spoken words that often co-occur with visual motion or emphasis) and their associated head gestures. We propose a statistical approach to automatically identify accentuated words in a collection of online videos from the same

T. Bickmore et al. (Eds.): IVA 2014, LNAI 8637, pp. 496–503, 2014.

speaker. We also present an analysis of the head motion patterns associated with these emphasized words, studying the variability and idiosyncrasy of these gestures. Our main research hypothesis is that some of the words will follow motion distribution different from the overall distribution, enabling us to identify these visually-accentuated words. Following a brief review of related work, section 3 describes our long-term vision. Our experiments and results are presented in Section 4 and 5. We conclude with future directions in Section 6. We will discuss the related works in the next section.

2 Related Work

Our research builds upon the previous literature and research on human gesture analysis and virtual human animation. Some of the original work on this topic used rule-based systems designed on general observations of human gestures [1, 2, 3]. Lee and Marsella created during their video analysis created a list of nonverbal behavior generation rules and used it for virtual human animation [5]. BEAT system developed by Cassell et al. uses plain text as input and based on priority values and linguistic analysis of the input text generates meaningful gestures and facial animation [13]. By focusing on behavior rules that would best generalize over a normal population, these approaches enabled automatic nonverbal behavior generation for virtual human.

Co-articulation of vocal and facial dynamics have also been studied alongside the relation between prosody features and certain gestures or gesture classes. Brand used a co-articulation model of vocal and facial dynamics to create realistically speaking animation [12]. Busso et al. created a dataset of videos and calculated rigid head motion. They used Hidden Markov Models for each emotional category they defined and synthesized a virtual human based on different emotions and prosody features [7].

More related to our current work, Stone et al. used a dataset of audio and motion captured segments of full body motion to recreate a specific person's gestures [6]. They use a set of simple grammar rules and match the gestures with the communicative function of the utterance. Neff et al. used an annotated dataset of two TV shows and created gesture profiles for each performer and later used these profiles in animation synthesis [4]. Their annotation scheme was based on a predefined gesture set and the customization for a specific individual was performed by directly modifying the statistics used to map gestures to semantic tags.

In contrast with prior work, our long-term vision covers the customization of both the timing of visual gestures as well as their appearance and dynamic. To reach this goal, we propose a novel approach which takes advantage of online multimedia content to automatically identify idiosyncratic gestures and their mapping to the verbal and prosodic content. As the first step towards this goal, we propose computational analysis of the relationship between head motion and spoken words to automatically quantify the nonverbal behaviors of a specific speaker.

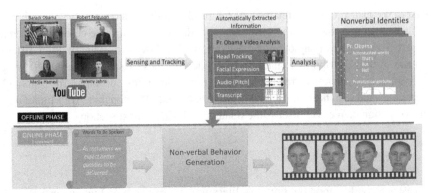

Fig. 1. An overview of our long-term vision for learning nonverbal identities from the web

3   Vision: Learning Nonverbal Identities from the Web

The long-term vision is to create a portfolio of *nonverbal identities* to help customize how virtual humans are animated. These nonverbal identities are computational representations of how a specific person gestures when speaking, including what words are usually emphasized, which gesture or facial expression is used to emphasize and how specific concepts or emotions are displayed by this speaker. To enable such large-scale diversity in computational representations of human nonverbal behaviors, we propose to take advantage of online multimedia content such as videos posted on YouTube to learn these nonverbal identities. These online websites are an almost infinite source of data since people love posting videos expressing their opinions about different topics.

Since many videos are often available for the same person (e.g., through a You-Tube channel) it is possible to get multiple examples from the same person. With HD webcams becoming popular and microphone quality increasing, we can get high quality data on a large-scale. Figure 1 shows an overview of our long-term vision where nonverbal identities are learned automatically from online videos and then used to animate a virtual human that resembles a specific person (or a mixture of nonverbal identities). This vision includes an offline phase where online videos are analyzed to learn the portfolio of nonverbal identities and an online phase where these identities are used to animate the virtual human. The experiments presented in the following section focus on the offline phase, looking at the visually accentuated words.

4   Experiments: Identifying Visually-Accentuated Words

As a first step towards learning nonverbal identities from the web, we designed a preliminary set of experiments to study the viability of this approach, focusing on a specific type of nonverbal behavior (head motion) and its relationship to the verbal content. As discussed in the previous section, we are particularly interested in visually-accentuated words and their related head gestures. Our primary goal with these experiments is to evaluate the feasibility of automatically extracting behavioral patterns from online videos (e.g., YouTube videos). As a secondary goal, we are interested to analyze the type of multimodal patterns identified in these online videos. In the following sub-sections, we present our approach for automatically crawling online videos, then present our techniques for automatic audio-visual feature extraction and finally describe our experimental methodology for our analysis.

Web Data Acquisition. Many online video sharing websites such as YouTube have a "channel" functionality where the same person (or company) can post multiple videos. These are particularly interesting in our case since we can easily gather multiple videos from the same person using these channels. In our experiments, we specifically used the White House Weekly Address video channel of President Barack Obama on YouTube. We developed a customized video web crawler which can find all videos of the same channel with all captions, audio and metadata of the online videos. This customized web crawler was augmented with a functionality to check if each download video contained only one person facing directly the camera. This functionality was optimized to work on a large-scale using CUDA and TBB. Our final dataset contained 196 videos of President Barack Obama, which represents more than 12 hours.

Audio-Visual Feature Extraction. An important aspect in our automatic multimodal feature extraction is the synchronization between information streams (text, audio and video). For the text modality, we took advantage of the captions associated to most YouTube videos. In fact, many videos posted on YouTube channels come with manually transcribed captions. Many companies are offering this service of manual transcription to YouTube video producers, simplifying our first step of speech transcription. To assure the synchronization of the text captions with the audio and video streams, we processed all videos using the P2FA forced alignment software [10]. This method allowed us to have exact timestamp for each spoken word. We assessed the quality of these word alignments on a subset of our dataset, showing good precision given the high quality recording of the audio stream.

Since we are interested in visual accentuation from the head motion, we automatically extracted head orientation from the video stream. For this step, we used the Intraface head pose tracker which returns a three dimensional rotation vector, representing the rotations around X, Y and Z axes [11]. These rotations can be interpreted as pitch, yaw and roll. These head orientation estimates were computed at 30Hz.

Methodology. The goal of our experiments is to study the interaction between spoken words and visual accentuations from head motions. To perform this analysis, we first created a dictionary of words spoken at least 50 times by President Obama. The stream of head orientation estimates was modified to compute the instantaneous head motion at each frame, keeping only the absolute value of this motion. This computation was performed for each rotation X, Y and Z. The multimodal analysis was performed by defining a time window of +/- 25 milliseconds around each instance of the words from our dictionary.

We are interested in automatically differentiating behavior patterns that are prototypical from the ones that are only happening by chance. As a first step in this direction, we propose to perform a statistical analysis to identify these recurring visual behaviors that are attached to specific verbal cues. To perform this analysis we hypothesize that the distribution of head motion happening during emphasized words is statistically different from the distribution of head motion over the whole interaction. To test this hypothesis, we perform student t-test analysis comparing all individual word with the overall distribution of head motion. This approach allows us to identify words with head motion patterns statistically different than the average spoken words. We can use the p-value returned by the statistical test as a measure of the uniqueness of this specific spoken word. This allowed us to identify the top visually accentuated words of President Obama for all three head rotations (pitch, yaw and roll). The following section describes our results and discussion.

Table 1. Top 10 words having lowest p-value in each rotation axis

	Rot. X	*Rot.Y*	*Rot. Z*
1	that's	not	but
2	but	all	that's
3	if	no	we
4	we	there's	I
5	I	the	it's
6	because	a	and
7	there's	across	why
8	so	just	so
9	don't	had	it
10	all	too	we're

5   Results and Discussion

Table 1 shows the top-ranked accentuated words by President Obama based on the head velocities around the X axis, the Y axis and the Z axis. The words presented in this table were ranked based on their p-value after the statistical test comparing them with the distribution of all words. A total of 155 words (including the words shown in Table 1) were shown to be statistically significant with $p<0.01$. This first result suggests that our multimodal analysis was able to automatically identify visually accentuated words. Another interesting result is the analysis of accentuated words per rotation axis. Words such as 'no' and 'not' are emerging for the rotation around Y axis which goes with our intuition that negative words should be accompanied by a head shake gesture. Words such as 'we' and 'I' are more significant around X and Z axes, which means either a gesture going vertically emphasizing himself (X axis) or tilting gesture including people around him. The number of significant words for the X, Y and Z rotations were 78, 85 and 91 respectively.

To better understand the head motion patterns accompanying these visually accentuated words, we plotted the average head rotational velocity around the X for 5 seconds before and after words from Table 1. Figure 2 shows these average graphs for three words: "don't", "because" and "but". We can see in all three cases an increase of the head motion around the word itself. It is important to notice that this head motion could be in either direction (e.g., going up or down for the rotation around the X axis).

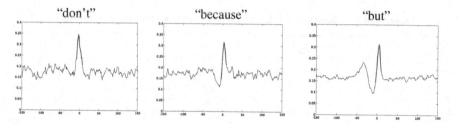

Fig. 2. Examples of the average motion plots (rotation around X axis, in degrees) for 3 top words from Table 1. The +/- 25 millisecond boundary of the specified word is drawn in red.

One interesting observation is the little dip right before the words "because" and "but". This is most likely a preparation phase right before the emphasis of these two spoken words. Even more interesting is the second bump before the word "but" which means that the speaker also emphasized a previous word before not moving and then emphasizing the word "but". During our analysis of the head motion patterns around this word "but", we observed that a significant proportion of these instances are preceded by a short pause. In fact, this is a typical behavior of President Obama who often pauses for a little while before making his strong point, using a word such as "but". These results show that our algorithms were able to identify such specific nonverbal behaviors of President Obama. This is a first step toward our long-term vision of automatically learning nonverbal identities of speakers based on their online videos.

We show in Figure 3 an example of a spoken sentence with below the direct head orientation around the X axis (i.e., pitch). We highlighted moments where the words "don't" were used. It is interesting to see that the head motion observed in Figure 2 is in fact a motion down for both instances. By segmenting these head motion instances we can start building a dictionary of prototypical head gestures and associate them with specific keywords. These behavioral rules can later be integrated in a generic nonverbal behavior generator to help customize it to a specific speaker.

6   Conclusion and Future Work

This paper introduced the long-term idea of learning prototypical nonverbal behaviors of a specific speaker from their online videos and use this information to customize the nonverbal behaviors of a virtual human. This automatic learning of *nonverbal identities* will allow us to create a portfolio of different speakers and enable more diversity in virtual human animations. As the first step towards this goal, we studied the relationship between head motion and spoken words to automatically identify visually accentuated words in online videos. Our results showed that we can automatically identify accentuated words for a specific speaker, showing interesting differences for head motion around the X, Y and Z axes.

... americans who still don't have jobs, but for the millions more who still don't have the right job ...

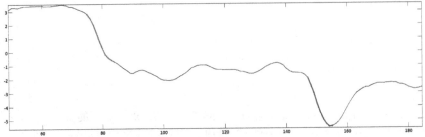

Fig. 3. Shows orientation around the X axis (pitch) for a specific spoken utterance. Two instances of the word "don't" are highlighted, showing in both case a motion downward

This first proof of concept opens up the way to many research directions analyzing online multimedia content to quantify human nonverbal behaviors. As one interesting next step, we plan to create a complete representation of not only the visually accentuated words but also include a dictionary of prototypical head gestures for each individual. We plan to evaluate the effectiveness of our virtual human animation method by studying how people perceive the virtual human gestures and if they are able to differentiate or even recognize specific person just from their customized virtual humans.

Acknowledgements. This material is based upon work supported by the National Science Foundation under Grant No. IIS-1118018 and the U.S. Army Research, Development, and Engineering Command (RDECOM). The content does not necessarily reflect the position or the policy of the Government, and no official endorsement should be inferred.

References

1. Cassell, J., Pelachaud, C., Badler, N., Steedman, M., Achorn, B., Douville, B., Prevost, S., And Stone, M.: Animated conversation: Rule-based generation of facial expression, gesture and spoken intonation for multiple conversational agents 413–420 (1994)
2. Decarlo, D., Stone, M., Revilla, C., And Venditti, J.J.: Specifying and animating fa-cial signals for discourse in embodied conversational agents. Computer Animation and Virtual Worlds 15(1), 27–38 (2004)
3. Bergmann, K., And Kopp, S.: Increasing the expressiveness of virtual agents: auto-nomous generation of speech and gesture for spatial description tasks. In: Proceedings of The 8th International Conference on Autonomous Agents and Multiagent Systems-, vol. 1, pp. 361–368 (2009)
4. Neff, M., Kipp, M., Albrecht, I., And Seidel, H.-P.: Gesture modeling and animation based on a probabilistic recreation of speaker style. ACM Transactions on Graphics 27(1), 5 (2008)

5. Lee, J., Marsella, S.C.: Nonverbal behavior generator for embodied conversational agents. In: Gratch, J., Young, M., Aylett, R.S., Ballin, D., Olivier, P. (eds.) IVA 2006. LNCS (LNAI), vol. 4133, pp. 243–255. Springer, Heidelberg (2006)
6. Stone, M., Decarlo, D., Oh, I., Rodriguez, C., Stere, A., Lees, A., Bregler, C.: Speaking with hands: Creating animated conversational characters from recordings of human performance. In: Proc. SIGGRAPH 2004, pp. 506–513 (2004)
7. Busso, C., Deng, Z., Grimm, M., Neumann, U., And Narayanan, S.: Rigid head motion in expressive speech animation: Analysis and synthesis. IEEE Transactions on Audio, Speech, and Language Processing 15(3), 1075–1086 (2007)
8. Albrecht, I., Haber, J., Peter Seidel, H.: Automatic generation of non-verbal facial expressions from speech. In: Proc. Computer Graphics International 2002, pp. 283–293 (2002)
9. Levine, S., Krähenbühl, P., Thrun, S., And Koltun, V.: Gesture controllers. In: ACM SIGGRAPH 2010 papers, SIGGRAPH 2010, pp. 124:1–124:11. ACM, New York (2010)
10. Yuan, J., Liberman, M.: Speaker identification on the SCOTUS corpus. In: Proceedings of Acoustics, pp. 5687–5690 (2008)
11. Xiong, X., De la Torre, F.: Supervised descent method and its applica-tions to face alignment. In: 2013 IEEE Conference on Computer Vision and Pattern Recognition (CVPR). IEEE (2013)
12. Brand, M.: Voice puppetry. In: Proceedings of the 26th Annual Conference on Computer Graphics and Interactive Techniques, SIGGRAPH 1999, pp. 21–28. ACM Press/Addison-Wesley Publishing Co., New York, NY, USA (1999)
13. Cassel, J., Vilhjálmsson, H., And Bickmore, T.: BEAT: The Behavior Expression Animation Toolkit. In: Proc. SIGGRAPH 2001, pp. 477–486 (2001)

Maintaining Continuity in Longitudinal, Multi-method Health Interventions Using Virtual Agents: The Case of Breastfeeding Promotion

Zhe Zhang[1], Timothy Bickmore[1], Krissy Mainello[2], Meghan Mueller[3], Mary Foley[4], Lucia Jenkins[5], and Roger A. Edwards[2]

[1] College of Computer and Information Science, Northeastern University, Boston, MA, USA
{zessiez,bickmore}@ccs.neu.edu
[2] Bouvé College of Health Sciences, Northeastern University, Boston, MA, USA
{k.mainello,ro.edwards}@ neu.edu
[3] Northeastern University, Boston, MA, USA
meghanlmueller@gmail.com
[4] Melrose Wakefield Hospital, Hallmark Health, Melrose, MA, USA
mfoley@hallmarkhealth.org
[5] Baby Café USA, Wakefield, MA, USA
luciansla@aol.com

Abstract. Virtual agents can provide a sense of continuity in applications that span long periods of time and incorporate diverse activities, media, and modalities. We describe the design of a virtual lactation educator - agent that promotes breastfeeding in three settings, across different time spans, using a range of media and counseling techniques. The agent provides "interpersonal continuity of care" that is important in many areas of medicine. The results of a pilot study and an ongoing clinical trial are presented.

Keywords: Relational agent, embodied conversational agent, breastfeeding, medical informatics, health informatics.

1 Introduction

Many health interventions require multiple contacts with users over extended periods of time to be effective. Health behavior change interventions, such as walking promotion or smoking cessation, can often take months or years of sustained coaching to succeed, even when the behaviors involved are relatively simple. Some health interventions, however, require not only sustained effort over time but the use of a wide range of counseling and instructional techniques, media, and intervention modalities. For example, the promotion of self-care management for newly-diagnosed individuals with diabetes typically requires education about the disease, instruction in self-inspection techniques (foot exams to prevent ulcers resulting from diabetic neuropathy), and longitudinal behavior change counseling on diet, exercise, and medication adherence. Such longitudinal, multi-method and multi-modal interventions are

T. Bickmore et al. (Eds.): IVA 2014, LNAI 8637, pp. 504–513, 2014.
© Springer International Publishing Switzerland 2014

particularly challenging to automate, because of the range of topics to be covered, the range of pedagogical and persuasive techniques that must be leveraged, the changing needs of users over time, and the need to maintain user engagement over the months or years required.

Breastfeeding promotion is another example of a health behavior that requires such a longitudinal multi-faceted intervention [1]. The intervention should start prenatally by educating women about the advantages of breastfeeding, motivating them to begin breastfeeding immediately after birth, and providing them with basic information about how to breastfeed and where to find additional information. Immediately following the birth of their babies, women need critical information about how to get started breastfeeding, help troubleshooting common problems, and the means for contacting a lactation consultant should significant problems arise. Once they transition home, women need information on a wide range of topics related to breastfeeding, sustained motivation for continuing breastfeeding in the face of common obstacles, help tracking their behavior and outcomes, and a mechanism for alerting clinicians if significant problems arise. Each of these elements may be best delivered through a different type of media, from text and images, dialogue, and graphs to video clips demonstrating different breastfeeding techniques.

Virtual agents may be a particularly well-suited medium for delivering such complex interventions, given their ability to provide a persistent, continuous presence across computing platforms, across time, and across different intervention modalities. In addition to functioning as a breastfeeding counselor, an agent can also play the role of instructor, cheerleader, and confidant, and use a wide range of media in its counseling sessions with users, while maintaining the user-agent dialogue and relationship as an anchor during the months-long intervention. In medicine, such "interpersonal continuity of care" across visits has been shown to be a significant determinant of patient satisfaction and health outcomes [2].

In this paper we describe our experience developing a virtual agent that promotes breastfeeding from the third trimester to six months after birth, across a range of computing platforms and use sites, and using a range of pedagogical and motivational techniques and media. We first describe the importance of breastfeeding, and previous work in automating breastfeeding promotion, before discussing our development methodology, and the design of our agent and intervention. We then present the results of a pilot study and preliminary results from an ongoing clinical trial before concluding.

2   The Importance of Breastfeeding

There are many health benefits of breastfeeding for both mothers and babies. According to the American Academy of Pediatrics, infants who receive any breast-feeding experience 23% lower risk of inflammation of the middle ear, 64% lower risk of gastroenteritis, 40% lower risk of Type 2 diabetes, 31% lower risk of inflammatory bowel disease as well as a 15-30% reduction of adolescent and adult obesity rates in infants who were breastfed. In addition, a 35% lower risk of SIDS is found in infants who receive any breastfeeding longer than 1 month. Additional health benefits accrue when intensity and duration of breast-feeding increases. For example, infants who are exclusively breastfed for the first 3 months of life have a 42% lower risk of developing atopic dermatitis, an inflammatory skin disorder, as well as a 30% reduction in risk of developing Type 1 diabetes and a 40% lower risk of asthma when the atopic family history is positive (26% when family history is negative). Breastfeeding at 6 months results in a 63% lower risk of upper respiratory tract infection and a 20% lower risk in childhood leukemia [22].

There are also numerous health benefits to mothers who breastfeed their infants. For example, breastfeeding moms have less postpartum bleeding, experience lower rates of postpartum depression and have lower rates of breast and ovarian cancers [22]. Although evidence remains inconclusive, there are studies that have shown women who breastfeed return to pre-pregnancy weight faster than moms who do not breastfeed their newborns. In addition, women who have breastfed for a cumulative period of 12-23 months have a significant reduction in hypertension, hyperlipidemia, cardiovascular disease and diabetes [3].

For maximum health benefits, the current World Health Organization (WHO) and American Academy of Pediatrics (AAP) recommend that women breastfeed their infants exclusively for the first 6 months of life and up to 1 year or longer if mutually desired by the mother and child. Although there have been several initiatives aimed at improving exclusive breastfeeding rates in the US, including the Healthy People national disease prevention goals in 2000, 2010 and 2020 and a 2011 Surgeon General's Call to Action to Support Breastfeeding, a significant disparity in breastfeeding rates persists in the US. In 2013 the percentage of women who reached the current AAP and WHO recommendation was only 16.4% nationwide [4].

3   Related Work

Several virtual agents have now been developed to support longitudinal interactions with users, and several studies on longitudinal effects and continuity have been conducted. Many of the longitudinal applications have been in the health domain [5, 6, 7], including interventions for women's preconception health [5], but also in game-playing and education [8]. Studies have explored methods for maintaining longitudinal engagement [23], and assessing the sense of continuity when an agent changes form or moves from one body to another [24].

Several hundred non-automated breastfeeding interventions have now been evaluated, with generally positive outcomes [9]. A few automated systems have been developed to promote breastfeeding among mothers. Most of the interventions developed to date have been educational materials deployed on static web pages or multimedia CD-ROMs ([10, 11]). Joshi, et al, describe a bilingual touch-screen tablet-based intervention to promote breastfeeding. However, the system is not a longitudinal intervention (designed for single contact use), and has not been evaluated in a clinical trial (only formative usability testing results are reported) [12]. Emrick describes the development of "Latch Master", an iPhone game designed to teach mothers about correct breastfeeding positions and latching, although no evaluation is reported [13].

4   Design of a Virtual Agent for Breastfeeding Promotion

The primary support for breastfeeding mothers is face-to-face counseling along with paper-based information materials. However, the effectiveness of such support is limited by several major issues. Professionals are not always able to spend a sufficient amount of time with each mother going through necessary information. Lack of conformity in recommended guidelines and advice also impedes mothers' perception of high-quality information. By using virtual agents, an entire consultation can be virtually simulated where mothers are free to spend as much time as needed interacting with the agents to absorb knowledge and resolve concerns. We developed a virtual agent to promote and support breastfeeding among new mothers. The agent is designed to interact with mothers at three time points:

1. Prenatally, during the third trimester, typically in the obstetrician's office, on a tablet computer. The overall objective of this module of the intervention is to motivate women to choose to breastfeed—by emphasizing the health benefits for the baby and the mother—and to provide information on what to expect and how to get started with the initial breastfeeding attempts.

2. Perinatally, immediately following birth, in woman's room in the maternity unit of the hospital, either on a wheeled computer kiosk or a tablet computer. The objective of this module of the intervention is to provide "breastfeeding 101" information on how to get started, to provide initial tracking capability (number of feeds, number of soiled diapers), and to provide referral to a human lactation consultant if needed.

3. Postnatally, once a woman leaves the hospital and returns home, for the following six months, accessed daily over the web. This overall objective of this module is to promote adherence to the CDC-recommended six months of exclusive breastfeeding, and to provide women with time-based information needed by breastfeeding mothers.

The virtual agent was developed to play the role of a virtual lactation educator. Our development methodology involved initially videotaping sample counseling sessions with an International Board Certified Lactation Consultant. This was followed by several months of meetings of the interdisciplinary team to work through the overall design of the system and the specific dialogue scripts and media content used in each part of the intervention.

The virtual agent's appearance was designed based on feedback from user testing with new mothers (Figure 1). The agent is rendered in a web-based Unity plugin, using the LiteBody framework [14], with speech output produced on the server with a commercial speech synthesizer. Dialogues are scripted using a custom hierarchical transition network-based scripting language. Agent nonverbal conversational behavior is generated using BEAT [15], and includes beat (baton) hand gestures and eyebrow raises for emphasis, gaze away behavior for signaling turn-taking, and posture shifts to mark topic boundaries, synchronized with speech. User input is obtained via multiple choice selection of utterances [16].

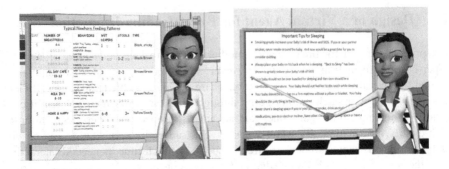

Fig. 1. Virtual Breastfeeding Promotion Agent

4.1   Intervention Methods, Modalities, and Media

A wide range of intervention methods and media is used in the agent-based breast-feeding intervention, including:

Agent Dialogue. Conversation with the agent is the primary communication modality used in the system, and the overall intervention is framed as a series of conversations with a virtual lactation consultant. The agent uses a number of counseling techniques to educate and motivate the user, including techniques from Motivational Interviewing to motivate [17], and social cognitive techniques to maintain adherence (goal setting, positive reinforcement, problem solving). In addition to therapeutic dialogue, social dialogue and empathy were used to establish rapport and therapeutic alliance with the agent to increase adherence [18]. Additional media were typically introduced to support dialogue (Figure 1).

Educational Content. All three interventions used text and images to provide additional educational content, outlines of topics under discussion, and digital versions of paper forms the agent could explain to the user (Figure 1).

Demonstration Videos. A variety of short video clips were used in the system to demonstrate different breastfeeding positions, hand expression, the "birth crawl" and other physical behaviors that would be very difficult to describe in speech and static images.

Longitudinal Tracking. The perinatal system helps women track the number of breast-milk feedings and soiled diapers to gage their baby's progress while in the hospital. The postnatal system tracks the baby's weight and plots it against norms so that the mother can be reassured that their infant is getting enough nourishment (Figure 2) Significantly underweight babies are automatically reported to study personnel for follow-up.

Time-Based Content. The postnatal module uses a complex schedule of topics that the agent introduces to mothers based on the age of their infant (Figure 3). Topics are designed and delivered daily for the first two weeks, weekly from the third week to the eighth week, and monthly from the third month towards the end of the six-month intervention. Since we cannot control how frequently mothers access the system, strategies were devised for "timing out" of topics that may no longer be relevant, and prioritization among multiple accrued topics.

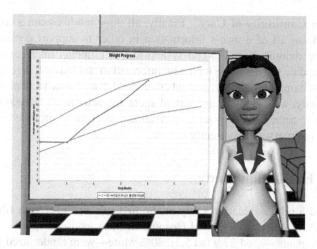

Fig. 2. Agent Showing Infant Weight Chart

Topic	Day 8	Day 9	Day 10	Day 11	Day 12	Day 13	Day14/ Week 2	Week 3	Week 4	Week 5	Week 6	Week 7	Week 8	Month 3	Month 4	Month 5	Month 6
Needing to be held constantly					M												
Sleepy baby							Q										
Night time nursing*		M					Q		Q					M			
Leaking	M							Q									
bottling									M				Q				
Partner back to work							Q										
Pumping basics/breastmilk storage				M				x	Q		Q			Q			
nipple shield					Q						Q			Q			
calming (fussiness)					Q				Q	Q	Q						
crying (1-3 weeks) (3-6 weeks)				M			Q	Q				Q					
thrush							M						Q				
mastitis or plugged milk duct								M			Q						
sleeplessness										M							
Appropriate pacifier use post discharge									M					Q			
choosing a breastpump				M			x		Q								
Working										M			Q	Q			
Child care arrangements								M					Q	Q			
Infant behaviors at breast											M			M	Q		Q
Starting solids															M	Q	Q
breastfeeding in public							M				Q					Q	
early social support																	
social support		M						x	Q	Q	Q			Q			
multiparous mother-specific									M			Q					
baby's development			M				x		Q	Q					Q	Q	
teething															M		Q
Mother's emotions immediately postpartum*							Q										
Typical output (as part of script)								M			M			Q			
nursing strike												Q		Q	Q		
growth spurt							M	Q			M			M	Q	Q	Q

Fig. 3. Excerpt of Educational Breastfeeding Topic Schedule after the first week of the six-month intervention M = Mandatory topic (user must hear, otherwise offered as optional); c/s = C-section delivery (vs. vaginal)

Adaptive Interactions. The postnatal module is designed to transition mothers from their hospitalization to their postnatal care. The interactive content is adapted based on a mother's personal progress and her prior interactions with the agent. To avoid overwhelming users, we only focus on two mandatory topics in each interaction but allow flexibility for users to be able to review other optional topics.

Homework Assignments. The postnatal module also integrates a certain number of homework assignments that were designed to help the mother obtain support in the community. The agent plays a role to convey the importance of the community support in breastfeeding behavior and introduce the related assignments to mothers.

Interpersonal Continuity of Care. Finally, all three modules use a common database that contains all of a user's information in order to support continuity of care across the nine months of end-to-end system use. A clinician interface allows study personnel to update the database with new information, such as the date and time of a birth, a baby's name and gender, and whether the delivery was vaginal or C-section. Most importantly, we used the same virtual agent character in all three systems, along with dialogue to refer back to prior conversations, in order to provide users with the perception of interpersonal continuity of care.

5   Pilot Evaluation Study

We conducted a pilot evaluation study of the first two modules with fifteen women who delivered at Melrose-Wakefield Hospital in Massachusetts (previously reported in [19]). Participants—aged 27.9 (sd 5.7), 80% white—were randomized to the agent-based intervention or standard care. Overall satisfaction with the agent was rated 5.7 on a 7-point scale (1=not at all satisfied, 7=very satisfied). On a 7-point scale assessing subjects' overall confidence in the agent's ability to help, mean scores were 5.9 for the prenatal module and 6.7 for the perinatal module. Those in the intervention group demonstrated significantly greater intent to exclusively breastfeed following their interaction with the prenatal module (p<.05), and significantly greater breastfeeding knowledge following interaction with the perinatal module (p<.05), compared to the control group.

6   Ongoing Clinical Trial

We are currently conducting a randomized controlled trial to evaluate all three modules of the breastfeeding promotion agent. As in the pilot, we are comparing women who interact with the agent to a second group randomized to receive standard care at Melrose-Wakefield Hospital in terms of their initiation and duration of exclusive breastfeeding. We are also interested to explore the impact of the intervention on mothers' attitude towards breastfeeding and their confidence in breastfeeding.

6.1   Measures

Self-report measures are administered at the end of the first two weeks after delivery, at the end of two months, and at the end of six months. Confidence in breastfeeding is measured for both intervention group and control group using the 14-item Breastfeeding Self-Efficacy Scale Short-Form (BSES-SF) [20]. Intervention participants also complete two additional questionnaires about their satisfaction with the Agent and their attitude towards the Agent, assessed using a modified version of the Working Alliance Inventory [21]. Intervention participants' use of all three modules is assessed from database and log file analysis.

The system also enables tracking of when a breastfeeding mother starts to supplement and why. This information will provide the basis for subsequent generations of the agent and what content might be needed to help her continue to breastfeed.

6.2   Procedure

Participants are recruited through Melrose-Wakefield Hospital and peripheral obstetrics-gynecology offices. Women were required to be pregnant and in the third trimester either with their first baby or a subsequent baby if they did not reach their breastfeeding goals with their previous children. Women were excluded if they indicated frequent use of alcohol during pregnancy, use of street drugs, pregnant with twins or more and known medical complications or high-risk pregnancies.

A particular challenge in this study is providing a computer-based intervention to patients in the hospital given that we do not know what day they will arrive for delivery. Study staff in the hospital monitored Labor and Delivery to determine when enrolled patients were admitted in labor. When a subject participating in the study was identified as being admitted, study staff visited them on the birth day of her baby to complete questionnaires and provide access to the Agent. Study staff are monitoring use and following-up with mothers if any "red flags" are noted. Institutional Review Board approval was obtained from both Northeastern University and MWH. All subjects provided the informed consent and they were compensated for their time.

6.3   Preliminary Clinical Trial Results

The study is ongoing. A total of thirty-two women have been recruited to date, out of a target of 60, with twenty randomized into the agent group. Participants to date are aged 19 to 40 (mean 31.4), are 75.9% white, 75.9% are currently married, and 72.4% have high levels of computer literacy.

Eighteen of the intervention participants completed the prenatal module of the system, rating their satisfaction with agent moderately high (average 5.2 on a composite scale of 1= negatively satisfied to 7 = positively satisfied) and attitude towards the agent above neutral (average 4.1 on a composite scale of 1= negative attitude to 7 = positive attitude).

Seven of the intervention participants have already given birth, and have interacted with the agent in the labor and delivery floor of the hospital, and are currently using the postnatal module at home. These seven participants have had a total of 124 (range 4 to 31 each) conversations with the agent in the postnatal system thus far.

7   Conclusions and Future Work

Preliminary results from the pilot study and the clinical trial in progress are promising, and use of the perinatal module has been very high giving us confidence that the breastfeeding promotion agent can have a real impact on postnatal breastfeeding practice.

One of the challenges of breastfeeding is that the needs of the baby, the needs of the mother, and the circumstances of the mother-baby dyad change substantially from birth to six months. These needs also vary significantly from one dyad to another. Hence, the capability for the agent to adapt and adjust the content and nature of its counseling is one of the distinguishing features of this system. The creation of the mandatory topics, suggested topics, and a library of topics also enables more persona-lized breastfeeding promotion.

It is also important for continuity of education and care to have an ongoing connec-tion with healthcare providers; this system enables that through participant log-in data submissions and recommendations to contact a provider based on the user's res-ponses. The agent's non-judgmental style can be especially effective for helping mothers feel comfortable about reporting their feelings as a new mother. Because breastfeeding involves health, medical, and non-medical aspects, our system provides a cohesive way to address a range of topics and direct the mother to appro-priate sources of assistance as well.

Despite the very complex nature of the longitudinal intervention we designed, the virtual agent provides a persistent, continuous presence across the disparate aspects of the system. Bringing a new baby home can be very stressful, and mothers can have significant anxiety about breastfeeding for the first time. Many new mothers are not sure if they are breastfeeding correctly or whether their baby is getting enough to eat, since they cannot see the milk consumed. We hope the virtual agent provides a sense of stability, reliability and comfort during this stressful but exciting time.

Acknowledgments. Thanks to Juan Fernandez and other members of the Relational Agents Group at Northeastern for their assistance in developing the system. This work is supported by grants from the Hood Foundation and Northeastern University.

References

1. McInnes, R., Chambers, J.: Supporting breastfeeding mothers: Qualitative synthesis. Jour-nal of Advanced Nursing 62, 407–427 (2008)
2. Saultz, J., Lochner, J.: Interpersonal Continuity of Care and Care Outcomes: A Critical Review. Ann Family Medicine 3, 159–166 (2005)
3. Section on Breastfeeding: Breastfeeding and the use of human milk. Pediatrics 129, e827–e841 (2012)
4. http://www.cdc.gov/breastfeeding/data/NIS_data/index.htm
5. Bickmore, T., Silliman, R., Nelson, K., Cheng, D., Winter, M., Henaulat, L., Paasche-Orlow, M.: A Randomized Controlled Trial of an Automated Exercise Coach for Older Adults. Journal of the American Geriatrics Society 61, 1676–1683 (2013)
6. Bickmore, T., Schulman, D., Sidner, C.: Automated Interventions for Multiple Health Be-haviors Using Conversational Agents. Patient Education and Counseling 92, 142–148 (2013)
7. Bickmore, T., Puskar, K., Schlenk, E., Pfeifer, L., Sereika, S.: Maintaining Reality: Rela-tional Agents for Antipsychotic Medication Adherence. Interacting with Computers 22, 276–288 (2010)

8. Leite, I.: Using adaptive empathic responses to improve long-term interaction with social robots. User Modeling, Adaption and Personalization, 446–449 (2011)

9. Haroon, S., Das, J., Bhutta, Z.: Breastfeeding promotion interventions and breastfeeding practices: a systematic review. BMC Public Health 13, S20 (2013)

10. Labarère, J., Gelbert-Baudino, N., Laborde, L., Arragain, D., Schelstraete, C., François, P.: CD-ROM-based program for breastfeeding mothers. Matern Child Nutr. 7, 263–272 (2011)

11. Giglia, R., Binns, C.: The Effectiveness of the Internet in Improving Breastfeeding Outcomes: A Systematic Review. J. Hum. Lact (2014)

12. Joshi, A., Wilhelm, S., Aguirre, T., Trout, K., Amadi, C.: An Interactive, Bilingual Touch Screen Program to Promote Breastfeeding Among Hispanic Rural Women: Usability Study. JMIR Research Protocols 2, e47 (2013)

13. http://surf-it.soe.ucsc.edu/node/153

14. Bickmore, T., Schulman, D., Shaw, G.: DTask and liteBody: Open source, standards-based tools for building web-deployed embodied conversational agents. In: Ruttkay, Z., Kipp, M., Nijholt, A., Vilhjálmsson, H.H. (eds.) IVA 2009. LNCS, vol. 5773, pp. 425–431. Springer, Heidelberg (2009)

15. Cassell, J., Vilhjálmsson, H., Bickmore, T.: BEAT: The Behavior Expression Animation Toolkit. In: Conference BEAT: The Behavior Expression Animation Toolkit, pp. 477–486 (2004)

16. Bickmore, T., Picard, R.: Establishing and Maintaining Long-Term Human-Computer Relationships. ACM Transactions on Computer Human Interaction 12, 293–327 (2005)

17. Miller, W., Rollnick, S.: Motivational Interviewing: Preparing People for Change. Guilford Press, New York (2002)

18. Bickmore, T., Gruber, A., Picard, R.: Establishing the computer-patient working alliance in automated health behavior change interventions. Patient Educ. Couns. 59, 21–30 (2005)

19. Edwards, R.A., Bickmore, T., Jenkins, L., Foley, M., Manjourides, J.: Use of an Interactive Computer Agent to Support Breastfeeding. Maternal and Child Health Journal 17(10), 1961–1968 (2013)

20. Dennis, C., Faux, S.: Development and psychometric testing of the Breastfeeding Self-Efficacy Scale. Research in Nursing Health 22, 399–409 (1999)

21. Horvath, A., Greenberg, L.: Development and Validation of the Working Alliance Inventory. Journal of Counseling Psychology 36, 223–233 (1989)

22. US Department of Health and Human Services. The Surgeon General's call to action to support breastfeeding (2011)

23. Bickmore, T., Schulman, D., Yin, L.: Maintaining Engagement in Long-term Interventions with Relational Agents. International Journal of Applied Artificial Intelligence 24(6), 648–666 (2010)

24. Koay, K.L., Syrdal, D.S., Walters, M.L., Dautenhahn, K.: A user study on visualization of agent migration between two companion robots. Human-Computer Interaction 13 (2009)

Towards a Dyadic Computational Model of Rapport Management for Human-Virtual Agent Interaction

Ran Zhao, Alexandros Papangelis, and Justine Cassell

ArticuLab, Carnegie Mellon University, 5000 Forbes Ave, Pittsburgh, PA, USA

Abstract. Rapport has been identified as an important function of human interaction, but to our knowledge no model exists of building and maintaining rapport between humans and conversational agents over the long-term that operates at the level of the dyad. In this paper we leverage existing literature and a corpus of peer tutoring data to develop a framework able to explain how humans in dyadic interactions build, maintain, and destroy rapport through the use of specific conversational strategies that function to fulfill specific social goals, and that are instantiated in particular verbal and nonverbal behaviors. We demonstrate its functionality using examples from our experimental data.

1 Introduction

Rapport, a feeling of connection and closeness with another, feels good, but it also has powerful effects on performance in a variety of domains, including negotiation [15], counseling [19] and education [4]. As agents increasingly take over tasks such as those described above, we maintain that it is important to evoke a feeling of rapport in people interacting with those agents so as to improve their task collaboration – and recognize rapport in people interacting with agents so as to know when the system has been successful. It turns out, however, that what constitutes rapport-evoking and rapport-signaling behavior varies widely. For example, our prior work [22] demonstrated that, in pairs of friends tutoring one another, rudeness had a positive social function and was correlated with learning. In pairs of strangers, however, the opposite function and correlation was found. These results indicate that long term rapport (such as one might find among friends) may have an effect on rapport signaling behavior (such as polite vs. rude language). While prior work [e.g., 20] has confirmed that some rapport-signaling behavior such as attentiveness is capable of enhancing task performance,there do not exist computational models to tell us how that rapport-signaling behavior should change over the course of a long-term collaboration between a human and an agent. One obstacle to models of this sort is the fact that, as [3] has written, "rapport is a social construct that must be defined at the level of a dyad or larger group." Dyadic processes of this sort have traditionally posed challenges to modeling since, as Kelley *et al*, 1983 [as cited in 8] have described, a change in the state of one partner will produce a change

T. Bickmore et al. (Eds.): IVA 2014, LNAI 8637, pp. 514–527, 2014.

in the state of the other. We believe that prior attempts have not sufficiently distinguished between the social functions that lead to rapport, the conversational and behavioral strategies that play a role in those social functions, and the observable phenomena that make up those strategies. Rapport is sometimes experienced on a first meeting but most often it must be built and maintained – or it will be destroyed. Drawing these distinctions has also allowed us to move toward an implementable computational architecture, described in a separate paper in this same volume [23], that takes into account both participants' cognitions, intentions, actions and beliefs, and their interplay, within one person and across the dyad.

In what follows we first review prior literature from the social sciences on the components that make up the experience of rapport, the way people assess rapport in others, and the goals and strategies people use to build, maintain and destroy rapport. Drawing all of these components together, we next propose a model for rapport enhancement, maintenance, and destruction in human-human and human-agent interaction. Throughout we rely on a rich background of literature across the social sciences, as well as on data [33] from our own research into peer tutoring between dyads of friends and of strangers across several months. These data have been annotated for verbal and nonverbal behaviors, as well as for relevant conversational strategies. Our contributions in this work are twofold: (1) an analysis of the social functions and conversational strategies that go into building, maintaining and breaking rapport; (2) a computationally viable dyadic model of rapport over time built from that analysis.

2   Theoretical Framework for Rapport Management

[30]'s work on the changing nonverbal expression of rapport over the course of a relationship has had significant impact on the development of virtual agents. They provide an actionable starting point by outlining the experience of rapport as a dynamic structure of three interrelating behavioral components: positivity, mutual attentiveness and coordination. Behavioral positivity generates a feeling of friendliness between interactants; mutual attentiveness leads to an experience of connectedness; and behavioral coordination evokes a sense of "being in synch". The work posits that the relative weights of those components change over the course of a relationship; the importance of mutual attentiveness remains constant, while the importance of positivity decreases and that of coordination increases.

While [30]'s work is predicated on a dual level of analysis - what they call "molecular" and "molar," researchers in virtual agents have relied more on the molecular level, meaning that they have translated [30]'s components directly into observable behavioral expression or action. [30], however, propose that it is the molar level that is more predictive - that is, that theory should attend to the conversational strategies and goals of communication that interactants use to be positive, be attentive and to coordinate. In fact, they suggest that "initial encounters are rigidly circumscribed by culturally acceptable and stereotypical behavior" while, after some time, "rather than following more culturally-defined communication conventions, they would develop their own conventions and show more diversity in the ways they communicate thoughts to one another." This aspect of their work has largely been ignored in subsequent computational approaches to rapport. In the development of agent models and an architecture to realize them, however, this leaves us less than well-informed about what the agents should do. How do we determine what is meant by "stereotypical behavior" or "more diversity in the ways they communicate"? How should we represent the goals of two interactants and conversational strategies to fulfill the goals? In the current work, then, we discuss a broad range of literature that allows us to understand the kinds of strategies that interactants use in rapport management, and the kinds of goals and functionality those interactants intend. As we do so, we pay particular attention to the dyadic nature of these constructs, and how they change over the course of a relationship. Our review focuses on 3 top-level goals that make up rapport - **face management, mutual attentiveness**, and **coordination** - and some of the subgoals that achieve those top-level goals - such as *becoming predictable, appreciating the other's true self*, and *enhancing the other's face*. We also describe many of the conversational strategies that achieve those goals - `initiating mutual self-disclosure, adhering to behavioral expectations or norms`, and so forth. While we believe that something like the experience of rapport is probably universal and perhaps even that the subgoals of face, attentiveness, and coordination as important contributors to rapport might also be (somewhat) universal, there is no doubt that the sub-sub-goals and conversational strategies differ in different sociocultural contexts. Here, for the purposes of the discussion, we adduce evidence from our own data collection with teenage middle-class Americans, and that context therefore serves as our object of study. We hope, however, that in outlining an approach to building this kind of dyadic model of rapport, we will have opened the way to discussions of other contexts, and that other strategies and goals will be thereby be discovered.

Spencer-Oatey [26] offers an alternative approach to [30]'s to conceptualizing the strategies and behaviors that contribute to rapport, and we find it more complete and more convincing for our purposes. She points out that rapport management comprises the task of increasing rapport, but also maintaining, and destroying it. In her perspective, each of these tasks requires management of face which, in turn, relies on behavioral expectations, and interactional goals. Our data support the tremendous importance of face, as the teens alternately praise and insult one another, all the while hedging their own positive performance on the algebra task in order to highlight the performance of the other. The data also contain numerous examples of mutual attentiveness and coordination as putative input into rapport management, but we found it difficult to code positivity independently of its role in face. Our formulation below, therefore, posits a tripartite approach to rapport management, comprising mutual attentitiveness, coordination, and face management.

Face Management: [10] define positive face as, roughly, a desire by each of us to be approved of. They posit that politeness functions to avoid challenging that desire, as well as to boost the other's sense of being approved, while *face-threatening acts* (FTA) challenge face. [27], however, points out that this definition ignores the interpersonal nature of face, and she defines "identity face" as the desire to be recognized for one's positive social identity, as well as one's individual positive traits. In this context, FTAs can challenge one's sense of self or one's identity in the social world. On the flip-side, *face-boosting acts* can create increased self-esteem in the individual, and increased interpersonal cohesiveness - or rapport - in the dyad. Of course [26] points out that what constitutes politeness, other face-boosting acts, and FTAs, is not fixed, and is largely a subjective judgement about the social appropriateness of verbal and non-verbal behaviors. She attributes these judgments about social appropriateness to our "sociality rights and obligations" - how we feel entitled to be treated based on the behaviors we expect from others – which in turn derive from sociocultural norms, including the relative power and status of the two members of the dyad, and interactional principles. Fulfilling these rights and obligations induces a feeling of being approved and, in turn, increases rapport.

What, however, are these sociocultural norms and interactional principles? A key aspect of the theory laid out here is that *behavioral expectations* (the instantiation of "sociality rights and obligations") are allied with sociocultural norms early in a relationship, and become more interpersonally determined as the relationship proceeds. Thus, the stranger dyads in our data spend a fair amount of time agreeing with one another when they first meet, in ways that fit upper middle class politeness norms (when asked what he wants to be when he grows up, one teen responds "I kind of want to be a chef" to which the other politely responds "I'd think about that too"). Friends, on the other hand, are less likely to demonstrate polite responses (one teen asks the other "wait why do you have to keep your hat on" to which the other responds "it's [his neck] not supposed to be in the sun" and receives in reply "yeah it's really swollen and ugly"). In both cases while the behavioral expectations have changed (politeness has been replaced by teasing), the fact of meeting them continues to be rapport-increasing.

How does one learn enough about the other to adapt behavioral expectations? **Mutual attentiveness** is an important part of the answer, as [30] have described. Mutual attentiveness may be fulfilled by providing information about oneself through small talk [11] and self-disclosure [21]. Social penetration theory [29] describes the ways in which, as a relationship deepens, the breadth and depth of the topics disclosed become wider and deeper, helping the interlocutor to gain common ground as a basis for an interpersonally-specific set of behavioral expectations. Self-disclosure, however, plays another role in rapport-building, as when successful it is reciprocal [14] – self-disclosure in our data is most often met with reciprocal self-disclosure at a similar level of intimacy. This kind of mutual responsiveness signals receptivity and appreciation of another's self-disclosure [14] and the very process enhances **coordination** among the participants (much as we argued is the case for small talk [11]), likewise increasing a sense of rapport. The goal of coordination as a path to rapport is also met by verbal and nonverbal synchrony [34], and this is common in our own data.

In addition, while self-disclosure is not always negative, it may be, and this is a way to challenge one's own face, and thereby boost the face of the other. For that reason it is common in rapport management. In our own data, for example, strangers quickly began to share superficial negative facts about themselves, such as their presumed poor performance on the algebra pre-test at the beginning of the session. When met with a self-disclosing utterance at the same level of intimacy and with the same negative valence ("oh my gosh I could not answer like half of those"), the interlocutors increased mutual gaze and smiling, and proceeded to more intimate topics, such as their poor performance at keeping their pets alive. In fact, [9] found that in a negotiation setting not reciprocating negative self-disclosure led to decreased feelings of rapport. [31] point out the role of humor in rapport; it is a particularly interesting rapport management strategy as it too follows behavior expectations, whereby generally-accepted humor is successful early in the relationship, and humor that violates sociocultural norms may be successful as a strategy to increase liking and rapport only later in the relationship. In our data from teenagers, this rule is only sometimes observed, and the effect of humor that violates behavior expectations is swift and negative.

Self-disclosure, then, serves multiple goals in rapport management. Yet another is to reveal aspects of one's "true self" as a way of indicating one's openness to being truly seen by the other, and hence one's availability for rapport. According to [24], the "true-self" is composed of important aspects of one's identity that are not always validated in one's daily life. People are highly motivated to make these important aspects of identity a 'social reality' - to have these attributes acknowledged by others so that they become authentic features of their "self-concept" [1]. This explains why interlocutors engage in self-disclosure - perhaps even why rapport is sought in interactions with strangers.

Based on the literature surveyed above, it is clear that mutual attentiveness to, and learning about and adhering to, the behavioral expectations of one's interlocutor is helpful in building rapport. Initially, when interactants are strangers, without any knowledge of their interlocutor's behavioral expectations, they adhere to a socioculturally-ratified model (general expectations established as appropriate in their cultural and social milieu). This may include behaving politely and in accordance with their relative social roles. As the relationship proceeds, interlocutors increasingly rely on knowledge of one another's expectations, thereby adhering to a shared and increasingly interpersonally-specific set of sociality rights and obligations, where more general norms may be purposely violated in order to accommodate each other's behavioral expectations.

Why, however, might two interactants violate sociocultural norms when others around them are adhering to those norms? [2] suggests that people have an unconscious motivation to affiliate themselves to a group, which drives them to participate in social activities and search for long-term relationships. The fact of violating sociocultural norms may in fact reinforce the sense that the two belong in the same social group and this may enhance their unified self-image [28] through reinforcing the sense of in-group connectedness through a comparison with other individuals who don't know these specific rules of behavior. This is supported by our own findings on peer tutoring, whereby rudeness predicts learning gain [22]. We know that rapport between teacher and student increases learning. When tutor and tutee are strangers, their behavior complies with sociocultural norms. Impoliteness may reduce the learning gain in strangers by challenging rapport through violating those sociocultural behavioral expectations. When tutor and tutee are friends, however, they have knowledge of one another's behavioral expectations and are thus able to follow interpersonal norms and sacrifice sociocultural norms. Rudeness, may be a part of the interpersonal norms. It may also be a way to cement the sense that the two are part of a unified group, and different from those around them. The topics they are rude about may also serve to index commonalities between the two, as referring to shared experience also differentiates in-group from out-group individuals.

3 Towards a Computational Model of Rapport Management

The literature review above, while not allowing each component sub-goal or strategy the space it deserves, provides a sense of the complexity, but also of the mundane nature of rapport management between people. We wish to be seen and known the way we truly are, and we want the way we are to be approved; we desire affiliation with a social group; we are more comfortable when the behavior of our interlocutors matches our expectations; we wish for the success of our interpersonal and our task goals. These common sense and everyday goals work together to lead us to desire rapport, and to build it, even with strangers, and to put effort into maintaining it with friends and acquaintances.

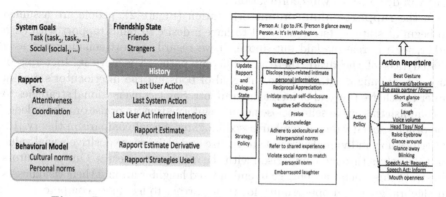

Fig. 1. Dyadic state (left) and Strategy/Action repertoire (right)

In order to represent these goals and desires in a computational model, we must take into account the fact that while rapport is dyadic, it nevertheless depends on the cognition, actions, beliefs and intentions of each interlocutor, and on the perception by each interlocutor of these aspects of the mind of the other interlocutor. In the computational model, therefore, we represent the state of each participant, and of that participant's perception of the state of the interlocutor, which enables us to reason about the cognition and rapport orientation (enhancement, maintenance, destruction) of the dyad, based on observable behaviors. Immediately after each dialogue turn, we represent the participants' modified self-images and their assessment of the modification of their interlocutor's self-image and, based on this reasoning, the sub-goals they wish to achieve, and the consequent appropriate strategy for the next dialogue turn. More specifically, Figure 1(left) presents the *dyadic state*, which may be updated after each user's turn or incrementally. Figure 1(right) displays how a user and system state leads to a choice of *Strategy* and then of *Action* (although the latter is beyond the scope of the current paper). Of course, in order to allow rapport state monitoring and management, we need to detect the goals and conversational strategies of the interlocutors on the basis of the behaviors we observe them engaging in, and we need to assess their contribution to each rapport orientation. Below, for rapport enhancement, maintenance and destruction we list, from the perspective of the agent trying to achieve those goals, the strategies and their contribution to the series of sub-goals and interrelating behavioral components of rapport we laid out above - face, mutual attentiveness, coordination. The conversational strategies enumerated here are no doubt not exhaustive. However they include all phenomena found in the literature that were also represented in our data. To give a more complete sense of many of the possible "response pairs" (the conversational strategy of one interlocutor and the strategy it is met with by the other interlocutor) and their effect on the four behavioral components, we provide a more complete set here: http://tinyurl.com/dyadic-rapport. For instance, if a speaker discloses topic-related personal information and the listener deploys the same strategy, both face and coordination will be updated. If a speaker initializes self-disclosure but the listener verbally attacks the speaker, face will decrease, as will coordination.

In the **rapport-enhancement** orientation (Figure 2), people are assumed to begin at state T_1 (stranger) and to have a desire to build rapport with each other, for the reasons laid out above. If we regard rapport-enhancement as a shared task of the dyad, there are different paths to achieve it. In terms of face, people might establish the sub-goal of boosting the interlocutor's face in order to achieve the goal of increasing rapport. Some conversational strategies to accomplish this are to self-disclose negative information, to praise or acknowledge the other's social value, or embarrassed laughter. Social comparison theory [16] describes how individuals are able to realize and claim more positive social value for themselves through comparison with the other's weaknesses. Our peer tutors illustrate this when they engage in embarassed laughter around their weaknesses in algebra, giving an opportunity for their partner to feel more competent.

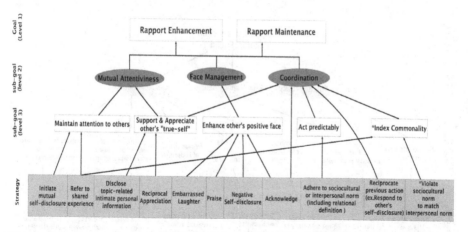

Fig. 2. Social Functions and Conversational Strategies for Rapport Enhancement and Maintenance

As described above, predictability is a core part of coordination. In order to achieve this sub-goal, interactants adhere to behavior expectations. At the initial state T_1, the expectations are guided by sociocultural norms which include the obligation to engage in social validation of the interlocutor's self-disclosures, and to reciprocate with similarly intimate self-disclosure. This also functions to signal attentiveness to the interlocutor. In fact, initiating mutual self-disclosure is a compelling strategy for learning about an individual at the initial stage of the relationship as well as for signaling attentiveness. In our data we also observed that peers often demonstrate mutual attentiveness by referring to past shared experience. As well as increasing common ground, acknowledging and reciprocating reference to previous experience function to increase coordination.

In the **rapport-maintenance** orientation (Figure 2), people are assumed to begin at state T_2 (Acquaintance) and have a desire to maintain the current harmonious relationship. Those marked with (*) refer to rapport maintenance only. Typically, friends have some knowledge of each other's behavioral expectations and in order to maintain high rapport, dyads mark their affiliation with one another, and their shared membership in a social identity group. Indexing commonality strengthens connectedness between in-group members. Compared to stranger peers, friend peers refer to more intimate shared experiences. Moreover, contrary to the sociocultural norms that govern behavior during rapport enhancement, friends may violate sociocultural norms to match their interlocutor's behavioral expectations for example, through rudeness to one another or swearing, both of which were common among friends in our corpus.

In the two orientations just described, we presented strategies for building and maintaining rapport with our interlocutor, and it's hard to imagine instances in which a virtual agent might want to challenge rapport. However, the **rapport-destruction** orientation (Figure 3) is useful in the sense that detecting it will help us choose appropriate rapport "recovery" strategies. Here people are assumed to begin at state T_2 and have a desire to destroy or challenge the

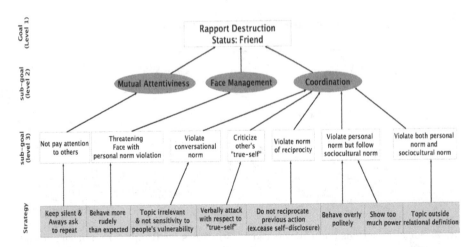

Fig. 3. Social Functions and Conversational Strategies for Rapport Destruction

current harmonious relationship with their friends. According to the rapport management perspective [27], even though some FTAs in politeness theory do not diminish the listener's positive social value, there still exist some highly FTAs. For instance, challenging one's friends during peer tutoring could be seen as a way of showing rapport, while physically or verbally attacking without reason ruins rapport due to the lack of justification for those actions, meaning that this behavior is too rude to fit expectations of any kind.

In this orientation, people pay no attention to learning about their interlocutor's behavioral expectation. Strategies to achieve this include keeping silent or continually asking others to repeat themselves. Although friends' actions are mainly guided by interpersonal norms, Derlega [14] suggests that people, even in close relationships, should follow several sociocultural norms with respect to self-disclosure. In particular, reciprocity, interactional and conversational norms and social validation of the "true-self" remain important over the long term. Ceasing self-disclosure is a strategy to violate reciprocity. An interlocutor could also try to attack the vulnerability of the self-discloser by scoffing at the content or responding with an irrelevant remark. Furthermore, they could verbally attack or neglect the self-disclosure's "true-self" [24] instead of reciprocally appreciating. As we mentioned before, self-disclosure is successful when dyadic. Thus, all of the strategies above do not only violate the sociocultural norms but also block the road to reciprocal self-disclosure. Another way to break rapport is to violate interpersonal norms while following sociocultural norms. For instance, suddenly behaving too politely to one's friend may lead to awkwardness and a reduced feeling of coordination. Suddenly changing demonstration of power or status would have the same effect. Last, one could violate both personal and sociocultural norms, by talking about a topic that does not match the relationship definition of the dyad (for instance, a student choosing to discuss sexual information with an advisor).

3.1 Examples from Corpus Data

In order to demonstrate the functioning of the computational model, six examples are taken from our data, collected in [33]. In this experiment, 12 dyads of 12-15 year old students (half boys and half girls, half friends and half strangers) tutor each other in algebra over a period of 5 weeks. Table 1(left) shows how dyads of strangers interact early in the 5-week period. Table 1(right), shows dyads of friends. Labels indicate how the computational model would generate the same output, based on our annotations of the data for nonverbal behavior and for conversational strategies such as disagreement and agreement, politeness and rudeness, and on- and off-task talk (while we continue to annotate the data for additional phenomena, Cohen's Kappa inter-rater reliability for all annotations to date is between 0.7 and 0.8). Note that while the data serve here to adduce evidence for the goals and strategies of rapport management in this age group and this task context, in other work we have pursued a data-driven approach to analyzing the relationship between the conversational strategies and

Table 1. Stranger examples (left) and Friend examples(right) session, where s is a rapport strategy, t_d is topic depth and R is dynamics of rapport. During the first session, most topics are discussed in shallow depth, while during the second, more personal information is being disclosed.

Stranger-Example 1

P1: b equals nineteen over nine
$[s_1 = N/A, t_d = 1]$
P2: {laughter} good job
$[s_2 = praise, t_d = 1]$
R=Increase

Stranger-Example 2

P1:I suck at negative numbers
$[s_1 = negative\ self\text{-}disclosure,\ t_d = 1]$
P2: it's okay so do I
$[s_2 = reciprocate\ self\text{-}disclosure,\ t_d = 1]$
R=Increase

Stranger-Example 3

P1: x equals sixty-four over three
$[s_1 = N/A, t_d = 1]$
P2: yep
$[s_2 = acknowledge,\ t_d = 1]$
R=Increase

P1: x all right thanks .. all right
$[s_1 = adhere\ to\ sociocultural\ norm,\ t_d = 1]$
P2: it was a complicated one
$[s_2 = face\text{-}boosting\ acknowledgment,\ t_d = 1]$
R=Increase

Friend-Example 1

P1: are there any girls you like
$[s_1 = elicit\ self\text{-}disclosure,\ t_d = 3$
more personal topic]
P2: all of them are not the best looking
$[s_2 = reciprocate\ self\text{-}disclosure, t_d = 3]$
R=Increase

Friend-Example 2

P1:remember you went to Connecticut
$[s_1 = Refer\ to\ shared\ experience, t_d = 2]$
P2:that was just to visit my cousin
$[s_2 = disclose\ topic\text{-}related\ intimate$
personal information, $t_d = 2]$
R=Increase

Friend-Example 3

P1: silly goose that's a backwards two
$[s_1 = violate\ sociocultural\ norm\ to\ adhere$
to interpersonal norm, $t_d = 1]$
P2:two
$[s_2 = N/A,\ t_d = 1]$
R=Increase

observable behaviors (or actions) [33]. We continue to pursue an analysis of those data by using hand annotation as ground truth for the automatic assessment of rapport through multimodal analysis. That automatic detection will serve as input to the dialogue system.

4   Related Work

A number of prior papers have addressed the issue of rapport, or related notions such as trust, friendship, and intimacy, between people and virtual agents. Some have looked at what we have referred to as "instant rapport" [13] where a sense of connection is not acquired but instantaneous, and some have addressed the building of rapport over time. An early paper [12] used prior work in sociolinguistics and social psychology to develop a computational model of trust, and a computational architecture to establish trust between a person and virtual agent. The system, however, did no assessment of the user's level of trust, and only built trust through verbal behavior - primarily small talk. While successful in building trust - particularly with extroverts - a subsequent paper [5] demonstrated the need for incorporating nonverbal behavior into the model. Since then, Bickmore and his colleagues have gone on to develop a model that describes strategies for an agent to build a relationship with a user over time.

Until recently, much like the early work described above, these systems have primarily engaged in a set of predetermined conversational strategies without associated updates in underlying goals or representations of the user or the user-system dyad [inter alia 32]. While not always successful at promoting rapport, these strategies have had positive effects on the non-dyadic construct of engagement [6]. More recently [7] has relied on accommodation theory to design conversational strategies intended to generate discourse that matches a user's level of intimacy, and to increase intimacy. The prior goal was met but not the latter, perhaps because, as the authors themselves indicate, the model of intimacy was quite simplistic, without the kinds of goals, subgoals, and conversational strategies laid out here. On the other hand, accommodation theory provided a successful means for assessing the user's level of intimacy, which bears keeping in mind for future work. Following on from this work, [25] developed a planning algorithm that keeps track of the intimacy level of the user, and produces session plans that target both relational and task goals. The activity planning approach seems promising, however the session plans appear to be made up of activities that are appropriate at a particular level of closeness rather than activities that have been shown specifically to *increase* closeness. Our approach, whereby conversational strategies target sub-goals that specifically manage rapport, might be more successful at moving the system and user further along on the relational continuum.

An alternative approach is represented by the work of Gratch and colleagues [17,18], who target immediate rapport in the service of implementing a sensitive listener. In this work, the level of goals and conversational strategies are avoided, and instead the agent attemps to elicit the experience of rapport by working at the level of observable phenomena - coordinating its nonverbal behavior to the human user. Rather than treating rapport as a dyadic or interpersonal construct, they address it similarly to other display functions and perhaps not surprisingly, as with other engaging displays, they have found increased user engagement. Most recently they have extended this approach to the analysis of the nonverbal behaviors that accompany intimate self-disclosure [19]. However, by not taking into account the relative roles of the two interlocutors, and the nature of their relationship, they have ignored the significant difference in conversational strategies between interlocutors with different levels of power in the relationship. In contrast to the prior work described here, our work distinguishes between the dyad's goals (overarching goals such as "create rapport" or sub-goals such as "index commonality"), their conversational strategies (such as "violate sociocultural norms through rude talk" or "initiate self-disclosure") and the observable verbal and nonverbal phenomena that instantiate those phenomena (such as mutual eye gaze, embarassed laughter, or insults). This tri-partite distinction allows us to generate the same behaviors (insults, for example) in different contexts (early or late in the relationship) to achieve different goals (destroy rapport or enhance it). The unit of analysis of the computational model we present is the dyad, with system state updates impacting the model of the user, and of the user's model of the system, and particular weight placed on intrinsically dyadic constructs such as reciprocity.

5   Conclusion and Future Work

In this article, leveraging a broad base of existing literature and a corpus of data of friends and strangers engaging in peer tutoring, we have made steps towards a unified theoretical framework explaining the process of enhancing, maintaining and destroying rapport in human to human interaction. Based on this framework we have designed a computational model of rapport that can be applied to interactions between humans and virtual agents. In turn, that computational model allows us to make first steps towards a dyadic computational architecture for a virtual agent. A first sketch of the details necessary to realize this work computationally is described in a sister paper to this one, also published in this volume [23], in which we suggest reinforcement learning as an approach to learning behavioral expectations, rapport strategies, and dialogue act policies.

The potential benefits of such a dyadic approach to rapport management between human and virtual agent are numerous, including the fact that increased rapport leads to better task performance by humans [4,15,19], and could therefore lead to more effective virtual agent tutors and counselors, among other roles. It should be noted that in the current paper we have traced the relationship between rapport management goals and sub-goals and their associated conversational strategies. We have occasionally described how a conversational strategy is instantiated by a set of observable verbal and nonverbal actions but we have not formalized that step of the process, which will form the content of future work (currently in process, as described in [33]). That future work will also serve as ground truth against which our computational model will be evaluated. We then plan to implement the model and architecture in a virtual peer tutoring application. Foreseeable challenges include recognition of the human users' rapport strategies (which may span several dialogue turns or interleave with other strategies) in order to correctly update our model as well as react in the appropriate fashion, and to develop an appropriate domain-specific user model for the algebra tutoring that interacts appropriately with the rapport management. Some of these issues evoke core AI challenges, such as representing many aspects of the mental state of participants. Nevertheless, we believe that here we have made the first step towards a dyadic and more realistic computational model of rapport. We expect the future challenges to be substantial, but rewarding, as we begin to model those aspects of human-human interaction that are not only helpful to human-agent collaboration, but also sustain aspects of what we cherish most in being human.

Acknowledgments. The authors would like to thank Zhou Yu for her contribution to this work, as well as the other students and staff of the ArticuLab. This work was partially supported by the R.K. Mellon Foundation, and NSF IIS.

References

1. Bargh, J.A., McKenna, K.Y., Fitzsimons, G.M.: Can you see the real me? activation and expression of the "true self" on the internet. Journal of Social Issues 58(1), 33–48 (2002)
2. Baumeister, R.F., Leary, M.R.: The need to belong: desire for interpersonal attachments as a fundamental human motivation. Psychological Bulletin 117(3), 497 (1995)
3. Bernieri, F.J., Gillis, J.S.: Judging rapport: Employing brunswik's lens model to study interpersonal sensitivity. In: Interpersonal sensitivity: Theory and measurement, pp. 67–88 (2001)
4. Bernieri, F.J., Rosenthal, R.: Interpersonal coordination: Behavior matching and interactional synchrony. In: Fundamentals of Nonverbal Behavior, p. 401 (1991)
5. Bickmore, T., Cassell, J.: Social dialogue with embodied conversational agents. In: Advances in Natural Multimodal Dialogue Systems, pp. 23–54. Springer, Heidelberg (2005)
6. Bickmore, T., Pfeifer, L., Schulman, D.: Relational agents improve engagement and learning in science museum visitors (2011)
7. Bickmore, T., Schulman, D.: Empirical validation of an accommodation theory-based model of user-agent relationship (2012)
8. Bickmore, T.W., Caruso, L., Clough-Gorr, K., Heeren, T.: it's just like you talk to a friend' relational agents for older adults. Interacting with Computers 17(6), 711–735 (2005)
9. Bronstein, I., Nelson, N., Livnat, Z., Ben-Ari, R.: Rapport in negotiation the contribution of the verbal channel. Journal of Conflict Resolution 56(6), 1089–1115 (2012)
10. Brown, P., Levinson, S.: Universals in language usage: Politeness phenomena. questions and politeness: Strategies in social interaction, ed. by e. goody, 56–311 (1978)

11. Cassell, J., Bickmore, T.: Negotiated collusion: Modeling social language and its relationship effects in intelligent agents. User Modeling and User-Adapted Interaction 13(1-2), 89–132 (2003)
12. Cassell, J., Bickmore, T., Billinghurst, M., Campbell, L., Chang, K., Vilhjalmsson, H., Yan, H.: Embodiment in conversational interfaces: Rea (1999)
13. Cassell, J., Gill, A.J., Tepper, P.A.: Coordination in conversation and rapport (2007)
14. Derlega, V.J., Metts, S., Petronio, S., Margulis, S.T.: Self-disclosure. Sage Publications, Inc. (1993)
15. Drolet, A.L., Morris, M.W.: Rapport in conflict resolution: Accounting for how face-to-face contact fosters mutual cooperation in mixed-motive conflicts. Journal of Experimental Social Psychology (1), 26–50 (2000)
16. Festinger, L.: A theory of social comparison processes. Human Relations 7(2), 117–140 (1954)
17. Gratch, J., Okhmatovskaia, A., Lamothe, F., Marsella, S., Morales, M., van der Werf, R.J., Morency, L.-P.: Virtual rapport (2006)
18. Huang, L., Morency, L.-P., Gratch, J.: Virtual rapport 2.0 (2011)
19. Kang, S.-H., Gratch, J., Sidner, C., Artstein, R., Huang, L., Morency, L.-P.: Towards building a virtual counselor: modeling nonverbal behavior during intimate self-disclosure (2012)
20. Karacora, B., Dehghani, M., Krämer-Mertens, N., Gratch, J.: The influence of virtual agents' gender and rapport on enhancing math performance (2012)
21. Moon, Y.: Intimate exchanges: Using computers to elicit self-disclosure from consumers. Journal of Consumer Research 26(4), 323–339 (2000)
22. Ogan, A., Finkelstein, S., Walker, E., Carlson, R., Cassell, J.: Rudeness and rapport: Insults and learning gains in peer tutoring (2012)
23. Papangelis, A., Zhao, R., Cassell, J.: Towards a computational architecture of dyadic rapport management for virtual agents. In: Bickmore, T., Marsella, S., Sidner, C. (eds.) IVA 2014. LNCS, vol. 8637, pp. 320–324. Springer, Heidelberg (2014)
24. Rogers, C.R.: Client-centered therapy. American Psychological Association (1966)
25. Sidner, C.: Engagement: Looking and not looking as evidence for disengagement. In: Workshop at HRI 2012 (2012)
26. Spencer-Oatey, H.: (im) politeness, face and perceptions of rapport: unpackaging their bases and interrelationships (2005)
27. Spencer-Oatey, H.: Culturally speaking: Culture, communication and politeness theory. Continuum Int. Publishing Group (2008)
28. Tajfel, H., Turner, J.C.: An integrative theory of intergroup conflict. The Social Psychology of Intergroup Relations 33, 47 (1979)
29. Taylor, D.A., Altman, I.: Communication in interpersonal relationships: Social penetration processes (1987)
30. Tickle-Degnen, L., Rosenthal, R.: The nature of rapport and its nonverbal correlates. Psychological Inquiry 1(4), 285–293 (1990)
31. Treger, S., Sprecher, S., Erber, R.: Laughing and liking: Exploring the interpersonal effects of humor use in initial social interactions. European Journal of Social Psychology 43(6), 532–543 (2013)
32. Vardoulakis, L.P., Ring, L., Barry, B., Sidner, C.L., Bickmore, T.: Designing relational agents as long term social companions for older adults (2012)
33. Yu, Z., Gerritsen, D., Ogan, A., Black, A., Cassell, J.: Automatic prediction of friendship via multi-model dyadic features (August. 2013)
34. Zanna, M.P.: Advances in experimental social psychology, vol. 31. Elsevier (1999)

Agent-User Concordance and Satisfaction with a Virtual Hospital Discharge Nurse

Shuo Zhou[1], Timothy Bickmore[1], Michael Paasche-Orlow[2], and Brian Jack[2]

[1] College of Computer and Information Science, Northeastern University, Boston, MA, USA
{zhous06,bickmore}@ccs.neu.edu
[2] Boston University School of Medicine, Boston Medical Center, Boston, MA, USA
mpo@bu.edu, brian.jack@bmc.org

Abstract. User attitudes towards a hospital virtual nurse agent are described, as evaluated in a randomized clinical trial involving 764 hospital patients. Patients talked to the agent for an average of 29 minutes while in their hospital beds, receiving their customized hospital discharge instructions from the agent and a printed booklet. Patients reported very high levels of satisfaction with and trust in the nurse agent, preferred receiving their discharge instructions from the agent over their human doctors and nurses, and found the system very easy to use. Perceived similarity to the agent was a significant determiner of liking, trust, desire to continue, and working alliance, although perceived similarity was unrelated to racial concordance between patients and the agent.

Keywords: Relational agent, embodied conversational agent, medical informatics, health informatics, hospital discharge.

1 Introduction

Several studies have shown the positive effects of racial concordance between virtual agents and users on user satisfaction in laboratory or educational settings. However, none of these studies have determined whether these effects hold in real-world professional settings in which topics of significant gravity are discussed, such as medical consultations in a hospital. Although positive effects of concordance in human patient-provider interactions have also been demonstrated [1-4], it is unknown whether these effects would hold for virtual agents that are designed to counsel users about their health. It is possible that—given the importance of medical topics being discussed, or the distractions and stress in a real-world environment such as a hospital—subtle factors such as the apparent race, gender, and age of a virtual agent are irrelevant.

As part of a large clinical trial to evaluate a virtual agent that plays the role of a hospital discharge nurse, we investigated whether racial concordance effects would still hold in a hospital setting. Few virtual agents have been evaluated in real-world professional settings such as hospitals. User reactions to virtual agents in laboratory settings always raise the issue of ecological validity; whether the experimental results would continue to hold in an uncontrolled work environment with study participants who are not college students.

T. Bickmore et al. (Eds.): IVA 2014, LNAI 8637, pp. 528–541, 2014.

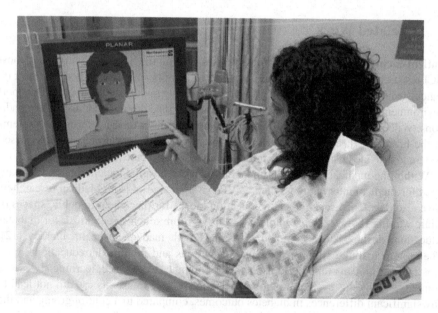

Fig. 1. Virtual Hospital Discharge Nurse System

The hospital discharge process can be very complex and is the source of many medical errors. The average patient in our trial is discharged with ten medications and multiple follow up appointments. Approximately 20% of patients discharged from hospitals in the U.S. suffer adverse events and are re-hospitalized within 90 days, and approximately one third of these complications are preventable [5]. Among the leading reasons cited for these preventable complications are inadequate patient health literacy [6], patient lack of understanding of how to take their medications or of medication side effects, and low patient adherence to treatment regimens. The poor preparation of patients for hospital discharge is highlighted by studies showing that less than half of discharged patients know their diagnosis or the purpose of their medications [7].

We present the results of a clinical trial in which 764 hospital patients were randomized to be discharged by a virtual nurse agent (N=376, Figure 1) or standard procedure (N=388). Patients in the virtual nurse condition were further randomized to talk to a virtual agent that was designed to appear African American or Caucasian. In addition to assessing racial concordance objectively, we also asked patients to rate how similar they felt they were to the agent. We hypothesized that:

H1. Racial concordance would be a significant predictor of perceived similarity with the virtual agent.

H2. Perceived similarity would be a significant predictor of satisfaction with and trust in the virtual agent.

2   Related Work

Patient-facing Hospital Information Systems. Within the hospital environment, most HCI research has been clinician-centric, although there is an emerging body of work on patient-facing systems. Bers, *et al.* provided immersive multi-user collaborative support environments for pediatric patients with renal and cardiac diseases [8], and other conditions. Wilcox, reports a series of design studies for patient-facing information systems in the hospital [9], and a subsequent pilot usability study of a prototype tablet-based system to provide hospital patients information about their care [10].

Within the medical community there are many in-hospital patient interfaces developed for medical interventions, such as VR-based analgesia [11]. Medical researchers have also developed several health education kiosks for placement in public spaces or clinic waiting rooms. One example is a waiting room touch screen kiosk for diabetes education, designed to accommodate patients with inadequate health literacy [12]. The system featured simplified navigation buttons and multimedia educational content and testimonials tailored to users' prior computer experience, learning styles and ethnicity. While this system was found to be fairly easy to use, its use did not lead to any significant differences in diabetes outcomes, compared to a control group, and the authors did not describe what design features they specifically included to address health literacy issues.

User-Agent Concordance. Baylor et al. conducted studies on the impact of racial and gender concordance between virtual agents and users in an educational application [13]. In one study, they developed several animated agents for an intelligent tutoring system that varied in race and gender. Study participants were 139 teachers enrolled in an introductory technology education class. Results indicated that teachers rated the agents of their own race more engaging and affable (p<.05). A follow-up study investigated what kind of virtual agent students would choose to work with. African American students selected African American characters more frequently, while white students preferred the white agents (p<.001). When asked why they made their choices, African American students often indicated that they wanted an agent that they could "better relate to" in terms of ethnicity and gender.

Persky et al. conducted a study on the effects of racial concordance between study subjects and simulated doctor agents that provided personalized cancer risk information. Subjects who interacted with a racially concordant virtual doctor were more accurate in their risk perceptions than those who interacted with a non-concordant virtual doctor, and this effect was amplified among current smokers [14].

3   The Virtual Hospital Discharge Nurse

The virtual discharge nurse system was developed over a course of three years by a multi-disciplinary design team comprised of HCI researchers, doctors and nurses, a health literacy expert, and programmers and animators [15]. The virtual nurse is deployed on a touch screen computer on a mobile kiosk that allows for patient education at the patient's hospital bedside (Figure 1). The kiosk consists of a wheeled base, a 4' tall stand and an articulated arm. The arm allows the screen to be positioned and tilted in front of a patient accommodating their mobility whether they are lying or sitting up in bed, or sitting in a chair.

The agent spends approximately half an hour with each patient before they leave the hospital, reviewing the layout and contents of the patient's discharge instruction booklet. The paper booklet is given to patients before their conversation with the agent, and the agent reviews a digital version of the booklet in the interface, so that patients can follow along with the agent's explanation in their paper booklets. The discharge conversation covers the patient's primary diagnosis, medications, follow-up appointments, and self-care procedures the patient will need to manage once they leave the hospital. The agent is also designed to talk with patients once a day, every day they are in the hospital, communicating all of the information that is known at that time about their diagnosis and post-discharge self-care regimen, in order to reinforce the information as much as possible. Dialogues were designed that describe 2,254 medicines—including brief descriptions, warnings, and side effects—in addition to the 48 most common diagnoses in the hospital.

The agent also tested patient understanding of key points using short "open book" tests during the interaction with a few multiple-choice questions. If a patient failed these tests, the agent helped them locate the information in their booklet. If the patient failed a subsequent comprehension test, or requested additional information about any part of the booklet, a report was printed with the patient's information needs for a human nurse to follow up with before the patient went home.

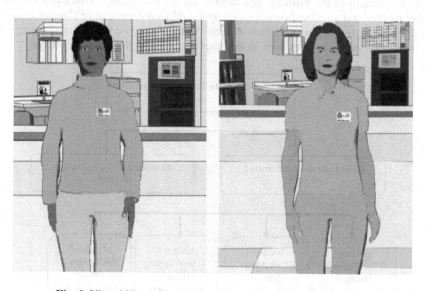

Fig. 2. Virtual Nurse Characters, African American and Caucasian

The virtual agent is driven by a hierarchical transition-network based dialogue model that uses template-based text generation. The agent speaks using a synthetic voice, and displays animated nonverbal behavior (hand gestures, posture shifts, facial expressions, etc.) in synchrony with the speech, including deictic gestures towards a digital version of the patient's discharge instructions [16]. User contributions to the conversation are made by touching utterance option buttons on the touch screen display that are dynamically updated for each user speaking turn. Utterance option buttons are used to avoid any potential inaccuracy in this sensitive medical scenario.

Two female nurse characters were designed—one middle-aged Caucasian and one middle-aged African American—to better match the patient demographic at the Boston Medical Center where the clinical trial was conducted, and to improve acceptability of the agent (Figure 2). We originally designed eight character models of both genders and different ethnic groups, and conducted a survey of 32 hospital patients to select the two most acceptable characters. We also conducted surveys to select the synthetic voice that patients felt best matched each character from among a set of available commercial voices, and to determine given names for the characters.

4   Randomized Clinical Trial

We conducted a clinical trial to evaluate the Virtual Nurse system, with participants randomized between the Virtual Nurse and standard care in the hospital. The trial was conducted at Boston Medical Center, a 547 bed safety net hospital that serves an urban, 84% minority, traditionally underserved population. The patient population at Boston Medical center consists of 43% African American, 29% white, 19% Hispanic or Latino, and other races. In addition to the primary trial randomization, intervention group patients were further randomized to either be discharged by the African American or Caucasian agent, and to either have a single interaction with the Virtual Nurse on the day of discharge, or one interaction every day they were in the hospital, including the day of discharge.

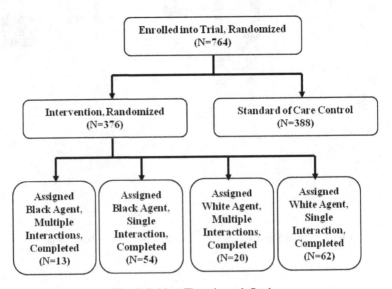

Fig. 3. Subject Flow through Study

4.1   Clinical Trial Methods

Participants. Figure 3 shows the flow of patients in this study and Table 1 shows the demographic breakdown. In total, 764 participants were recruited in this study and retained for analysis. All participants were patients admitted to a general medicine floor of Boston Medical Center, and 50.8% were female, aged 18 to 90 years old (mean=49). Among all participants, 52.6% were African American, 29.1% were Caucasian, and 11.4% were Hispanic.

Table 1. Demographics of Intervention Subjects who Completed Surveys (Education: <HS: less than high school, HS: high school, >HS: more than high school)

Variable		All N=149	Black Agent N=67	White Agent N=82	p
Sex (Female)	N (%)	71 (47.7)	26 (38.8)	45 (54.9)	0.07
Age	Mean (SD)	49.6 (13.1)	48.9 (12.7)	50.1 (13.5)	0.59
Race	Black, N(%)	81 (54.4)	34 (50.8)	47 (57.3)	0.15
	White, N(%)	40 (26.8)	23 (34.3)	17 (20.7)	
	Other, N(%)	28 (18.8)	10 (14.9)	18 (22.0)	
Education	<HS, N(%)	41 (27.5)	16 (23.9)	25 (30.5)	0.45
	HS, N(%)	50 (33.6)	26 (38.8)	24 (29.3)	
	>HS, N(%)	52 (34.9)	23 (34.3)	29 (35.4)	
Married	N (%)	35 (23.5)	14 (20.9)	21 (25.6)	0.63
Health Literacy (Inadequate)	N (%)	74 (49.7)	31 (46.3)	43 (52.4)	0.56

Measures. Health literacy (an individual's ability to read and follow written medical instructions) was assessed at intake using the REALM instrument [17], in addition to computer literacy (single self-report item with 1="I've never used a computer." to 4="I'm an expert."), and demographics (age, gender, race). Immediately following their interaction with the agent, participants completed a self-report questionnaire assessing working alliance (trust and belief in working with the agent to achieve a therapeutic outcome [18], scores ranging from 1-7), as well as the single scale item questions in Table 2.

Table 2. Self-Report Items Completed after Agent Interaction ("Elizabeth" is the agent's name)

Question	Anchor 1	Anchor 7
How satisfied were you with Elizabeth?	Not at all	Very satisfied
How easy was talking to Elizabeth?	Easy	Difficult
How much would you like to continue working with Elizabeth?	Not at all	Very much
How much do you like Elizabeth?	Not at all	Very much
How would you characterize your relationship with Elizabeth?	Complete stranger	Close friend
How much do you trust Elizabeth?	Not at all	Very much
How much do you feel that Elizabeth cares about you?	Not at all	Very much
Would you rather have talked to your doctor or nurse than Elizabeth?	definitely prefer doctor or nurse	definitely prefer Elizabeth
How likely is it that you will follow Elizabeth's advice?	Not at all likely	Very likely
How similar do you feel that you are to Elizabeth?	Very different	Very similar

4.2   Results

Among the intervention group, 302 participants actually interacted with the agent, and 149 completed all questionnaires. Among these 149 patients, 116 had only a single interaction at the time of discharge, while 33 had multiple interactions during their hospital stay (up to 5 sessions)(Figure 3). The large number of patients who did not complete all study tasks was due to the challenging logistics of the study. Patients could not use the final discharge system until they had been approved for hospital discharge (an event we had no control over), the time between this approval and when patients could actually leave was highly variable, and patients were anxious to get home. The combination of these factors led to a large number of patients who were enrolled in our study leaving the hospital before we could configure the agent, run the interaction, and collect all measures.

Overall, patients reported very high satisfaction with the agent (median="very satisfied"), very high ease of use (median="very easy"), and high working alliance with the agent (median=6, IQR=1.9). Participants in general liked the agent (median="like agent very much"), and trusted the agent (median="trust agent very much")(Figure 4). For the question whether they preferred to talk to the agent or their doctor or nurse, 49 out of 135 participants who answered this question clearly indicated that they preferred the agent, while only 33 indicated they preferred a human (Figure 5). Participants' answers were recorded based on a 7-point scale (Table 2), with 4 being neutral. Any answer higher than 4 was recorded as preference towards the agent.

Bivariate correlations among measures are shown in Table 3. Since most measures are single scale items, non-parametric tests are used throughout [19].

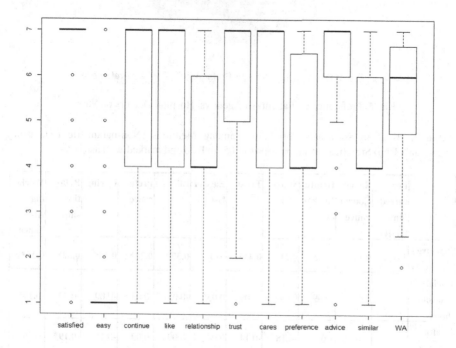

Fig. 4. Boxplots (showing range, 1st, 2nd, 3rd quartiles) of Self-Report Measures WA = Working Alliance Bond Inventory Subscale Score

Racial Concordance. We created a racial concordance index by scoring '1' if both the agent and the user were African American, or both the agent and user were not African American, '0' otherwise. There was no significant relationship between this measure and perceived similarity, Mann-Whitney U=1085, n.s. There was a significant relationship between concordance and working alliance, Mann-Whitney U=2761, p=.03, in which patients with racial concordance scored significantly lower compared to discordant patients. However, concordance was unrelated to any other measure (Table 3).

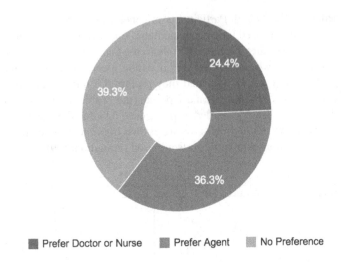

■ Prefer Doctor or Nurse   ■ Prefer Agent   ▨ No Preference

Fig. 5. Preference by Patients of Agent vs. Hospital Doctors or Nurses

Table 3. Bivariate Spearman Correlations among Measures (Non-parametric tests using Spearman's Rho) Significant relationships (p<.05) in bold and marked with asterisk

	Perceived Similarity	Racial Concordance	Health Literacy	Satisfied	Trust	Ease of Use	Liking	Preference	Caring	Relationship	Working Alliance
Perceived Similarity	1.0	0.14	-0.15	**0.21***	**0.41***	-0.13	**0.37***	**0.37***	**0.34***	**0.32***	**0.35***
Racial Concordance		1.0	-0.09	0.04	-0.09	0.03	-0.05	-0.03	-0.09	-0.02	**-0.19***
Health Literacy			1.0	**-0.18***	-0.14	0.04	-0.09	-0.09	-0.15	**-0.19***	-0.09
Satisfied				1.0	0.37*	**-0.39***	**0.42***	0.13	**0.26***	**0.23***	**0.31***
Trust					1.0	**-0.26***	**0.44***	**0.31***	**0.52***	**0.33***	**0.57***
Ease of Use						1.0	**-0.28***	-0.03	**-0.28***	-0.09	**-0.22***
Liking							1.0	**0.33***	**0.50***	**0.47***	**0.54***
Preference								1.0	**0.27***	**0.36***	**0.39***
Caring									1.0	**0.48***	**0.61***
Relationship										1.0	**0.35***
Working Alliance											1.0

Perceived Similarity. We investigated relationships between patient-rated perceived similarity with the agent and other outcome measures using Spearman's rho non-parametric correlation tests. Several significant relationships emerged. Patients who perceived higher similarity with the agent reported higher working alliance (rho=.35, p<.001), higher satisfaction (rho=.21, p<.05), greater desire to continue working with the agent (rho=.25, p<.05), greater liking of the agent (rho=.37, p<.001), greater trust in the agent (rho=.41, p<.001), a closer relationship with the agent (rho=.32, p=.001), and felt the agent cared more about them (rho=.34, p<.001), compared to patients reporting lower similarity with the agent. Patients who reported higher similarity with the agent also said they were more likely to follow the agent's advice upon hospital discharge (rho=.19, p=.07), and preferred receiving their discharge instructions from the agent (rho=.37, p<.001) compared to other patients.

Literacy. We also investigated relationships between computer literacy, health literacy, and attitudes towards the agent. We found a significant relationship between computer literacy and satisfaction with the agent, consistent with previous findings [20]. Patients with low computer literacy rated higher satisfaction compared to those with high computer literacy (Mann-Whitney U=3028.5, p=.003). Furthermore, patients with low computer literacy rated the agent higher on ease of use compared to other patients (Mann-Whitney U=2109.5, p=.01).

We also found effects of health literacy on participants' perceived relationship with the agent. Low health literacy patients reported closer relationships with the agent (Mann-Whitney U=3417, p=.02) and greater perceptions of feeling cared for by the agent (Mann-Whitney U=3200.5, p<.08) compared to high health literacy patients.

Using a non-parametric ANOVA [21], we also found significant main effect of health literacy on trust (p=.007) and a marginally significant interaction between health literacy and number of interactions with the agent (single vs. multiple) on trust (p=.08). In general, low health literacy participants trusted the agent more, and trust in the agent increased after more interactions with the agent, but only for patients with low health literacy (Figure 6).

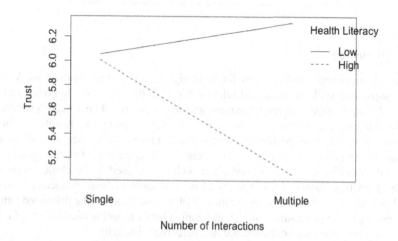

Fig. 6. Effect of Health Literacy and Number of Interactions on Trust in Nurse Agent

Number of Interactions. We also investigated relationships between the number of interactions a patient had with the nurse agent and their perceptions of the agent. We found that the more interactions a patient had, the closer their reported relationship (Mann-Whitney U=1571.5, p=.06).

4.3   Factors Predicting Perceived Similarity with the Agent

Given the number of significant correlations between perceived similarity and other measures, we sought to understand what patient factors predicted their assessment of similarity. We conducted a linear regression of patient demographic factors onto perceived similarity. The predictors included: racial concordance, gender, age, education level, and computer literacy. Results are shown in Table 4. Although none of the coefficients are significantly different from zero, gender, age, and racial concordance are trending. Female patients, older patients, and those who were racially concordant with the agent tended to rate their similarity higher.

Table 4. Regression Model of Patient Demographics on Perceived Similarity with Agent Multiple model $R^2 = 0.095$

Factor	Coefficient	P
(Intercept)	3.073	0.006
Gender	-0.624	0.106
Age	0.026	0.115
Education	-0.039	0.703
Racial Concordance	0.698	0.070
Computer Experience	0.032	0.898

4.4   Discussion

In general, perceived similarity was found to significantly affect patients' working alliance, satisfaction, liking, trust, and relationship with the agent. We hypothesized that the racial-concordance between the patient and the agent would be a major predictor of perceived similarity, but this hypothesis was not supported by our results. Although trending was found in our preliminary linear model, racial concordance was not strongly correlated with perceived similarity. The trending for correlation between gender and perceived similarity can be explained since both agents used in the clinical trial were female characters. Trending for age could be explained as both characters were designed as middle-aged. Racial concordance slightly contributed to the perceived similarity according to the preliminary model, although a better model is needed to explain the relationship between racial concordance and perceived similarity.

Patients who reported higher similarity with the agent were more likely to prefer receiving their discharge instructions from the agent compared to other patients. Among all patients who answered the question about preference, 36.3% (N=49) said they would prefer the agent, 24.4% (N=33) preferred doctor or nurse, and 39.3% (N=53) indicated no preference. More than one-third of the participants who answered this question clearly indicated that they preferred the agent. Interviews with patients in the pilot study [15] provide some insight into why patients preferred the virtual nurse. Patients liked that the agent took as much time as was needed to go through all the details of the discharge booklet, and that the agent checked to make sure the patient understood what was being described:

- "I prefer Louise, she's better than a doctor, she explains more, and doctors are always in a hurry."
- "It was just like a nurse, actually better, because sometimes a nurse just gives you the paper and says 'Here you go.' Elizabeth explains everything."
- "Sometimes doctors just talk and assume you understand what they're saying. With a computer you can go slow, go over things again and she checks that you understand."

The clinical scenario of care transition and hospital discharge in which we placed the system may be particularly stressful for patients. The level of satisfaction participants had with our system may have been accentuated due to a high level of dissatisfaction participants feel with their health providers in this scenario. We did not measure dissatisfaction with human providers and did not explore in this study the extent to which perceived similarity with the agent might reflect perceived alienation from the human providers.

5   Conclusions and Future Work

We found many signification correlations between patients' perceived similarity to a virtual discharge nurse agent and their satisfaction with and preference for the agent. Thus, H2 was strongly supported. Surprisingly, perceived similarity was not strongly related to racial concordance, as predicted. Thus, H1 was not supported. Perceived similarity was related to a few other factors (such as a patient's age and gender) but the overall fit of the model was very poor, indicating there are yet unknown factors that lead patients to rate a virtual nurse agent as being similar to themselves. Possible factors include: the appearance of the agent (dress, hairstyle, apparent educational level and socioeconomic status), the qualities of the synthetic speech (accent, apparent personality, apparent ethnic or cultural background), similarity in health status and affective state, and differing interpretations of the role and status of the agent (same as a human vs. a computer program vs. a cartoon character). The exploration of these factors remains an open research problem.

Patients also reported a high level of trust in the agent, and this may have superseded any effects of racial concordance. Elements of the system, such as social talk, empathy, and engaging users to check comprehension, may have instilled trust despite the complexity of the material. This, together with the importance and volume of the information conveyed, may overwhelm the relatively subtle effects of agent appearance.

The results presented indicate that perceived similarity to a virtual agent is important in many serious task settings, and serve as a partial guide for the design of future virtual agents and their applications.

In our ongoing work we are developing a version of the virtual nurse that is persistent throughout a patient's hospital stay, and is equipped with a range of sensors so that it is aware of events in the hospital room. This "Hospital Buddy" is being designed to help patients communicate with their providers, manage their sleep, and track their symptoms while in the hospital [22].

Acknowledgments. Thanks to the many members of the Re-Engineered Discharge project team at Boston Medical Center and the Relational Agents Group at Northeastern University for their contributions to this work. This work was supported by grants from the NIH National Heart Lung and Blood Institute and the Agency for Healthcare Research and Quality.

References

1. King, W., Wong, M., Shapiro, M., Landon, B., Cunningham, W.: Does racial concordance between HIV-positive patients and their physicians affect the time to receipt of protease inhibitors? Journal of General Internal Medicine 19, 1146–1153 (2004)
2. Gordon, H., Street, R., Sharf, B., Souchek, J.: Racial differences in doctors' information-giving and patients' participation. Cancer 107, 1313–1320 (2006)
3. LaVeist, T., Nuru-Jeter, A., Jones, K.: The association of doctor-patient race concordance with health services utilization. J. Public Health Policy 24, 312–323 (2003)
4. Saha, S., Komaromy, M., Koepsell, T., Bindman, A.: Patient-physician racial concordance and the perceived quality and use of health care. Archives of Internal Medicine 159, 997–1004 (1999)
5. Forster, A., Murff, H., Peterson, J., Gandhi, T., Bates, D.: The Incidence and Severity of Adverse Events Affecting Patients after Discharge from the Hospital. Annals of Internal Medicine 138 (2003)
6. Baker, D., Parker, R., Williams, M., Clark, S.: Health literacy and the risk of hospital admission. J. Gen. Intern. Med. 13, 791–798 (1998)
7. Makaryus, A., Friedman, E.: Patients' understanding of their discharge treatment plans and diagnosis at discharge. Mayo. Clin. Proc. 80, 991–994 (2005)
8. Bers, M., Ackermanntt, E., Cassell, J., Donegan, B., Gonzalez-Heydrichttt, J., DeMaso, D., Strobeckerfi, C., Lualditi, S., Bromleytt, D., Karlint, J.: Interactive Storytelling Environments: Coping with Cardiac Illness at Boston's Children's Hospital. In: Conference Interactive Storytelling Environments: Coping with Cardiac Illness at Boston's Children's Hospital (1998)
9. Wilcox, L., Gatewood, J., Morris, D., Tan, D., Feiner, S., Horvitz, E.: Physician Attitudes about Patient-Facing Information Displays at an Urban Emergency Department. In: Proceedings of AMIA, Washington, DC (2010)
10. Vawdrey, D., Wilcox, L., Collins, S., Bakken, S., Feiner, S., Boyer, A., Restaino, S.: A Tablet Computer Application for Patients to Participate in Their Hospital Care. In: American Medical Informatics Association (AMIA) Annual Meeting, Washington, DC, pp. 1428–1435 (2011)

11. Hoffman, H., Seibel, E., Richards, T., Furness, T., Patterson, D., Sharar, S.: Virtual reality helmet display quality influences the magnitude of virtual reality analgesia. J. Pain 7, 843–850 (2006)

12. Gerber, B.S., Brodsky, I.G., Lawless, K.A., et al.: Implementation and Evaluation of a Low-Literacy Diabetes Education Computer Multimedia Application. Diabetes Care 28, 1574–1580 (2005)

13. Baylor, A., Shen, E., Huang, X.: Which Pedagogical Agent Do Learners Choose? The Effects of Gender and Ethnicity. In: E-Learn (World Conference on E-Learning in Corporate, Government, Healthcare, & Higher Education), Phoenix, AZ (2003)

14. Persky, S., Kaphingst, K., Allen, V., Senay, I.: Effects of patient-provider race concordance and smoking status on lung cancer risk perception accuracy among African-Americans. Annals of Behaviroal Medicine 45, 308–317 (2013)

15. Bickmore, T., Pfeifer, L., Jack, B.W.: Taking the Time to Care: Empowering Low Health Literacy Hospital Patients with Virtual Nurse Agents. In: Conference Taking the Time to Care: Empowering Low Health Literacy Hospital Patients with Virtual Nurse Agents (2009)

16. Bickmore, T., Pfeifer, L., Yin, L.: The Role of Gesture in Document Explanation by Embodied Conversational Agents. International Journal of Semantic Computing 2, 47–70 (2008)

17. Davis, T., Long, S., Jackson, R., et al.: Rapid estimate of adult literacy in medicine: a shortened screening instrument. Fam. Med. 25, 391–395 (1993)

18. Horvath, A., Greenberg, L.: Development and Validation of the Working Alliance Inventory. Journal of Counseling Psychology 36, 223–233 (1989)

19. Carifio, J., Perla, R.: Resolving the 50-year debate around using and misusing Likert scales. Medical Education 42, 1150–1152 (2008)

20. Bickmore, T., Pfeifer, L., Byron, D., Forsythe, S., Henault, L., Jack, B., Silliman, R., Paasche-Orlow, M.: Usability of Conversational Agents by Patients with Inadequate Health Literacy: Evidence from Two Clinical Trials. Journal of Health Communication 15, 197–210 (2010)

21. Wobbrock, J., Findlater, L., Gergle, D., Higgins, J.: The Aligned Rank Transform for Nonparametric Factorial Analyses Using Only ANOVA Procedures. In: Human Factors in Computing Systems, CHI (2011)

22. Bickmore, T., Bukhari, L., Vardoulakis, L.P., Paasche-Orlow, M., Shanahan, C.: Hospital buddy: A persistent emotional support companion agent for hospital patients. In: Nakano, Y., Neff, M., Paiva, A., Walker, M. (eds.) IVA 2012. LNCS, vol. 7502, pp. 492–495. Springer, Heidelberg (2012)

Author Index